900 Questions:
An Interventional Cardiology
Board Review

900 Questions:
An Interventional Cardiology Board Review

EDITORS

Debabrata Mukherjee, MD

Associate Professor of Medicine
Director, Cardiac Catheterization Laboratories
Gill Foundation Professor of Interventional Cardiology
Gill Heart Institute and Division of Cardiovascular Medicine
University of Kentucky
Lexington, Kentucky

Leslie Cho, MD

Director, Women's Cardiovascular Center
Medical Director, Preventive Cardiology and Rehabilitation
Department of Cardiovascular Medicine
Cleveland Clinic Foundation
Cleveland, Ohio

David J. Moliterno, MD

Professor and Vice-Chairman of Medicine
Chief, Cardiovascular Medicine
Jefferson Morris Gill Professor of Cardiology
Gill Heart Institute and Division of Cardiovascular Medicine
University of Kentucky
Lexington, Kentucky

Donna A. Gilbreath

Managing Editor
Gill Heart Institute and Division of Cardiovascular Medicine
University of Kentucky
Lexington, Kentucky

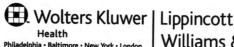

Wolters Kluwer
Health
Philadelphia · Baltimore · New York · London
Buenos Aires · Hong Kong · Sydney · Tokyo

Lippincott
Williams & Wilkins

Acquisitions Editor: Frances R. DeStefano
Managing Editor: Nicole Dernoski
Project Manager: Jennifer Harper
Senior Manufacturing Manager: Benjamin Rivera
Marketing Manager: Angela Panetta
Design Coordinator: Risa Clow
Production Services: Laserwords Private Limited, Chennai, India
Printer: Victor Graphics, Inc.

© 2007 by LIPPINCOTT WILLIAMS & WILKINS, a Wolters Kluwer business
530 Walnut Street
Philadelphia, PA 19106 USA
LWW.com

Library of Congress Cataloging-in-Publication Data

900 questions : an interventional cardiology board review / editors,
  Debabrata Mukherjee ... [et al.].
    p. ; cm.
  ISBN-13: 978-0-7817-7349-2
  ISBN-10: 0-7817-7349-0
  1. Heart—Diseases—Treatment—Examinations, questions, etc. 2. Cardiovascular system—Diseases—Treatment—Examinations, questions, etc. I. Mukherjee, Debabrata.
II. Title: Nine hundred questions.
  [DNLM: 1. Cardiovascular Diseases—Examination Questions. 2. Cardiovascular Diseases—therapy—Examination Questions. WG 18.2 Z9991 2007]
  RC683.8.N564 2007
  616.1'20076—dc22
                                                            2006027893

"To my parents, for their infinite patience, love, and understanding, who continue to be my source of inspiration, and to my wonderful wife, Suchandra, for her love and support"

Debabrata Mukherjee

"To Nathaniel and Benjamin, my sons and suppliers of life's important questions, and to Judith, my wife and partner in finding the answers"

David J. Moliterno

Preface

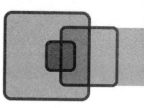

Insightful questions have been used through the ages as a metric to assess one's knowledge, but when coupled with carefully delivered answers they can become a powerful teaching tool. This book of questions and annotated answers covering the field of interventional cardiology is meant to serve as a helpful resource for individuals preparing for the interventional cardiovascular medicine board examination as well as for clinicians who wish to perform an in-depth self-assessment on individual topics or the full spectrum. The book has many key features, which we believe will make the reader successful in passing the boards and improving clinical practice.

Of foremost importance, the areas covered are relevant not only to the day-to-day practice of interventional cardiology, but have also been patterned in scope and content to the actual board examination. The book begins with several chapters dedicated to the anatomy and physiology associated with interventional cardiology and the pathobiology of atherosclerosis and inflammation. This corresponds to the 15% of the board examination targeting material in basic science. The subsequent chapters focus on the essential interventional pharmacotherapy of antiplatelets, anticoagulants, and other commonly used medications in the catheterization laboratory and outpatient setting for patients with atherosclerosis. These chapters correspond to the next 15% of the boards centering on pharmacology. A similar-sized 15% of the board examination is directed toward imaging, and the book includes specific chapters on radiation safety, catheterization laboratory equipment and technique, contrast agents, and intravascular ultrasound. The two largest areas of the examination, each covering 25% of the content, include case selection–management and procedural techniques. The review book dedicates 25 chapters to comprehensively cover these areas. Finally, we have included chapters for the miscellaneous remaining areas covered by the board examination, including peripheral vascular disease, ethics, statistics, and epidemiology, as well as a chapter directed at improving test-taking skills.

Also essential to the quality and appropriateness of the questions and annotated answers is the expertise of the chapter authors. We are fortunate to have assembled the "who's who of academic interventional cardiology". The 59 contributing authors from leading medical centers around the world have over 4,600 articles cited in PubMed. We are greatly indebted to these authors who are recognized both for their interventional expertise and for their teaching skills. In the end, the true value of this textbook is not only the relevance of the questions, the outstanding quality of the authors, but also the value of the annotated answers. The text includes 910 questions and 254 figures and tables. The corresponding answers have been appropriately detailed to provide relevant facts and information as well as up-to-date journal citations.

The practice of interventional cardiology is exciting, rewarding, and a privilege each of us enjoys. Likewise, it has been our privilege to work with the superb contributors, our colleagues in interventional cardiology, as well as the editorial team at the University of Kentucky and Lippincott Williams and Wilkins. It is our personal hope that you will enjoy this book and that it will be a valuable resource to you in passing the board examination and providing the highest quality care possible to your patients.

DEBABRATA MUKHERJEE, MD
LESLIE CHO, MD
DAVID J. MOLITERNO, MD

Contributors

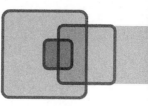

Robert J. Applegate, MD
Director, Cardiovascular Training Program
Wake Forest University School of Medicine
Winston-Salem, North Carolina

Joseph Babb, MD
Professor of Medicine
Department of Internal Medicine, Cardiology Division
Brody School of Medicine
East Carolina University;
Director, Cardiac Catheterization Laboratories
Pitt County Memorial Hospital
Greenville, North Carolina

Thomas M. Bashore, MD
Professor of Medicine
Division of Cardiovascular Medicine;
Director, Fellowship Training Program
and Adult Congenital and Valvular Disease Program
Duke University Medical Center
Durham, North Carolina

Matthew C. Becker, MD
Fellow in Cardiovascular Disease
Department of Cardiovascular Medicine
Cleveland Clinic Foundation
Cleveland, Ohio

Deepak L. Bhatt, MD
Associate Professor of Medicine
Staff, Cardiac, Peripheral, and Carotid Intervention
Department of Cardiovascular Medicine
Cleveland Clinic Foundation
Cleveland, Ohio

David C. Booth, MD
Endowed Professor Medicine
Gill Heart Institute and
Division of Cardiovascular Medicine
University of Kentucky;
Chief of Cardiology
Lexington VA Medical Center
Lexington, Kentucky

Sorin J. Brener, MD
Associate Professor of Medicine
Department of Medicine
Case Western Reserve University;
Staff Physician
Department of Cardiovascular Medicine
Cleveland Clinic Foundation
Cleveland, Ohio

Ivan P. Casserly, MD
Assistant Professor of Medicine
Cardiology Division
University of Colorado;
Director of Interventional Cardiology
Denver VA Medical Center
Denver, Colorado

Leslie Cho, MD
Director, Women's Cardiovascular Center
Medical Director, Preventive Cardiology
and Rehabilitation
Department of Cardiovascular Medicine
Cleveland Clinic Foundation
Cleveland, Ohio

Antonio Colombo, MD
Chief of Invasive Cardiology
Università Vita-Salute
and San Raffaele Scientific Institute
and Columbus Hospitals
Milan, Italy

Harold L. Dauerman, MD
Professor of Medicine
University of Vermont;
Director, Cardiovascular Catheterization Laboratories
Fletcher Allen Health Care
Burlington, Vermont

Steven R. Daugherty, PhD
Assistant Professor of Psychology
Assistant Professor of Preventive Medicine
Rush Medical College
Chicago, Illinois

Stephen G. Ellis, MD

Professor of Medicine
Department of Cardiovascular Medicine
Cleveland Clinic Lerner College of Medicine
Case Western Reserve University;
Director, Cardiac Catheterization Laboratories
Cleveland Clinic Foundation
Cleveland, Ohio

Nezar Falluji, MD, MPH

Clinical Instructor
Gill Heart Institute
Division of Cardiovascular Medicine
University of Kentucky
Lexington, Kentucky

David P. Faxon, MD

Director of Strategic Planning
Department of Medicine
Brigham and Women's Hospital;
Professor of Medicine
Department of Medicine
Harvard Medical School
Boston, Massachusetts

Joel A. Garcia, MD

Interventional Cardiology and Research Fellow
Department of Cardiology
University of Colorado
Denver, Colorado

Thomas Gehrig, MD

Cardiology Fellow
Division of Cardiovascular Medicine
Duke University Medical Center
Durham, North Carolina

Bernard Gersh, MB, ChB, DPhil

Professor of Medicine
Cardiology Diseases
Mayo Clinic College of Medicine
Rochester, Minnesota

John C. Gurley, MD, MBA

Professor of Medicine
Director, Interventional Cardiology Fellowship
Gill Heart Institute
Division of Cardiovascular Medicine
University of Kentucky
Lexington, Kentucky

Hussam Hamdalla, MD

Assistant Professor of Medicine
Gill Heart Institute and
Division of Cardiovascular Medicine
University of Kentucky
Lexington, Kentucky

Robert A. Harrington, MD

Professor of Medicine
Director, Cardiovascular Clinical Trials
Co-Director, Cardiovascular Research
Duke Clinical Research Institute
Department of Medicine, Division of Cardiology
Duke University Medical Center
Durham, North Carolina

Howard C. Herrmann, MD

Professor of Medicine
Cardiovascular Division
University of Pennsylvania School of Medicine;
Director, Interventional Cardiology and Cardiac
Catheterization Laboratories
Hospital of the University of Pennsylvania
Philadelphia, Pennsylvania

L. David Hillis, MD

Professor and Vice Chair
Department of Internal Medicine
University of Texas Southwestern Medical Center
Dallas, Texas

Alice K. Jacobs, MD

Professor of Medicine
Department of Medicine, Section of Cardiology
Boston University School of Medicine;
Director, Cardiac Catheterization Laboratories
and Interventional Cardiology
Boston Medical Center
Boston, Massachusetts

John Lynn Jefferies, MD, MPH

Assistant Professor
Adult and Pediatric Cardiology
Baylor College of Medicine
Divisions of Adult Cardiovascular Diseases
and Pediatric Cardiology
Texas Children's Hospital
Texas Heart Institute at St. Luke's Episcopal Hospital
Houston, Texas

Hani Jneid, MD

Division of Cardiology
Massachusetts General Hospital
and Harvard Medical School
Boston, Massachusetts

Dominique Joyal, MD

Interventional Cardiology Fellow
Cardiology Division
Loyola University Medical Center
Maywood, Illinois

David E. Kandzari, MD

John B. Simpson Assistant Professor of Interventional
Cardiology and Genomic Sciences
Division of Cardiology
Department of Medicine
Duke University Medical Center
Durham, North Carolina

Samir Kapadia, MD

Associate Professor of Medicine
Cleveland Clinic Lerner College of Medicine
of Case Western Reserve University;
Director, Interventional Cardiology Fellowship
Department of Cardiovascular Medicine
Cleveland Clinic Foundation
Cleveland, Ohio

Juhana Karha, MD

Fellow, Cardiovascular Medicine
Department of Cardiovascular Medicine
Cleveland Clinic Foundation
Cleveland, Ohio

Morton J. Kern, MD

Clinical Professor of Medicine
Associate Chief of Cardiology
Department of Cardiology
University of California Irvine
Orange, California

Richard A. Lange, MD

Professor of Medicine
Chief of Clinical Cardiology
Johns Hopkins University
Baltimore, Maryland

Bruce E. Lewis, MD

Professor of Medicine
Associate Director, Interventional Cardiology
Loyola University Medical Center
Maywood, Illinois;
Chief, Cardiology Division
St. Joseph Hospital
Chicago, Illinois

Ferdinand Leya, MD

Cardiology Department
Loyola University Medical Center
Maywood, Illinois

Andrew O. Maree, MD

Interventional Cardiology Fellow
Division of Cardiology
Massachusetts General Hospital;
Instructor, Department of Medicine
Harvard Medical School
Boston, Massachusetts

J. Jeffery Marshall, MD

Medical Director
Cardiac Catheterization Laboratory
Northeast Georgia Heart Center
Gainesville, Florida

Telly A. Meadows, MD

Cardiology Fellow
Department of Cardiovascular Medicine
Cleveland Clinic Foundation
Cleveland, Ohio

Bernhard Meier, MD

Professor of Medicine
Chairman, Department of Cardiology
University Hospital Bern
Bern, Switzerland

David J. Moliterno, MD

Professor and Vice-Chairman of Medicine
Chief, Cardiovascular Medicine
Jefferson Morris Gill Professor of Cardiology
Gill Heart Institute and
Division of Cardiovascular Medicine
University of Kentucky
Lexington, Kentucky

Pedro R. Moreno, MD

Director, Interventional Cardiology Research
Mount Sinai Hospital;
Associate Professor
Department of Medicine
Mount Sinai School of Medicine
New York, New York

Douglass A. Morrison, MD

Cardiology Department
University of Arizona
Tucson, Arizona

Debabrata Mukherjee, MD

Associate Professor of Medicine
Director, Cardiac Catheterization Laboratories
Gill Foundation Professor of Interventional Cardiology
Gill Heart Institute and
Division of Cardiovascular Medicine
University of Kentucky
Lexington, Kentucky

Brahmajee K. Nallamothu, MD, MPH

Assistant Professor of Medicine
Interventional Cardiologist
Department of Internal Medicine
University of Michigan Health System
Ann Arbor, Michigan

Craig R. Narins, MD

Assistant Professor of Medicine
Division of Cardiology
University of Rochester School of Medicine
Rochester, New York

Zoran S. Nedeljkovic, MD

Assistant Professor of Medicine
Department of Medicine, Section of Cardiology
Boston University School of Medicine;
Interventional Cardiologist
Boston Medical Center
Boston, Massachusetts

Michael R. Nihill, MBBS

Professor of Clinical Pediatrics
Department of Pediatrics
Baylor College of Medicine;
Associate in Pediatric Cardiology
Department of Cardiology
Texas Children's Hospital
Houston, Texas

Alan W. Nugent, MBBS

Assistant Professor of Pediatrics
Baylor College of Medicine;
Pediatric Cardiologist
Texas Children's Heart Center
Texas Children's Hospital
Houston, Texas

Ann O'Connor, MD

Instructor in Medicine
Section of Cardiology
Department of Medicine
University of Chicago
Chicago, Illnois

Igor F. Palacios, MD

Physician
Cardiac Unit
Massachusetts General Hospital
Boston, Massachusetts

Karen S. Pieper, MS

Senior Statistician
Duke Clinical Research Institute
Department of Medicine, Division of Cardiology
Duke University Medical Center
Durham, North Carolina

Marco Roffi, MD

Lecturer in Cardiology
Zurich Medical School;
Staff Cardiologist
University Hospital
Zurich, Switzerland

Christopher L. Sarnoski, MD

Cardiology Fellow
Division of Cardiovascular Medicine
University of Vermont
Burlington, Vermont

Paul Sorajja, MD

Assistant Professor of Medicine
Mayo Clinic College of Medicine
Rochester, Minnesota

Amy L. Seidel, MD

Interventional Cardiology Fellow
Division of Cardiovascular Medicine
Emory University School of Medicine
Atlanta, Georgia

Steven R. Steinhubl, MD

Associate Professor of Medicine
Director of CV Education and Clinical Research
Gill Heart Institute and
Division of Cardiovascular Medicine
University of Kentucky
Lexington, Kentucky

Eric J. Topol, MD

Professor of Genetics
Department of Genetics
Case Western Reserve University
Cleveland, Ohio

Thomas T. Tsai, MD
Cardiology Fellow
Department of Internal Medicine
University of Michigan
Ann Arbor, Michigan

E. Murat Tuzcu, MD
Professor of Medicine
Department of Cardiovascular Medicine
Cleveland Clinic Lerner College of Medicine
Case Western Reserve University;
Vice Chairman
Department of Cardiovascular Medicine
Cleveland Clinic Foundation
Cleveland, Ohio

Christopher Walters, MD
Cardiology Fellow
Gill Heart Institute
Division of Cardiovascular Medicine
University of Kentucky
Lexington, Kentucky

Peter Wenaweser, MD
Attending Physician
Department of Cardiology
University Hospital Bern
Bern, Switzerland

Christophe A. Wyss, MD
Cardiology Fellow
University Hospital
Zurich, Switzerland

Khaled M. Ziada, MD
Assistant Professor of Medicine
Gill Heart Institute
Division of Cardiovascular Medicine
University of Kentucky;
Director, Cardiac Catheterization Laboratories
Lexington VA Medical Center
Lexington, Kentucky

Contents

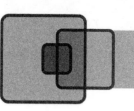

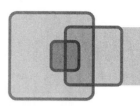

1

Vascular Biology

Pedro R. Moreno

Questions

1 All of the following statements regarding the American Heart Association (AHA) classification for early atherosclerosis are true, *except*:

(A) The type I lesion is proteoglycan rich and prone to develop atherosclerosis
(B) The type II lesion is characterized by foam cell infiltration and may regress
(C) The type III lesion is characterized by pools of intracellular lipid and collagen
(D) Early lesions are flat, asymptomatic, and do not obstruct the lumen

2 All of the following statements regarding advanced atherosclerosis are true, *except*:

(A) Vasa vasorum neovascularization is increased in ruptured plaques
(B) Thin-cap fibroatheromas are characterized by cap thickness <65 μm, macrophages, and large lipid core
(C) Extravasation of red blood cells (RBCs) within plaques increases lipid core expansion
(D) Plaque rupture is most frequently symptomatic, leading to acute coronary events

3 All of the following statements regarding advanced atherosclerosis are true, *except*:

(A) Coronary calcification is a predictor of future coronary events
(B) Coronary calcification always reflects advanced disease by histologic criteria
(C) Plaque erosion is more frequently seen in smokers
(D) Chronic stable angina lesions are frequently healed ruptured plaques

(E) Plaque rupture more frequently occurs at the center of the fibrous cap

4 All of the following statements are true, *except*:

(A) Nonobstructive lesions are the most frequent cause of acute myocardial infarction (MI)
(B) Obstructive lesions can evolve into complete occlusion silently
(C) The individual risk for plaque progression to complete occlusion is higher in nonobstructive lesions
(D) Vulnerable plaques are located predominately in the proximal segments of the coronary arteries

5 All of the following statements are true, *except*:

(A) Plaque rupture may occur simultaneously in two different arteries
(B) Plaque healing after rupture is mediated by smooth muscle cell (SMC) production of collagen III
(C) SMCs are responsible for weakening the fibrous cap
(D) T lymphocytes increase proteolytic activity and decrease collagen synthesis

6 All of the following statements are true, *except*:

(A) Inflammation precipitates plaque rupture and thrombosis
(B) Collagen is the most thrombogenic substrate after plaque rupture
(C) Inflammation promotes neovascularization
(D) Macrophages are the main source of metalloproteinases in the plaque

7 All of the following statements are true, *except*:

(A) The main source of plaque neovessels is the vasa vasorum

(B) C-reactive protein (CRP) is produced in the liver as a proinflammatory response to interleukin-6 (IL-6)

(C) CRP has been found within the plaque at the lipid core

(D) CRP has intrinsic atherogenic properties stimulating foam cell formation

(E) CRP has been found to be an independent predictor for events only in univariate analysis

8 All of the following statements about inflammation are true, *except*:

(A) Patients with unstable angina and increased inflammation have a higher risk for subsequent events

(B) Randomized trials have shown no benefit for steroids in unstable angina

(C) Leukocytosis is an independent predictor for future events

(D) The beneficial effects of acetylsalicylic acid (ASA) in primary prevention are independent of CRP levels

9 All of the following statements are true, *except*:

(A) Remodeling preserves the lumen area and protects from heart attacks

(B) Positive remodeling is most frequently seen in unstable syndromes

(C) Positive remodeled plaques have more macrophages

(D) Plaques can grow up to 40% area stenosis without significantly obstructing the lumen

10 All of the following statements are true, *except*:

(A) Coronary thrombosis in unstable angina is predominately platelet rich

(B) Deep-vein thrombosis in pulmonary embolism (PE) is predominately fibrin rich

(C) Coronary thrombosis in ST-elevation myocardial infarction (STEMI) is a combination of platelet-rich and fibrin-rich thrombus

(D) Natural anticoagulants include protein C, protein S, and tissue factor pathway inhibitor (TFPI)

(E) The plasminogen-activator inhibitor-1 (PAI-1) system is decreased in patients with diabetes

11 Metalloproteinases are relevant for the following, *except*:

(A) Positive remodeling, by digesting the internal elastic lamina

(B) Plaque angiogenesis, by mediating tunnelization of neovessels

(C) Plaque rupture, by digesting the collagen of the fibrous cap

(D) Myocardial salvage by preventing expansion and remodeling

12 Monocyte-derived macrophages are involved in the following, *except*:

(A) Foam cell formation

(B) Matrix metalloproteinases (MMPs) expression

(C) Tissue factor expression

(D) Plaque regression

13 Which of the following statements is *true* regarding the lipid core?

(A) Is composed of cholesterol crystals and collagen

(B) The predominant cell is the SMC

(C) Can be identified as a green structure on polarized microscopy using the picrosirius red stain

(D) Is the most potent thrombogenic substrate of human atherosclerotic plaques

14 Which of the following statements is *true* regarding the fibrous cap?

(A) It is composed of collagen and SMCs

(B) It is located at the base of the plaque, in contact with the internal elastic lamina

(C) It can be easily quantified by intravascular ultrasound

(D) It is the major source of neovessels in human atherosclerosis

15 Which of the following statements is *false* regarding vulnerable plaques?

(A) They are located predominately in the proximal segments of coronary arteries

(B) They are mostly lipid rich, with increased macrophage infiltration

(C) They exhibit positive remodeling

(D) They can be identified by angioscopy, showing a white surface

16 Which of the following statements is *true* regarding plaques undergoing erosion?

(A) They are more frequently seen in hypercholesterolemic, postmenopausal women

(B) They are mostly calcified plaques

(C) They are associated with positive remodeling

(D) They commonly exhibit a thick, SMC-rich fibrous cap

17 Which of the following statements is *true* regarding atherosclerotic mast cells?

(A) They produce nitric oxide
(B) They are increased in rupture plaques
(C) They are located mostly in the tunica media
(D) They are known as potent thrombogenic cells

18 Which of the following statements is *false* regarding plaque rupture?

(A) It occurs more frequently in lipid-rich plaques
(B) It may occur simultaneously in multiple coronary vessels
(C) It may occur more than once in the same plaque
(D) Increased macrophage activity in ruptured plaques is related to decreased macrophage apoptosis

19 Which of the following statements is *false* regarding diabetes?

(A) It is associated with increased atherosclerotic burden
(B) Diabetic coronary plaques have increased macrophage infiltration
(C) It is associated with increased thrombogenicity
(D) Macrophage receptor for advanced end-glycation products (RAGE) is downregulated

20 Which of the following statements is *false* regarding vessel wall inflammation?

(A) T cells are less frequently found when compared with macrophages
(B) Plaque inflammation is associated with increased neovascularization
(C) Cell-adhesion molecules (vascular cell adhesion molecule [VCAM], intercellular adhesion molecule [ICAM]) are mostly expressed in the endothelium and less expressed in plaque neovessels
(D) It is reduced after lipid-lowering therapy

21 Which of the following is *not* an independent predictor of positive remodeling?

(A) Inflammation
(B) Calcification
(C) Medial atrophy
(D) Cigarette smoking

22 Which of the following statements is *false* regarding intraplaque hemorrhage?

(A) It is associated with increased neovascularization
(B) It is associated with symptomatic carotid disease
(C) RBC extravasation stimulates lipid core expansion
(D) It downregulates macrophage CD163 receptor

(E) It increases the production of reactive oxygen species

23 Which of the following statements is *false* regarding plaque neovascularization?

(A) It is increased in ruptured plaques
(B) It is associated with inflammation
(C) Hypoxic factor-1α triggers plaque angiogenesis
(D) Most neovessels communicate with the vessel lumen to nurture the base of the plaque

24 Which of the following statements is *false* regarding SMC proliferation after stent deployment?

(A) It is increased in diabetic lesions after bare metal stenting
(B) It is characterized by increased production of collagen I
(C) It is associated with inflammation
(D) It is reduced after complete endothelialization
(E) It is associated with increased cell apoptosis

25 Which of the following statements is *false* regarding coronary thrombosis in unstable angina and non–ST-elevation myocardial infarction (NSTEMI)?

(A) It is more frequently mediated by plaque rupture rather than erosion
(B) It is associated with distal embolization, predominately composed of cholesterol crystals and necrotic debris
(C) Thrombosis reduces embolization and facilitates intervention
(D) It is associated with increased circulating tissue factor particles and cell apoptosis

26 Which of the following statements is *false* regarding plaque regression?

(A) It follows an eccentric pattern, reducing plaque volume before improving the lumen
(B) It can be obtained by aggressive lipid-lowering therapy
(C) It improves the lumen and therefore reduces coronary events
(D) It is associated with reverse lipid transport from the plaque to the liver

27 Which of the following statements is *false* regarding symptomatic, nonculprit plaque progression 1 year after percutaneous coronary revascularization?

(A) It can be as high as 12% per year in patients with three-vessel coronary disease
(B) It is higher in patients with diabetes
(C) It is higher in patients younger than 65 years
(D) Most patients present with acute coronary syndrome (ACS)
(E) Statins are protective

Answers and Explanations

1 **Answer C.** The AHA classification for early lesions (*Arterioscler Thromb.* 1994;14:840–856) defines the type III lesion as characterized by pools of *extracellular lipid and collagen.*

2 **Answer D.** Plaque rupture more frequently is asymptomatic. Symptomatic plaque rupture is the exception and not the rule.

3 **Answer E.** Plaque rupture more frequently occurs at the shoulders, not the center of the fibrous cap (*Lancet.* 1989;2:941–944).

4 **Answer C.** The individual risk for plaque progression to complete occlusion is lower in nonobstructive lesions (<5%) when compared with obstructive lesions (24%) (*J Am Coll Cardiol.* 1993;22:1141–1154).

5 **Answer C.** SMCs are responsible for strengthening, not weakening of the fibrous cap (*J Am Coll Cardiol.* 1998;32:283–285).

6 **Answer B.** Collagen is not the most potent thrombogenic substrate of the plaque. Lipid core is by far much more thrombogenic than any other plaque substrate (*J Am Coll Cardiol.* 1994;23:1562–1569).

7 **Answer E.** CRP has been found to be an independent predictor for events in univariate and multivariate analysis (*N Engl J Med.* 2005;352:20–28).

8 **Answer D.** The beneficial effects of ASA in primary prevention are closely related to CRP levels (*N Engl J Med.* 1997;336:973–979). In patients with the lowest quintile of CRP, ASA does not prevent cardiovascular events (13% reduction when compared with placebo; $p =$ not significant). However, in patients with the highest quintile of CRP, ASA prevents cardiovascular events (53% reduction when compared with placebo; $p < 0.0001$).

9 **Answer A.** Remodeling preserves the lumen, but does not protect from heart attacks. It is actually increased in plaques in patients with acute coronary events (*Circulation.* 2000;101:598–603).

10 **Answer E.** PAI-1 is increased in diabetic plaques (*Circulation.* 1998;97:2213–2221).

11 **Answer D.** Metalloproteinases do not salvage myocardium. On the contrary, MMPs are associated with expansion and remodeling of the ventricle after MI (*Circulation.* 2002;105:753–758).

12 **Answer D.** Macrophages are associated with plaque progression, not plaque regression.

13 **Answer D.** The lipid core is the most potent thrombogenic substrate of human atherosclerotic plaques (*J Am Coll Cardiol.* 1994;23:1562–1569).

14 **Answer A.** The fibrous cap is composed of collagen and SMCs.

15 **Answer D.** On angioscopy, vulnerable plaques are associated with a glistening yellow color. Stable plaques are white (*Am Heart J.* 1995;130:195–203).

16 **Answer D.** Plaque erosion is associated with a thick, SMC-rich fibrous cap (*Circulation.* 1996;93:1354–1363).

17 **Answer B.** Mast cells are increased in ruptured plaques (*J Am Coll Cardiol.* 1998;32:606–612).

18 **Answer D.** Macrophage activity in plaque rupture is mediated by increased apoptosis (*J Am Coll Cardiol.* 2005;46:937–954).

19 **Answer D.** Diabetes atherosclerosis is characterized by upregulation of RAGE (*Atherosclerosis.* 2006;185:70–77).

20 **Answer C.** Cell-adhesion molecule expression is two to three times higher in plaque neovessels than in the luminal endothelium (*J Clin Invest.* 1993;92:945–951).

21 **Answer D.** The independent predictors of plaque remodeling include inflammation, calcification, and medial atrophy (*Circulation.* 2002;105:297–303). Cigarette smoking is associated with plaque erosion but not positive remodeling.

22 **Answer D.** Intraplaque hemorrhage upregulates macrophage CD163 receptor, increasing inflammation and foam cell formation (*Atherosclerosis.* 2002;163:199–201).

23 **Answer D.** Most neovessels are derived from adventitial vasa vasorum and do not communicate with the lumen. Only a minority of plaque neovessels originates from the lumen (*Hum Pathol.* 1995;26:450–456).

24 **Answer B.** SMC proliferation after stent deployment is characterized by increased production of collagen III, not collagen I.

25 **Answer C.** Coronary thrombosis in unstable angina and NSTEMI is mediated by platelet-rich thrombus (*J Am Coll Cardiol.* 2005;46:937–954). Thrombosis activates platelets and may be harmful in ACS (*Circulation.* 1994;90:69–77).

26 **Answer C.** Plaque regression follows an eccentric pattern, initially improving the plaque burden associated with positive remodeling. Most importantly, plaque regression is associated with a significant reduction of new plaque formation, preventing plaque rupture, and reducing acute coronary events (*J Am Coll Cardiol.* 2005;46:937–954).

27 **Answer E.** Nonculprit plaque progression is a major cause of recurrent events within the first year of percutaneous coronary intervention (PCI), increasing from 4% in single vessel up to 12% in three-vessel coronary artery disease (CAD). Independent predictors include diabetes, unstable syndromes at presentation and age <65 years. Up to 65% present with ACS, and 9% present with total occlusion. Of note, statins were not protective against rapid progression within the first year (*Circulation.* 2005;111:143–149).

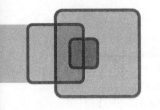

2

Anatomy and Physiology

Richard A. Lange and L. David Hillis

Questions

1 Pressure recordings from the coronary catheter tip during catheter engagement in the coronary ostium and withdrawal (see arrow) into the aorta indicate:

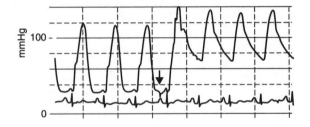

(A) Collateral coronary flow
(B) Obstruction of antegrade coronary flow by the catheter
(C) Anomalous origin of a coronary artery
(D) Severe aortic stenosis

2 Left ventriculography in the 30 degree right anterior oblique (RAO) projection shows a "button" projecting from the aortic root (see following figure). This suggests the patient has:

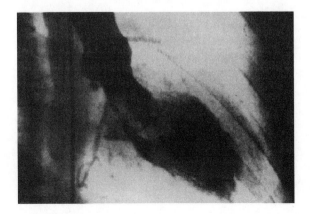

(A) Occlusion of the proximal right coronary artery (RCA)
(B) Ulceration in the proximal ascending aorta
(C) Anomalous origin of the left circumflex artery
(D) Focal aortic root dissection

3 Which of the following projections allows the operator to best visualize a proximal left circumflex stenosis?

(A) 30 degree RAO
(B) 30 degree RAO, 30 degree cranial
(C) 60 degree left anterior oblique (LAO), 30 degree cranial
(D) 30 degree RAO, 30 degree caudal

4 In what percentage of individuals does the left circumflex coronary artery provide the blood flow to the sinoatrial node?

(A) 90%
(B) 60%
(C) 40%
(D) 10%

5 What percentage of individuals with a bicuspid aortic valve have a left dominant coronary circulation?

(A) 1%
(B) 10%
(C) 30%
(D) 50%

6 In order to obtain a "spider view" to better visualize the left main, proximal left anterior descending (LAD) and left circumflex views, the radiographic technician should be directed to position the image intensifier:

(A) 15 degree RAO, 30 degree cranial
(B) 30 degree RAO, 30 degree caudal
(C) 50 degree LAO, 35 degree cranial
(D) 50 degree LAO, 20 degree caudal

7 In clinical practice, the severity of coronary stenosis is estimated from visual inspection of the coronary angiogram. Compared with quantitative coronary angiography, visual estimation of coronary stenosis usually:

(A) Underestimates the severity of stenosis by 20%
(B) Underestimates the severity of stenosis by 10%
(C) Overestimates the severity of stenosis by 20%
(D) Provides similar results

8 Impaired vasodilator reserve is first noted when the coronary luminal diameter narrowing (e.g., stenosis) is:

(A) 50%
(B) 60%
(C) 75%
(D) 90%

9 Coronary angiography demonstrates a mid-right coronary stenosis in which there is penetration of contrast material without perfusion. This would be characterized as:

(A) Thrombolysis in myocardial infarction (TIMI) 0 flow
(B) TIMI 1 flow
(C) TIMI 2 flow
(D) TIMI 3 flow

10 What is a Kugel's artery?

(A) Anomalous origin of the LAD coronary artery from the pulmonary artery
(B) Coronary arteriovenous fistula
(C) Conus artery branch
(D) Right-to-right collateral (from proximal to distal RCA through the atrioventricular (AV) node branch)

11 A 50% luminal diameter narrowing (e.g., stenosis) on coronary angiography corresponds to a cross-sectional area narrowing of:

(A) 50%
(B) 60%
(C) 75%
(D) 90%

12 Endothelial dysfunction can be identified by:

(A) Reduced coronary sinus blood levels of endothelial-derived relaxing factor (EDRF) and nitric oxide (NO)
(B) Inability to vasodilate in response to intracoronary nitroprusside
(C) Vasoconstrictor response to intracoronary acetylcholine
(D) Luminal irregularities on coronary angiography

13 All of the following are characteristic of a hemodynamically significant coronary stenosis, *except*:

(A) A myocardial fractional flow reserve (FFR) <0.90
(B) An impaired phasic pattern of phasic coronary flow distal to the stenosis with diastolic to systolic ratio <1.5
(C) Impaired coronary hyperemic flow (less than two times basal values)
(D) A translesional pressure gradient >30 mm Hg

14 Flow from which coronary artery or arteries is represented by great cardiac vein flow?

(A) LAD
(B) Left circumflex
(C) LAD and left circumflex
(D) RCA

15 Which of the following is *not* true of coronary flow reserve (CFR)?

(A) It is computed as hyperemic flow velocity divided by basal mean flow velocity
(B) It can be used to assess the physiologic significance of the stenosis in the epicardial coronary vessels
(C) Normal CFR is 2.5 to 5
(D) Maximal hyperemia is attained with intracoronary injections of adenosine, papaverine, or acetylcholine

16 All of the following are true regarding coronary vascular resistance, *except*:

(A) In the absence of stenosis, R1 (epicardial vessels) resistance is trivial
(B) The R2 (prearteriolar) vessels are responsible for most of the total coronary resistance
(C) The R3 (arteriolar and intramyocardial) vessels are regulated by neurogenic and local control
(D) Left ventricular (LV) hypertrophy and diabetes can impair microcirculatory (R3) resistance

17 CFR measurements obtained through thermodilution catheter (e.g., Webster catheter) are typically:

(A) Lower than values obtained with Doppler guidewire

(B) Higher than values obtained with Doppler guidewire

(C) Similar to values obtained with Doppler guidewire

18 The correct formula for determining myocardial oxygen consumption (MVO_2) from the coronary arterial or venous flow (Q), arterial oxygen content (AoO_2), and coronary sinus oxygen content (CSO_2) is:

(A) $MVO_2 = Q/(AoO_2 - CSO_2)$

(B) $MVO_2 = Q \times (AoO_2 - CSO_2)$

(C) $MVO_2 = (AoO_2 - CSO_2)/Q$

(D) Unable to calculate with the data provided

19 The "abbreviated" form of the Gorlin formula (so-called, Hakki equation: valve area (cm^2) = flow (L per minute)/$\sqrt{\text{peak-to-peak pressure gradient}}$) is often used to estimate valve area in patients with valvular stenosis referred for catheterization. It may be inaccurate in which of the following circumstances:

(A) Bradycardia (heart rate <60 bpm) or tachycardia (heart rate >60 bpm)

(B) Valve area <1.0 cm^2

(C) High cardiac output

(D) Low transvalvular gradient

20 In which of the following circumstances does the use of an LV–Ao pullback pressure to assess aortic valve area yield inaccurate results?

(A) Low (<35 mm Hg) transvalvular gradient

(B) Atrial fibrillation

(C) Postventriculography

(D) All the above

21 Coronary venous oxygen saturation is typically:

(A) 30%

(B) 50%

(C) 65%

(D) 80%

22 Which of the following is *not* true of corrected TIMI frame counts (CTFCs)?

(A) TIMI frame counts should be performed on angiograms obtained at 30 frames per second

(B) The frame rate required for full opacification of the LAD is 1.7 times longer than the RCA or left circumflex vessels

(C) In patients successfully treated with thrombolysis, a CTFC of <20 frames per second is associated with a high risk of adverse events

(D) Prolonged CTFC 4 weeks after myocardial infarction (MI) is associated with impaired infarct-related arterial flow at 1 year

23 Which of the following coronary artery anomalies does *not* course between the aorta and pulmonary artery?

(A) Anomalous origin of the LAD artery from the right cusp

(B) Anomalous origin of the left circumflex artery from the right cusp

(C) Anomalous origin of the RCA from the left cusp

(D) Anomalous origin of the left main from the right cusp

24 All of the following are true regarding coronary blood flow, *except*:

(A) Coronary α_1-adrenergic receptor stimulation causes vasodilatation

(B) Stimulation of the parasympathetic nervous system results in vasoconstriction

(C) Stimulation of B_1 receptors in the coronary arterioles leads to vasodilatation

(D) Stimulation of B_2 receptors in the coronary arterioles leads to vasodilatation

Answers and Explanations

1 **Answer B.** The pressure recording shows "ventricularization," in which diastolic pressure is reduced but systolic pressure is preserved. Normally, the catheter tip pressure and the sidearm pressure are similar. If an ostial coronary stenosis is present, engagement of the catheter may obstruct antegrade blood flow and cause ventricularization of the catheter pressure waveform (*Am Heart J.* 1989;118: 1160–1166).

2 **Answer C.** The most common coronary anomaly is origin of the left circumflex artery from the right sinus of Valsalva. This can often be visualized during left ventriculography (30 degree RAO projection) as a "dot" or "button" projecting from the aortic root as the left circumflex courses posterior to the aorta (*Circulation* 1974;50:768–773, *Ann Thorac Surg.* 1997;63:377–381).

3 **Answer D.** In the 30 degree RAO projection, one is looking down the AV plane, in which the left circumflex artery resides. Because the proximal portion of the vessel is foreshortened in this view, caudal angulation needs to be applied to unforeshorten it. In the other angles listed, the proximal left circumflex is either foreshortened or overlapped by other vessels.

4 **Answer C.** The sinus node artery originates from the left circumflex artery in 40% of individuals and as a proximal branch from the RCA in 60%, regardless of whether the patient is right or left dominant.

5 **Answer C.** In the general population, only 10% of individuals are right dominant (e.g., the posterior descending artery arises from the distal left circumflex artery). However, 30% of patients with a bicuspid valve are left dominant (*Am J Cardiol.* 1978;42: 57–59).

6 **Answer D.** The LAO caudal view projects the LAD upward from the left main in the appearance of a spider and permits improved visualization of the left main and the proximal bifurcation.

7 **Answer C.** Visual estimation of coronary stenosis is subject to significant operator variability and a systematic form of "stenosis inflation," in which the operator's estimate of diameter stenosis is approximately 20% more severe than that measured by quantitative coronary angiography (*Circulation* 1990;82:2231–2234). Therefore, a stenosis that measures 50% is typically called 70%.

8 **Answer A.** A 50% reduction in lumen diameter (hence, a 75% reduction in cross-sectional area) is "hemodynamically significant" in that it reduces the three- to fourfold CFR (*N Engl J Med.* 1994;330:1782–1788). The ability to increase flow during vasodilator stimulus is impaired when luminal diameter is reduced 50% and abolished when the stenosis is >70%.

9 **Answer B.** As initially defined by the TIMI investigators (*N Engl J Med.* 1985;312:932–936), TIMI 0 flow represents no perfusion, TIMI 1 flow represents penetration of contrast material without perfusion (e.g., contrast material is visualized beyond the area of obstruction but fails to opacify the entire distal coronary bed), TIMI 2 flow represents partial perfusion (contrast material visualized in the coronary distal to the obstruction), and TIMI 3 flow represents complete perfusion.

10 **Answer D.** A Kugel's artery passes from either the proximal right or left coronary artery down along the anterior margin of the atrial septum to anastomose with the AV node branch of the distal RCA to provide blood supply to the posterior circulation (*Tex Heart Inst.* 2004;31:267–270, *Am Heart J.* 1950; 40:260–270.)

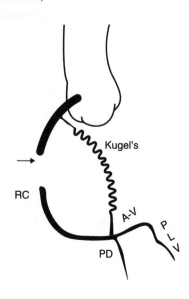

11 **Answer C.** A 50% stenosis represents a 75% narrowing in cross-sectional area (see figure).

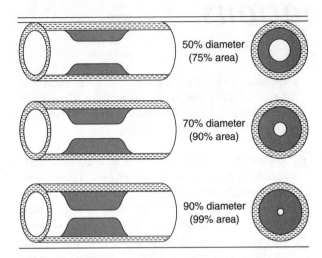

50% diameter
(75% area)

70% diameter
(90% area)

90% diameter
(99% area)

12 **Answer B.** Endothelial dysfunction results in reduced levels of EDRF and NO locally; however, they have a very short half-life, so that changes in local concentration cannot be detected in the coronary sinus circulation. Nitroprusside is an endothelium-independent vasodilator, whereas acetylcholine is an endothelium-dependent vasodilator. Nitroprusside induces vasodilation by acting directly on the vascular smooth muscle. Acetylcholine causes vasodilation if the endothelium is intact and vasoconstriction if the endothelium is absent or dysfunctional. Normal coronary arteries on angiography do not exclude endothelial dysfunction.

13 **Answer A.** An FFR >0.75 is associated with the absence of exercise-induced myocardial ischemia and a low incidence of clinical events (*J Am Coll Cardiol.* 1998;31:841–847, *Circulation* 1995;92:39–46).

14 **Answer A.** Approximately two thirds of the LAD blood flow drains into the great cardiac vein. The great cardiac vein becomes the coronary sinus at the point where the oblique vein of Marshall (a left atrial venous remnant of the embryonic left-sided superior vena cava). Great cardiac vein flow represents primarily LAD venous effluent, whereas coronary sinus flow represents a mixture of LAD and left circumflex flow.

15 **Answer D.** CFR is the hyperemic flow (or velocity) divided by the basal flow (or velocity) and normally ranges from 2.5 to 5. A reduction in CFR occurs with hemodynamically significant stenosis (>50% luminal diameter narrowing). Maximal hyperemia is attained with intracoronary

injections of dipyridamole, adenosine, or papaverine (not acetylcholine). Intracoronary acetylcholine may cause vasodilation if the endothelium is normal or vasoconstriction if the endothelium is absent or dysfunctional.

16 **Answer B.** In the absence of stenosis, the R3 vessels (arteriolar and intramyocardial) are responsible for 40% to 50% of total coronary resistance, the R2 vessels (prearteriolar) are responsible for 25% to 35%, and the R1 (epicardial) vessels contribute little to coronary resistance.

17 **Answer A.** CFR by thermodilution catheter is substantially smaller than a Doppler-derived measurement (*J Am Coll Cardiol.* 1992;20:402–407). With thermodilution, CFR is typically 2 to 3; with Doppler it is 2.5 to 5.

18 **Answer B.** According to the Fick principle, the uptake of a substance (e.g., oxygen or MVO_2) is the product of flow (Q) and the arteriovenous concentration difference of the substance ($AoO_2 - CSO_2$). Therefore, $MVO_2 = Q \times (AoO_2 - CSO_2)$.

19 **Answer A.** At extremes of heart rate (<60 bpm or >100 bpm), the Hakki equation should not be used to estimate valve area, as it may be inaccurate (*Kardiologiia* 1991;31:40–44).

20 **Answer D.** Nonsimultaneous measurement of LV and aortic pressures may be inaccurate when the transvalvular gradient is low (*Am Heart J.* 1992;123:948–953), the systolic pressure is fluctuating (e.g., atrial fibrillation), or LV systolic function is depressed immediately after administration of contrast material.

21 **Answer A.** At rest, transmyocardial oxygen extraction is nearly maximal, with coronary venous oxygen saturation (25% to 35%) being lower than other venous circulations in the body.

22 **Answer C.** CTFC in coronary vessels without stenosis is approximately 20 frames. In the TIMI 4, 10A, and 10B thrombolysis trials, a CTFC <20 in the infarct-related artery was associated with a low risk for adverse outcomes, whereas CTFCs between 20 and 40 frames per second showed a higher risk of adverse events (*Circulation* 1999;99:1945–1950, *Am Heart J.* 1989;117:665–679).

23 **Answer B.** The most common coronary anomaly is origin of the left circumflex artery from the right proximal RCA or sinus of Valsalva (top panel), from which it courses posterior to the aorta. With the anomalous RCA (middle panel) or LAD (bottom panel), the vessel may course anterior to the pulmonary artery or between the aortic root and the pulmonary artery, which is associated with sudden cardiac death.

24 **Answer A.** The balance between β-adrenergic stimulation (leading to coronary vasodilatation) and α-adrenergic stimulation (leading to vasoconstriction) determines coronary blood flow. Stimulation of the parasympathetic nervous system releases acetylcholine which leads to epicardial vasodilation. B_2 receptors are located in the myocardium and their stimulation increases contractility.

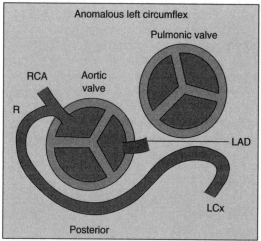

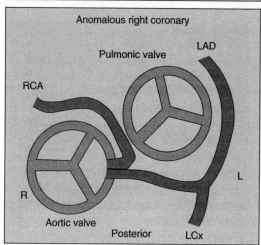

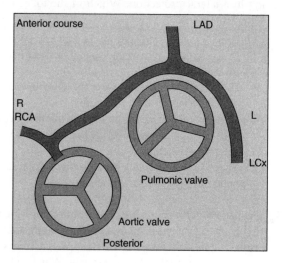

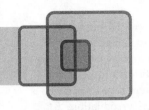

3

Radiation Safety, Equipment, and Basic Concepts

John C. Gurley

Questions

1 Which of the following statements regarding fluoroscopy in the modern cardiac catheterization laboratory is *true*?

(A) Modern catheterization laboratories have reduced the potential for x-ray exposure to patients and operators

(B) The x-ray exposure for fluoroscopy is much lower than the exposure for diagnostic cineangiography

(C) Most reports of radiation skin injury due to fluoroscopy occurred before 1996 and were linked to improperly calibrated, analog imaging equipment

(D) The federal government limits the maximum allowable fluoroscopic exposure rate to 10 R/min, a rate that is below the known threshold for skin burns

2 The interventional cardiologist shown in the following figure wishes to minimize his own radiation

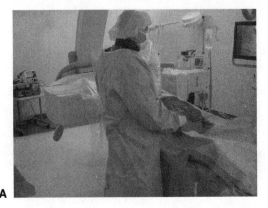

A

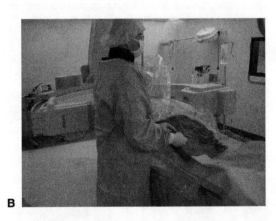

B

exposure during a procedure that will require imaging in a lateral projection. Which of the following statements is *true*?

(A) Panel B is preferred because the principal source of scatter radiation is positioned farthest from the operator

(B) Panel A is preferred because the x-ray beam is directed away from the operator

(C) There is no difference as long as the distances between the x-ray tube, patient, and image receptor are held constant

(D) There is no difference because the x-ray beam penetrates the same thickness of tissue

3 The patient in the following photograph complained to his family physician about an uncomfortable "rash" on his right lower back that appeared 3 weeks after he was hospitalized for chest pain. Which of the following statements is *true*?

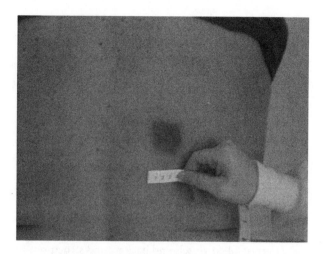

(A) The photograph illustrates a stochastic effect of radiation
(B) The photograph illustrates a deterministic effect of radiation
(C) The delayed appearance makes radiation skin injury unlikely
(D) This type of injury is very unpredictable

4 The following images were obtained from the same patient, with the same radiographic equipment. The image on the left has a grainy appearance, whereas that on the right is smoother and sharper. Which of the statements best explains the difference?

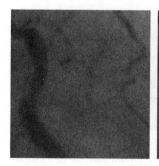
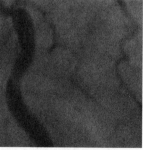

(A) The image on the left was acquired with an excessively high milliampere (mA) setting
(B) The one on the right has been electronically processed with an edge enhancement filter
(C) The speckled appearance of the image on the left could have been improved by decreasing the pulse width
(D) The image on the right is visually superior because it was made with a larger dose of x-rays
(E) The image on the left indicates that the charge-coupled device (CCD) camera is out of focus and should be recalibrated by the service technician

5 The arteriogram shown in the following figure was obtained with digital subtraction technique, which eliminates background structures and enhances the visibility of contrast-filled vessels. Which of the following statements about digital subtraction angiography and radiation is *true*?

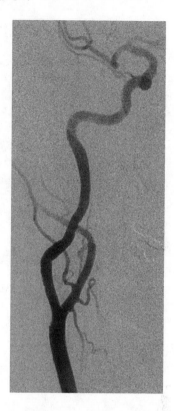

(A) A principle advantage of digital subtraction technique is that each frame delivers a reduced dose of radiation to the patient
(B) Compared to cardiac "cine" acquisitions, each frame of a subtraction study delivers a much larger dose of radiation to the patient
(C) Digital subtraction is a form of postprocessing that does not influence patient dose
(D) Subtraction technique can enhance low-quality images obtained with very low x-ray exposure settings

6 Which of the following statements about tube filament current (mA) is correct?

(A) Doubling the mA will decrease the patient dose rate by 50%
(B) Doubling the mA will increase the patient dose rate by 50%
(C) Doubling the mA will double the patient dose rate
(D) Doubling the mA will quadruple the patient dose rate

7 The following images illustrate the use of collimation during coronary arteriography. Which of the following statements about collimation is *false*?

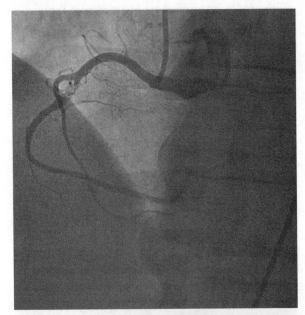

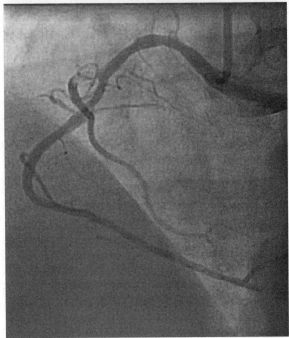

(A) Collimation reduces the skin entrance dose
(B) Collimation reduces x-ray exposure everywhere in the room
(C) Collimation improves image quality
(D) As a means of reducing x-ray exposure, collimation is superior to selecting a smaller field of view (higher magnification) that just encompasses the area of interest

8 Which of the following statements is *true* about the function of the grid?

(A) The grid is applied to the surface of the x-ray tube
(B) The grid reduces the radiation dose received by the patient
(C) The grid improves image quality
(D) The grid should be removed when imaging larger patients

9 The following images depict coronary arteriograms obtained from two different patients, utilizing the same radiographic equipment. In panel A, the arteries are well opacified, with excellent contrast between contrast-filled vessels and background structures. In panel B, the arteries are not as dark and they do not stand out as well against the background. Which of the following statements best explains the difference?

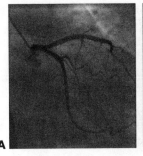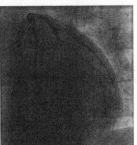

A   B

(A) The operator injected less contrast agent in panel B, so fewer iodine atoms are available to absorb x-rays
(B) A higher mA setting was used in panel B
(C) A shorter pulse width was used in panel A
(D) A higher peak kilovoltage (kVp) setting was used in panel B

10 A 23-year-old woman has developed pulmonary edema during her second trimester of pregnancy. Echocardiography demonstrates critical rheumatic mitral stenosis, and the patient is now referred for balloon valvotomy. Which of the following statements is *true* regarding radiation exposure during pregnancy?

(A) Pregnancy is an absolute contraindication to cardiac fluoroscopy
(B) The procedure can be performed safely as long as proper shielding is applied to the abdomen and pelvis
(C) The radiation hazard to the fetus is very small, and shielding is not necessary
(D) The most likely adverse effect is intrauterine growth retardation because rapidly growing

tissues are extremely sensitive to small doses of ionizing radiation

11 Modern cardiac fluoroscopy systems display values for "air kinetic energy released to matter (KERMA)" and "dose area product (DAP)." Interventional cardiologists should understand what these values mean. Which of the following statements is *true*?

(A) Air KERMA estimates the skin dose and can be used to predict the risk of radiation skin injury

(B) DAP is a valuable measure of total x-ray exposure because it cannot be manipulated by collimation or any other operator-controlled variable

(C) Air KERMA is a measure of scatter radiation in the air surrounding the image receptor (intensifier or flat detector)

(D) Air KERMA and DAP are instantaneous values that should never be used to infer the skin dose or the total absorbed dose

12 The operator in the following photograph has selected the right radial approach to coronary arteriography for an obese patient with a very large abdominal pannus. Which of the following statements about this situation is *false*?

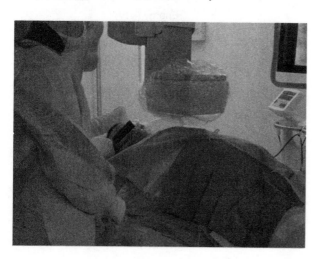

(A) He should obtain eye protection and a radiation shield and stand back as far as possible because the x-ray exposure levels needed to penetrate this heavy patient will increase exponentially with patient thickness

(B) He has lowered the table as far as possible; this will minimize the risk of radiation skin injury

(C) He should expect low-quality images

(D) He should utilize a large field of view (low magnification) and minimize panning

(E) It is unethical to perform the procedure on an extremely obese patient in whom large doses

of x-ray will be needed to generate low-quality images

(F) He should add "skin burns" to the consent document

13 The operator controls several factors that significantly influence radiation exposure and image quality. Among these are table height, tube position, and image detector position. In the following photograph, the image detector (*arrow*) is positioned well above the patient's chest. Which of the following statements is *true*?

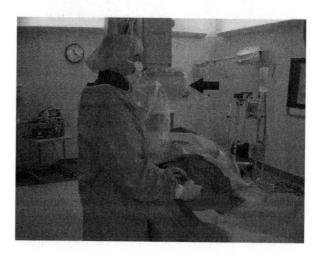

(A) The operator has placed an air gap between the patient and the image detector to reduce his dose of scatter radiation

(B) The operator has placed an air gap between the patient and the image detector to improve image quality

(C) The operator should lower the detector to the patient's chest in order to reduce the skin entrance dose

(D) The operator should lower the table as much as possible to minimize the skin entrance dose

14 Which of the following statements about radiation safety terminology is *true*?

(A) The unit of measure for the quantity of radiation absorbed is the Roentgen (R)

(B) ALARA is the adjusted lifetime average of radiation accumulated

(C) The unit of measure for the quantity of radiation absorbed is the Gray (Gy)

(D) The unit of measure for radiation exposure is the Sievert (Sv)

15 Which of the following statements about the device shown in the following figure is *true*?

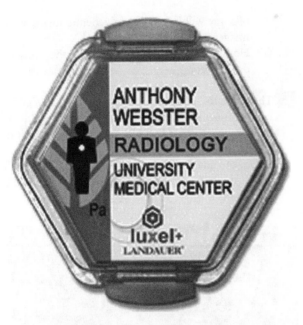

(A) If a single film badge is worn, it should be placed under the apron at waist level
(B) If a single film badge is worn, it should be placed on the outside of the apron at waist level
(C) If a single film badge is worn, it should be placed on the outside of the thyroid collar on the side closest to the source of scatter radiation
(D) Acceptable readings indicate that the operator is using safe radiologic practices
(E) This device protects the operator against cumulative doses of radiation that are above the threshold for stochastic effects

16 The following photograph depicts a flat-detector catheterization laboratory. Which of the following statements about this technology is *false*?

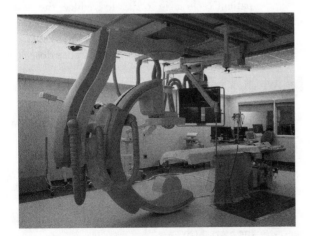

(A) Flat-panel detectors and image intensifiers are similar in that they both require a fluorescent phosphor to convert x-rays into visible light

(B) Flat-panel systems use a conventional x-ray tube
(C) Flat-panel systems typically deliver 30% to 50% less x-ray exposure than image intensifier–based systems
(D) Flat detectors are solid-state devices, whereas image intensifiers use a large vacuum tube
(E) Flat-panel detectors require a high-speed CCD video camera

17 The following three plots depict the energy spectra of x-rays produced by a typical cardiac fluoroscopy unit. In each case, the dashed line represents a change that has been made to the settings. Which of the following statements is *true*?

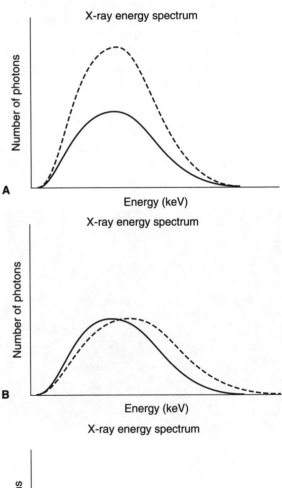

(A) The dashed line in A indicates that kVp has been increased

(B) The dashed line in B indicates that mA has been increased

(C) The dashed line in B indicates that the pulse width has been increased

(D) The dashed line in C indicates that the beam has been hardened by placing copper or aluminum filters over the output port of the x-ray tube

18 In the following illustration, a dotted line has been superimposed on the plot of photon energies produced by a typical cardiac fluoroscopy unit. Which of the following statements about this dotted line is *true*?

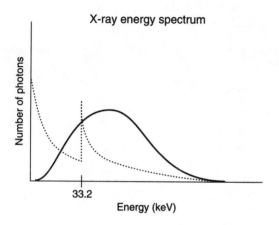

X-ray energy spectrum

(A) The spike in the dotted line depicts characteristic x-rays originating from the K shell of the tungsten atom

(B) The spike in the dotted line depicts the bremsstrahlung effect

(C) The dotted line depicts the absorption spectrum of iodine, with an absorption peak at 33.2 keV

(D) The spike in the dotted line depicts Compton scatter, which peaks at 33.2 keV

(E) The dotted line illustrates how copper beam filters reduce skin dose by eliminating x-rays with energies above 33.2 keV

19 Time, distance, and shielding are the three variables that determine exposure to scatter radiation during catheterization procedures. Which of the following statements about shielding is *false*?

(A) Lead aprons typically provide the equivalent of 0.5-mm lead thickness and block >90% of scatter radiation

(B) Lead eyeglasses reduce radiation exposure to the lens by approximately 35%

(C) Operators who find leaded glasses uncomfortable can utilize a transparent, movable shield to provide good protection

(D) A transparent, movable shield should be placed between the operator and the face of the image intensifier or flat-panel detector

(E) Assistants can reduce their exposure to scatter radiation by standing behind the primary operator

20 Which of the following statements about occupational exposure to x-rays in the cardiac catheterization laboratory is *false*?

(A) The lifetime risk of developing cancer in the United States is approximately 20%

(B) A career in interventional cardiology can be expected to measurably increase the risk of developing cancer

(C) A reasonable annual dose limit for an interventional cardiologist is 50 mSv

(D) Background radiation delivers an equivalent dose of approximately 3 to 4 mSv per year

(E) Cataract is a major occupational hazard for interventional cardiologists

21 The following is a schematic diagram of a simple x-ray tube, along with a plot of the energy it produces. Which of the following statements is *true*?

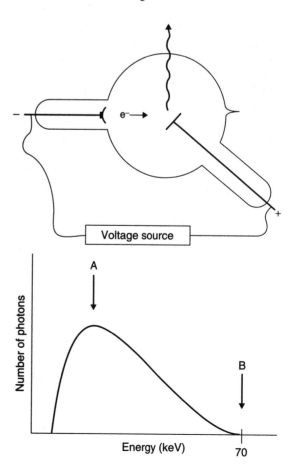

(A) *Arrow* A marks the kVp of the x-ray tube
(B) The x-rays were made with a peak filament current of 70 mA
(C) *Arrow* B indicates the power rating of the tube
(D) Up to 70,000 V was applied to this tube

22 Which of the following statements is *true* regarding safe operation of x-ray equipment by the physician during cardiac catheterization?

(A) Selecting 15 frames per second instead of 30 frames per second will cut the dose rate exactly in half
(B) An interventional cardiologist who constantly switches "fluoro" on and off every time he glances at his hands is not reducing x-ray exposure as expected; this is due to a power surge at start-up
(C) Virtual collimators do not reduce x-ray doses as effectively as standard lead collimators
(D) Each person in the room is responsible for his or her own radiation safety

23 A 56-year-old man has been referred to you for a second attempt at catheter-based repair of a chronic, total circumflex artery occlusion. He had not seen a physician until 1 week ago, when he presented with heart failure and angina. During the past week, he underwent diagnostic coronary arteriography, an unsuccessful percutaneous coronary intervention, and successful implantation of a biventricular defibrillator. The transfer records note hyperglycemia and obesity (weight 329 pounds). You realize that two of the three procedures performed during the past week probably involved prolonged fluoroscopy, so radiation skin injury is a very real possibility. Before beginning another procedure, which of the following should you do?

(A) Examine the back of the chest for signs of hair loss (epilation)

(B) Examine the back of the chest for signs of telangiectasia
(C) Examine the back of the chest for signs of dermal atrophy or necrosis
(D) Examine the back of the chest for signs of moist desquamation
(E) None of the above

24 The following image is a radiograph of a line pair phantom that can be used by radiation physicists and service technicians to measure high-contrast spatial resolution. Which of the following statements about calibration and maintenance is *false*?

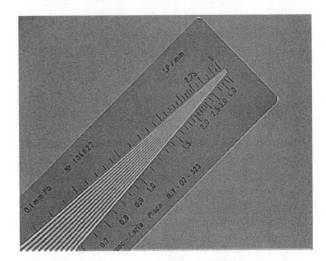

(A) The physicist and service technician should strive for the best possible image quality
(B) Image quality and dose measurements are still necessary for modern flat-detector systems
(C) A physicist should measure radiation levels and image quality parameters on a regularly scheduled basis
(D) Image quality can be improved by simply increasing the dose

Answers and Explanations

1 Answer B. In recent years, the scope and complexity of interventional procedures has expanded greatly. Although it is true that refinements to imaging systems have reduced x-ray exposure rates, the greater duration of therapeutic procedures has actually *increased* the potential for radiation exposure to patients and operators.

The x-ray exposure rates for fluoroscopy are typically 15 to 20 times lower than those used for diagnostic ("cine" mode) acquisitions. Nevertheless, during interventional procedures, most x-ray exposure to patients and operators comes from fluoroscopy. Procedures that utilize only fluoroscopy are capable of delivering skin doses sufficient to cause severe burns.

The recognition that diagnostic x-ray systems can cause skin injury to patients is a relatively recent phenomenon. The first U.S. Food and Drug Administration (FDA) advisory was published in 1994 and the first reports of radiation skin necrosis due to fluoroscopy did not appear in the medical literature until 1996. (www.fda.gov/cdrh/fluor.html. 2006, *Radiographics*. 1996;16: 1195–1199) Even modern, properly calibrated systems are capable of causing radiation skin injury. The risk is greatest with prolonged or repeated procedures, heavy patients, and when body parts are positioned close to the x-ray tube.

The FDA limits the maximum exposure rate for diagnostic fluoroscopy, but this does not guarantee patient safety. Body parts that are positioned close to the x-ray tube (such as the arm in a lateral projection) can receive much more than the calibrated 10 R/min limit. Prolonged exposures can further increase the risk of injury.

2 Answer A. Scatter radiation is the main source of exposure to the operator, to laboratory staff, and to patient body parts outside the x-ray beam. Most scatter to the operator originates from the beam entry point, where incoming x-rays strike the table and body surface. In panel B, the source of scatter is farther from the operator, so exposure is reduced as predicted by the inverse square law. In addition, the patient's body is positioned as a shield between the source of scatter and the operator. By choosing panel B, this operator can estimate a 10-fold reduction in personal exposure.

The primary beam is collimated, by law, to the size of the image receptor. Therefore, the operator in these illustrations would not be exposed to the primary beam.

3 Answer B. Stochastic effects pertain to deoxyribonucleic acid (DNA) injury that may increase the probability of genetic defects or cancer at some point in the future. Theoretically, even a single x-ray photon can induce DNA injury in a single cell that leads to fatal lymphoma 20 years later. A greater exposure and one of a longer duration will increase the probability of a stochastic effect, but there is no safe threshold and the consequences are unpredictable. Cancer caused by a single x-ray photon is just as bad as cancer caused by millions of photons.

Deterministic effects pertain to cell injury that occurs shortly (hours to months) after a threshold dose of radiation is exceeded. Skin injury is the most common deterministic effect of diagnostic x-ray exposure. Because skin cells divide continuously, they are susceptible to injury from large doses of radiation that can occur at the beam entrance port. The injury becomes apparent weeks to months after exposure, when cells lost by normal desquamation are no longer replaced. Because of the delay, patients and physicians may not even suspect the cause.

The photograph illustrates radiation skin injury from fluoroscopy used during a percutaneous coronary intervention. The size and location indicate that the operator worked in the right anterior oblique (RAO) projection and utilized square collimators. This type of injury can progress for months, sometimes leading to deep, nonhealing ulcers that require grafting. It is important to know that deterministic effects are predictable, and therefore preventable.

4 Answer D. The background granularity of the image on the left is known as "quantum mottle." It is due to random variation in the distribution of x-ray photons striking the image detector, and it is most apparent when very few photons are available to generate an image. The images obtained through night-vision goggles are grainy for the same reason—few light photons. X-rays and visible light are both forms of electromagnetic radiation, with energy carried in discrete packets or quanta.

Quantum mottle is a form of noise that degrades the detectability of vessel edges and low contrast structures. Increasing the tube filament current (mA) or the pulse width would generate more x-ray photons and thereby suppress quantum mottle. Small amounts of x-ray are used during fluoroscopy, whereas larger amounts of x-ray are used to produce archive quality images such as the one on the right.

Quantum mottle does not indicate a lack of focus or any other problem with the equipment. In fact, the ability to appreciate quantum mottle should reassure the operator that the fluoroscopic dose settings are appropriately low.

The image on the left was obtained with "low-dose" fluoroscopy, whereas that on the right was obtained in the "cine" acquisition mode. The difference in x-ray dose to the patient and operator was approximately 40-fold.

5 Answer B. In digital subtraction angiography, a non–contrast-filled (mask) image is subtracted from a contrast-filled (live) image. Constant densities, such as bone, are neutralized, leaving only the contrast column. The pattern created by random noise is different on the mask and live images, so subtraction accentuates the noise inherent in low-dose images. To suppress noise, each frame of a subtraction study requires a substantially larger dose of radiation than is needed for a cardiac cine frame. A typical subtraction study can deliver more than 10 times the dose per frame to the patient. Scatter exposure to the operator and room staff is increased commensurately. Subtraction studies are usually acquired at low frame rates of 1 to 6 per second, but this only partially mitigates the higher dose per frame. Subtraction cannot create image detail that was not present in the original image.

6 Answer C. Tube filament current (mA) is directly proportional to the number of x-ray photons being produced. Doubling the mA will double the patient's skin entry dose and it will also double the amount of scatter radiation for operators and room staff.

7 Answer A. Collimators are lead shutters that restrict the size and shape of the x-ray beam as it leaves the tube. The amount of radiation exiting the tube is directly proportional to the *area* of the beam.

The uncollimated beam used to create the image on the left exposes tissues outside the area of interest to useless radiation. This creates scatter radiation that unnecessarily exposes the operator, patient, and room staff. Scatter that reaches the detector fogs the desirable portion of the image, reducing contrast and overall image quality.

The exposed area of the collimated image on the right is less than half of the uncollimated image. This means that exposure for everyone in the room is less than half of what it would be without collimation.

Although collimation reduces the area of skin exposed, it does not reduce the dose absorbed by skin cells within the irradiated area. In some cases, tight collimation can actually increase the skin dose (this happens if the collimator blades fall within the sampling area for automatic brightness compensation).

8 Answer C. The antiscatter grid is a plate-like device that attaches to the face of the image intensifier or flat detector. It functions like the slats of a Venetian blind, allowing straight-line rays from the x-ray tube to pass through while blocking tangentially directed scatter rays. The grid improves image quality by reducing the fogging effect of scatter, but it does so at the expense of increased patient doses. The grid can more than double the entrance doses received by the patient. Because small children and very thin adults produce little scatter, removing the grid can reduce patient exposure without compromising image quality. This might be important in cases in which the operator wishes to minimize radiation exposure to sensitive areas such as the breast.

9 Answer D. The difference in image quality stems from the greater thickness and density of tissue that must be penetrated in panel B. The image in panel A was obtained from an average-sized patient, in a shallow RAO projection, with lung as the background. The image in panel B was obtained from a large patient, in a cranial projection, with the spine as the background.

When steep projections are used in large patients, the generator control system automatically increases the kVp, often to >90 kVp, in an attempt to maintain image brightness. This produces more energetic photons that are able to penetrate tissues better. Unfortunately, many of these photons are too energetic to be absorbed by the iodine, which has a K-edge absorption peak at 33.2 keV.

It does appear that the iodine concentration is too low in panel B, but the same contrast medium was used and both arteries were well injected. The problem is not the concentration of iodine, but rather that iodine is transparent to high-energy photons. The washed-out image is characteristic of a high kVp.

10 Answer C. Pregnancy is not a contraindication to necessary cardiac catheterization procedures. External shielding is useless because the fetus is not exposed to the primary beam, only to scatter radiation originating from the mother's chest, and most of this scatter is absorbed by the abdominal viscera. The very small doses of radiation reaching the pelvis would not be expected to cause cell damage (a deterministic effect) leading to intrauterine growth retardation. However, even the smallest dose of ionizing radiation could increase the future risk of malignancy in an unpredictable manner. Fetuses and newborns are known to be at least an order of magnitude more susceptible to radiation-induced malignancy than adults, so the risk is not entirely theoretical. (*Med Phys.* 2001;28: 1543–1545, Committee on the Biological Effects of Ionizing Radiation. *National research council: health effects of exposure to low levels of ionizing radiation.* 1990).

The operator should discuss the very small cancer risk with the patient and utilize the smallest amount of radiation needed to conduct the procedure safely. The operator should limit the beam to the chest and utilize fluoroscopy instead of cine mode acquisition whenever possible.

11 Answer A. The transfer of x-ray energy to tissues is estimated with an air-filled ionization chamber placed within the beam, inside the x-ray tube housing. The KERMA is then calculated for a point that approximates the location of the skin surface when the heart is at the isocenter. The cumulative air KERMA displayed on the monitor, in units of Gray, can be a very good substitute for skin dose, which is difficult to measure directly. This assumes a typical table height and a single projection. Air KERMA will overestimate the skin dose when multiple projections are utilized because the dose spreads over several different entry ports. It will underestimate the skin dose and the risk of injury whenever body parts are placed close to the x-ray tube.

DAP is the air KERMA multiplied by the beam cross-sectional area. The cumulative DAP is a good measure of the total amount of radiation absorbed by the patient. It is also a good indicator of total room exposure. Collimation reduces beam area, DAP, total patient dose, and room exposure.

12 Answer B. Shielding and distance are highly effective methods of reducing operator exposure. Because the intensity of scatter radiation is inversely proportional to the square of the distance from the source, one step backward can reduce exposure tenfold.

To produce an image, x-rays must penetrate the patient and enter the detector. Because absorption increases exponentially with increasing tissue thickness, obese patients require far greater input levels of radiation.

In obese patients, the generator control computer will automatically increase the kVp in an attempt to maintain image brightness, and this will reduce image contrast. It may also increase the pulse

width, which can blur moving vessels. These effects, along with increased scatter, will markedly degrade the image quality. This operator should select a large field of view and avoid panning if possible. This will minimize the skin entry dose, keep kVp to a minimum, maximize image contrast, and minimize motion blur.

The operator cannot deny this patient a necessary procedure, but he must be responsible for balancing the risks and benefits. For most patients, the potential for radiation skin injury is so low that a discussion of risk is not necessary. However, for interventional procedures in extremely obese patients, the operator should probably discuss the possibility of skin injury.

Lowering the table as much as possible would place the skin entry in the most concentrated portion of the x-ray beam. This would markedly increase the skin dose and the risk of skin injury.

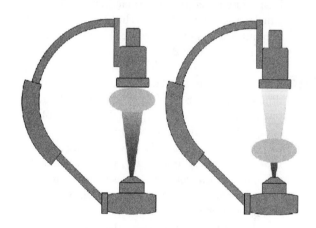

The above figures illustrate what happens when the table is lowered as much as possible. A smaller area of skin is exposed to more intense radiation.

13 Answer C. The table height and detector position are key determinants of x-ray exposure, and both are under the operator's control. The x-ray beam diverges and becomes less intense as it leaves the tube, just like a beam of light diverges and becomes less intense as it leaves a flashlight.

Raising the detector, as shown in the photograph, forces the generator control computer to increase x-ray output to compensate for lost image brightness. This markedly increases the patient skin dose, as well as the scatter dose absorbed by everyone in the room. The computer also increases the kVp, which diminishes image contrast. The detector should always be placed as close to the patient as possible.

Lowering the table will place the patient's skin in the most concentrated portion of the x-ray beam, increasing skin dose rates. This is why some medical x-ray tubes have spacers to keep body parts away from the intense beam. Spacers must never be removed.

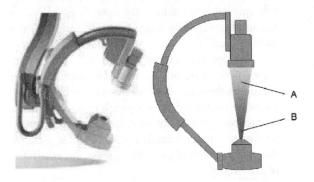

The above images depict how an x-ray beam diverges and becomes less intense with distance from the source. The left panel is a photograph of a typical image intensifier–based cardiac system. The right panel is a schematic diagram showing how the beam at point A is less likely to cause skin injury than the same beam at point B.

14 Answer C. It is useful to think of radiation in three dimensions: intensity of exposure, absorption, and biological effect. An analogy is the transfer of heat energy that occurs when one briefly passes a hand through a candle flame. The brief exposure to intense heat transfers very little energy, which is insufficient to injure tissue. Prolonged exposure to warm air on a summer day can cause heat stroke, a profound whole-body effect.

The unit used to measure the *intensity* of x-ray exposure is the Roentgen (R). Simplistically, this value tells you whether you are dealing with a candle flame or with warm air. The intensity of radiation diminishes with the square of the distance from the source (inverse square law). This is why distance is an excellent way to minimize operator exposure. If you know that you are dealing with a candle flame, it is best not to put your hand too close. Unfortunately, operators cannot see or feel x-rays. This is why cardiac fluoroscopy systems have instrumentation that displays the intensity of radiation.

The concentration of radiation at a given location can be determined by exposing some material to x-rays, then measuring the KERMA. Catheterization laboratory x-ray machines use air as material. They count ionizations in a chamber with a known volume of material (air) and then calculate air KERMA.

Absorbed dose refers to the concentration of energy transferred to tissue, and the unit of measure for *absorption* is the Gray (Gy). In cardiac

fluoroscopy, this is an important measure of the potential risk of skin injury.

The Sievert (Sv) is a measure of the whole-body biological effect of one or more absorbed doses. This value can be used to estimate the long-term risk of cancer in an operator.

ALARA is an acronym for as low as reasonably achievable. It is the guiding principle for everyone who uses x-rays.

15 Answer C. This is a film badge type of dosimeter that records the accumulated dose of scatter radiation over a period of time. Ideally, two badges should be worn, one on the thyroid collar and one under the apron at waist level. If a single badge is used, it should be placed on the outside of the thyroid collar on the side closest to the source of scatter radiation. Acceptable readings do not indicate safe practice. An operator who performs a limited number of procedures can expose his patient and his room staff to unnecessary radiation while recording low badge readings. There is no threshold for stochastic effects, including genetic defects and cancer. A badge will not protect anyone. The best protection is a good understanding of radiation safety.

16 Answer C. Flat detectors and image intensifiers utilize phosphors that convert x-ray photons into faint scintillations of visible light. Early fluoroscopists looked directly at the phosphor in darkened rooms, but this delivered high radiation doses to the eyes and caused cataracts. Image intensifiers brighten the image with a large photomultiplier tube, to the point where it can be captured with a video camera and displayed on a television monitor. With flat detectors, the input phosphors are bonded directly to photodiode arrays that convert the visible light into digital signals.

Both systems use a conventional x-ray tube and similar x-ray exposure levels. Because flat detectors are solid-state devices, they tend to be smaller and lighter, and their performance is more stable over time. Flat-panel catheterization systems are rapidly replacing image intensifier–based systems.

17 Answer D. An increase in filament current (mA) increases the number of photons produced without altering the distribution of photon energies, as depicted in panel A. An increase in kVp shifts the energy spectrum toward the right, increasing the proportion of high-energy photons (panel B). Because high-energy photons are more likely to penetrate the patient, they are less likely to be absorbed and therefore less likely to deposit their energy into tissues. Low-energy photons are absorbed by the skin at the beam entry point; they deposit all their energy into tissues and do not contribute to an image. Obviously, the higher-energy photons are desirable for imaging, but only to a point. High-energy photons are poorly absorbed by iodine, so they produce low contrast arteriograms. Copper and aluminum filters are routinely utilized to absorb the low-energy x-rays that would contribute to skin dose but not to image production. The effect is illustrated in panel C.

18 **Answer C.** The black line represents the energy *emission* spectrum of an x-ray tube. The dotted line represents the x-ray *absorption* spectrum of iodine. A sudden jump in absorption occurs when the photon energy is just above the binding energy of the K-shell electron of the iodine atom. The process is known as *photoelectric absorption*. Iodine is a good agent for contrast angiography because it is relatively nontoxic and has a K-shell binding energy of 33.2 keV, which is close to the peak of the output spectrum of medical x-ray machines. Barium has a K edge of 37.4 keV, so it would make a good contrast agent if it were not toxic.

X-rays are produced when electrons emitted from the cathode are accelerated into a tungsten target. When a high-speed electron approaches a dense, positively charged tungsten nucleus, it is deflected and slowed, and its kinetic energy is released in the form of an x-ray photon. These photons are called *bremsstrahlung* or *braking x-rays*. Almost all the x-rays produced by a medical x-ray machine are bremsstrahlung rays.

A few of the high-speed electrons that interact with the target cause the ejection of orbital electrons from shells close to the tungsten nucleus. When an electron from a higher shell drops down to fill the void, the difference in binding energy between the two shells is released in the form of an x-ray photon. These x-rays always have the same wavelength, which is *characteristic* of the target metal and the specific shells involved. The production of bremsstrahlung and characteristic x-rays is illustrated in the following figures.

Bremsstrahlung x-rays

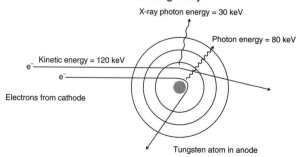

Characteristic x-rays

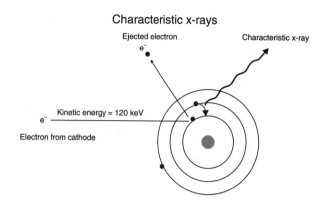

It is apparent that many of the x-rays produced by a fluoroscopy unit have energies that are either too low to penetrate the patient or too high to be absorbed by iodine. Copper filters screen out the low-energy photons that would contribute to skin dose but have no imaging value. An ideal x-ray beam for angiography would contain photons in the range between 30 and 70 keV.

Compton scattering occurs when the incoming x-ray photon energies are much greater than the electron binding energies in body tissues. The incoming photon transfers enough energy to completely eject an electron from its atom; it then continues as a lower-energy x-ray in a different direction (to conserve momentum of the system). Most of the scatter radiation in a catheterization laboratory comes from Compton interactions.

19 **Answer C.** A movable acrylic shield should be part of every catheterization laboratory. Because most scatter radiation originates from the area where the x-ray beam first strikes the patient's chest wall, the shield should be positioned between the beam entry port and the operator's face. It is important to remember that scatter radiation comes from the patient, not from the image detector. A well-positioned acrylic shield will reduce exposure to the operator's eyes, chest, and thyroid by 90%. An assistant who stands in the "shadow" of the primary operator can reduce his or her exposure by two methods. First, the increased distance alone can reduce exposure by 90% compared to the primary operator (inverse square law). Second, scatter rays must penetrate the body of the operator plus two layers of lead worn by the operator. This can be expected to attenuate the scatter beam by >99%.

20 **Answer E.** The lifetime risk of cancer in the United States is approximately 20%. The cumulative occupational dose acquired during a busy interventional career can be projected to increase that risk by 3% to 4%. Although no amount of radiation can be considered safe, the generally accepted annual dose limit is 50 mSv. To place this amount in perspective, average background radiation delivers 3 to 4 mSv per year.

Cataract formation is a deterministic effect of x-ray exposure that depends on a threshold dose and dose rate. Early fluoroscopists who looked directly into the x-ray beam received large doses of radiation in a short period, and they did develop cataracts. With modern equipment, the risk of developing a cataract is probably very low. Even so, eye protection is a reasonable precaution.

21 **Answer D.** This type of x-ray tube was used in the late 1890s by Roentgen and other pioneers to produce amazingly high-quality radiographs. Electrons from the cathode are accelerated by a high voltage until they collide with the metal anode. The maximum voltage across the tube determines the maximum energy of the x-ray photons produced. In this example, the 70,000 V peak (70 kVp) produces x-rays with energies up to 70 keV.

Modern cardiovascular tubes utilize the same principle, with a few refinements to increase the output of x-rays. The cathode consists of a white-hot filament that boils off the large quantities of electrons needed to make large amounts of x-rays. The anode consists of a rotating tungsten disk that absorbs and dissipates heat much better than a stationary target, which would quickly melt if used for cardiac angiography.

X-ray production is very inefficient. Only approximately 1% of the electrical energy delivered to the tube is converted into x-rays; the remaining 99% is converted to heat that must be dissipated. For years, heat dissipation was a major technical challenge for cardiovascular x-ray tubes. The problem has largely been solved by liquid cooling systems that work like automobile radiators.

22 **Answer A.** Most cardiac systems now operate at 15 frames per second. Thirty frames per second are sometimes used for pediatric patients with high heart rates and for ventricular wall motion studies.

Limiting the beam-on time is one of the most effective methods of reducing radiation exposure. The operator should *never* make x-rays unless he is looking directly at the monitor and prepared to work. Live fluoroscopy should never be used when an operator is manipulating equipment under direct vision, and it should never be used when contemplating the next move. "Last image hold" and "fluoro replay" features provide the same information without unnecessary radiation.

Virtual collimators are software-generated lines on the last recorded image. They allow the operator to position the collimators without stepping on the "fluoro" pedal. They are an excellent way to minimize radiation exposure.

The physician in charge is responsible for the radiation safety of everyone in the room. The operating physician must be knowledgeable enough to recognize and correct unsafe practices.

23 **Answer E.** Because of his obesity, this patient will receive substantially increased skin entry doses during cardiac fluoroscopy. The recent exposures will lower the threshold for skin injury with the next procedure. Diabetes may further increase the susceptibility to skin injury. In addition to discussing the risks and benefits, and considering the alternatives to another fluoroscopic procedure, this operator should examine the patient carefully for signs of radiation skin injury.

All the answers list deterministic effects of radiation. However, hair loss does not appear until 3 weeks after the exposure, and the latent period is even longer for desquamation (4 weeks), dermal atrophy or necrosis (3 months), and telangiectasia formation (1 year). Erythema can develop within hours to days.

24 **Answer A.** The objective of cardiac fluoroscopy is not to make the best possible image, but rather to strike a balance between image quality and dose. A good image contains some degree of noise. To achieve this objective, a regularly scheduled testing program is necessary for all fluoroscopy systems. Older image intensifier systems are especially susceptible to loss of contrast that can be partially compensated by increasing the input dose.

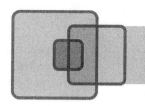

4

Inflammation and Arterial Injury

Christopher L. Sarnoski and Harold L. Dauerman

Questions

1 After coronary stenting, which of the following cell types would *not* be part of the initial injury response?

(A) Platelets
(B) Lymphocytes and macrophages
(C) α-Actin positive smooth muscle cells
(D) Neutrophils

2 How does arterial injury caused by angioplasty differ from injury due to drug-eluting stent (DES) placement?

(A) Negative remodeling may be a major factor in DES-related healing
(B) DESs abolish the early phases of platelet activation and inflammatory cytokine increases
(C) Polymer coating of the stent limits migration of smooth muscle cells
(D) Both neointimal hyperplasia and negative remodeling play major roles in the long-term healing response to balloon angioplasty

3 All of the following may contribute to arterial injury and inflammation, *except*:

(A) Stent coating with selected polymers/drugs
(B) Increased stent strut thickness and specific geometric factors
(C) Stent deployment with struts in contact with damaged media or lipid core
(D) Stent deployment with struts in contact with fibrous plaque

4 Panel A of the following figure is a histopathologic section from a rabbit artery stented with polymer and

a high dose of paclitaxel. Panel B is from an artery stented with polymer alone. How did this high dose of paclitaxel influence the healing response?

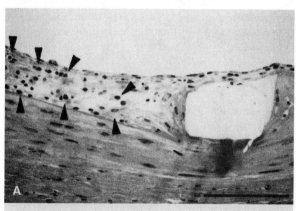

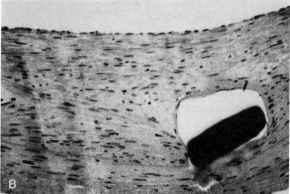

Circulation. 2001;104:473–479.

(A) Decreased intimal hyperplasia in the paclitaxel-polymer coated stent

(B) Increased inflammatory reaction in the polymer-only stent

(C) Decreased intimal hyperplasia in the polymer-only stent

(D) Persistent fibrin deposition in the polymer-only stent

5 The following figure shows a histopathologic analysis 1 day after implantation of a coronary stent. What does the asterisk in panel B demonstrate?

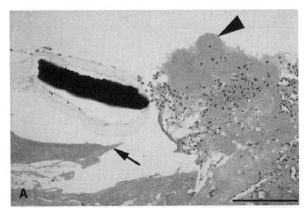

Circulation. 1999;99:44–52.

(A) Platelet-rich thrombus

(B) Lipid-rich vulnerable plaque

(C) Site of stent strut

(D) Fibrous plaque

6 Late stent thrombosis after drug-eluting stenting has been associated with which of the following?

(A) Warfarin anticoagulation in addition to dual antiplatelet therapy

(B) A localized, hypersensitivity (eosinophilic, giant cell) reaction to the polymer

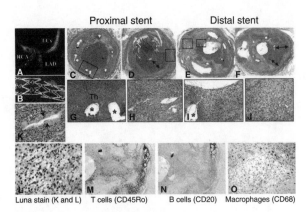

Luna stain (K and L) T cells (CD45Ro) B cells (CD20) Macrophages (CD68)

Circulation. 2004;109:701–705.

(C) Implantation of DESs in ST-elevated myocardial infarction (STEMI)

(D) Geographic miss during DES implantation

7 A patient develops acute chest pain and electrocardiogram (EKG) changes within 1 minute of stent implantation. What type of arterial injury is shown just distal to the stent?

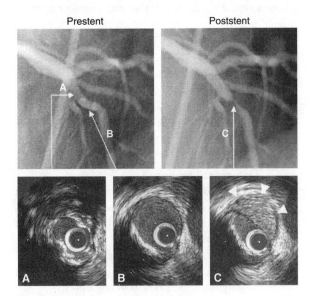

Circulation. 2002;105:2037–2042.

(A) Acute intramural hematoma

(B) Intraprocedural stent thrombosis

(C) Spontaneous rupture of distal lipid-rich plaque

(D) Acute platelet-rich thrombus due to stent-mediated hypersensitivity

8 Arterial injury due to stenting induces a systemic inflammatory response. The following figure shows the systemic rise of which inflammatory marker after stenting?

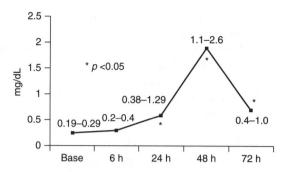

Am J Cardiol. **1998;82:515–518.**

(A) Serum amyloid-A
(B) C-reactive protein (CRP)
(C) Soluble CD40 ligand (sCD40L)
(D) Interleukin (IL)-6

9 The pre–percutaneous coronary intervention (PCI) level of which systemic marker of inflammation is associated with subsequent adverse cardiac events?

(A) Soluble intercellular adhesion molecule-1 (sICAM-1)
(B) IL-6
(C) IL-10
(D) sCD40L

10 Which level of CRP before PCI has been associated with increased risk of adverse events after stenting?

(A) 1.0 mg/dL to 3.0 mg/dL
(B) >3.0 mg/dL
(C) >10 mg/dL
(D) >3.0 mg/dL but only in patients with coexisting diabetes mellitus

11 Platelet activation after arterial injury promotes an inflammatory response through the following mediators:

(A) sCD40L
(B) P-selectin
(C) T cells
(D) All of the above

12 Activated macrophages, recruited after arterial injury, secrete which systemic mediators of inflammation?

(A) CRP
(B) sCD40L
(C) IL-1 and IL-6
(D) P-selectin

13 Platelet-leukocyte clusters may form in acute coronary syndromes and after PCI. Which event is unlikely to be related to platelet-leukocyte aggregates?

(A) Stent thrombosis
(B) Restenosis
(C) Contrast-induced nephropathy
(D) Periprocedural rise in creatine kinase-MB (CK-MB)

14 Arterial injury leads to a cascade of platelet activation followed by local and systemic inflammation. The following figure demonstrates vasoconstriction occurring after exercise in a patient who had received a sirolimus stent >6 months before the stress test. Which answer is incorrect?

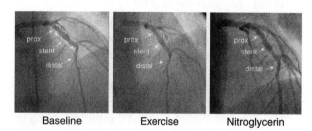

Baseline   Exercise   Nitroglycerin

J Am Coll Cardiol. **2005;46:231–236.**

(A) The patient might also have abnormal flow-independent dilation of the brachial artery
(B) The patient might also have abnormal flow-mediated dilation of the brachial artery
(C) DESs lead to delay in endothelial regeneration after injury
(D) Sirolimus or polymer may have an impact on endothelial function even after stent endothelialization

15 The following figure demonstrates similar DES-induced and bare metal stent (BMS)-induced systemic inflammation after PCI. If inflammation after arterial injury is important in developing restenosis, what best explains the 50% to 80% reduction in restenosis with DESs?

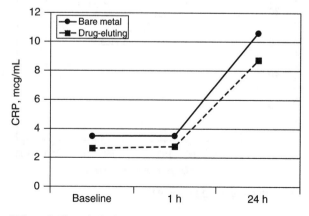

J Thromb Thrombolysis. **2005;19:87–92.**

(A) DES decreases initial and chronic platelet activation compared with BMS

(B) DES decreases the early systemic inflammatory response to stenting compared with BMS

(C) DES decreases the systemic inflammation occurring between 24 hours and 9 months after stenting

(D) DES decreases the local, but not systemic, impact of stenting on inflammation

16 An enhanced systemic inflammatory response may occur after PCI for cardiogenic shock. This inflammatory response may lead to:

(A) Upregulation of nitric oxide synthase leading to vasodilation and hypotension

(B) Severe vasoconstriction, thereby resulting in a decreased cardiac output

(C) A down regulation of nitric oxide synthase leading to pulmonary edema

(D) Upregulation of natriuretic peptides leading to hypotension through excessive diuresis

17 All of the following drugs have been shown to have a potential positive impact on the acute inflammatory response after PCI, *except*:

(A) Atorvastatin

(B) Clopidogrel

(C) Abciximab

(D) β-Blockers

18 In the IMPRESS (Immunosuppressive Therapy for the Prevention of Restenosis After Coronary Artery Stent Implantation) randomized trial, prednisone or placebo was given for 45 days after bare metal stenting with a reduction in 6-month cardiovascular event rates. What was the key entry requirement to be randomized in this trial?

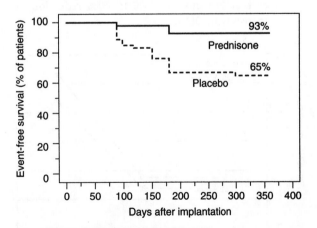

J Am Coll Cardiol. 2002;40:1935–1942.

(A) Elevated preprocedural levels of soluble CD40 after stenting

(B) High risk for restenosis based on presence of diabetes mellitus

(C) Elevated preprocedural levels of CRP

(D) A persistently elevated CRP level 72 hours after stenting

19 Which of the patients undergoing PCI may benefit the most from preprocedural clopidogrel administration?

(A) Patients at lower risk for inflammation as defined by a CRP level of <1.0

(B) Patients with a heightened inflammatory status as defined by an elevated CRP level before the PCI

(C) Patients undergoing PCI for stable angina, but not for acute coronary syndromes

(D) Patients with a heightened inflammatory status as defined by sCD40L

20 Eptifibatide and tirofiban have clearly shown to have which effects after PCI?

(A) Decreased intimal hyperplasia through a direct effect on macrophage accumulation

(B) Decreased intimal hyperplasia through inhibition of smooth muscle cell hyperplasia

(C) Decrease the rise of CRP and IL-6 levels in the first 24 hours after PCI compared with heparin alone

(D) Decreased platelet aggregation and the incidence of periprocedural myonecrosis

Answers and Explanations

Answer C. Coronary stenting is a model for arterial injury, and the healing response proceeds in phases. Phase 1 is de-endothelialization followed by deposition of platelets and fibrin. Through platelet activation and cytokine increases, acute inflammatory cells are then recruited in the first few days after stenting. Phase 2 involves release of growth factors from platelets and leukocytes, driving proliferation and migration of smooth muscle cells and long-term inflammatory cells. Phase 3 (weeks to months after injury) is characterized by the migration of α-actin positive smooth muscle cells into the neointima, extracellular matrix deposition, and re-endothelialization of the stent (*Circulation.* 2004;110:940–947, *Circulation.* 1999;99:44–52, *J Am Coll Cardiol.* 2000;35:157–163, *Arterioscler Thromb Vasc Biol.* 2002;22:1769–1776).

Answer D. All forms of arterial injury lead to platelet activation, inflammation, and smooth muscle cell–mediated chronic healing. Paclitaxel and sirolimus decrease the amount of neointimal hyperplasia compared with bare metal stenting, but the underlying polymer has no favorable effect on the healing process. All stents in general abolish two adverse components of the healing response: An acute decrease in vessel diameter (recoil), and a chronic decrease in the external elastic membrane dimension (negative remodeling). Incomplete stent apposition may rarely occur as part of the healing process after stenting. This is related to positive remodeling during the healing process and does not contribute to restenosis after bare metal or drug-eluting stenting (*J Am Coll Cardiol.* 1995;26:720–724, *Circulation.* 1999;99:44–52, *Circulation.* 1997;96:475–483, *Circulation.* 2003;107:2660–2663, *Circulation.* 2005; 111:900–905).

Answer D. The inflammatory response to stent-mediated arterial injury determines adverse healing responses. Among the factors that may increase inflammation and restenosis are (a) certain polymers/drugs, (b) stent strut thickness and geometric factors, and (c) medial injury or lipid core penetration by stent struts. Deployment of stents in fibrous plaque without causing medial damage reduces the inflammatory response to stenting (*Circulation.* 2002;105:2974–2980, *J Am Coll Cardiol.* 2003; 41:1283–1288, *Circulation.* 2004;110:3430–3434, *Circulation.* 2005;111:900–905, *Circulation.* 2002;106: 2649–2651).

Answer A. Paclitaxel successfully reduced the thickness of intimal hyperplasia in panel A, as compared with polymer alone. At this high dose of paclitaxel, though, the inflammatory response is augmented (*arrowheads*) as compared with polymer alone. Adverse events possibly related to chronic inflammation, and delayed healing due to high dose paclitaxel were seen with the QuaDS QP-2 stent. Similar adverse clinical events were not seen when using the different polymer/paclitaxel dosing regimen of the TAXUS-IV trial (*Circulation.* 2001;104: 473–479, *N Engl J Med.* 2004;350:221–231, *Circulation.* 2002;106:2649–2651).

Answer C. Both panels show the acute response to arterial injury. In panel A, platelet-rich thrombus (*arrowhead*) is seen. Numerous acute inflammatory cells are also present within the thrombus; focal fibrous cap disruption is also demonstrated (*arrow*). In panel B, the asterisk shows the site of the stent strut with associated fibrin-rich thrombus (*arrowheads*). Fibrous plaque (p) is present below the strut (*Circulation.* 1999;99:44–52).

Answer B. The major cause of DES thrombosis is early cessation of dual antiplatelet therapy. But case reports demonstrate rare hypersensitivity reactions after implantation of Cypher DESs, which may be associated with stent thrombosis. While other causes of hypersensitivity reactions may occur (i.e., clopidogrel or aspirin allergies), the pathologic specimen shown in the figure demonstrates an eosinophilic reaction at the site of the stent strut in a patient suffering a fatal stent thrombosis (panels E, K, and L). This could be due to either drug or polymer, but early drug elution suggests that an allergic reaction to the permanent polymer may have been implicated in this case of late stent thrombosis (*JAMA.* 2005;293:2126–2130, *Circulation.* 2004;109:701–705).

Answer A. Arterial injury can manifest itself angiographically immediately after stent deployment. Causes of acute vessel closure in the stent era include intraprocedural stent thrombosis, extensive dissection, or intramural hematoma formation.

Intramural hematoma complicates approximately 7% of PCI procedures and the angiogram may show stenosis, dissection, or even a normal appearance. On intravascular ultrasonography, intramural hematomas are crescent-shaped, homogenous, hyperechoic areas with an entry site from dissection into the media (*Circulation.* 2004;109:2732–2736, *Circulation.* 2002;105:2037–2042).

8 Answer B.   The most extensively studied systemic marker of inflammation is CRP; the magnitudes of pre-PCI and post-PCI levels of CRP have been associated with adverse events after stenting. The systemic rise in CRP levels after injury is fairly slow, with no rise appreciated until at least 24 hours after PCI. The slow systemic rise of CRP levels after stenting is most consistent with production of CRP primarily in the liver and a downstream role of this cytokine in response to injury (*Am J Cardiol.* 2003;91:1346–1349, *Circulation.* 2001;104:992–997, *Am J Cardiol.* 1998;82:515–518, *Eur Heart J.* 2000;21:1152–1158).

9 Answer D.   sCD40L is released by activated platelets. It may promote several proinflammatory mediators. Adverse early and late events have been associated with elevated preprocedural levels of CRP and sCD40L (*Circulation.* 2002;106:896–899, *Circulation.* 2003;108:2776–2782, *Eur Heart J.* 2004;25:1679–1687).

10 Answer B.   The same levels shown to confer an independent risk in the general population (CRP >3.0 mg/dL) have also been implicated in predicting 30-day and longer term adverse events after PCI. The significance value of pre-PCI or post-PCI CRP levels in predicting restenosis in the DES era, though, is very much in doubt given the low event rates regardless of the CRP status (*Am Heart J.* 2003;145:693–699, *J Am Coll Cardiol.* 1999;34:1512–1521, *Circulation.* 2001;104:992–997, *Am J Cardiol.* 2005;95:1238–1240, *J Thromb Thrombolysis.* 2005;19:87–92).

11 Answer D.   Thrombosis and inflammation are related events after arterial injury. While the initial injury response may promote thrombosis through platelet activation and fibrin deposition, activated platelets then initiate the inflammatory cell response through both localized and systemic sCD40L and cytokine activation (*Am J Cardiol.* 2004;93:6–9, *Circulation.* 2002;106:896–899, *J Thromb Haemost.* 2005;3:312–320).

12 Answer C.   CRP is an acute-phase reactant produced by the liver. IL-6 is the main hepatic stimulus for CRP production and is produced by macrophages. CRP in turn stimulates further production of inflammatory cytokines such as IL-1, IL-6, and tumor necrosis factor-α (TNF-α) by macrophages. P-selectin is stored in the α granules of platelets. CD40 ligand, a transmembrane protein, was originally identified on CD4$^+$ T cells, and was recently found on activated platelets. Both membrane-bound and soluble forms of this ligand may interact with CD40, which are expressed on vascular cells resulting in a variety of inflammatory responses (*Circulation.* 2002;106:896–899, *Circulation.* 1999;100:614–620, *Am Heart J.* 2003;145:563–566).

13 Answer D.   The relationship between arterial injury, inflammation, and adverse events has been examined for both early events (30 day) and late events (restenosis). Platelet activation and inflammation after PCI, as measured by cytokines or platelet–leukocyte aggregates, may influence stent thrombosis, periprocedural infarction, and restenosis. Glycoprotein IIb/IIIa inhibitors reduce periprocedural infarction through both platelet aggregation inhibition and, possibly, post-PCI inflammation. Of the three glycoprotein IIb/IIIa inhibitors, only abciximab binds to both platelets and leukocytes and therefore may directly inhibit the formation of leukocyte–platelet aggregates that could cause microvascular obstruction and periprocedural MI (*Am Heart J.* 2003;145:693–699, *J Am Coll Cardiol.* 2001;38:1002–1006, *J Thromb Haemost.* 2005;3:312–320, *Circulation.* 2001;104:163–167, *Am Heart J.* 2003;145:563–566, *J Am Coll Cardiol.* 1999;34:1420–1426).

14 Answer A.   Flow-mediated dilation of the brachial artery reflects systemic endothelial dysfunction while flow-independent dilation reflects smooth muscle function. Patients have abnormal endothelial function early after PCI, but it is somewhat surprising that abnormal endothelial function can be seen >6 months after DES placement. As sirolimus is no longer present on the stent at that time, the etiology of this longer term endothelial function is unclear but may in part explain the rare occurrence of late stent thromboses (*Am J Cardiol.* 2004;94:1420–1423, *Eur Heart J.* 2006;27:166–170, *J Am Coll Cardiol.* 2005;46:231–236).

15 Answer D.   While prior literature has suggested that the post-PCI rise of cytokines is predictive of restenosis, this has not been confirmed in the DES era. In fact, it appears that systemic cytokine rise after PCI is marked and similar for both DESs and BMSs. No difference in platelet activation has been shown for various stent types. Given the markedly lower restenosis rates for DESs, it is likely local drug delivery works through local suppression of inflammation and smooth muscle cell migration despite a similar systemic inflammatory response (*Am Heart J.* 2005;150: 344–350, *Am J Cardiol.* 2005;95:1238–1240, *Am J Cardiol.* 1998;82:515–518, *J Thromb Thrombolysis.* 2005;19:87–92).

16 Answer A. Cardiogenic shock has traditionally been thought of as massive myonecrosis leading to reduced cardiac output and compensatory vasoconstriction. In the SHOCK trial, though, systemic vascular resistance was not markedly elevated in most cardiogenic shock patients. Newer evidence suggests that a shock induces a systemic inflammatory response leading to nitric oxide synthase overproduction. This leads to inappropriate vasodilation and may play an important role in the refractory hypotension associated with cardiogenic shock (*Eur Heart J.* 2003;24:1287–1295, *Circulation.* 2003;107:2998–3002).

17 Answer D. Atorvastatin, clopidogrel, and abciximab may blunt the inflammatory response after PCI as a mechanism of their beneficial impact on PCI. Abciximab blunted the rise of CRP and IL-6 levels after PCI in a subset of patients in the EPIC trial. Clopidogrel may attenuate the increased risk associated with PCI among patients with high CRP levels. Similarly, statin therapy before PCI seems to have the most benefit among patients with the highest level of pre-PCI inflammation. While none of these systemic medications clearly impact long-term healing (stent restenosis), local applications of statin drugs may be promising given their potential effects on inflammation and smooth muscle cell migration (*Circulation.* 2003;107:1750–1756, *Am J Cardiol.* 2001;88:672–674, *Am J Cardiol.* 2002;90:786–789, *Cardiovasc Res.* 2005;68:483–492, *Circulation.* 2001;104:163–167, *Circulation.* 2003; 107:1123–1128).

18 Answer D. The IMPRESS trial hypothesized that patients with persistent inflammation after PCI would benefit from anti-inflammatory therapy. Eighty-three patients undergoing successful bare metal stenting with CRP levels of >0.5 mg/dL measured 72 hours after the procedure were randomized to receive oral prednisone or placebo for 45 days. As shown in the figure, this trial supports the importance of inflammation after bare metal stenting by demonstrating decreased events in the prednisone group. As 93% event-free survival can also be seen with drug-eluting stenting without prednisone, it is not clear whether adjunctive oral steroids would be beneficial in the current era (*N Engl J Med.* 2004;350:221–231, *J Am Coll Cardiol.* 2002;40:1935–1942).

19 Answer B. In addition to inhibiting platelet aggregation, clopidogrel may have an impact on inflammation after PCI. One mechanism of clopidogrel benefit on inflammation may be through decreased expression of P-selectin after clopidogrel administration. P-selectin may play a key role in activation of TNF-α as well as other cytokines. Therefore, treatment with clopidogrel before PCI may be especially beneficial among patients with heightened inflammatory status as defined by the CRP level (*Am J Cardiol.* 2001;88:672–674, *J Am Coll Cardiol.* 2004;43:162–168, *J Am Coll Cardiol.* 2003;41:45A).

20 Answer D. Glycoprotein IIb/IIIa inhibitors decrease platelet aggregation and periprocedural myonecrosis. While the EPIC trial suggests that abciximab decreased the rise of CRP and IL-6 levels after PCI as compared with heparin alone, there is little data to suggest that eptifibatide or tirofiban significantly suppress the inflammatory response to PCI. It is possible that the inferiority of tirofiban compared with abciximab in TARGET (do Tirofiban And Reopro Give similar Efficacy Trial) may relate to both the inadequate tirofiban dosing and the lack of tirofiban anti-inflammatory effects. None of the glycoprotein IIb/IIIa inhibitors have been clearly shown to prevent intimal hyperplasia and stent restenosis (*Am J Cardiol.* 2003;91:1346–1349, *Am Heart J.* 2003;145:693–699, *J Am Coll Cardiol.* 2004;43:162–168, *Am Heart J.* 2003;146:S1–S4, *Am J Cardiol.* 2003;91:334–336, *N Engl J Med.* 2001;344:1888–1894).

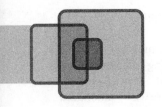

5

Antiplatelet, Antithrombotic, and Thrombolytic Agents

David J. Moliterno

Questions

1 Which of the following factors associated with coagulation is *not* released from activated platelets?

(A) Fibrinogen
(B) Adenosine diphosphate (ADP)
(C) Tissue plasminogen activator (tPA)
(D) Plasminogen activator inhibitor-1 (PAI-1)
(E) Platelet factor 4 (PF4)

2 In the GUSTO-I (Global Utilization of Streptokinase and Tissue plasminogen activator for Occluded Arteries) trial, ischemic events and bleeding events were correlated with the activated partial thromboplastin time (aPTT) 12 hours after heparin therapy was initiated. The investigators described an optimal therapeutic range for aPTT where the risk of death and moderate or severe bleeding was lowest. This range (from point a to point b in the following figures) was found to be:

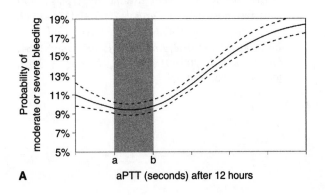

A

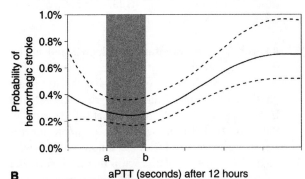

B

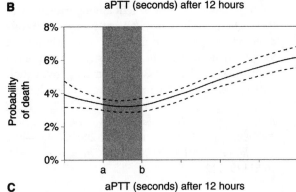

C

Circulation. 1996;93:870–878.

(A) 40 to 60 seconds
(B) 50 to 70 seconds
(C) 70 to 90 seconds
(D) None of the above

3 Pharmacotherapies known to reduce the occurrence of death or myocardial infarction (MI) among patients with non–ST-segment elevation myocardial infarction (NSTEMI) include all of the following, *except*:

(A) Aspirin
(B) Clopidogrel
(C) Unfractionated heparin
(D) Low-molecular-weight heparin
(E) IIb/IIIa antagonists
(F) Fibrinolytic agents

4 Unfractionated heparin affects several factors in the coagulation cascade. What is the effect of heparin on levels of tissue factor pathway inhibitor (TFPI)?

(A) Increased
(B) Unchanged
(C) Decreased

5 Which of the following statements is *false* concerning IIb/IIIa inhibitors?

(A) Bleeding is infrequent although it usually occurs in hollow organs (gastrointestinal, genitourinary, and vascular)
(B) Severe thrombocytopenia occurs in approximately 1% of patients
(C) Thrombocytopenia is more frequent with abciximab, especially with early repeat administration
(D) Thrombolysis in myocardial infarction (TIMI) major bleeding is increased by approximately 1% when using a IIb/IIIa inhibitor, and this is predominately due to an increase in intracranial hemorrhage

6 A 47-year-old white man was found to have a positive stress test result on preoperative evaluation. He underwent successful implantation of a drug-eluting stent (TAXUS) into the left anterior descending coronary artery. Approximately 6 weeks later, you are contacted by the patient's orthopaedic surgeon who wishes to proceed with a planned knee surgery. Your recommendations are:

(A) Proceed with planned surgery, but discontinue clopidogrel at least 5 days in advance
(B) Admit the patient to hospital, discontinue clopidogrel, and begin intravenous eptifibatide
(C) Discontinue clopidogrel and after 2 days admit the patient to hospital for fondaparinux injections
(D) Postpone surgery for at least 4 months

7 The most commonly present hypercoagulable state in westernized countries is:

(A) Antiphospholipid antibody syndrome
(B) Protein C deficiency
(C) Protein S deficiency

(D) Factor V Leiden mutation
(E) Lupus anticoagulant

8 As compared with second- and third-generation fibrinolytic agents, which of the following statements regarding streptokinase is *false*?

(A) Streptokinase is less fibrin specific
(B) Streptokinase is an indirect activator of plasminogen
(C) Streptokinase is the most fibrinogenolytic of the agents
(D) Streptokinase has the shortest half-life

9 A 69-year-old Hispanic woman is referred to you for preoperative assessment. She is planning to have a thyroid mass removed. Her past medical history is remarkable for successful placement of a stent in her right coronary artery approximately 8 years ago. Five years ago she had aortic valve replacement using a St. Jude prosthesis. As part of her evaluation, a stress echocardiography was performed. This revealed anterolateral ischemia at a moderate workload. Her protime-international normalization ratio (INR) is 2.9. Which of the following plans should be implemented for her to undergo coronary angiography?

(A) Admit the patient to hospital, discontinue warfarin, and begin bivalirudin
(B) Discontinue warfarin 3 days before outpatient catheterization and measure the protime-INR on the day of planned catheterization
(C) Continue warfarin and use a 5-F diagnostic coronary artery catheter
(D) Administer fresh frozen plasma on the day of planned catheterization
(E) Admit the patient to hospital, discontinue warfarin, and begin enoxaparin

10 Which of the following is *not* an absolute contraindication for thrombolytic therapy?

(A) Active menses
(B) Hemorrhagic stroke >1 year earlier
(C) Suspected aortic dissection
(D) Intracranial arteriovenous malformation
(E) Recent, severe head trauma

11 Which of the following factors at presentation *least* strongly predicts 30-day mortality following ST-elevation myocardial infarction (STEMI)?

(A) Age
(B) History of hypertension
(C) MI location
(D) Killip class
(E) Heart rate on presentation

12 Platelet aggregability is affected by numerous factors (thrombin, epinephrine, ADP) including hypertriglyceridemia. Which of the following lipoproteins is associated with a lowered platelet aggregability?

(A) High density lipoprotein (HDL)
(B) Low density lipoprotein (LDL)
(C) Very low density lipoprotein (VLDL)
(D) Lipoprotein(a)
(E) Apolipoproteins E (apoE)

13 Which of the following is *not* true regarding the actions of thrombin?

(A) Converts fibrinogen to fibrin
(B) Activates factors V and XII
(C) Causes normal endothelium to vasoconstrict
(D) Stimulates platelet aggregation

14 Which of the following is *false* considering the activated clotting time (ACT)?

(A) An agent, such as kaolin or diatomaceous earth, stimulates the intrinsic pathway of coagulation
(B) Currently available measures of the ACT have been developed to assess anticoagulation produced by unfractionated heparin
(C) The ACT is unaffected by most coagulation factor deficiencies such as hemophilia
(D) The ACT is similar for arterial and venous blood samples

15 Which of the following practices in interventional cardiology has reduced the occurrence of bleeding associated with percutaneous coronary intervention (PCI)?

(A) Using weight-based heparin dosing
(B) Decreasing arterial sheath size
(C) Removing sheaths on the same day of the procedure
(D) Avoiding the use of heparin postprocedure
(E) All of the above

16 The average relative risk reduction for the 30-day occurrence of death/MI in patients with acute coronary syndrome (ACS) receiving a IIb/IIIa inhibitor as medical therapy in addition to aspirin and heparin is:

(A) <10%
(B) 10% to 20%
(C) 20% to 30%
(D) >30%

17 As the ACT increases among patients receiving heparin with a glycoprotein IIb/IIIa inhibitor, the occurrence of ischemic events:

(A) Gradually increases
(B) Remain largely unchanged
(C) Gradually decreases

18 Factors important in assessing whether patients being treated with enoxaparin have adequate anticoagulation during percutaneous coronary revascularization include all of the following, *except*:

(A) Timing of last enoxaparin dose
(B) The current ACT
(C) The dose of enoxaparin
(D) The number of subcutaneous doses of enoxaparin received
(E) The estimated creatinine clearance

19 Which of the following statements regarding heparin-induced thrombocytopenia (HIT) is *true*?

(A) The diagnosis of HIT is a clinical one and should be suspected when the platelet count is below 150,000 per mm^3 or has decreased 50% from baseline
(B) The likelihood of HIT substantially increases for patients receiving heparin for ≥ 4 days
(C) Patients with HIT can be safely treated with low-molecular-weight heparin
(D) A and B
(E) All of the above

20 Advantages that low-molecular-weight heparins have over unfractionated heparins include all of the following, *except*:

(A) Bind less to plasma proteins, thereby producing a more consistent effect
(B) Have better subcutaneous absorption
(C) Do not require anticoagulant monitoring
(D) Can be used safely in patients with heparin–PF4 antibodies
(E) Have a several-fold longer half-life

21 As compared with unfractionated heparin, the use of enoxaparin in several large-scale clinical trials of medical therapy for unstable angina has lowered the incidence of death or MI in the first 4 to 6 weeks by:

(A) 0%
(B) 5% to 10%
(C) 10% to 15%
(D) 15% to 20%

22 Major bleeding, as defined by the TIMI study criteria, has occurred at what rate in recent randomized PCI trials?

(A) 1%
(B) 2% to 4%
(C) 6% to 8%
(D) >10%

[23] Reasonable measures to decrease bleeding complications among patients receiving IIb/IIIa inhibitors include all *except*:

(A) Giving clopidogrel after the coronary intervention procedure is completed
(B) Using smaller arterial access sheaths
(C) Targeting lower ACT values by using a lower bolus dose of heparin
(D) Removing vascular access sheaths on the same day as the procedure

[24] Which of the following statements regarding abciximab is *false*?

(A) The plasma half-life is approximately 10 to 15 minutes
(B) Approximately three-fourths of the total abciximab dose is given in the initial bolus
(C) Using a standard dose of abciximab, the ratio of drug to IIb/IIIa receptor is 2:1
(D) The dose should be adjusted for patients with renal insufficiency

[25] Which of the following is *true* regarding thrombocytopenia associated with abciximab?

(A) The occurrence of thrombocytopenia is roughly doubled among patients receiving repeat dosing of abciximab within a 2-week interval
(B) Thrombocytopenia can be quickly predicted with a simple laboratory test before abciximab administration
(C) Although infrequent, severe thrombocytopenia can often be detected within 2 hours of drug administration
(D) The nadir platelet count usually occurs 4 to 6 days after receiving abciximab
(E) A and C

[26] PCI trials testing IIb/IIIa inhibitors have used a 30-day composite endpoint of death, MI, and urgent target vessel revascularization (TVR). What percentage of this composite endpoint is accounted for by MI?

(A) 20%
(B) 40%
(C) 60%
(D) 80%

[27] For which of the following does abciximab have a class III indication?

(A) Left main coronary artery stenting
(B) As medical therapy among patients with ACS
(C) Angioplasty in patients older than 90 years
(D) Percutaneous coronary revascularization among patients with recent stroke

[28] Which of the following drugs has the shortest half-life?

(A) Unfractionated heparin
(B) Low-molecular-weight heparin
(C) Lepirudin
(D) Bivalirudin
(E) Argatroban

[29] The maximal clinical benefit of a 300 mg loading dose of clopidogrel in a *post hoc* analysis of the CREDO (Clopidogrel for the Reduction of Events During Observation) trial was found to be:

(A) 2 hours
(B) 6 hours
(C) 15 hours
(D) 24 hours
(E) 96 hours

[30] Clinically relevant antibodies can form to all of the following drugs, *except*?

(A) Unfractionated heparin
(B) Low-molecular-weight heparin
(C) Argatroban
(D) Lepirudin
(E) Abciximab

[31] Which antithrombin is potentially safer among patients with severe renal insufficiency or worsening renal function?

(A) Unfractionated heparin
(B) Low-molecular-weight heparin
(C) Lepirudin
(D) Argatroban
(E) Bivalirudin

[32] Which anticoagulant is represented in the following figure?

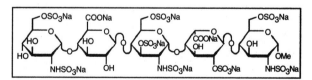

With permission from *Therapeutic strategies in thrombolysis.* 2006;123–144.

(A) Unfractionated heparin
(B) Enoxaparin
(C) Fondaparinux
(D) Bivalirudin
(E) Eptifibatide

33 A 73-year-old white woman weighing 62 kg undergoes an uneventful percutaneous coronary revascularization procedure by you. Because she had an ACS and evidence of residual thrombus in the culprit lesion, procedural abciximab was utilized. Following the procedure, the patient is found to be hypotensive and tachycardiac and a retroperitoneal hemorrhage is diagnosed. Which of the following measures would be the next step in her treatment to reverse the effects of abciximab?

(A) Administer intravenous protamine
(B) Request fresh frozen plasma from the blood bank
(C) Intravenous bolus of cryoprecipitate
(D) Transfuse random donor platelets
(E) Transfuse single donor platelets

Answers and Explanations

1 Answer C. Many factors associated with coagulation, inflammation, or cell repair and growth are released from platelets. Most factors either accelerate coagulation or promote inflammation. Platelets do not contain tPA, but rather release PAI-1 (the natural inhibitor of tPA) when activated.

2 Answer B. Granger et al. found this optimal therapeutic range, which fortunately minimized both ischemic and bleeding events. Before this study, a number of investigators and clinicians used a therapeutic range of 60 to 85 seconds. Since this manuscript, most subsequent studies and clinicians have chosen 50 to 70 seconds. In the GUSTO-II trial, a 20% increase in the dose of heparin resulted in a 5 to 10 second higher aPTT as compared with results from the GUSTO-I trial. This increase in aPTT was associated with a doubling in the rate of intracranial hemorrhage among patients treated with thrombolytic therapy (*Circulation.* 1996;93:870–878).

3 Answer F. Placebo-controlled trials have shown many antiplatelet and antithrombin therapies to reduce death or MI among patients with NSTEMI. Several studies, including TIMI-IIIB, showed patients with NSTEMI–ACS receiving fibrinolytic therapy to have a worse outcome—primarily a higher rate of MI.

4 Answer A. Unfractionated heparin affects coagulation factors in the intrinsic, extrinsic, and common pathways of coagulation. The extrinsic pathway, including tissue factor and factor VII, is affected by unfractionated heparin since it increases levels of TFPI.

5 Answer D. Although TIMI major bleeding is increased by approximately 1%, this is not due to an increase in intracranial hemorrhage. Intracranial hemorrhage occurs in 0.1% of patients undergoing PCI, and this is not particularly increased with the use of IIb/IIIa inhibitors.

6 Answer D. The need for surgery in the early weeks to months following drug-eluting stent placement is a vexing problem. No prospective data are available. On the other hand, it is well recognized that premature discontinuation of adequate antiplatelet surgery markedly increases the risk for stent thrombosis. In one large-scale registry, it was found that premature antiplatelet therapy discontinuation was associated with a hazard ratio of 90% for stent thrombosis (*JAMA.* 2005;293:2126–2130).

7 Answer D. This genetic defect is present in roughly 6% of the population. Most thrombotic events from this deficiency are venous, although arterial thrombosis does infrequently occur.

8 Answer D. Streptokinase, a first-generation fibrinolytic agent, is least fibrin specific and also depletes fibrinogen levels the greatest. As such, patients have a longer time of coagulation abnormality and hence do not require early heparin administration. Separately, streptokinase has an intermediate half-life (20 minutes) as compared with tPA which has the shortest half-life (5 minutes).

9 Answer B. The patient's stent placement was done many years before so there is no particular concern for stent thrombosis. Likewise, the mechanical valve was placed long enough earlier that the suture line should be well healed. Although the patient could be admitted to hospital and a heparin or other antithrombin therapy initiated, this may not be cost-effective. Rather, this patient could receive outpatient enoxaparin or since the patient's INR is 2.9, it is also reasonable to simply discontinue the warfarin (Coumadin) and measure the protime-INR on the third morning. If the patient's INR still remains >1.5, using a particularly small arterial sheath and/or possibly an arteriotomy closure device could be considered.

10 Answer A. The absolute contraindications for thrombolytic therapy are solely centered on life-threatening bleeding such as intracranial hemorrhage. Any history of previous hemorrhagic stroke is an absolute contraindication. Active internal bleeding is considered a contraindication except for menses.

11 Answer B. All these factors are independent predictors of 30-day mortality. A history of hypertension, however, represents <1% of predictive models for mortality. MI location and heart rate are each roughly 10 times more powerful predictors than hypertension. In fact, most of the predictive factors for 30-day mortality can be assessed by the ambulance driver or triage nurse before the patient's arrival at the hospital.

12 **Answer A.** The elevation of most lipid and lipoprotein levels is associated with increased platelet aggregation. Triglyceride-rich lipids increase a number of procoagulant factors and increase blood viscosity. On the other hand, HDL reduces PAI-1, and high levels of HDL inhibit platelet aggregability (*Atherosclerosis.* 1998;140:271–280).

13 **Answer C.** Among the primary activities of thrombin is causing the conversion of fibrinogen to fibrin. Thrombin does activate a number of other coagulation pathway factors including V, VIII, and XII as it autoamplifies its production. Normal endothelium, in response to thrombin, releases tPA and also vasodilates. Abnormal endothelium vasoconstricts (through endothelin) in response to thrombin. Another important activity of thrombin is that it is one of the most potent stimulators of platelet aggregation.

14 **Answer C.** The ACT initiates the intrinsic pathway of coagulation. The commercially available assays are almost exclusively designed for measuring therapeutic levels of unfractionated heparin. The assay is poorly sensitive to most factor Xa inhibitors and low-molecular-weight heparins. The ACT can measure the extent of anticoagulation from direct thrombin inhibitors, although it is less accurate than other assays. Clinically important coagulation factor deficiencies, such as with hemophilia, substantially prolong the ACT as well as other clotting time assays.

15 **Answer E.** The rate of major bleeding in randomized clinical trials and in practice has substantially decreased over the last decade from 2%–4% to <1%. Many changes in practice have resulted in this decrease in bleeding despite the use of multiple anticoagulants (aspirin, clopidogrel, IIb/IIIa inhibitors, and potent antithrombins).

16 **Answer B.** The average relative risk reduction among large-scale clinical trials considering a 30-day occurrence of death or MI among patients with ACS is 12%. The range is 10% to 30% with most data suggesting the relative risk reduction with medical therapy to be 10% to 20%. In these older trials, patients did not receive clopidogrel as standard therapy for ACS. The benefit of IIb/IIIa inhibitors is likely reduced among patients adequately treated with thienopyridine, although this has not been formally tested.

17 **Answer B.** As compared with heparin alone when increasing ACT is associated with an ischemic event rate which slowly decreases, the rate of ischemic events among patients receiving heparin with a glycoprotein IIb/IIIa inhibitor is largely unchanged from an ACT in the range of approximately 200 to 400 seconds.

18 **Answer B.** Several factors are important when deciding if a patient remains adequately anticoagulated from enoxaparin. These include the amount of enoxaparin given and the number of hours since this last dose. Likewise, patients who have received only one subcutaneous dose of enoxaparin will be therapeutic for a shorter interval than patients who have reached steady state following several subcutaneous doses. It is also important whether the patient has received intravenous or subcutaneous enoxaparin. The ACT is an unreliable measure of the extent of anticoagulation provided by enoxaparin. Since the primary excretion for low-molecular-weight heparins is renal, the creatinine clearance can have an important influence on the extent and duration of anticoagulant effect.

19 **Answer D.** The suspicion and diagnosis of HIT should be made near solely on clinical grounds. Laboratory-based assays for HIT can be diagnostic, but should be confirmatory. While unfractionated heparin is more likely than low-molecular-weight heparin to cause HIT, all heparins can cause and exacerbate HIT. The mechanism of HIT is antibody generation in response to a heparin–platelet factor complex. This antibody formation usually takes exposure to several days of heparin to occur.

20 **Answer D.** Low-molecular-weight heparins provide several advantages over unfractionated heparin since they bind less to the endothelium, plasma proteins, and macrophages thereby providing a more consistent effect. They are also better absorbed subcutaneously and have a longer half-life. Although low-molecular-weight heparins are less likely to cause formation of heparin-induced platelet antibodies than unfractionated heparin, both agents are unsafe once antibodies are formed, and a direct thrombin inhibitor should be used instead.

21 **Answer D.** A meta-analysis combining data from ESSENCE (Efficacy and Safety of Subcutaneous Enoxaparin in Non-Q-wave Coronary Events) and

TIMI-11B showed that the 43-day incidence of death or nonfatal MI was reduced by 17%.

22   Answer A. The TIMI major bleeding definition has been used for many years in thrombolytic therapy trials as well as in percutaneous revascularization trials. For several reasons, including the fact that TIMI major bleeding has occurred in only approximately 1% of patients with recent PCI, more clinically relevant bleeding definitions have been defined and used in several studies such as REPLACE-2. The REPLACE-2 major bleeding definition, as compared with the TIMI major bleeding definition, includes transfusion of ≥2 units of packed red blood cell, observed blood loss with >3 g per dL Hgb blood loss, and retroperitoneal hemorrhage.

23   Answer A. The primary measures by which vascular bleeding events have decreased in the setting of IIb/IIIa inhibitor use center around using lower bolus doses of heparin and removing the arterial access sheaths the same day as the procedure (as opposed to leaving them overnight). Clopidogrel should be given preprocedure when possible.

24   Answer D. Abciximab is largely cleared by the reticuloendothelial system and not by the kidney. Therefore, the dose does not need to be adjusted for renal insufficiency. This is in contrast to the small-molecule IIb/IIIa inhibitors.

25   Answer E. Thrombocytopenia associated with abciximab (*Semin Thromb Hemost.* 2004;30:569–577) occurs very quickly, and therefore it is recommended that a platelet count be performed 2 hours after drug administration. There is no quick laboratory test to predict thrombocytopenia caused by abciximab. The occurrence of severe thrombocytopenia among patients receiving abciximab is approximately 2%, and this occurrence is doubled (4%) among patients who receive repeat administration of abciximab within 2 weeks. Severe thrombocytopenia secondary to abciximab administration should prompt immediate drug discontinuation and future avoidance.

26   Answer D. Periprocedural MI accounts for nearly 90% of the 30-day composite of ischemic endpoints. In current practice, death and urgent TVR each occur in fewer than 1% of patients.

27   Answer B. While there are a number of reasons not to use abciximab, using it as medical therapy alone among patients with ACS is a class III indication. This distinction is given because of the results of GUSTO-IV trial (*Lancet.* 2001;357:1915–1924), which showed

no benefit but rather a nonsignificant increase in adverse events among patients receiving abciximab alone (without PCI) for ACS.

28   Answer D. While unfractionated heparin can have a half-life as short as 30 minutes among patients with high rates of creatinine clearance, the half-life ranges from 30 to 60 minutes. Bivalirudin has the consistently shortest half-life of these drugs, and it is approximately 20 to 25 minutes. The other direct thrombin inhibitors have half-lives of approximately 60 minutes (*Am Heart J.* 2003;146:S23–S30).

29   Answer D. While no prospective large-scale study has been completed to discern the exact time interval required to receive maximal benefit from a clopidogrel loading dose, a *post hoc* analysis from the CREDO trial observed the maximal separation of the adverse event curves between the group of patients pretreated with placebo and those receiving a 300 mg loading dose to occur maximally at 24 hours. No statistically significant difference was seen in the clinical outcome until after 15 hours. At this time point, a 59% reduction in the ischemic event rate was noted relative to placebo (*J Am Coll Cardiol.* 2006;47:939–943).

30   Answer C. Both unfractionated heparins and fractionated or low-molecular-weight heparins, by interacting with PF4, can lead to antibody formation. Abciximab, having a protein-antibody structure can act as an antigen and cause antibody formation. Hirudin and lepirudin are polypeptides and may lead to relevant antibody formation; whereas, argatroban is a synthetic arginine derivative and has not been found to cause antibody formation.

31   Answer D. For the heparins and lepirudin the primary mode of excretion is renal, and therefore these agents if needed for chronic administration should be avoided in patients with compromised or worsening renal function. Bivalirudin has several modes of excretion including nonrenal mechanisms, and is therefore safer than lepirudin. On the other hand, argatroban is metabolized in the liver and excreted in the feces (*Pharmacotherapy.* 2000;20:318–329).

32   Answer C. The diagram shows a 5-sugar unit entity, namely, a pentasaccharide (fondaparinux).

33   Answer D. Abciximab being a monoclonal antibody avidly binds to platelet receptors. Protamine would be a useful treatment to reverse the effects of heparin, however, it will have no effect on abciximab. Administering cryoprecipitate or plasma products will be of little to no value because of the mechanism of abciximab binding. Rather, transfusion of platelets will provide additional IIb/IIIa receptors to facilitate appropriate coagulation. In addition, abciximab can migrate among platelets and the transfused platelets will aide in decreasing the number of abciximab molecules on the originally affected platelets, thereby allowing their earlier recovery. Single donor platelets reduce alloimmunization and should be considered for individuals who need repeated transfusion or are candidates for bone marrow transplantation. Random donor platelets are easier to obtain and can be transfused faster.

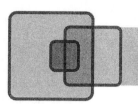

6

Inotropes, Antiarrhythmics, Sedatives, and Lipid-Lowering Agents

J. Jeffrey Marshall and David J. Moliterno

Questions

1 A 74-year-old white man with a history of hypertension presents 2 hours after the onset of substernal chest pressure. His electrocardiogram (EKG) is shown in the upper part of the following figure. He is seen in the emergency department and then taken to the catheterization suite for coronary angiography and possible direct angioplasty. You insert a 6 Fr sheath into the right femoral artery and a 7 Fr sheath into the right femoral vein. After injecting the right coronary artery, the nurse notifies you of a rapid heart rate as shown in the lower part of the following figure. The aortic pressure is noted to be 74/48 mm Hg and the patient does not respond to questions. What is the best treatment?

(A) Immediate lidocaine 100 mg IV bolus
(B) Electrical cardioversion
(C) Convert the rhythm with rapid atrial pacing
(D) Start diltiazem 10 mg IV bolus and 5 mg per hour
(E) Load with IV amiodarone 150 mg

2 The vascular endothelium produces a number of vasoactive molecules. Which of the following is *not* produced by the endothelium?

(A) Nitrous oxide
(B) Prostacycline
(C) Thromboxane
(D) Endothelin

3 Which of the following is *true* regarding the advantages of vasopressin over dopamine in resuscitation following cardiac arrest?

(A) All vasopressin receptors cause intense vasoconstriction thereby increasing systemic vascular resistance (SVR) more potently than dopamine
(B) Vasopressin increases SVR, the chronotropic and inotropic state of the myocardium, whereas dopamine only increases SVR
(C) Vasopressin receptors in the brain mediate vasodilatation, and vasopressin receptors in the periphery mediate vasoconstriction thereby preserving cerebral perfusion

RHYTHM STRIP: II
25 mm/sec:1 cm/mV

(D) Reflex vasoconstriction from vasopressin-induced bradycardia increases the effect on SVR making it a more potent vasoconstrictor than dopamine

4 Methergine is used as the "gold standard" vasoactive agent for the diagnosis of coronary artery spasm. Which of the following is most correct about methergine?

(A) Methergine is a vasopressin agonist that directly activates the coronary vascular smooth muscle in patients prone to coronary artery spasm

(B) Methergine causes coronary vasoconstriction by upregulating thromboxane production in abnormal vascular endothelium but not in arterial segments with normal endothelium

(C) Methergine stimulates abnormal vascular endothelium to produce large amounts of endothelin, causing vasoconstriction

(D) Methergine is a serotonin receptor agonist that causes vasodilation if normal endothelium is present but vasoconstriction in the presence of unhealthy endothelium

5 Nitric oxide has many physiologic effects on vascular endothelium and the underlying smooth muscle. Which of the following is *not* correct about nitric oxide?

(A) Inhibition of platelet aggregation

(B) Decreases cyclic guanosine monophosphate (cGMP) in the adjacent vascular smooth muscle cells

(C) Inhibition of neutrophil adhesion

(D) Inhibits adhesion molecule production by vascular endothelial cells

6 Which of the following is an endothelium-dependent vasodilator?

(A) Nitric oxide

(B) Serotonin

(C) Verapamil

(D) Nitroglycerine

(E) Adenosine

7 Which of the following are *true* regarding the angiographic no-reflow phenomenon?

(A) Endothelial cell edema is not a contributor to no-reflow

(B) Reactive oxygen species play a significant role in no-reflow

(C) Vasodilators like verapamil and sodium nitroprusside improve survival in patients with no-reflow

(D) The presence of no-reflow alone is not an independent predictor of mortality in patients with acute myocardial infarction

(E) Direct stenting reduces the incidence of no-reflow in acute myocardial infarction

8 Which one of the following statements about anaphylactoid reactions from contrast media and its treatment is most correct?

(A) Anaphylactoid reactions to contrast media occur in slightly more than 1% of all patients undergoing selective coronary angiography

(B) Urticaria should be immediately treated with subcutaneous (SQ) epinephrine

(C) Angioedema should be treated with 0.3 mL of 1:1,000 IV bolus

(D) Cardiogenic shock should be treated with 10 μg per minute IV epinephrine followed by a drip of 1 to 4 μg per minute IV as needed

(E) Intravenous steroid injection is effective in ameliorating the acute hemodynamic effects of contrast-mediated anaphylactoid reactions

9 A 58-year-old African American woman is found unresponsive, on the floor. Seizure activity is noted and she is incontinent of urine. She regains consciousness within 90 seconds and is complaining of indigestion. She is brought to the emergency department by ambulance. When you evaluate her she is chest pain free, but subsequently develops shortness of breath and complains of palpitations. An EKG or rhythm strip is performed. Rhythm strips are shown in the following figure. Which response best reflects the electrocardiographic findings for this case?

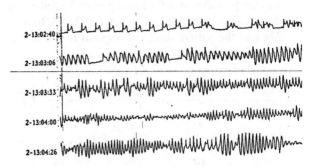

(A) No treatment is necessary

(B) This rhythm is due to myocardial ischemia

(C) This rhythm is due to an old myocardial infarct

(D) An atrioventricular (AV) (reciprocating) bypass tract is present

(E) An AV nodal bypass tract is present

10 A 42-year-old Caucasian woman is found unresponsive. She quickly regains consciousness and is complaining of shortness of breath. When evaluated in the emergency department she is chest pain free, but continues to complain of shortness of breath and palpitations. An EKG or rhythm strip is performed. Rhythm strips are shown in the following figure. Which response best reflects the electrocardiographic findings for this case?

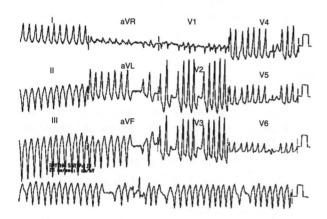

(A) No treatment is necessary
(B) This rhythm is due to myocardial ischemia
(C) This rhythm is due to an old myocardial infarct
(D) An AV (reciprocating) bypass tract is present
(E) An AV nodal bypass tract is present

11 A 73-year-old man is found poorly responsive in the locker room of a health club. He is brought to the emergency department by ambulance. On evaluation he is chest pain free, but complains of palpitations and lightheadedness. An EKG or rhythm strip is performed. Rhythm strips are shown below. Which response best reflects the electrocardiographic findings for this case?

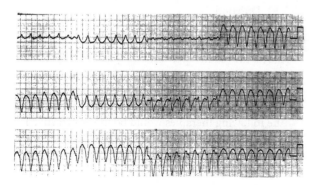

(A) No treatment is necessary
(B) This rhythm is due to myocardial ischemia
(C) This rhythm is due to an old myocardial infarct
(D) An AV (reciprocating) bypass tract is present
(E) An AV nodal bypass tract is present

12 A 67-year-old woman resident at an in-patient physical rehabilitation center is found unresponsive on the floor of her room. Seizure activity is noted and she is incontinent of urine. She is taken to the nearest emergency department, and upon evaluation she complains of chest, back, and abdominal muscle pain. Rhythm strips are shown in the following figure. Which response best reflects the electrocardiographic findings for this case?

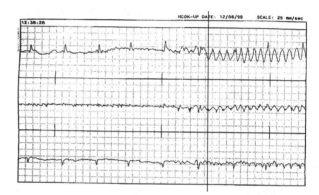

(A) No treatment is necessary
(B) This rhythm is due to myocardial ischemia
(C) This rhythm is due to an old myocardial infarct
(D) An AV (reciprocating) bypass tract is present
(E) An AV nodal bypass tract is present

13 The 5-year follow-up to the bypass angioplasty revascularization investigation (BARI) study showed that rather than restenosis at the percutaneous transluminal coronary angioplasty (PTCA) site, or bypass graft closure at the surgical site, the development of new blockages was a leading cause for recurrent coronary artery disease and symptoms. As such, it is crucial following percutaneous coronary interventions to aggressively treat all lipid abnormalities. Lipoprotein(a) (Lp[a]) is highly associated with coronary artery disease. Which of the following drugs most effectively lowers Lp(a)?

(A) Pravastatin
(B) Simvastatin

(C) Policosanol

(D) Fenofibrate

(E) Rosuvastatin

14 An 84-year-old woman undergoes left heart catheterization and diagnostic angiography following a large myocardial infarction. The night before the procedure she was anxious and had difficulty sleeping. She received 15 mg of flurazepam orally. The morning of the catheterization she received 25 mg of diphenhydramine orally. Near the time her femoral arterial sheath was placed she complained of back pain and received 5 mg of morphine sulphate intravenously. She was also given some additional lidocaine at the puncture site to better achieve local anesthesia. Over the next several minutes her oxygen saturation was noticed to decrease to <80% and it was difficult to arouse her. Her vital signs were stable except that her respiratory rate was decreased. The next appropriate step would be to administer:

(A) Midazolam

(B) Atropine

(C) Naloxone

(D) Flumazenil

(E) Metoclopramide

15 Atropine is used in the cardiac catheterization laboratory particularly among patients who are experiencing reflex bradycardia and/or hypotension. Which of the following statements are *true* for the use of atropine in the cardiac catheterization laboratory?

(A) It should be used with caution among patients with a seizure disorder since it lowers the threshold at which seizures occur

(B) It should be used with caution among patients with asthma since it increases the risk of bronchospasm

(C) It should be used among patients who experience a decrease in heart rate by >10 bpm with ionic contrast

(D) It should be used in small doses (<0.4 mg) especially among patients with diabetes

(E) It should be given in large doses (>2 mg) among patients with a large body mass index (>30)

(F) All of the above

(G) None of the above

16 On your morning rounds you plan to discharge a 67-year-old man who had been admitted yesterday with unstable angina. He underwent successful angioplasty and drug-eluting stent placement. You notice that his fasting cholesterol profile reveals the total cholesterol to be 272, triglycerides 318, high-density lipoprotein (HDL) 34, and low-density lipoprotein (LDL) 191. You also notice that the rounding house officer has already written prescriptions for the discharge medications. Which of the following prescriptions for this patient's cholesterol would you be *least* supportive of?

(A) Niaspan (niacin)

(B) WelChol (colesevelam)

(C) Crestor (rosuvastatin)

(D) Lopid (gemfibrozil)

(E) Pravachol (pravastatin)

17 Protamine sulfate reverses nearly all the anticoagulant effect of unfractionated heparin and reverses roughly 60% of the effect of low-molecular-weight heparin. Several factors are known to increase the risk of severe allergic reaction to protamine. These include all of the following, *except*:

(A) Use of Neutral Protamine Hagedorn (NPH) insulin

(B) Allergy to fish

(C) Previous administration of protamine

(D) Use of amiodarone

(E) Vasectomy

18 An 81-year-old man with a creatinine clearance of 20 mL per minute needs to undergo coronary angiography. Angioplasty and direct stent placement are successful; however, the patient develops worsening renal insufficiency and atrial fibrillation. Which antiarrhythmic medication would be the best treatment for this patient at this time?

(A) Sotalol

(B) Propafenone

(C) Flecainide

(D) Mexilitene

(E) Dofetilide

19 The patient above ultimately develops end-stage renal failure requiring chronic dialysis. Since profanone has a relatively long half-life (up to 36 hours in patients with slow metabolism) it is unattractive for use among patients undergoing dialysis. Which of the following therapies would be more attractive for long-term prophalyxis against atrial fibrillation in this patient?

(A) Sotalol

(B) Dofetilide

(C) Amiodarone
(D) Quinidine

20 Which of the following lipid-lowering therapies has no or very limited affect on warfarin metabolism?

(A) Ezetimibe
(B) Cholestyramine
(C) Fenofibrate
(D) Simvastatin

Answers and Explanations

1 **Answer B.** This is an ischemic rhythm, as evidenced by the upper figure. The lower figure shows a tracing of Torsade de Pointes that is associated with hypotension and reduced mental status (the patient does not respond to your question). In this scenario the best treatment is direct current cardioversion to immediately restore sinus rhythm. Although lidocaine and amiodarone are advanced cardiac life support (ACLS) drugs of choice for hemodynamically stable ventricular tachycardia (VT) the goal here is to rapidly convert the patient to a more stable rhythm. Diltiazem would be contraindicated.

2 **Answer A.** Prostacycline and thromboxane are products of cyclo-oxygenase and are produced by the vascular endothelium. Endothelin is a protein produced by the endothelium and is one of the most potent vasoconstrictors known. Nitric oxide is a free radical produced by the constitutive enzyme endothelial nitric-oxide synthase (eNOS) in normal endothelial cells in nonpathologic situations. There is also an inducible form of nitric-oxide synthase—inducible nitric-oxide synthase (iNOS)—that can be rapidly induced by a number of pathologic or inflammatory processes including ischemia-reperfusion injury, and the sepsis syndrome. Nitric oxide is the putative endothelium-derived relaxing factor (EDRF) that is also a neurotransmitter in the brain, and one of the principal mediators of flow-dependent vasodilation. Nitrous oxide is an inhaled anesthetic and is not produced by the endothelium.

3 **Answer C.** Vasopressin receptors in the brain are mediators of endothelium-dependent cerebral vasodilation. In the periphery, vasopressin receptors mediate vasoconstriction. This combination of peripheral vasoconstriction and cerebral vasodilation are an ideal hemodynamic combination for resuscitation and vasopressin has been recommended as an alternative agent to dopamine by the Emergency Cardiac Care committee in ACLS protocols. Dopamine, in the doses suggested by ACLS recommendations, increases SVR and the chronotropic state of the heart by stimulating α and β receptors.

4 **Answer D.** Methergine is a serotonin receptor agonist and has effects on both the vascular endothelium and the vascular smooth muscle. When the vascular endothelium is healthy, methergine produces vasodilation through an endothelium-dependent (nitric oxide-mediated) mechanism that overpowers the direct vasoconstrictor effects on the vascular smooth muscle. However, if the endothelium in coronary artery segments is unhealthy, methergine stimulation does not result in increased amounts of endothelium-dependent vasodilators and the direct vasoconstrictor action on the vascular smooth muscle is unopposed; thereby causing "spasm" in that coronary artery segment. Methergine has no effect on vasopressin receptors, thromboxane or endothelin. Additionally, endothelin is a protein, not a small molecule, and it takes much more time for its production due to translation, transcription, and secretion of protein products from endothelial cells.

5 **Answer B.** Nitric oxide diffuses rapidly from endothelial cells into the surrounding vascular smooth muscle cells and increases production of cGMP, which initiates a cascade of events leading to vascular smooth muscle relaxation. Nitric oxide is a potent inhibitor of platelet aggregation in conjunction with endothelial-derived prostacycline. Nitric oxide also inhibits adhesion of neutrophils by at least two mechanisms: Nitric oxide production reduces expression of adhesion molecules in normal vascular endothelium and it also has a direct effect on neutrophils preventing adhesion.

6 **Answer B.** Nitric oxide is the *product* of the endothelium being stimulated by an endothelium-dependent vasodilator like acetylcholine or serotonin. Therefore nitric oxide is an endothelium-independent vasodilator. Indeed, the nitrate-based, endothelium-independent vasodilators used in clinical practice (like sodium nitroprusside and nitroglycerine produce nitric oxide spontaneously or enzymatically) which acts directly on vascular smooth muscle. A healthy endothelium is not needed for nitrates or the active molecule nitric oxide to cause vasodilation. Calcium channel blockers and adenosine have mechanisms of action that are also independent of the vascular endothelium.

7 **Answer B.** No-reflow is a complex pathophysiologic phenomenon that was first described in animal models of ischemia-reperfusion injury. As oxygen is reintroduced following anoxia, reactive oxygen species like superoxide anion, hydroxyl radical, and hydrogen peroxide cause free radical-mediated cell injury. Endothelial cell edema, capillary plugging with neutrophils, platelet plugs, and eventually red cells all contribute to the no-reflow seen angiographically. Microvascular vasospasm, atheroembolic debris, and endothelial dysfunction also participate in the no-reflow phenomenon. No reflow is most likely to occur in coronary vein graft intervention and in patients with acute myocardial infarction. It occurs in 1% to 4% of all percutaneous interventions. Useful medical therapies (i.e., intracoronary vasodilators) include Verapamil, adenosine, diltiazem, papaverine, nicardipine, and sodium nitroprusside. There is a suggestion in the literature that "combination therapy" with adenosine and nitroprusside is better than adenosine alone. Finally, infusion of vasodilators into the distal vascular bed, instead of through the guide catheter, using a pulse spray method may also improve angiographic outcome. However, angiographic improvement does not alter morbidity and mortality. (*Catheter Cardiovasc Interv.* 2004;61: 484–491, *Am Heart J.* 2003;145: 42–46).

8 Answer D. In cardiogenic shock from contrast-mediated anaphylactoid reactions, IV epinephrine should be administered in bolus doses of 10 µg every minute until a desired restoration in blood pressure is accomplished. A 10 mL syringe of 10 µg per mL epinephrine can be prepared by diluting 0.1 mL of 1:1,000 or 1 mL of 1:10,000 in 10 mL of 0.9% NS. If continued epinephrine support is needed, then a drip at 1 to 4 µg per minute by continuous infusion may be given. In large databases of complications in the catheterization laboratory, anaphylactoid reactions occur in <0.5% of patients undergoing coronary angiography. Steroids should be administered to patients having anaphylactoid reactions, but this does not affect the acute hemodynamic disturbances. It takes several hours for steroids to be effective but acute administration may reduce the possibility of delayed recurrent symptoms that may occur as late as 48 hours after the index episode. For minor or moderate anaphylactoid reactions epinephrine can be administered SQ. The dose for this is 0.3 mL of 1:1,000 every 15 minutes up to a total dose of 1 mL. Minor reactions such as isolated urticaria can be treated with diphenhydramine 25 to 50 mg IV. (*Catheter Cardiovasc Interv* 1995;34: 99–104).

9 Answer B. This is classic Torsade de Pointes that is seen following ST-segment elevation in the first line of the rhythm strip. Polymorphic VT is an ischemic rhythm and often degenerates into ventricular fibrillation, which is seen intermittently in this rhythm strip. The mechanism of ischemic

ventricular rhythms is not known with certainty, but has molecular origins in free radical production from ischemia-reperfusion injury that damages cell membranes, ion pumps, enzymes and other cellular organelles leading to cell damage and arrhythmias.

10 Answer D. This is a wide complex, irregularly, irregular rhythm that is most consistent with atrial fibrillation with aberrancy due to conduction over a bypass tract. This is a rhythm that should never be treated with AV nodal blocking drugs because it could accelerate conduction over the bypass tract and lead to hypotension and life threatening sequelae.

11 Answer C. This is a wide complex, regular rhythm most consistent with VT. This regular, sustained VT is most likely due to reentrant phenomenon that is strongly suggestive of prior myocardial scarring from an old myocardial infarction. The anatomic mechanisms responsible for sustained, monomorphic VT are very different from the acute, ischemic mechanisms responsible for Torsade de Pointes.

12 Answer A. Note in the upper tracing at the right-hand edge, that the previous R–R intervals appear to be imbedded in the "wide complex tachycardia." This is an example of artifact mimicking VT.

13 Answer D. The levels of Lp(a) are relatively consistent throughout an individual's lifetime. They increase after menopause, and the levels can be somewhat lowered with estrogen therapy. 3-Hydroxy-3-methylglutaryl coenzyme A (HMG Co-A) reductase inhibitors do not affect the levels of Lp(a). Niacin and fibric acid derivatives have been shown to modestly lower Lp(a) levels.

14 Answer C. This elderly woman is at risk for excess sedation, especially with polypharmacy. She is showing signs of respiratory depression. This is quite unlikely to be due to the flurazepam she received the evening before. Midazolam would only intensify any respiratory depression and metoclopramide would have no effect. The best next step would be to administer naloxone and reverse the effects of the intravenous morphine. At the same time, the patient should be given supplemental oxygen.

15 Answer G. Atropine is a very valuable drug in the cardiac catheterization laboratory and can quickly reverse the bradycardia and hypotension sometimes associated with infarction, ischemia, and inappropriate vagle tone. Atropine causes bronchodilation rather than constriction and it should not be used in particularly low doses or particularly high doses because it may result in inappropriate effects. For example, particularly small doses can produce a paradoxic effect, whereas particularly large doses in a single administration can also produce a paradoxic effect or excessive tachycardia. An appropriate first dose is 0.5 to 1.0 mg intravenously.

16 Answer B. This patient clearly has a marked elevation in the LDL cholesterol, and the goal should be to reduce this to well under 100, and preferably under 80. Each of the drugs will lower LDL cholesterol somewhat. The greatest effect will be with the statins. WelChol (colesevelam) will only lower LDL cholesterol approximately 15%, and, it is contraindicated in patients who already have elevated triglycerides to the level this patient has.

17 Answer D. Each of the factors listed is associated with an increased risk of reaction to protamine, which is a fish-derived (salmon testes) product. There is no known relationship between amiodarone use and protamine reaction. The risk of having a severe allergic reaction to protamine among patients who use NPH insulin is approximately 2%; whereas, among patients undergoing cardiac catheterization who have not received NPH insulin in the past, risk is approximately 0.1%. (*Cathet Cardiovasc Diagn.* 1991;23:164–168).

18 Answer B. Dofetilide and sotalol are excreted by a renal mechanism and should be cautiously used in patients with severe or worsening renal function. Encainide, flecainide, mexilitene, and propafenone undergo important hepatic metabolism and have a minor component of renal elimination. The route of elimination for propafenone is almost entirely hepatic. As such, it is very reasonable to treat this patient with propafenone. It can be used successfully not only in acute atrial fibrillation but also as a prophalactic agent to prevent recurrent atrial fibrillation.

19 Answer C. Most of these drugs are somewhat or minimally affected by dialysis. Amiodarone is a good therapy for prophylaxis against recurrent atrial fibrillation, has a long biologic half-life, and is least affected by dialysis. It would be a very reasonable choice in this patient.

20 Answer A. Many lipid-lowering therapies affect the hepatic cytochrome systems or bowel function, both of which can affect the metabolism of warfarin. Ezetimibe is not known to affect either hepatic metabolism of warfarin or vitamin k production in the gut (*Clin Pharmacokinet.* 2005;44:467–494).

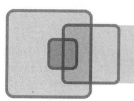

7

Guiding Catheter Selection for Coronary Interventions

Bruce E. Lewis and Dominique Joyal

Questions

The importance of a thorough understanding of guiding catheter shapes and sizes commercially available for percutaneous interventional treatment of various coronary lesions is underscored by the statement that cardiologists should not undertake a coronary intervention until they have performed an absolute minimum of 1,000 diagnostic angiograms underscores the importance of understanding catheter shapes and coronary anatomy (including both common and uncommon coronary anomalies). A thorough understanding of both normal and anomalous coronary anatomy will only be achieved after years of experience. However, certain basic principles can be learned early in one's career. The goal of this chapter is to familiarize the reader with basic guide catheter principles and to expose the reader to interventional approaches to more common coronary anomalies. Although a minority of questions on a formal interventional board are expected to examine concepts pertinent to the utilization of guide catheters, the foundation of interventional cardiology remains a thorough understanding of guide catheter selection and the application of guide catheter selection to specific coronary anatomy.

1 All of the following catheter selections can be expected to reliably provide backup for coronary interventions on the left coronary artery with significant tortuosity or calcification, *except*:

(A) XB3.5
(B) EBU4
(C) AL2
(D) JL4
(E) None of the above

2 Guide catheter selections appropriate for treatment of lesions located in an anomalous circumflex that arises from the right coronary cusp are most likely achieved with all the following catheters, *except*:

(A) JR4
(B) Multipurpose A curve
(C) Short right JR4
(D) The Leya catheter (which is a left Amplatz 1 or 2 modified with an anterior deflection of the distal catheter tip)
(E) All of the above can be useful for cannulation of the anomalous circumflex

3 Catheters that can be used to treat the anomalous right coronary artery (RCA) originating from the left coronary cusp include all of the following, *except*:

(A) JR4
(B) The Leya family of catheters
(C) The Judkins left family of catheters
(D) The left Amplatz family of catheters
(E) None of the above

4 Treatment of left anterior descending (LAD) lesions that are located in the mid and distal segments of the LAD through a tortuous left internal mammary artery (LIMA) are most likely to be managed effectively with:

(A) 100 cm IM catheter
(B) 90 cm IM catheter
(C) Right Judkins 100 cm catheter
(D) Right Judkins 90 cm catheter
(E) None of the above

5 The "crushed" stent technique, which has been described for the treatment of bifurcation of lesions, involves the simultaneous introduction of a primary stent in the parent vessel and a secondary stent in the side branch. The following guide catheter selection provides the minimum diameter required to accomplish a "crushed" stent technique using any commercially available drug-eluting stent (DES) in the United States.

(A) A 6 French standard lumen guide catheter
(B) A 7 French standard lumen guide catheter
(C) An 8 French standard diameter lumen catheter
(D) A 7 French large lumen diameter catheter
(E) An 8 French large lumen diameter catheter

6 Common guider strategies that can be employed to treat right coronary posterolateral branch lesions that are observed to be quite distal from the right coronary origin include all of the following, *except*:

(A) "Deep seating" of a 6 French JR 4 catheter into the mid or distal RCA because of the trauma transmitted to the vessel wall
(B) Use of an AL1 standard guiding catheter to cannulate the proximal RCA and provide extra backup because the left Amplatz shape does not fit the right coronary
(C) Use of an AL2 guiding catheter to cannulate the proximal RCA and provide extra backup because only the AL1 shape can be used to cannulate the right coronary
(D) Use of the hockey stick shape to provide extra backup
(E) Use of a JR4 guiding catheter in the standard ostial right position

7 The largest rotablator burr that can be delivered through a standard 8 French Cordis catheter is a:

(A) 1.5-mm burr
(B) 1.75-mm burr
(C) 2-mm burr
(D) 2.15-mm burr
(E) 2.25-mm burr

8 The largest rotablator burr size that will fit through a 6 French standard Cordis guide catheter is a:

(A) 1.25-mm burr
(B) 1.5-mm burr
(C) 1.75-mm burr
(D) 2.0-mm burr
(E) 2.15-mm burr

9 A patient is transferred from an outpatient diagnostic center where 5 F diagnostic catheters were used to identify a 70% LAD lesion. When you cannulate the left main with your guiding catheter, ventricularization is noted as shown in the following figure. Appropriate responses to the observation of ventricularization encountered on routine coronary intervention during cannulation of the left coronary system using a 6 French guiding system include all of the following, *except*:

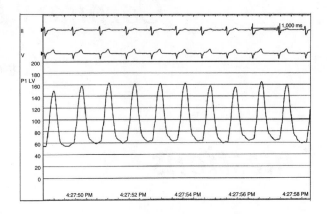

(A) Repositioning the guiding catheter to reevaluate the wave form and assess catheter tip relationships
(B) Proceeding with the coronary intervention because ventricularization is frequently seen during cannulation of the left main coronary artery
(C) Performing a more thorough evaluation of the coronary tree using intravascular ultrasound (IVUS)
(D) All of the above
(E) None of the above

10 Prolonged radial artery cannulation is associated with compromise of the radial artery occlusion rates in what percentage of patients?

(A) 2% to 10%
(B) 10% to 15%
(C) 15% to 20%
(D) 25% to 30%
(E) None of the above

11 A common complication associated with the radial artery approach is occlusion of the radial artery. This occurs in the following percentage of cases when procedures are *not* prolonged:

(A) <1%
(B) 1% to 2%
(C) 2% to 10%
(D) 10% to 20%
(E) >20%

12 Legitimate concerns that should be considered when selecting larger lumen guide catheters over smaller lumen guide catheters include all of the following, *except*:

(A) Increased potential for trauma at the ostium of the artery selected for intervention
(B) Larger defect at the access site for sheath introduction and consequent delayed ambulation
(C) Contrast volume
(D) All of the above
(E) A and B

13 Extreme tortuosity of the iliac system and aorta will often present problems with cannulation of both the right and the left coronary artery. The most efficient technical maneuver that can overcome peripheral and aortic tortuosity includes:

(A) After sheath introduction, immediate use of the 0.038 "stiff" wire for negotiation of the tortuosity
(B) Use of the coated wire (e.g., glide wire) to negotiate the tortuosity and enter the ascending aorta
(C) Use of an 0.068 Arani wire after the sheath has been inserted and advancing the Arani wire into the ascending aorta, followed by advancing the guide catheter over the Arani wire
(D) Initial negotiation of the tortuosity with a glide coated wire or soft wire followed by advancing the guide catheter into the ascending aorta. The coated wire or soft wire can then be removed and a stiffer 0.038 wire placed into the guide to facilitate further advancement of the guiding catheter into the appropriate coronary cusp and cannulation of the appropriate coronary artery
(E) None of the above

14 The observation of a damped waveform in the following figure seen on hemodynamic monitoring can be managed by all of the following maneuvers, *except*:

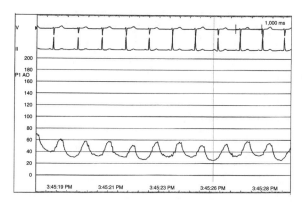

(A) Reposition the catheter to ensure that the guiding catheter tip is not against the vessel wall
(B) Flush the guiding catheter
(C) Flush the transducer tubing

(D) Change to a catheter with side holes
(E) Select a smaller French catheter

15 During prolonged and difficult catheter manipulation, secondary to a tortuous iliac system while attempting to cannulate the RCA with a JR4 guide, the waveform shown in the following figure is noticed. A common cause of this waveform is:

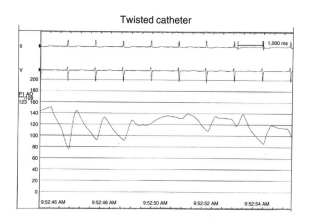

(A) Kinking of the guide catheter
(B) Stripping of the stent off the balloon delivery catheter
(C) Thrombus within the catheter lumen
(D) Air in the catheter lumen
(E) All of the above

16 Treatment of lesions in the distal RCA through saphenous vein grafts to the right system are usually accomplished with all of the following, *except*:

(A) Multipurpose A (MPA)
(B) Short tip Judkins right
(C) Right coronary bypass (RCB)
(D) Left coronary bypass (LCB)
(E) None of the above

17 Aorta-coronary saphenous vein grafts that are anastomosed to the LAD and circumflex are most commonly cannulated with each of the following, *except*:

(A) JR4
(B) Hockey stick
(C) JL4
(D) LCB
(E) Amplatz left

18 Which of the statements regarding catheters used for the radial approach is true?

(A) Judkins catheter should not be used
(B) For the right radial approach, the Judkins left catheter should be 0.5 cm larger than what would be selected for the femoral approach

(C) For the right radial approach, the Judkins left catheter should be 0.5 cm smaller than what would be selected for a femoral approach

(D) For the right radial approach, Judkins right catheter should be 0.5 cm smaller than what would be selected for the femoral approach

(E) For the left radial artery, Judkins right catheter should be 0.5 cm smaller than would be selected for the femoral approach

19 The following guide catheter choice will usually provide the most reliable backup when treating saphenous vein grafts to the left coronary artery:

(A) JL4
(B) No torque right
(C) LCB
(D) Short right Judkins
(E) Hockey stick

20 Your junior partner encounters difficulty in cannulating the left main for treatment of an LAD lesion in a 5 ft. 2 in., 120 pound, 58-year-old, Asian woman. Your assessment of a JL4 guide catheter shows the JL4 catheter tip to consistently fall in the left cusp inferior to the take-off of the left main origin. You would advise your partner to select which of the following catheters:

(A) JL5
(B) Reposition the JL4
(C) JL 3.5
(D) Amplatz 2
(E) Amplatz 3

21 Your partner has just completed a diagnostic cath on a 59-year-old juvenile onset diabetic patient who presented with a 3-month history of severe exertional angina. The anomalous right artery cannulation was extremely difficult and required multiple catheters and test injections to locate but the RCA was free of significant disease. Multiple catheters and test injections were also required to image the left coronary artery, which had a minimally diseased circumflex but a severe stenosis at a calcified LAD diagonal bifurcation. Both the LAD and diagonal serve large territories of myocardium. The LV angiogram demonstrated normal LV function. Your plan for this patient would include:

(A) Proceed with "crush" stent technique on the LAD diagonal system

(B) Proceed with the intervention using a stent on the LAD and protect the diagonal with a curve

(C) Proceed with the intervention on the LAD but forgo wire protection of the diagonal

(D) Postpone the intervention

(E) Treat the patient medically

22 The importance of the evaluation of hemodynamic waveforms during coronary intervention cannot be overemphasized. Many young operators tend to focus on the angiographic image and ignore the hemodynamic clues of pressure tracing. The pressure waveforms can alert the interventionalist to catheter position (e.g., migration to the ventricle during difficult RCA interventions), dangerous anatomy (e.g., left main stenosis), and unstable hemodynamics (e.g., hypotension and hypertension). Match the following waveforms with the correct answer:

(A)

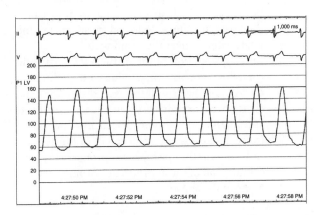

(B)

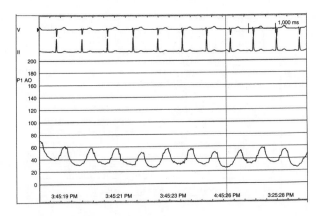

(C)

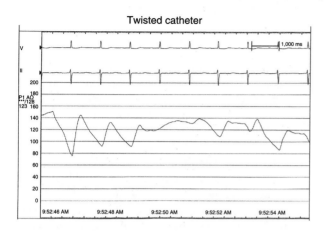

(E)

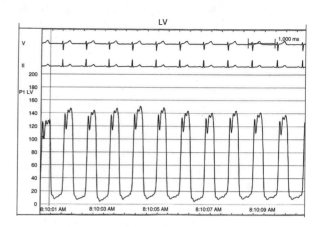

(D)

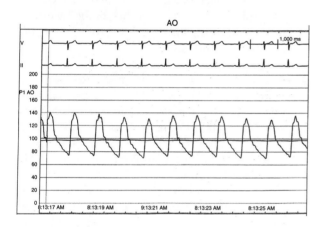

1. Catheter kinking
2. Damping
3. Normal aortic waveform
4. Normal ventricular waveform
5. Ventricularization

Answers and Explanations

1 **Answer D.** The Amplatz catheter shape, the XB family of curves (Cordis), and the EBU family of curves (Medtronic) all provide excellent backup for delivery of stents and/or larger devices such as rotablator and AngioJet. The JL4 shape provides only modest backup and frequently operators rely on catheter manipulation or support wires to complete even straightforward interventions when a left Judkins guider is used.

2 **Answer D.** The "Leya" catheter is a left Amplatz shape specifically modified to cannulate anomalies of the RCA that arise from the left coronary cusp. The anomalous circumflex is the most common coronary anomaly encountered during coronary angiography (prevalence 0.37%) and, therefore, it is important to understand the catheter options that can be used to cannulate these vessels. The MPA curve and short right Judkins will usually provide coaxial support for the anomalous circumflex that originates from the right coronary cusp (*Cathet Cardiovasc Diagn.* 1987;13:407–410, *Cathet Cardiovasc Diagn.* 1990;21:28–40).

3 **Answer A.** The anomalous right originating from the left coronary cusp is often very challenging to cannulate. Standard left catheters (JL3.5, JL4, JL5, AL I, AL II) can often be utilized. However, the "Leya" catheters will usually simplify cannulation and provide excellent backup. The Leya catheter is an AL I or AL II with an anterior flair of the distal tip of the catheter. One significant concern regarding treatment of the anomalous RCA is when the course of the vessel is between the pulmonary artery and aorta. This anomalous course can be associated with sudden death, especially in young athletes, and has been reported to be the second most common cardiac abnormality associated with death in young athletes. Careful preprocedural clinical evaluation must be applied to these patients (*Cathet Cardiovasc Diagn.* 1989;16:16–18, *Catheter Cardiovasc Interv.* 2003;60:382–388, *Hum Pathol.* 1999;30:595–596).

4 **Answer B.** When standard shaft length balloons and stents are used for treatment of distal LAD lesions through the LIMA, the most common technical limitation is the balloon catheter shaft length. The "shorter" 90 cm LIMA guide will allow access to distal LAD lesions with standard balloon lengths (135 cm shaft length). A second option is to select a longer balloon shaft length (e.g., 150 cm shaft length).

5 **Answer E.** Simultaneous introduction of two stents through a guiding catheter should generally be accomplished by using the smallest French size that will provide adequate catheter lumen to both introduce the two stents and visualize vessel landmarks during stent deployment. The guide catheters that provide an inner lumen diameter of 0.088 inches for the Cypher stent and 0.081 inches for the Taxol stent will usually satisfy these criteria (*J Am Coll Cardiol.* 2005;46:1446–1455).

6 **Answer E.** Answers A–D are all acceptable solutions when distal RCA branch lesions clinically warrant intervention. Deep seating of smaller French guide catheters is frequently used to overcome distal delivery problems, but does carry a small risk of proximal vessel dissection. Both the AL1 and AL2 can be used to cannulate the RCA and usually provide excellent backup. Care must be taken to ensure coaxial guide position when applying left Amplatz curves to the RCA to both avoid catheter tip ostial dissections and wire dissections when passing the wire through the guide catheter tip (*Cathet Cardiovasc Diagn.* 1986;12:189–197, *Cathet Cardiovasc Diagn.* 1990;19:58–67).

7 **Answer D.** An essential component in planning for a rotablation case is the assessment of the maximum burr size anticipated as necessary to complete the case. The operator should then select a guide catheter that can accommodate the largest burr anticipated for completion of the case.

8 **Answer C.** Physicians who have had a significant experience with the rotablator will generally know the maximum burr size that is compatible with various guide catheters. Younger interventionalists should familiarize themselves with the following table and consider posting the table in their cath lab (*The manual of interventional cardiology.* 2001;14–17).

Guide catheter selection

Burr Diameter (mm)	Burr Diameter (inches)	Guide Catheter ID (inches)
1.25	0.049	0.053
1.50	0.059	0.063
1.75	0.069	0.073
2.00	0.079	0.083
2.15	0.085	0.089
2.25	0.089	0.093
2.38	0.094	0.098
2.50	0.098	0.102

9 Answer B. The use of smaller 4, 5 and 6 F diagnostic catheters can result in an incomplete assessment of ostial lesions. Smaller catheter sizes can result in both underfilling of the coronary and can mask hemodynamic clues such as ventricularization of the pressure waveform. Ventricularization of the waveform is usually a hybrid of a ventricular waveform and an aortic pressure tracing. Ventricularization can be a sign of significant left main disease and should be carefully assessed before proceeding with a scheduled intervention. Withdrawal of the catheter tip may reveal that the catheter was selectively engaged in a branch of the left main and reassure the interventionalist that no significant left main disease is present. IVUS could also be used to evaluate the left main. A cross sectional area of <6 mm would strongly suggest consideration for bypass surgery (*J Am Coll Cardiol.* 2005;45:204–211, *Am Heart J.* 1989;118:1160–1166).

10 Answer D. Prolonged interventional procedures performed through a femoral artery access are associated with higher complication rates. Radial arteries are generally smaller diameter vessels with reduced distal flow and, therefore, prolonged radial artery procedures are at increased risk for vascular access complication and radial artery compromise in 25% to 30% of cases. This observation suggests that complex cases may be better treated from a femoral approach when feasible (*Catheter Cardiovasc Interv.* 1999;46: 173–178).

11 Answer C. The findings of a pulseless radial artery following transradial approach are reported in 2% to 10% of patients. However, because of the dual blood supply to the hand, this rarely leads to ischemic sequela. An Allen test should be performed before any radial artery cannulation to ensure an adequate ulnar supply in the event of radial artery occlusion. The radial approach is often avoided when complex interventions (e.g., Percutaneous Transluminal Coronary Rotational Ablation [PTCRA]) are anticipated, which

may require larger lumen guide catheters (*Catheter Cardiovasc Interv.* 1999;46:173–178, *Cathet Cardiovasc Diagn.* 1997;40:156–158).

12 Answer D. Larger lumen catheters require larger introducer sheaths and carry an increased potential for complication at the puncture site as well as the origin of the target vessel. Larger lumen catheters require a larger volume of contrast to fill the catheter and are associated with higher contrast loads. Care should be taken to limit contrast loads in patients with underlying renal dysfunction when larger diameter catheters are needed (*Cathet Cardiovasc Diagn.* 1991;23:93–99).

13 Answer D. Multiple maneuvers are frequently required to overcome tortuosity of the iliac artery and aorta. All of the guide catheter support wires described in the answers can be used; however, stiff wires run the risk of dissection in tortuous vessels and, therefore, a safer approach is to use a softer wire or coated wire to negotiate the tortuosity and advance the guide into the thoracic aorta and then exchange to stiffer wires to both straighten the guide catheter and strengthen the system with an improved catheter "torque."

14 Answer B. Understanding the cause of a damped waveform in a given patient is critical for the interventionalist to prevent potentially life-threatening complications. Damping can occur from deep cannulation of the guide catheter and as a result the catheter tip can rest against the vessel wall. Repositioning the catheter may correct a damped image on hemodynamic monitoring and prevent possible catheter-induced injury from injection into the vessel wall. Flushing the guide catheter could be dangerous because damping of the waveform could also occur with thrombus, air or atheroma inside the catheter. Flushing any of these foreign bodies could result in embolism and significant clinical deterioration. Air in the transducer system could cause a damped waveform and time should be taken to reflush the transducer. Smaller vessels (often co-dominate small diameter right coronary arteries) will result in damping and this can be overcome by choosing a smaller diameter catheter or switching to side holes (*Practical angioplasty.* 1993:53).

15 Answer A. Thrombus or air in the catheter lumen usually appears damped but retains some features of an aortic pressure tracing pattern. Guide catheter kinking is not uncommon during difficult RCA cannulations and is usually associated with near complete or complete loss of the usual aortic waveform. A kinked catheter is easily diagnosed by viewing the catheter under fluoroscopy and identifying the kinked catheter segment. Extreme kinking of the guide catheter can be easily addressed by counter torquing the guide in a rotation opposite to the rotation that caused the kink.

16 **Answer D.** Saphenous grafts to the RCA system usually have an inferior take off and arise from the anterior wall of the aorta. MPA, short tip right and RCB have a less acute curve just before the catheter tip and usually allow for cannulation. The LCB has a more acute angle and is usually not coaxial with the right-sided vein graft origin (*The manual of interventional cardiology.* 2001:14–17).

17 **Answer C.** Left coronary bypasses are frequently positioned lateral and superior in the aorta. The JR4 and LCB catheters will generally provide coaxial support when treating left-sided vein graft lesions. The Hockey stick and left Amplatz catheters will usually provide additional backup compared with the JR4 and LCB catheters. The JL4 shape does not fit vein grafts to the left system (*The manual of interventional cardiology.* 2001:14–17).

18 **Answer C.** When using a Judkins Left catheter from the right radial artery, the curve should be in general 0.5 cm smaller than the curve that would have been used from the femoral approach. When using a Judkins right catheter from the right radial artery, the curve should be in general 1 cm larger. When using the left transradial approach, no changes in curve size are usually needed.

19 **Answer E.** Again, the Hockey stick will generally provide the most reliable backup for treatment of vein grafts to the left coronary system.

20 **Answer C.** Smaller stature patients frequently require smaller catheter sizes during cannulation of the left main. Furthermore, downsizing Judkins left catheters is often helpful to selectively engage the LAD. The Amplatz 2 and 3 curves would more likely be useful in larger patients or hypertensive patients with elongated ascending aortas (*The manual of interventional cardiology.* 2001:14–17).

21 **Answer D.** The diagnostic procedure appears to have been technically challenging and the patient has already been exposed to a significant contrast load. The patient's 3-month history of angina suggests a subacute clinical course, and the patient could be safely observed while appropriate pharmacologic therapy and preinterventional hydration could be initiated before a potentially complex interventional procedure is initiated on the patient at risk for contrast-induced nephropathy. Resisting the occulostenotic reflex would also allow the patient to consider other revascularization options. The limitation of contrast volume should reduce the incidence of contrast-induced nephrotoxicity from 21% to 2% (*Am J Med.* 1989;86:649–652, *AJR Am J Roentgenol.* 1991;157:49–58).

22 **Answer A-5, B-2, C-1, D-3, E-4.**

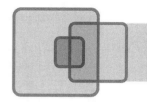

8

Intravascular Contrast Agents

Thomas T. Tsai and Brahmajee K. Nallamothu

Questions

1 Contrast agents are known to cause adverse effects. All of the following responses would be considered anaphylactoid reactions, *except*:

(A) Bronchospasm
(B) Bradycardia
(C) Angioedema
(D) Urticaria
(E) Cardiovascular collapse

2 Which of the following is *true* regarding the mechanism of contrast media anaphylactoid reactions?

(A) They are due to immunoglobulin E (IgE)-mediated degranulation of mast cells
(B) They are due to chemokine release from memory T-cells, which cause degranulation of mast cells
(C) They involve iodine binding of vitronectin receptor and basophil degranulation
(D) They involve degranulation of circulating basophils and tissue mast cells by direct complement activation

3 A 63-year-old woman suffered bronchospasm during diagnostic coronary angiography with a high-osmolar contrast agent 2 years ago. She presents for repeat coronary angiography secondary to angina and a positive stress test. What is the likelihood of another reaction when reexposed to a nonionic low-osmolar contrast agent?

(A) <1%
(B) <10%
(C) <25%
(D) <50%

4 All of the following are clear indications for using low-osmolar contrast agents for coronary angiography, *except*:

(A) Severe coronary artery disease (e.g., left main disease)
(B) Severe emphysema
(C) Severe aortic stenosis
(D) Moderate-to-severe left ventricular dysfunction

5 Side effects of high-osmolar contrast agents such as a transient decrease in systolic blood pressure, flushing, bradycardia, and nausea are thought to be mediated by what properties?

(A) Hypertonicity
(B) Sodium concentration
(C) Iodine-mediated vasodilatation
(D) Low viscosity

6 Studies suggest that low-osmolar nonionic contrast agents compared with high-osmolar contrast agents reduce the incidence of which of the following adverse effects?

(A) Thrombotic complications
(B) Bradyarrhythmias
(C) Postprocedure renal failure
(D) Anaphylactoid reactions
(E) A and B
(F) B, C, and D

7 What is the incidence of life-threatening reactions to contrast agents?

(A) 1:100
(B) 1:1,000

(C) 1:100,000

(D) 1:1,000,000

8 A 52-year-old man with a history of asthma and hypertension receives his first injection of contrast for his diagnostic cardiac catheterization. He immediately develops bronchospasm, laryngeal edema, and hypotension. Immediate treatment should begin with:

(A) 1 mg of 1:10,000 epinephrine intravenous boluses every minute until pressure is restored

(B) 10 mg of 1:10,000 epinephrine intravenous boluses every minute until pressure is restored

(C) 0.1 mg of 1:10,000 epinephrine intravenous boluses every minute until pressure is restored

(D) 0.01 mg of 1:10,000 epinephrine intravenous boluses every minute until pressure is restored

(E) None of the above

9 Match the following intravascular contrast agents with the appropriate statement:

(A) Diatrizoate (Hypaque, Renografin, Angiovist)

(B) Iohexol (Omnipaque)

(C) Ioxaglate (Hexbrix)

(D) Iodixanol (Visipaque)

1. A nonionic, iso-osmolar agent

2. An agent with serum osmolality typically six times that of blood

3. A nonionic, low-osmolar agent that is water-soluble

4. An ionic, low-osmolar agent with a dimeric structure

10 Which of the following patients has the highest risk of developing contrast-associated nephropathy following cardiac catheterization and/or percutaneous coronary intervention (PCI)?

(A) A 72-year-old woman with diabetes mellitus and a serum creatinine of 2.0 mg per dL who presents with ST-elevation myocardial infarction and hypotension

(B) A 48-year-old man without diabetes mellitus and a serum creatinine of 2.6 mg per dL undergoing elective PCI

(C) An 80-year-old man with diabetes mellitus and a serum creatinine of 1.0 mg per dL who is also taking metformin

(D) A 45-year-old woman with a history of a solitary kidney and a serum creatinine of 0.9 mg per dL who is undergoing a right- and left-heart catheterization for a suspected atrial septal defect

11 Potential strategies for reducing the risk of contrast-associated nephropathy in high-risk patients include all of the following, *except*:

(A) Pre- and posthydration with half-normal saline at the time of the procedure

(B) Limiting the volume of intravascular contrast used

(C) Maintaining urine flow rates of 150 mL per hour with close hemodynamic monitoring and the use of fluid loading, dopamine, and furosemide

(D) Oral N-acetylcysteine (NAC) following the procedure

(E) Use of nonionic, iso-osmolar contrast

12 The mechanism by which intravascular contrast is believed to cause nephropathy is:

(A) Direct cellular toxicity to renal tubular cells resulting in acute tubular necrosis (ATN)

(B) Hypoxic injury due to localized hemodynamic alterations including renal vasoconstriction

(C) Neither

(D) Both

13 In a 70-kg patient with a baseline creatinine of 2.0 mg per dL who is undergoing cardiac catheterization and PCI, there should be attempts to limit the contrast dose to:

(A) 70 mL

(B) 105 mL

(C) 175 mL

(D) 210 mL

14 Patients with contrast-associated nephropathy typically have all of the following occur during their clinical course with the *exception* of:

(A) An early rise in serum creatinine usually within 4 days

(B) Recovery of serum creatinine within 2 weeks

(C) Transient need for renal replacement therapy with hemodialysis

(D) Urinalysis with active sediment showing "granular" muddy casts

15 Contrast-associated nephropathy can be differentiated from atheroembolic renal failure most clearly by:

(A) Absence of cutaneous findings like livedo reticularis

(B) Absence of peripheral eosinophilia or eosinophiluria

(C) Recovery of serum creatinine within 2 weeks

(D) Presence of a normal urinalysis

16 Typical doses of contrast agents for left ventriculography and thoracic aortography during routine cineangiography include:

(A) 30 to 40 mL injected at a rate of 10 mL per second and 80 to 100 mL injected at a rate of 40 mL per second, respectively

(B) 30 to 40 mL injected at a rate of 10 mL per second and 40 to 60 mL injected at a rate of 20 mL per second, respectively

(C) 20 to 30 mL injected at a rate of 5 mL per second and 20 to 40 mL injected at a rate of 20 mL per second, respectively

17 Methods for limiting toxicity from contrast agents during peripheral angiography include:

(A) Use of trace subtract fluoroscopy (i.e., road mapping)

(B) Use of interactive mode in run-off studies of the lower extremities with a single bolus injection

(C) Use of nontraditional agents like gadolinium and carbon dioxide

(D) A and B

(E) A, B, and C

Answers and Explanations

1 Answer B. With intracoronary injection of contrast agents, transient bradycardia may occur within 5 to 10 seconds, particularly in the right coronary artery, and subside quickly. All other answers are considered anaphylactoid reactions associated with mass cell activation (*Grossman's cardiac catheterization, angiography, and intervention.* 2006:52–53).

2 Answer D. Contrast media can cause direct complement activation with the degranulation of basophils and mast cells. This is considered an "anaphylactoid" reaction (*Ann Pharmacother.* 1994;28:236–241).

3 Answer A. Even without pretreatment using steroids and histamine blockers, the incidence of severe cross-reactions between ionic and nonionic contrast agents is extremely low (*J Am Coll Cardiol.* 1993;21:269–273).

4 Answer B. Severe emphysema is not an indication for low-osmolar contrast agents. All other conditions listed in the preceding text make patients more susceptible to the hemodynamic effects associated with high-osmolar contrast agents.

5 Answer A. The physiologic and adverse effects of high-osmolar contrast agents are largely a result of the hypertonicity and calcium chelating properties of these compounds (*Grossman's cardiac catheterization, angiography, and intervention.* 2006:31–33).

6 Answer F. Low-osmolar nonionic contrast agents are better tolerated by patients and produce fewer episodes of bradycardia, transient hypotension, renal dysfunction, and both mild and serious anaphylactoid reactions. There are no clear differences in the incidence of thrombotic complications (*Grossman's cardiac catheterization, angiography, and intervention.* 2006:31–33).

7 Answer C. Fatal reactions to contrast agents are rare and are most often quoted as being between 1:75,000 and 1:170,000 procedures (*Radiology.* 1990;175:621–628).

8 Answer D. Hemodynamic collapse that is suspected to be due to an anaphylactoid reaction needs to be treated aggressively. A dose of 0.01 mg of 1:10,000 epinephrine is 10 μg (micrograms). The epinephrine is administered IV as 10 μg boluses every minute until pressure is restored. Central access is preferred for delivery.

9 Answer A-2, B-3, C-4, D-1. Diatrizoate is an older ratio-1.5 ionic compound (3 atoms of iodine for every ion), which is associated with more side effects than low- and iso-osmolar agents due to its marked hypertonicity. Iohexol is a ratio-3 ionic compound nonionic, low-osmolar agent, whereas ioxaglate is a ratio-3 ionic compound with a unique dimeric structure. Iodixanol is newer ratio-6 compound that is nonionic and water-soluble. It is very well tolerated and may be associated with less allergic side effects and nephrotoxicity than even low-osmolar agents.

10 Answer A. Risk factors for contrast-associated nephropathy include preexisting chronic renal insufficiency, diabetes mellitus, advanced age, hemodynamic instability, intra-aortic balloon pump placement, congestive heart failure, anemia, volume depletion, and the volume of contrast used. The 72-year-old woman has several of these risk factors (*J Am Coll Cardiol.* 2004;44:1393–1399). In addition, it is likely that a serum creatinine of 2.0 mg per dL represents a more substantial decline in glomerular filtration rate in an elderly woman than a higher serum creatinine in a younger (and presumably larger) man. Metformin does not increase the risk of contrast-related nephropathy, but its continued use in that setting is contraindicated.

11 Answer D. Oral NAC has been shown to be beneficial in some studies if begun 1 day before the injection of intravascular contrast (*Lancet.* 2003;362:598–603). In one study, intravenous NAC reduced the incidence of contrast-associated nephropathy when given immediately before cardiac catheterization (*J Am Coll Cardiol.* 2003;41:2114–2118). The other strategies have been shown to be beneficial including the option of maintaining urine flow rates using close hemodynamic monitoring (*J Am Coll Cardiol.* 1999;33:403–411). Other potentially beneficial strategies include use of sodium bicarbonate infusions, ascorbic acid, and hemofiltration. Strategies that do not work are the use of routine mannitol or furosemide and fenoldopam.

12 Answer D. The precise pathophysiology of contrast-associated nephropathy is largely unclear. Direct cellular injury and hypoxic injury from renal vasoconstriction from intravascular contrast have been postulated as potentially important mechanisms that result from hyperosmolality.

13 Answer C. Although Cigarroa et al. proposed using 5 mL per body weight (kg)/serum creatinine to determine the maximum-allowable contrast dose (MACD) before the advent of modern contrast agents (*Am J Med.* 1989;86:649–652), recent studies suggest that the incidence of dialysis is substantially reduced when contrast doses are under this threshold (*Am J Cardiol.* 2002;90:1068–1073).

14 Answer C. Contrast-associated nephropathy typically occurs immediately following the procedure with an early peak in serum creatinine followed by complete recovery within 1 to 3 weeks. Urinalysis at this time is consistent with ATN and shows active sediment with "granular" casts. The need for hemodialysis is a rare but important complication (*Semin Nephrol.* 1998;18:551–557).

15 Answer C. Although cutaneous findings and peripheral eosinophilia or eosinophiluria should raise suspicions for atheroembolic renal failure, they are not consistently present. Skin findings occur in 50% of patients and peripheral eosinophilia is transient and may be difficult to document. The most consistent clinical finding that favors contrast-associated nephropathy is recovery within 2 weeks. A continuously increasing serum creatinine 3 to 8 weeks following the procedure raises suspicions of atheroembolic renal failure. Active sediment may be present in the urine of patients with either disease (*Medicine Baltimore.* 1995;74:350–358).

16 Answer B. Adequate visualization of the left ventricle and thoracic aorta requires rapid delivery of large amounts of contrast agents through power injectors. Typical rates for these procedures are listed in 'B', but these may be modified on the basis of the heart size or cardiac output, the catheter being used (e.g., lower flow rates with end-hole catheters), or the use of digital subtraction imaging in the case of aortic imaging (*Grossman's cardiac catheterization, angiography, and intervention.* 2006:225–227, 263).

17 Answer E. All of the above techniques take advantage of the relatively static nature of many peripheral vascular structures. In road mapping and digital subtraction angiography (DSA), this static nature allows for the generation of baseline images in which radio-opaque structures (i.e., bone) are subtracted out. It also permits the interactive mode and limits the need for sequential static imaging of the lower extremity run-off. Finally, this static nature permits the use of nontraditional agents, but vascular imaging may be suboptimal (*Manual of peripheral vascular intervention.* 2005:36–38, 44–45).

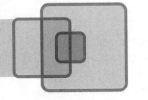

9

Elective Coronary Intervention

Douglass A. Morrison

Questions

Brief Review of the ACC/AHA/SCAI Guidelines, principles used in developing Questions and Answers for Board exams, and this chapter

The American College of Cardiology/American Heart Association (ACC/AHA) Guidelines form the basis of most Cardiology Board Exams. The Guidelines in percutaneous coronary intervention (PCI) were updated in 2005 (*Circulation.* 2006;113:156–175). The Guidelines in coronary artery bypass graft (CABG) surgery were updated in 2004 (*ACC/AHA 2004 Guideline Update.* 2004).

In an effort to avoid subjectivity, most exam questions focus on guideline recommendations that are either strongly *for* (Class I: Conditions for which there is evidence for and/or general agreement that a given procedure or treatment is beneficial, useful, and effective) or *against* (Class III: Conditions for which there is evidence and/or agreement that a procedure/treatment is not useful/effective and in some cases may be harmful). Specific *clinical subsets* used by the PCI guidelines include asymptomatic ischemia or Canadian Cardiovascular Society (CCS) Class I or II (CCS Table 17 in PCI Guideline update), CCS Class III angina, unstable angina (UA)/non–ST-elevation myocardial infarction (NSTEMI), and ST-elevation myocardial infarction (STEMI), which includes failed fibrinolysis, facilitated PCI, rescue PCI, and cardiogenic shock.

Patients may move from one clinical subset to the other over the course of their lives. Because patients with STEMI are generally taken to PCI emergently (meaning 90 minutes or less, if possible), and those with UA/NSTEMI are taken emergently and/or urgently (either this day or this hospital admission), neither group is ordinarily encompassed under the heading "elective PCI," the topic of this chapter. STEMI and UA/NSTEMI are covered in Chapters 10, 11, 35, and 37 of this volume. There is likely some overlap of this chapter with Chapters 34

(Chronic stable angina: ACC/AHA Guidelines) and 36 (PCI: ACC/AHA Guidelines). Hopefully, this will provide repetition of important concepts.

The generic approach to determining whether to revascularize, and if so, by CABG versus PCI, is summarized in PCI Guideline Table 18, which means: Start with the potential benefit to the patient, and then integrate potential risk to the patient in these decisions. The best evidence of benefit or risk comes from randomized clinical trials (RCT) and forms the basis for most A levels of evidence. In general, tables of RCTs are provided in the respective guidelines. The benefits of PCI versus medical therapy in stable patients are summarized in PCI Guideline update Table 12; the benefits of PCI versus CABG in stable patients are summarized in Guideline update Table 11. In the interpretation of these data tables *there is essentially no RCT data supporting the application of PCI to patients with stable angina or asymptomatic silent ischemia, for the purposes of reducing death, myocardial infarction (MI), and/or stroke.* Accordingly, and especially given the ever-growing literature that supports hard clinical outcome benefits of multiple classes of medical therapy (aspirin, thienopyridines, β-blockers, angiotensin-converting-enzyme inhibition (ACE-I) and/or angiotensin-receptor-blocking (ARB) agents, statins, and other lipid-lowering agents) for such patients, *a useful consideration is symptoms and/or ischemia, which persist after optimal medical therapy or "medically refractory."* Optimal medical therapy assumes risk factor modification, as well as the five categories of medications that have been shown to improve prognosis, and the categories shown to relieve angina (nitrates, calcium blockers, and β-blockers, plus the recently released metabolic agents).

The author opines that *the most common and best indication for revascularization among stable patients is* relief of medically refractory symptoms and/or ischemia. Both PCI and CABG effectively relieve symptoms and/or ischemia, but they have different strengths (particularly with regard to both completeness of relief of ischemia and durability of results) and weaknesses (primarily risks). The choice between CABG and PCI comes down to individual differences in both clinical and anatomic variables that impact both the utility and risks of the two methods. For example, because many chronic occlusions cannot be crossed with a wire, balloon, and/or stent, the presence of one or more potentially graftable, but likely uncrossable occlusions supplying important segments of myocardium, mitigate for CABG and against PCI. Conversely, the more emergent the need for revascularization (STEMI, hemodynamic, or electrical instability), the more PCI is favored. Many of the clinical risk factors for adverse outcome that favor consideration of PCI fall under the general heading of comorbidity, particularly severe neurologic or cerebrovascular, pulmonary, or hepatic comorbidities, which increase the risks of general anesthesia, heart-lung bypass, mechanical ventilation, and other supports needed to make CABG possible.

Both CABG and PCI have evolved. In the early days of balloon-only angioplasty (known affectionately as "plain-old balloon angioplasty" or POBA), a number of anatomic configurations were associated with both reduced likelihood of technical success (and attendant relief of ischemia), and increased likelihood of acute complications such as MI and/or emergent CABG, or even death. The combination of bare-metal stents (BMS) and dual-antiplatelet therapies were accompanied by increased acute success and reduced complications in many of these settings (in addition to the more highly emphasized effects on restenosis and long-term durability of results). It has appeared that these acute trends may be advancing still further with contemporary drug-eluting stents (DES); again, in addition to the benefit of reduced restenosis. *The point is that many anatomic considerations that were paramount in excluding POBA from consideration, such as small caliber, diffuse disease, major side branch, ostial lesions, saphenous vein-graft lesions with friable appearance or short total occlusions, are considerably less exclusive now.* For patients with medically refractory ischemia and clinical risk factors for adverse outcome with CABG, the decision between CABG and PCI can be considerably more dynamic. It is best made with appropriate input from both interventional cardiologists and surgeons working with patients and their families and advocates. To make the trip from trials and series to Guidelines to Board exams, and finally to individual patients requires integrating one's own experience with the specific anatomy (e.g., bifurcation disease with a large side-branch) and the specific clinical characteristics (e.g.,

limiting, stable angina with a large sestamibi defect in a patient with prior cerebrovascular accident [CVA] or "porcelain" aorta).

CASE #1 (FOR QUESTIONS 1–10): A 66-year-old man with exertional angina, is transferred to your institution for cardiac catheterization. His past medical history includes an MI and subsequent catheterization and three-vessel CABG, 9 years ago. He is currently taking aspirin and clopidogrel, Losartan and Diltiazem for hypertension, and simvastatin for hyperlipidemia. He is known to be less than perfectly compliant with his medical regimen, and he continues to smoke, despite multiple caregiver remonstrances. He has normal left ventricular systolic function by a recent echocardiogram, and his creatinine is chronically elevated in the range of 1.7 to 2.2 mg per dL. Although he gives no history of neurologic problems, a recent carotid Doppler study demonstrated bilateral high-grade internal carotid stenoses (80% to 99%). A recent sestamibi was interpreted as "multiple reversible defects over anterior and lateral walls suggestive of multivessel coronary artery disease (CAD)."

After vigorous prehydration with normal saline and bicarbonate, diagnostic angiography was performed with a total of 80 mL of x-ray contrast. The following findings were obtained:

■ Left internal mammary to left anterior descending (LAD) was widely patent with good anastomosis and good flow; there was approximately 70% eccentric stenosis of the native LAD shortly after insertion of the left internal mammary artery (LIMA) (see following figure).

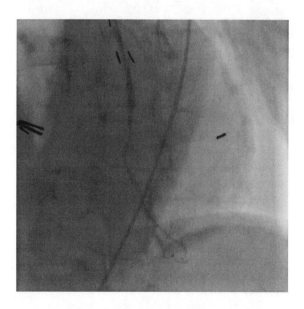

■ Saphenous vein graft (SVG) to the posterior descending was patent with a good distal anastomosis and good flow; the native vessel was <2.0 mm with additional discrete high-grade stenosis downstream from graft insertion (see following figure).

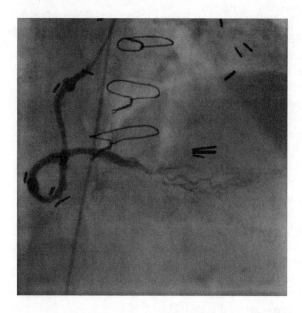

■ SVG to obtuse marginal was shaggy and irregular with angiographic suggestion of thrombus; there were both high grade lesions in the body of the SVG, and at the distal anastomosis; the native vessel was also small caliber (see following figure).

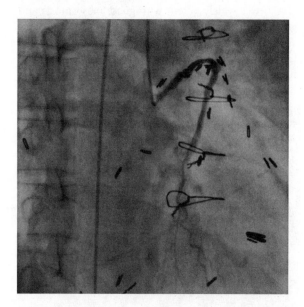

1 What clinical and anatomic features weigh against a reoperation (repeat CABG) in this patient?

(A) Patent internal mammary graft to the LAD artery
(B) Three patent grafts
(C) Bilateral severe carotid vascular disease
(D) Chronic renal insufficiency

(E) Risk of second CABG is approximately 3X higher than first CABG
(F) All of the above

2 What clinical and anatomic features weigh against PCI for this patient?

(A) Noncompliance causes concern for the use of dual antiplatelet therapy, if patient were to receive DES
(B) Noncompliance with statins and antihypertensive agents increases likelihood of adverse outcomes after PCI
(C) Chronic renal insufficiency increases risk of bleeding and restenosis
(D) Multivessel disease increases likely dye load (and attendant contrast-associated nephropathy) and restenosis likelihood
(E) SVG disease is associated with decreased likelihood of procedural success and increased likelihood of distal embolization with attendant morbidity and/or mortality
(F) All of the above

3 How soon is the creatinine likely to peak from the development of contrast-associated nephropathy?

(A) 1 day
(B) 2 days
(C) 3 days
(D) 5 days
(E) 1 week

4 Which of the following are established means (supported by one or more randomized trials) of reducing the likelihood of contrast-associated nephropathy?

(A) Hydration with normal saline
(B) Keeping contrast dose to a minimum (<125 mL)
(C) Fenoldopam
(D) N-acetyl cysteine
(E) Dopamine infusion in "renal perfusion" dose (<5 mics/kg/min)
(F) A and B
(G) A and D

5 With regard to PCI of the native LAD lesion in this patient, which of the following concepts is usually correct?

(A) PCI through the native LAD (were it possible) would be less likely to injure the internal mammary
(B) PCI of the distal LIMA-LAD anastomosis is one of the few anatomic settings where stents have *not* been shown to reduce restenosis

(C) Straightening of the LIMA with a PCI wire can produce pseudolesions

(D) With a regular length LIMA guide and a long internal mammary vessel, it is possible to "run out of catheter length" when trying to treat native LAD lesions

(E) All are correct

6 With regard to PCI of the SVG-obtuse marginal (OM) artery in this patient, which of the following concepts is likely to be correct?

(A) There is debate as to whether glycoprotein IIb/IIIa inhibitors will reduce the likelihood of distal embolization in this type of lesion

(B) RCT data supports the use of "distal protection" in old (>3 years) SVG lesions, "where technically feasible"

(C) The Transluminal Extraction Catheter (TEC) has been shown to reduce adverse events in this kind of lesion

(D) Thrombectomy devices have been shown to be superior to balloon angioplasty in SVG lesions

(E) Stents have been shown to be superior to balloon angioplasty in SVG lesions

(F) A, C, and E

(G) A, B, and E

7 With regard to PCI of the SVG-PDA in this patient, which of the following is likely to be correct?

(A) The posterior descending artery (PDA) is too small for even the smallest BMS

(B) This is not likely the source of anterior or lateral ischemia

(C) There is no "landing zone" for distal protection

(D) All are correct

8 What is the most evidence-based approach for this patient?

(A) Smoking cessation clinic, if he will go

(B) Repeat CABG

(C) PCI of the SVG-PDA and SVG-OM, with Percusurge Guardwire

(D) Optimize doses of β-blocker, ACE-I, and statins

(E) A and D

9 If you choose to call this Class II angina, refractory to medical management (which assumes patient compliance), what does the ACC/AHA/SCAI update to the PCI Guideline recommend at the Class I level (is recommended/should do)?

(A) PCI is reasonable in patients with CCS Class I or II angina with one or more significant lesions in one or two coronary arteries suitable for PCI with a high likelihood of success and a low risk of failure, morbidity, and mortality. The vessels to be dilated must subtend a moderate to large area of viable myocardium or be associated with moderate to severe ischemia

(B) PCI is reasonable for patients with CCS Class I or II angina, and recurrent stenosis after PCI with a large area of viable myocardium or high-risk criteria on noninvasive testing

(C) Use of PCI is reasonable for patients with CCS Class I and II angina and significant (>50%) left main stenosis who are candidates for revascularization but are not candidates for CABG

(D) None of the above

10 If you choose to call this Class II angina, refractory to medical management (which assumes patient compliance), what does the ACC/AHA/SCAI update to the PCI Guideline recommend at the Class III level (is not recommended/should not do)?

(A) Only a small area of viable myocardium at risk

(B) No objective evidence of ischemia

(C) Lesions that have a low likelihood of successful dilatation

(D) Mild symptoms that are unlikely to be related to myocardial ischemia

(E) Factors associated with increased morbidity or mortality

(F) Left main disease and eligibility for CABG

(G) Insignificant disease (<50% stenosis)

(H) All of the above

CASE #2 (FOR QUESTIONS 11–16): A 58-year-old man is referred for catheterization and likely revascularization. Three years ago, you performed right coronary artery stenting to treat an acute inferior/STEMI in this patient and he has subsequently done well on a medical regimen that included aspirin, metoprolol, and simvastatin; he does not smoke. After 3 days of severe chest pain he reported to his local hospital and was found to have anterior ST-segment elevation and positive troponins. Because >24 hours had passed from onset of symptoms he was given heparin, intravenous nitroglycerin, and eptifibatide, and because of continued pain he was transferred emergently. He is now pain free >4 days out; he is hemodynamically stable (normal sinus rhythm in the low 70s with blood pressure of 120/78 and respiratory rate of 18 and unlabored with 98% arterial saturation on 2 L, and has clear lung fields without jugular venous distension).

On angiography you demonstrate that his dominant right coronary artery is free of significant (>50%) narrowing and specifically that the proximal

BMS looks, in your words, "exquisite." The left main is smooth and not narrowed, but the proximal LAD has approximately 95% stenosis and appears to be approximately 2.0 mm; a significant diagonal branch follows the stenosis (see following figure). There is a large, tortuous ramus intermedius branch with approximately 70% discrete stenosis and a diminutive circumflex artery.

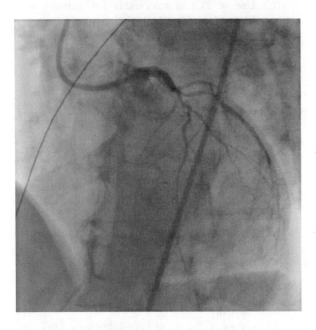

11 This patient presented as an STEMI who did not receive reperfusion (because of presentation >24 hours after pain onset). Which of the following are ACC/AHA/SCAI Class I indications (ought to) for PCI of post-STEMI patients who did not receive thrombolytics?

(A) Recurrent MI
(B) Spontaneous or provocable myocardial ischemia
(C) Cardiogenic shock or hemodynamic instability
(D) All of the above

12 The criteria for considering a patient's symptoms as "medically refractory" are continued symptoms and ischemia despite which of the following:

(A) Aspirin, unless contraindicated
(B) Clopidogrel, unless contraindicated
(C) β-Blocker in all post-MI and patients with congestive heart failure (CHF), unless contraindicated, and to blood pressure and heart rate targets
(D) ACE-I in all patients with left ventricular (LV) dysfunction, unless contraindicated, and to blood pressure targets

(E) Statins, unless contraindicated
(F) All of the above

13 This LAD lesion involves the takeoff of a diagonal branch. What are the two broad categories of approach to bifurcation lesions with stents? (And, what is the main caveat of one approach?)

14 What criteria favor attempting to stent only the main branch (mother)?

(A) Small caliber of daughter branch (<2.0 mm)
(B) Small territory of daughter (would not graft if sent for CABG)
(C) Extremely angulated takeoff of daughter
(D) All of the above

15 What types of two-vessel stenting have been used with DES for bifurcation lesions?

(A) V stenting
(B) Culotte stenting
(C) Y stenting
(D) T stenting
(E) Double-barrel stenting
(F) Crush stenting
(G) Reverse crush stenting
(H) All of the above

16 In the contemporary lesion risk classification, what feature of bifurcation lesions makes some of them high-risk?

CASE #3 (FOR 17–26): A 79-year-old man is transferred to your facility because of worsening exertional angina. His electrocardiogram (EKG) shows mild ST-depression and serial troponins were normal. He has a history of remote MI, hypertension, hyperlipidemia, and atrial fibrillation. Despite a regimen including aspirin, atenolol, isosorbide, statin, and lisinopril, he has chest pain at minimal activity. His resting heart rate is 60 beats per minute and blood pressure is 120/80.

Cardiac catheterization (see following figure) revealed a short left main with significant narrowing; ostial LAD stenosis >95% with a good downstream vessel, which wraps around apex and distal third of inferior wall; a large ramus branch that is unobstructed; a proximal, short (<20 mm) occlusion of the circumflex with left-to-left filling of a large obtuse marginal and distal circumflex branches; long chronic occlusion of mid right coronary with filling of posterolateral branch by left-to-right collaterals; and left ventricular ejection fraction (LVEF) approximately 0.40 by recent echocardiogram.

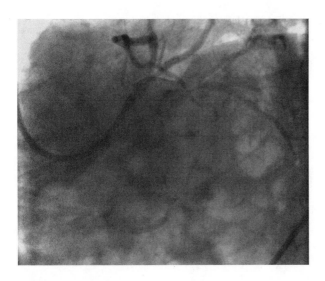

17 Relief of ischemia can be expected from which of the following (assuming technically successful):

(A) CABG
(B) Increased medical therapy
(C) PCI
(D) CABG or PCI
(E) Enhanced external counterpulsation (EECP)

18 Three-vessel coronary disease including ostial location of LAD stenosis favor CABG, but this elderly patient has a calcified ascending aorta, and serious concerns regarding adverse cerebral outcomes. Which of the following are risk factors for CABG associated CVA?

(A) UA
(B) Use of intra-aortic balloon counterpulsation
(C) Diabetes
(D) Known neurologic disease
(E) Proximal aortic atherosclerosis
(F) All of the above

19 Which risk factor is most important regarding post-CABG CVA (highest risk of peri-operative CVA)?

(A) UA
(B) Use of intra-aortic balloon counterpulsation
(C) Diabetes
(D) Known neurologic disease
(E) Proximal aortic atherosclerosis
(F) All of the above

20 What is the major pathophysiologic mechanism for post-CABG adverse cerebral outcomes?

(A) Nonpulsatile flow with cardiopulmonary bypass
(B) Carotid embolization
(C) Aortic embolization

21 In addition to the previously mentioned CVA risk factors, which of the following are associated with increased risk of CABG associated encephalopathy?

(A) Alcohol consumption
(B) Atrial fibrillation
(C) Hypertension
(D) Prior CABG
(E) Peripheral vascular disease
(F) CHF
(G) All of the above

22 If you decide to proceed with PCI in this patient, which artery is most likely to be responsible for this patient's symptoms? Or to put it another way, which artery can you least afford to leave alone if your objective is to relieve the patient's symptoms?

(A) LAD artery
(B) Ramus intermedius artery
(C) OM after the circumflex occlusion
(D) PDA

23 An acute occlusive syndrome of which artery is least likely to be tolerated without hemodynamic compromise?

(A) LAD artery
(B) Ramus intermedius artery
(C) OM after the circumflex occlusion
(D) PDA

24 What is the most important technical issue involved in treating the ostial LAD artery of this patient using PCI?

(A) Correct sizing of stent (neither over nor under)
(B) Guide catheter support or backup
(C) Guide wire stiffness
(D) Proper positioning of stent
(E) A and D
(F) All of above

25 In addition to choosing two or more close to orthogonal views which demonstrate the relationships of left main, LAD ostium, ramus ostium, and circumflex ostium, what else can you do to assess proper stent size and positioning?

(A) Intravascular ultrasound (IVUS)
(B) Flow wire
(C) Virtual histology with Volcano system
(D) 64 slice computed tomography (CT)

26 Which angiographic views are most likely to help assess the left main, LAD, and circumflex anatomic relationships?

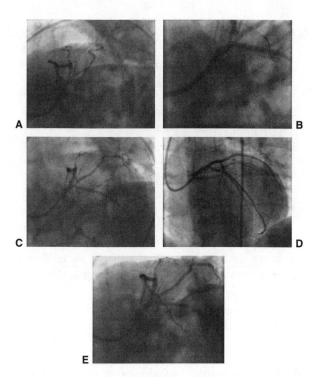

(A) Straight Anteroposterior (AP)
(B) LAO caudal
(C) Left lateral
(D) RAO cranial
(E) AP caudal
(F) A, B, and E
(G) A and C

27 Which of the following established medical therapies were used in the majority of patients in the three medical therapy versus CABG trials among patients with stable angina, and the two medical therapy versus CABG trials among patients with UA (VA Cooperative; National Heart, Lung, and Blood Institute [NHLBI])?

(A) Statins
(B) Aspirin
(C) ACE-I
(D) ARB
(E) Fibrates
(F) Clopidogrel
(G) None of the above

28 Patients with ischemic cardiomyopathy (defined in terms of LVEF <0.30) were excluded from all of the following trials, *except*:

(A) CASS
(B) BARI
(C) PAMI

(D) SIRIUS
(E) ARTS I

29 What proportion of screened patients was finally enrolled in the following trials of CABG versus PTCA: BARI, CABRI, EAST, GABI, ERACI I, and RITA?

(A) >75%
(B) >25%
(C) <10%

30 Diabetic patients with three-vessel CAD have been shown to have better long-term survival with CABG than balloon-only PTCA in which of the following prospective RCTs?

(A) BARI
(B) GABI
(C) ERACI
(D) EAST
(E) RITA
(F) BARI and EAST
(G) All of the above

31 In prospective RCT and/or meta-analyses, BMS (compared with PTCA) have been associated with statistically significant reductions in which of the following adverse outcomes?

(A) Survival
(B) MI
(C) Target-vessel revascularization (TVR)
(D) Major adverse cardiac outcomes (MACE)
(E) Survival + MI
(F) Both C and D

32 In prospective RCT and/or meta-analyses, DES (compared with BMS) have been associated with statistically significant reductions in which of the following adverse outcomes?

(A) Survival
(B) MI
(C) TVR
(D) MACE
(E) Survival + MI
(F) Both C and D

33 Risk factors for post-CABG mediastinitis include all of the following, *except*:

(A) Prior CABG
(B) Obesity
(C) Diabetes
(D) Use of bilateral internal thoracic arteries
(E) Antibiotic selection by cardiothoracic surgeons

34 Risk factors for post-CABG dialysis include all of the following, *except*:

(A) Advanced age
(B) History of CHF
(C) Prior CABG
(D) Renal disease
(E) Type 1 diabetes
(F) Number of major coronary arteries with >70% stenosis

35 Risk factors for contrast-associated nephropathy after PCI include all of the following, *except*:

(A) Total dye dose from procedure
(B) Multiple dye procedures within 1 week
(C) Diabetes
(D) Elevated creatinine before catheterization
(E) Number of coronary arteries with >70% stenosis

Answers and Explanations

1 **Answer F.** Both a patent LIMA and three patent grafts (to each major vascular territory: anterior, lateral, and inferior) reduce the potential benefit of a reoperation. The CABG Guideline lists the effect of reoperation in terms of operative mortality as threefold. Renal disease and cerebrovascular disease are risk factors for CABG mortality and cerebrovascular disease is an additional risk for cerebral morbidity with CABG (*Ann Thorac Surg.* 1994;57:27–32, *J Am Coll Cardiol.* 1996;28:1478–1487, *N Engl J Med.* 1996;335:1857–1863).

2 **Answer F.** A number of trials, notably intercoronary stenting and antithrombotic results (ISAR) and stent antithrombotic regimen study (STARS), demonstrated the superiority of dual antiplatelet therapy over aspirin alone or Coumadin as adjuncts to stenting. Failure to continue taking antiplatelet therapy is potentially a greater problem with DES, which inhibit endothelialization. In addition to the wealth of data showing hard outcome clinical benefits in patients with CAD with lipid-lowering and hypertension control, specific evaluation of post-PCI patients, as in the LIPS trial of statins, demonstrate the importance of ongoing medical management. Chronic renal insufficiency is a PCI risk factor for multiple reasons, including both increased bleeding diathesis and increased restenosis. SVG intervention is associated with increased risk of distal embolization, which is part of the rationale for "distal protection," and not necessarily ameliorated by glycoprotein IIb/IIIa inhibitors (PCI Guideline Table 10 and Section 3.5.6) (*Circulation.* 2001;103:1967–1971, *N Engl J Med.* 1998;339:1665–1671, *Am J Med.* 2000; 108:127–135, *J Am Coll Cardiol.* 2004;44:1393–1399, *J Am Coll Cardiol.* 2005;45:947–953, *N Engl J Med.* 1996;334:1084–1089, *Circulation.* 2003;108: 548–553).

3 **Answer D.** (*J Am Coll Cardiol.* 2002;39:1113–1119, *Circulation.* 2002;105:2259–2264, *Ann Intern Med.* 1986;104:501–504).

4 **Answer F.** (*Ann Intern Med.* 2003;139:123–136, *J Am Coll Cardiol.* 2004;44:1763–1771).

5 **Answer E.** (*J Am Coll Cardiol.* 2000;35:944–948).

6 **Answer G.** (*Circulation.* 2002;105:1285–1290, *Circulation.* 2002;106:3063–3067, *Circulation.* 2003;108: 548–553).

7 **Answer D.** (*Am J Med.* 2000;108:176–177).

8 **Answer E.** There is no RCT data to support survival benefit or MI reduction from either repeat CABG or PCI in a patient who has already had one or more CABG. PCI of both the SVGs to the circumflex and right coronary artery territories are unlikely to relieve the ischemia documented in the anterior distribution; accordingly, any PCI strategy should likely include the LAD artery stenosis. There is survival benefit data from RCTs of statins, beta-blockers, ACE-I, and smoking cessation (*Lancet.* 2002;360:7–22, *N Engl J Med.* 1998;339:1349–1357).

9 **Answer D.** A, B, and C are all Guideline Class II (maybe/maybe not) from section 5.1 patients with asymptomatic ischemia or CCS Class I or II angina. There are no Class I recommendations for PCI for patients with asymptomatic ischemia or CCS Class I or II angina. If that seems surprising, review the trials of medical therapy versus PCI, among patients with stable symptoms (*Lancet.* 1997;350:461–468, *Circulation.* 1997;95:2037–2043, *N Engl J Med.* 1992;326:10–16, *N Engl J Med.* 1999;341:70–76).

10 **Answer H.** All of these are Class III (should not) recommendations from the Guidelines, section 5.1 patients with asymptomatic ischemia or CCS Class I or II angina.

11 **Answer D.**

12 **Answer F.** (*BMJ.* 1994;308:81–106, *Circulation.* 1998;97:946–952, *Circulation.* 1998;97:2202–2212, *Prog Cardiovasc Dis.* 1985;27:335–371, *JAMA.* 1988; 260:2259–2263).

13 **Answer.** Single stent (main branch only) versus double stent ("mother and daughter"). The main caveat of the 2-stent approach to bifurcations is that all bifurcation stenting should be followed by "kissing balloon angioplasty" (*Catheter Cardiovasc Interv.* 2004;63:337–338, *Circulation.* 2004;109:1244–1249, *Am Heart J.* 2004;148:857–864, *J Am Coll Cardiol.* 2000;35:1145–1151).

14 Answer D. (*Eur Heart J.* 2004;25:895–897, *Catheter Cardiovasc Interv.* 2002;55:50–57).

15 Answer H. All of the above are correct. "Does one really need to know all of these techniques for either Boards or practice?" Perhaps not, but one does have to have a method that is likely to yield both good short-term and long-term results in patients with a large side branch, or else this becomes a reason to refer for CABG (*Am J Cardiol.* 1998;82:1418–1421, A8, *Am J Cardiol.* 1998;82:943–949, *Catheter Cardiovasc Interv.* 2003;60:145–151) (see also *Catheter Cardiovasc Interv.* 1997;41:197–199, *Catheter Cardiovasc Interv.* 1993;30:327–330, *Catheter Cardiovasc Interv.* 1996;39:320–326).

16 Answer. The inability to protect a large side-branch is one reason to consider the CABG and medical therapy alternatives (*J Interv Cardiol.* 2003;16:507–513, *Catheter Cardiovasc Interv.* 2000;50:411–412).

17 Answer D. Documentation that EECP relieves ischemia is lacking and patient is at limits of medical therapy. Both updated guidelines provide documentation of objective relief of ischemia with CABG and/or PCI (*Lancet.* 1995;346:1184–1189, *Circulation.* 1980;62:653–656).

18 Answer F. (*Am J Cardiol.* 1995;75:3C–8C).

19 Answer E. Proximal aortic atherosclerosis (*J Vasc Surg.* 1995;21:98–107; discussion 108–9, *Ann Thorac Surg.* 1985;40:574–581, *J Card Surg.* 1994;9:490–494, *N Engl J Med.* 1996;335:1857–1863).

20 Answer C. Aortic embolization (*Curr Opin Cardiol.* 1994;9:670–679, *JAMA.* 2002;287:1405–1412).

21 Answer G. (*ACC/AHA 2004 Guideline Update.* 2004).

22 Answer A. The LAD is the largest territory and provides collaterals to the OM and PDA!

23 Answer D. The LAD supplies the largest territory and currently has thrombolysis in myocardial infarction (TIMI) 3 flow, despite the high-grade lesion. The OM and PDA fill through collaterals, having al-ready been occluded; occlusions can be made worse if partially opened, but not if left alone.

24 Answer E. Over-sizing balloon or stent is associated with the higher likelihood of dissecting downstream LAD or worse, left main; under-sizing would increase risks of stent thrombosis and/or restenosis of vessel, which the patient cannot afford to lose; similarly missing the ostium with stent would increase risks of thrombosis and/or restenosis, and hanging stent out in left main would increase risks of thrombosis. The key to proper positioning of the stent is *being able to see*; that is, multiple well-selected views to open up pathology of interest.

25 Answer A. IVUS

26 Answer F.

27 Answer G. (*Circulation.* 1983;68:939–950, *N Engl J Med.* 1984;311:1333–1339, *N Engl J Med.* 1987;316:977–984, *Am J Cardiol.* 1976;37:896–902, *N Engl J Med.* 1988;319:332–337).

28 Answer C. Only trials of STEMI have routinely included patients regardless of some lower limit of left ventricular systolic function (*Circulation.* 1983;68:939–950, *N Engl J Med.* 1993;328:673–679, *N Engl J Med.* 2003;349:1315–1323, *N Engl J Med.* 2001;344:1117–1124) (BARI investigators *Circulation.* 1991;84:Suppl V:1–27).

29 Answer C. (*Lancet.* 1993;341:573–580, *Lancet.* 1995;346:1179–1184, *N Engl J Med.* 1994;331:1037–1043, *N Engl J Med.* 1994;331:1044–1050, *J Am Coll Cardiol.* 1993;22:1060–1067, *Am J Card.* 1995;75:1c–59c).

30 Answer F. (*Am J Cardiol.* 1995;75:3C–8C, *Lancet.* 1993;341:573–580, *Lancet.* 1995;346:1179–1184, *N Engl J Med.* 1994;331:1037–1043, *N Engl J Med.* 1994;331:1044–1050, *J Am Coll Cardiol.* 1993;22:1060–1067).

31 Answer F. (*N Engl J Med.* 1994;331:496–501, *N Engl J Med.* 1994;331:489–495).

32 Answer F. (*Lancet.* 2004;364:583–591, *N Engl J Med.* 2002;346:1773–1780, *N Engl J Med.* 2003;349:1315–1323, *N Engl J Med.* 2004;350:221–231).

33 Answer E. Antibiotic use with CABG has never been subjected to RCT, and likely never will (*Ann Thorac Surg.* 1990;49:179–186; discussion 186–7,

Ann Thorac Surg. 1987;44:173–179, *J Thorac Cardiovasc Surg.* 1996;111:1200–1207).

34 **Answer F.** (*Am J Med.* 1998;104:343–348, *Ann Intern Med.* 1998;128:194–203, *J Card Surg.* 1996;11:128–133; discussion 134–5).

35 **Answer E.** (*N Engl J Med.* 2003;348:491–499, *Lancet.* 2003;362:598–603, *J Am Coll Cardiol.* 2004;44:1763–1771, *N Engl J Med.* 1989;320:143–149, *N Engl J Med.* 1994;331:1416–1420, *Ann Intern Med.* 1986;104:501–504).

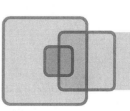

10

Percutaneous Coronary Intervention for Acute Coronary Syndromes

Christopher Walters and Steven R. Steinhubl

Questions

1 A 62-year-old man presents to the emergency room (ER) with complaints of newly onset waxing and waning chest pain over the past 4 hours. His initial electrocardiogram EKG is shown in the following figure. In deciding whether to initiate treatment with a glycoprotein IIb/IIIa receptor antagonist (and if so which agent to use) all of the following should influence your decision, *except*:

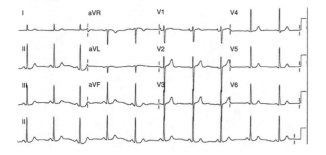

(A) Plans for a conservative or invasive management approach and the timing of any potential invasive approach

(B) Whether the patient has already received 600 mg of clopidogrel from the ER physician

(C) In the setting of a percutaneous coronary intervention (PCI), head-to-head trials have found all three available agents (abciximab, eptifibatide, and tirofiban) to be equally efficacious in decreasing peri-PCI thrombotic events

(D) Troponin status

2 For a patient presenting to the catheterization laboratory in the setting of a recent acute coronary syndrome, which of the following is *false* regarding the use of aspirin therapy?

(A) To minimize the risk of gastric bleeding, an enteric-coated aspirin should be used long-term

(B) Chewing 160 mg to 325 mg leads to complete antiplatelet effects within 15 to 20 minutes

(C) In placebo-controlled trials in acute coronary and PCI, aspirin decreases death and myocardial infarction (MI) rates by approximately 50%

(D) Patients who have aspirin allergy or intolerance should receive clopidogrel

3 An 87-year-old woman is transferred to your facility for catheterization and possible PCI after presenting with chest pain with ST-segment depressions and an elevated troponin level. Her creatinine level is 1.9 mg/dL and she weighs 58 kg. The patient is started on aspirin, 600 mg clopidogrel, enoxaparin, and eptifibatide. All of the following are independently associated with an increased risk of major bleeding, *except*:

(A) Renal dysfunction

(B) Female gender

(C) Previous coronary artery bypass graft (CABG)

(D) Advanced age

4 Which of the following is *true* regarding the use of clopidogrel in a patient presenting with acute coronary syndromes (ACSs)?

(A) A loading dose of at least 300 mg should be used

(B) Clinical outcomes in patients treated with clopidogrel are significantly worse in the setting of concomitant atorvastatin

(C) Doubling the loading dose and maintenance dose of clopidogrel has been shown to be more effective than standard therapy in high-risk patients

(D) A loading dose of clopidogrel is efficacious regardless of the time of dosing as long as it is before the percutaneous intervention

5 A 48-year-old man was admitted the previous day with a troponin-positive non–ST-segment elevation ACS and was started on enoxaparin 1 mg per kg subcutaneously. The patient is now in the catheterization laboratory preparing for coronary angiography and possible intervention. His last subcutaneous dose of enoxaparin was documented to have been given 5 hours earlier. Optimizing antithrombotic therapy in the setting of a possible PCI for this patient would require:

(A) Additional intravenous enoxaparin of 0.3 mg per kg

(B) 50 to 70 units per kilogram of unfractionated heparin (UFH) titrated to an ACT of >200 if a GPIIb/IIIa inhibitor is being used, and to an ACT of 300 if no GPIIb/IIIa inhibitor is planned

(C) No additional anticoagulant is necessary

(D) Further use of additional anticoagulant is based on whether a GPIIb/IIIa inhibitor is to be used

6 The Folts model was developed as a method to study thrombosis in the setting of a stenosed artery with endothelial damage, and therefore has been used as a means to study various therapeutic interventions to minimize thrombotic complications in the setting of an ACS or PCI. Key aspects of the Folts model include all of the following, *except*:

(A) A flow probe placed on the artery to measure cyclic flow reductions (CFRs)

(B) The ability to vary the severity of the arterial stenosis

(C) The inability of weaker antiplatelet agents such as aspirin to influence thrombosis in this model

(D) The ability to collect the coronary thrombus for histologic study

7 A 56-year-old diabetic woman is transferred directly to your catheterization laboratory in the setting of an anterior ST-segment elevation myocardial infarction (STEMI) treated with fibrinolytic therapy at an outside hospital. She has also been treated with aspirin, UFH, and 600 mg clopidogrel. Her ST segments have normalized, and she is pain free and hemodynamically stable. By the time you arrive the coronary angiography has already been completed by your partner and demonstrates the following:

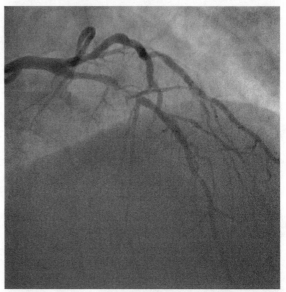

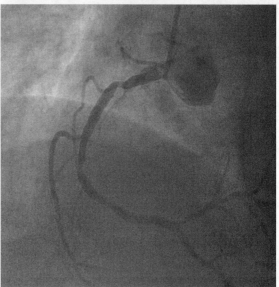

The optimal treatment approach to this patient would be:

(A) PCI with stenting of the left anterior descending (LAD) only

(B) PCI with stenting of the LAD and likely clinically significant right coronary artery (RCA) lesions

(C) Cardiothoracic surgery consults for urgent CABG surgery for this diabetic patient with multivessel disease

(D) Medical stabilization with plans to risk stratify before discharge

8 A 48-year-old man presents to your emergency department with substernal chest pain of 8 hours' duration. Despite increasing chest pain, the patient worked all day trying to ignore his discomfort. However, the pain increased while he was driving home, and he drove himself to the hospital. Initial EKG demonstrates normal sinus rhythm with ≤1 mm inferolateral ST-segment depression with evidence of left ventricular hypertrophy. The patient is administered sublingual nitroglycerin, a single dose of intravenous morphine and metoprolol, and oxygen by nasal canula. His pain slowly resolves. Initial cardiac enzymes are negative. Follow-up EKG shows resolution of the prior ST-segment depression. What is the best way to proceed with this patient at this point?

(A) Observe the patient in your chest pain unit, give the patient a proton pump inhibitor, and have the patient follow up with his phencyclidine (PCP) as long as you rule out MI, and the patient has no further chest pain

(B) Admit the patient to telemetry for medical treatment only, proceeding only to angiography if his chest pain recurs or enzymes become positive

(C) Admit the patient with plans to proceed to angiography only if he has a high-risk noninvasive evaluation

(D) Plan on proceeding to cardiac catheterization regardless of recurrence of chest pain, cardiac enzymes, or EKG changes

9 You are called to evaluate a 68-year-old man who presents with 2 hours of crushing substernal chest pain. Initial EKG shows 4-mm anterior ST-segment elevations consistent with acute anterior STEMI. Within 45 minutes of presentation, coronary angiography reveals a totally occluded mid-LAD with a long segment of apparent thrombus after the first septal perforator. The patient is hemodynamically stable. Because of the large thrombus burden, you consider whether rheolytic thrombectomy may

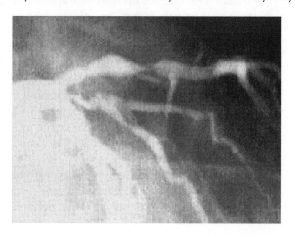

be beneficial in this patient. The patient's initial angiogram is shown in the following figure. Which of the following is *true* regarding thrombectomy in this setting?

(A) Thrombectomy in the setting of a large thrombus burden in anterior STEMI has been shown to improve the postprocedural TIMI flow rates in the infarct-related artery

(B) Overall major adverse cardiac events (MACE) rates are lower in the patients undergoing thrombectomy before definitive therapy in patients with inferior STEMI only

(C) Infarct size and mortality might be expected to be increased in patients undergoing thrombectomy before definitive therapy in patients with large anterior STEMI

(D) Thrombectomy in this setting only reduces the future incidence of target lesion revascularization

10 A 52-year-old man presents with a 2-week history of increasing exertional chest pain. His past medical history is significant for a 35-year history of ongoing tobacco use, hypertension, and "diet-controlled" diabetes mellitus. He undergoes coronary angiography followed by stenting of a circumflex stenosis. His postintervention course is unremarkable, and he is deemed ready for discharge 36 hours after his presentation. Secondary prevention goals for this patient include all of the following, *except*:

(A) Start drug therapy if blood pressure (BP) is >130/80 mm Hg

(B) Start β-blocker therapy if there are no specific contraindications before discharge

(C) Fasting lipid profiles should be delayed for >48 hours after a patient presents with an ACS (unstable angina [UA]/non–ST-elevation myocardial infarction [NSTEMI])

(D) Calculate body mass index (BMI) and encourage diet and exercise to achieve a BMI <30 kg per m²

11 A 68-year-old woman is sent to you for evaluation of chest pain. She is generally healthy, and has no history of hypertension, hyperlipidemia, or diabetes. She is a lifelong nonsmoker. She reports that over the last several months she has experienced chest pressure associated with exposure to cold, emotional stress, or briskly walking up inclines or stairs. She has undergone stress echocardiography, showing no discrete areas of stress-induced wall motion abnormalities after walking 8 minutes on Bruce protocol, with mild global hypokinesis of the left ventricle at rest. She is very concerned about her chest pain and wishes to have definitive coronary angiography performed. Catheterization reveals near normal coronary arteries angiographically, except for a discrete focal 50% stenosis in a posterolateral ventricular branch of a dominant RCA. What is the most appropriate course of action for this patient?

(A) Given the patient's concern, proceed with PCI to the focal lesion with a goal of improving her 5-year event-free survival from adverse cardiac events

(B) Proceed with PCI of the lesion with a goal of alleviating the patient's symptoms

(C) Do not proceed with PCI; rather repeat stress testing with nuclear scintigraphy for evaluation with a different modality

(D) Stop the diagnostic case with a goal of aggressive medical therapy as part of a comprehensive risk reduction strategy

12 A patient returns to your clinic for follow-up after you performed a PCI for single-vessel coronary artery disease (CAD) in the setting of an NSTEMI. He has done very well, and has had no evidence of recurrent angina or congestive heart failure (CHF). He is known to have normal left ventricular systolic function following the intervention. He asks about the benefit of future stress testing, and wonders if he should periodically have such a noninvasive evaluation performed. What should you tell him?

(A) Stress EKG is a simple and sensitive way to predict and identify the presence of restenosis following PCI

(B) All patients with documented CAD who undergo PCI should have yearly stress testing performed to evaluate functional capacity and to look for objective evidence of ischemia

(C) Stress testing in asymptomatic patients is indicated only for patients with high-risk features when trying to find objective evidence of ischemia

(D) Only the presence of recurrent symptoms justifies periodic stress testing in patients who have undergone PCI

13 A 72-year-old woman with known CAD presents to your office for routine follow-up. She underwent stenting for a focal RCA stenosis 5 months ago. Her BP is 145/85 and her pulse is 70 beats per minute. She is a known type 2 diabetic patient with a history of mild renal insufficiency. Today she complains of increasing frequency and severity of exertional substernal chest pain, Canadian Cardiovascular Society (CCS) Class II. Your preliminary diagnosis is UA perhaps related to in-stent restenosis of her previous stent. An early invasive strategy is a Class I indication in UA/NSTEMI patients who present with certain high-risk features. Which of the following characteristics places this patient in the high-risk group, thereby justifying the early invasive strategy?

(A) Age >70 years old

(B) History of diabetes

(C) BP >140/80

(D) Presence of renal insufficiency

(E) Recent PCI within the prior 6 months

14 Working in a rural underserved area, you see a 70-year-old man with no prior CAD who reports a 6-week history of increasing exertional chest pain and dyspnea. A stress echocardiogram is recommended. The patient walks 6 minutes on a Bruce protocol with mild chest pain and no EKG changes. The echo demonstrates focal anteroapical wall abnormality at peak exertion, with normal resting wall motion. With a diagnosis now of UA because of the recent onset of exertional angina and an abnormal finding on noninvasive ischemic evaluation, you suggest proceeding to cardiac catheterization and possible PCI. The local facility does not have on-site cardiac surgery, and the closest hospital with on-site surgery is 120 miles away. What is the most appropriate way to manage this patient?

(A) Proceed with catheterization, planning to proceed to PCI if indicated because you believe this would most likely be a lower risk coronary intervention if needed

(B) Proceed with catheterization, planning only to perform diagnostic coronary angiography

(C) Ask the patient whether he wants to proceed with PCI locally, knowing that there are potential increased risks

(D) Arrange for the procedure to be done at the nearest facility with on-site cardiac surgery

15 One of your long-term patients returns to see you in the clinic 1 month before his scheduled appointment because of chest pain at rest, and occasionally with exertion. He is known to have CAD and has had multiple PCIs in the past. In addition, he has been well-controlled medically from the standpoint of secondary prevention. His last catheterization was 1 year ago, demonstrating mild in-stent restenosis in a drug-eluting stent in a large diagonal branch. In your office his BP is 145/95 and pulse is 88. You advise repeat catheterization because of his history and the severity of his symptoms. Angiography reveals 40% to 50% in-stent restenosis of the diagonal stent, otherwise no hemodynamically significant disease is noted. A fractional flow reserve (FFR) performed across the lesion is 0.82. What is the most appropriate way to proceed with this patient?

(A) End the procedure and proceed with medical management to ensure the best possible control of risk factors, which may predispose the patient to ischemic chest pain

(B) End the procedure with plans for noninvasive nuclear stress testing in search of objective evidence of ischemia, which you suspect

(C) Given the severity of the patient's symptoms that you feel are highly suggestive of ischemia and without any other coronary culprit, proceed with PCI of the diagonal lesion

(D) Intravascular ultrasound (IVUS) the suspected lesion as you strongly suspect that the lesion is responsible for the patient's chest pain

16 You intend to perform an intervention on a complex left circumflex lesion in a 58-year-old man who presented 18 hours ago with a classic history of UA. His three sets of cardiac enzymes have been negative, and he has not had recurrence of his chest pain or dynamic EKG changes. You plan to use a glycoprotein IIb/IIIa inhibitor for the case. Which of the following

agents have been shown to be efficacious in reducing ischemic complications in patients with UA?

(A) Tirofiban
(B) Abciximab
(C) Eptifibatide
(D) All of the above

17 You are discharging a 68-year-old woman after having performed successful angioplasty and stenting (drug-eluting) 18 hours ago for UA. Which of the following is *correct* regarding long-term medical therapy plans upon discharge?

(A) Ticlopidine 250 mg orally twice daily in patients with aspirin allergies

(B) HMG Co-A reductase inhibitor and cardiac-prudent diet should be prescribed within 24 to 96 hours of admission in patients with LDL-C >100 mg per dL and should be continued on discharge

(C) Angiotensin-converting enzyme (ACE) inhibitor therapy for all patients if no specific contraindication is present

(D) Antihypertensive drug regimen sufficient to lower resting BP to <120/80 mm Hg as the goal

Answers and Explanations

1 Answer C. In the TARGET trial, abciximab was found to be superior to tirofiban in a PCI population with the greatest difference found in patients presenting with an ACS (*N Engl J Med.* 2001;344:1888–1894). There have been no head-to-head trials of eptifibatide versus the other agents. Abciximab is not recommended for use in a noninvasive approach or when a delayed (>24 hour) invasive approach is planned based on the GUSTO IV result that found no benefit of abciximab versus placebo in this population (*Lancet.* 2001;357:1915–1924). The addition of a Glycoprotein E IIb/IIIa antagonist to a 600 mg loading dose of clopidogrel was found to significantly reduce peri-PCI events compared with 600 mg loading dose of clopidogrel alone in the ISAR-REACT 2 trial, with the difference confined to troponin positive patients (*JAMA.* 2006;295:1531–1538). Finally, post hoc analysis of placebo-controlled trials of GPIIb/IIIa antagonists in ACS patients (CAPTURE, PRISM, and PARAGON-B) have consistently found a marked benefit for these agents in troponin positive patients, and no difference in outcomes compared with placebo in troponin negative patients (*N Engl J Med.* 1999;340:1623–1629, *Lancet.* 1999;354:1757–1762, *Circulation.* 2001;103:2891–2896).

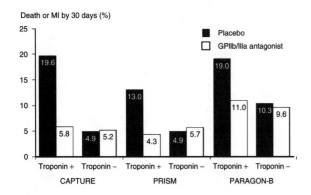

2 Answer A. Enteric-coating or buffered aspirin preparations do not appear to influence the risk of a major upper-gastrointestinal bleeding (*Lancet.* 1996;348:1413–1416). A wide range of aspirin doses, preparations, and methods of ingestion have been evaluated to determine the best way to achieve maximal antiplatelet activity in an acute setting. Chewing an aspirin or drinking solubilized aspirin (e.g., Alka-Seltzer) significantly shortens aspirin absorption and the onset of antiplatelet activity. A study

of 12 volunteers compared 325 mg of buffered aspirin, either chewed or swallowed, with Alka-Seltzer. Chewing the pill or drinking the solution resulted in maximal inhibition of serum TXB_2 production within 20 to 30 minutes of ingestion, whereas just swallowing the pill required approximately 60 minutes (*Am J Cardiol.* 1999;84:404–409.). In another study of 18 volunteers, chewing an 81 mg, 162 mg, or 324 mg aspirin pill led to equivalent reduction in TXB_2 production, but maximal inhibition within 15 minutes of ingestion was achieved only after the 162 mg and 324 mg doses (*Am J Cardiol.* 1994;74:720–723.) The results of these and other studies suggest that to achieve the maximal effects of aspirin rapidly (within approximately 15 minutes), at least 162 mg should be chewed and swallowed.

Four placebo-controlled trials found a consistent 50% or greater risk reduction in the combined endpoint of death or MI through the early initiation of aspirin therapy in patients with an NSTEMI ACS (*N Eng J Med.* 1983;309:396–403).

The American College of Cardiology (ACC)/ American Heart Association (AHA) guidelines recommend clopidogrel as an alternative to aspirin in all aspirin allergic or intolerant patients. (Available at: http://www.acc.org/clinical/guidelines/unstable/ unstable.pdf 2002).

3 Answer C. The best data evaluating the risk of in-hospital bleeding in an ACS population comes from an analysis of over 24,000 patients in the Global Registry of Acute Coronary Events (GRACE) (*Eur Heart J.* 2003;24:1815–1823). The analysis showed an incidence of major bleeding in 4.7% of the

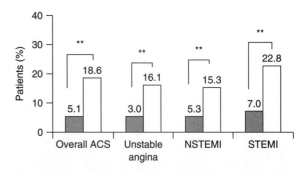

In-hospital Death Rates in Patients Who Developed (open bars) or Did Not Develop (closed bars) Major Bleeding (*J Am Coll Cardiol.* 2002;40:1531–1540.

NSTEMI population and identified four independent predictors of an increased risk of major bleeding: Advanced age, female gender, a history of bleeding, and renal insufficiency. As has been found in the subsequent studies, major bleeding was associated with a significant increase in mortality.

4 **Answer A.** The current ACC/AHA/ACS and PCI guidelines both recommend a 300 mg loading dose of clopidogrel, although the PCI guidelines suggest that a 600 mg loading dose can be considered. (Available at: http://www.acc.org/clinical/guidelines/unstable/unstable.pdf 2002, *Circulation.* 2006;113:e166–e286). Although some *ex vivo* studies have found that concomitant atorvastatin therapy influences the level of platelet function achieved with clopidogrel (some findings showed decreased platelet inhibition, others showed increased platelet inhibition), the bulk of the clinical data have found no clinically important interaction (*Circulation.* 2003;108:921–924). In the most recent PCI guidelines, a recommendation is made to consider doubling the maintenance dose of clopidogrel in high-risk patents if their measured inhibition of platelet aggregation is >50% (*Circulation.* 2006;113:e166–e286). At this time there are no clinical data to support the efficacy or safety of that recommendation. A 600 mg loading dose of clopidogrel has been shown to be equally efficacious if initiated 2 to 24 hours before the PCI (*J Am Coll Cardiol.* 2004;44:2133–2136), but for a 300 mg loading dose no benefit is found unless it is initiated >12 to 15 hours before the PCI (*J Am Coll Cardiol.* 2006;47:939–943).

5 **Answer C.** The pharmacokinetics of enoxaparin allow for what is generally considered to be therapeutic levels of anti-Xa activity within 30 to 60 minutes of a subcutaneous dose that is maintained for 8 hours (*Catheter Cardiovasc Interv.* 2003;60:185–193).

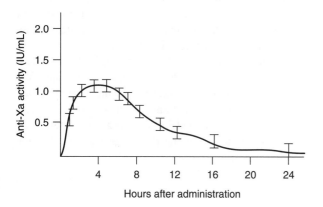

Therefore, it is recommended that no additional anticoagulant be given unless it has been 8 hours or more since their last dose, and in that case a booster dose of 0.3 mg per kg IV should be given. This was the peri-PCI treatment regimen utilized in the SYNERGY trial that involved over 10,000 high-risk ACS patients randomized to either enoxaparin or UFH (*JAMA.* 2004;292:45–54). Overall, the trial found no difference in efficacy between enoxaparin and UFH. One important outcome of SYNERGY was the knowledge that combined anticoagulant therapies (e.g., giving UFH to an enoxaparin-treated patient) was associated with a substantial increase in bleeding complications and no improvement in efficacy.

6 **Answer C.** John Folts developed an *in vivo* model of arterial stenosis, intimal damage and periodic thrombosis that is commonly referred to as the Folts model (*Circulation.* 1991;83(4):IV3–IV14). In this model, an animal (usually dog or pig) artery (usually coronary) is exposed and a flow probe is placed on it. Distal to the flow probe, the artery is injured with a vascular clamp to produce endothelial and/or medial injury. A plastic cylinder is then placed around the outside of the injured artery, producing a stenosis of varying severity. Acute platelet thrombus formation begins to occur at the area of stenosis that gradually leads to increased narrowing. This causes the coronary flow to decline, and eventually results in total cessation of flow when the artery is completely occluded. Following this, the thrombus will embolize with restoration of normal flow. This occurs repeatedly causing CFRs. When an antiplatelet agent (including aspirin) is used, CFRs can be reduced or completely eliminated.

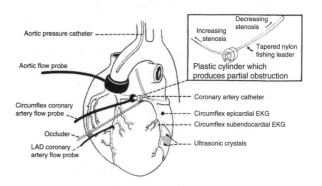

7 **Answer D.** The patient has multivessel disease with an angiographically severe LAD stenosis, but successful reperfusion following lytic therapy in the setting of an acute anterior STEMI. Emergent PCI is not indicated following thrombolysis and successful reperfusion as indicated in this patient by resolution of ST-segment elevation and restoration of normal flow in the LAD by angiography despite the presence of an angiographically severe lesion. The potential harm of routine PCI following thrombolytic therapy was confirmed recently in the ASSENT-4 study in which patients with STEMI randomized to lytics followed by PCI had significantly higher mortality than patients randomized to primary PCI alone (*Lancet.* 2006;367:569–578). Similarly, there is no clear indication for percutaneous treatment of this patient's RCA lesions at this time. In fact, the ACC/AHA guidelines make this a Class III recommendation even in the setting of a primary PCI, stating that a PCI should not be performed in a noninfarct artery at the time of primary PCI in patients without hemodynamic compromise (*J Am Coll Cardiol.* 2004;44:671). Urgent CABG is also contraindicated in patients with successful epicardial reperfusion and no mechanical complications.

8 **Answer D.** This situation must be tempered by the nuances of the patient presentation, and many would argue that the decision regarding when to proceed to catheterization varies from patient to patient. However, this patient presents with clear high-risk features, particularly dynamic EKG changes in the setting of anginal chest pain. As it is clear that an unstable coronary process must be evaluated, the essential part in decision making in this patient is determining whether one should pursue an "early invasive" or "early conservative" strategy. The early conservative strategy reserves coronary angiography for UA/NSTEMI patients who have evidence of recurrent ischemia or high-risk stress testing despite optimal and aggressive medical therapy. According to the 2002 Update of the ACC/AHA Guidelines for Management of Patients with Non-ST Elevation ACSs, an early invasive strategy in patients with high-risk features with coronary angiography and intervention is a Class I recommendation with level of evidence A (Available at: http://www.acc.org/clinical/guidelines/unstable/unstable.pdf 2002). In this guideline, high-risk features include:

- Recurrent angina/ischemia at rest or with low level activities despite intensive anti-ischemic therapy
- Elevated TnT or TnI
- New or presumably new ST-segment depression
- Recurrent angina/ischemia with CHF symptoms, an S_3 gallop, pulmonary edema, worsening rales, or new or worsening mitral regurgitation (MR)
- High-risk findings on noninvasive stress testing
- Depressed left ventricle (LV) systolic function (e.g., ejection function [EF] <0.40 on noninvasive study)
- Hemodynamic instability
- Sustained ventricular tachycardia
- PCI within 6 months
- Prior CABG

The guidelines go on to state that in the absence of these high-risk features in the setting of UA/NSTEMI, either the early invasive or conservative strategy is acceptable in hospitalized patients. Although the trial designs differed, the two most recent clinical trials comparing early invasive versus early conservative strategies in UA/NSTEMI patients were TACTICS-TIMI 18 and FRISC II. In TACTICS-TIMI 18, 2,200 patients with UA/NSTEMI were treated with aspirin, heparin, and an "upstream" GPIIb/IIIa inhibitor (tirofiban) (*N Engl J Med.* 2001;344:1879–1887). They were then randomized to an early invasive strategy including routine angiography within 48 hours, or a more conservative symptom-driven approach. In the latter, catheterization was performed only if the patient had recurrent ischemia or a positive stress test. Death, MI, or rehospitalization for ACS at 6 months occurred in 15.9% of the patients assigned to the invasive strategy versus 19.4% assigned to the more conservative strategy ($p = 0.025$). Death or MI was also reduced at 6 months (7.3% vs. 9.5%, $p < 0.05$). Interestingly, if the patient did not have high-risk features, the outcomes between the two groups were similar. In FRISC II, more than 3,000 patients were randomized in a 2×2 fashion with one arm being an early invasive versus early conservative approach (*Lancet.* 1999;354:708–715). At 6 months, death or MI occurred in 9.4% of the patients assigned to the invasive strategy and in 12.1% of those assigned to the noninvasive strategy ($p < 0.031$). During the first year the mortality rate in the invasive strategy group was 2.2% compared with 3.9% in the noninvasive strategy group ($p = 0.016$) (*Lancet.* 2000;356:9–16).

On the basis of these and other data, the current guidelines suggest an early invasive approach in UA/NSTEMI patients with certain high-risk features summarized in preceding text. Alternately, the compilation of the data suggests the following algorithm:

Feature	High Risk At Least One of the Following Features Must Be Present:	Intermediate Risk No High-Risk Feature but Must Have One of the Following:	Low Risk No High- or Intermediate-Risk Feature but May Have Any of the Following Features:
History	Accelerating tempo of ischemic symptoms in preceding 48 h	Prior MI, peripheral or cerebrovascular disease, or CABG, prior aspirin use	
Character of pain	Prolonged ongoing (>20 min) rest pain	Prolonged (>20 min) rest angina, now resolved, with moderate or high likelihood of CAD Rest angina (<20 min) or relieved with rest or sublingual NTG	New-onset or progressive CCS Class III or IV angina in the past 2 wk without prolonged (>20 min) rest pain but with moderate or high likelihood of CAD
Clinical findings	Pulmonary edema, most likely due to ischemia New or worsening MR murmur S_3 or new/worsening rales Hypotension, bradycardia, tachycardia Age >75 y	Age >70 y	
Electrocardiogram	Angina at rest with transient ST-segment changes >0.05 mV Bundle-branch block, new or presumed new Sustained ventricular tachycardia	T-wave inversions >0.2 mV Pathologic Q waves	Normal or unchanged EKG during an episode of chest discomfort
Cardiac markers	Elevated (e.g., TnT or TnI >0.1 ng/mL)	Slightly elevated (e.g., TnT >0.01 but <0.1 ng/mL)	Normal

[a]Estimation of the short-term risks of death and nonfatal cardiac ischemic events in unstable angina is a complex multivariable problem that cannot be fully specified in a table such as this; therefore, this table is meant to offer general guidance and illustration rather than rigid algorithms. MI, myocardial infarction; CABG, coronary artery bypass graft; CAD, coronary artery disease; NTG, nitroglycerin; EKG, electrocardiogram. Adapted from AHCPR Clinical Practice Guideline No. 10, Unstable Angina: Diagnosis and Management, May 1994. Braunwald E, Mark DB, Jones RH, et al. Unstable angina: diagnosis and management. Rockville, MD: Agency for Health Care Policy and Research and the National Heart, Lung, and Blood Institute, US Public Health Service, US Department of Health and Human Services; 1994; AHCPR Publication No. 94-0602.

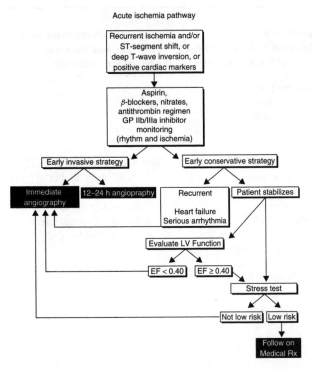

Acute ischemia pathway

(Adapted from Braunwald et al. Management of Patients with Unstable Angina and Non–ST-Segment Elevation Myocardial Infarction Update. http://www.acc.org/clinical/guidelines/unstable/incorporated/index.htm, 2006.)

With more studies, including the most recent ICTUS trial (*N Engl J Med.* 2005;353:1095–1104), which found no difference between an early invasive approach and an ischemia-guided approach, future recommendations may be refined.

9 Answer C. Expeditious restoration of coronary blood flow is the primary goal of all revascularization strategies, and time-to-reperfusion is the best correlate with most outcome measures in patients presenting with acute STEMI. Rheolytic thrombectomy was developed out of concern for protection of distal vessels and microvasculature when patients present with apparent large thrombus burden. In the VEGAS-1 and 2 trials, efficacy of thrombectomy in patients with STEMI and large thrombus burdens in vein grafts

was established. (*Am J Cardiol.* 2002;89:326–330). However, thrombectomy was compared with intracoronary infusion of urokinase, and the rates of adjunctive therapy such as glycoprotein IIb/IIIa inhibitor were low. In 2004, the AiMI trial sought to determine whether thrombectomy plus "definitive therapy" was superior to "definitive therapy" alone in patients presenting with anterior STEMI or large inferior STEMI (*Eur Heart J.* 2006;27:1139–1145). This trial was a multicenter, prospective, randomized and controlled trial that included 480 such patients presenting within 12 hours of symptom onset. Interestingly, the primary endpoint of final infarct size as measured by the SPECT imaging at 14 to 28 days was significantly larger in the subset of patients receiving thrombectomy. In addition to infarct size, mortality was also shown to be significantly higher in the thrombectomy arm (4.6% versus 0.8%; $p < 0.02$). Secondary endpoints including postprocedural TIMI flow and MACE (death, new Q wave MI, stroke, target lesion revascularization) showed no difference between the two treatment arms. Unlike VEGAS, patients with vein grafts were excluded in the AiMI trial, and the rate of GPIIb/IIIa use was much higher in AiMI (eptifibatide use >90%). The AiMI trialists concluded that their data do not support routine use of rheolytic thrombectomy in STEMI.

10 Answer C. As part of a comprehensive risk reduction strategy after PCI, the latest 2005 guideline update from the ACC/AHA/SCAI states that all post-MI and acute patients be started on β-blocker therapy before discharge if there are no specific contraindications (*Circulation.* 2006;113:e166–e286). In regard to drug therapy for hypertension for secondary prevention of events, it is recommended that therapy be initiated for individuals with BP >140/90 mm Hg. However, if patients have chronic kidney disease or diabetes, drug therapy should be started if BP is >130/80 mm Hg (*Circulation.* 2006;113:2363–2372). Although there has been historical controversy over when to obtain lipid profiles in patients presenting with ACSs, the published

Intervention Recommendations with Class of Recommendation and Level of Evidence	
Smoking: Goal Complete cessation. No exposure to environmental tobacco smoke.	■ Ask about tobacco use status at every visit. I (B) ■ Advise every tobacco user to quit. I (B) ■ Assess the tobacco user's willingness to quit. I (B) ■ Assist by counseling and developing a plan for quitting. I (B) ■ Arrange follow-up, referral to special programs, or pharmacotherapy (including nicotine replacement and bupropion). I (B) ■ Urge avoidance of exposure to environmental tobacco smoke at work and home. I (B)

	Intervention Recommendations with Class of Recommendation and Level of Evidence
Blood pressure control: Goal <140/90 mm Hg or <130/80 mm Hg if patient has diabetes or chronic kidney disease	For all patients: ■ Initiate or maintain lifestyle modification—weight control; increased physical activity; alcohol moderation; sodium reduction; and emphasis on increased consumption of fresh fruits, vegetables, and low-fat dairy products. I (B) For patients with blood pressure ≥140/90 mm Hg (or ≥130/80 mm Hg for individuals with chronic kidney disease or diabetes): ■ As tolerated, add blood pressure medication, treating initially with β-blockers and/or ACE inhibitors, with addition of other drugs such as thiazides as needed to achieve goal blood pressure. I (A) (For compelling indications for individual drug classes in specific vascular diseases, see Seventh Report of the Joint National Committee on Prevention, Detection, Evaluation, and Treatment of High Blood Pressure [JNC 7].)[a]

Lipid management: Goal LDL-C <100 mg/dL If triglycerides are ≥200 mg/dL, non-HDL-C should be <130 mg/dL[b]	For all patients:
	 ■ Start dietary therapy. Reduce intake of saturated fats (to <7% of total calories), *trans*-fatty acids, and cholesterol (to <200 mg/d). I (B)
	 ■ Adding plant stanol/sterols (2 g/d) and viscous fiber (>10 g/d) will further lower LDL-C.
	 ■ Promote daily physical activity and weight management. I (B)
	 ■ Encourage increased consumption of omega-3 fatty acids in the form of fish[c] or in capsule form (1 g/d) for risk reduction. For treatment of elevated triglycerides, higher doses are usually necessary for risk reduction. IIb (B)
	 For lipid management:
	 Assess fasting lipid profile in all patients, and within 24 hours of hospitalization for those with an acute cardiovascular or coronary event. For hospitalized patients, initiate lipid-lowering medication as recommended below before discharge according to the following schedule:
	 ■ LDL-C should be <100 mg/dL I (A), and
	 ■ Further reduction of LDL-C to <70 mg/dL is reasonable. IIa (A)
	 ■ If baseline LDL-C is ≥100 mg/dL, initiate LDL-lowering drug therapy.[d] I (A)
	 ■ If on-treatment LDL-C is ≥100 mg/dL, intensify LDL-lowering drug therapy (may require LDL-lowering drug combination[e]). I (A)
	 ■ If baseline LDL-C is 70 to 100 mg/dL, it is reasonable to treat to LDL-C <70 mg/dL. IIa (B)
	 ■ If triglycerides are 200 to 499 mg/dL, non-HDL-C should be <130 mg/dL. I (B), and
	 ■ Further reduction of non-HDL-C to <100 mg/dL is reasonable. IIa (B)
	 ■ Therapeutic options to reduce non-HDL-C are:
	   ■ More intense LDL-C-lowering therapy I (B), or
	   ■ Niacin[f] (after LDL-C-lowering therapy) IIa (B), or
	   ■ Fibrate therapy[g] (after LDL-C-lowering therapy) IIa (B)
	 ■ If triglycerides are ≥500 mg/dL[g], therapeutic options to prevent pancreatitis are fibrate[f] or niacin[f] before LDL-lowering therapy; and treat LDL-C to goal after triglyceride-lowering therapy. Achieve non-HDL-C <130 mg/dL if possible. I (C)

Physical activity: Goal 30 min, 7 d per wk (minimum 5 d per wk)	■ For all patients, assess risk with a physical activity history and/or an exercise test, to guide prescription. I (B) ■ For all patients, encourage 30 to 60 minutes of moderate-intensity aerobic activity, such as brisk walking, on most, preferably all, days of the week, supplemented by an increase in daily lifestyle activities (eg, walking breaks at work, gardening, household work). I (B) ■ Encourage resistance training 2 d per wk. IIb (C) ■ Advise medically supervised programs for high-risk patients (eg, recent acute coronary syndrome or revascularization, heart failure). I (B)

	Intervention Recommendations with Class of Recommendation and Level of Evidence
Weight management: Goal Body mass index: 18.5 to 24.9 kg/m^2 Waist circumference: men <40 in, women <35 in	■ Assess body mass index and/or waist circumference on each visit and consistently encourage weight maintenance/reduction through an appropriate balance of physical activity, caloric intake, and formal behavioral programs when indicated to maintain/achieve a body mass index between 18.5 and 24.9 kg/m^2. I (B) ■ If waist circumference (measured horizontally at the iliac crest) is ≥35 in. in women and ≥40 in. in men, initiate lifestyle changes and consider treatment strategies for metabolic syndrome as indicated. I (B) ■ The initial goal of weight loss therapy should be to reduce body weight by approximately 10% from baseline. With success, further weight loss can be attempted if indicated through further assessment. I (B)
Diabetes management: Goal HbA$_{1c}$ <7%	■ Initiate lifestyle and pharmacotherapy to achieve near-normal HbA$_{1c}$. I (B) ■ Begin vigorous modification of other risk factors (e.g., physical activity, weight management, blood pressure control, and cholesterol management as recommended above). I (B) ■ Coordinate diabetic care with patient's primary care physician or endocrinologist. I (C)

Antiplatelet agents/
anticoagulants:
	■ Start aspirin 75 to 162 mg/d and continue indefinitely in all patients unless contraindicated. I (A)
	  ■ For patients undergoing coronary artery bypass grafting, aspirin should be started within 48 hours of surgery to reduce saphenous vein graft closure. Dosing regimens ranging from 100 to 325 mg/d appear to be efficacious. Doses higher than 162 mg/d can be continued for up to 1 y. I (B)
	■ Start and continue clopidogrel 75 mg/d in combination with aspirin for up to 12 mo in patients after acute coronary syndrome or percutaneous coronary intervention with stent placement (≥1 mo for bare metal stent, ≥3 mo for sirolimus-eluting stent, and ≥6 mo for paclitaxel-eluting stent). I (B)
	  ■ Patients who have undergone percutanecus coronary intervention with stent placement should initially receive higher-dose aspirin at 325 mg/d for 1 mo for bare metal stent, 3 mo for sirolimus-eluting stent, and 6 mo for paclitaxel-eluting stent. I (B)
	■ Manage warfarin to international normalized ratio = 2.0 to 3.0 for paroxysmal or chronic atrial fibrillation or flutter, and in postmyocardial infarction patients when clinically indicated (e.g., atrial fibrillation, left ventricular thrombus). I (A)
	■ Use of warfarin in conjunction with aspirin and/or dopidogrel is associated with increased risk of bleeding and should be monitored closely. I (B)

Renin-angiotensin-aldosterone system blockers:	ACE inhibitors: ■ Start and continue indefinitely in all patients with left ventricular ejection fraction ≤40% and in those with hypertension, diabetes, or chronic kidney disease, unless contraindicated. I (A) ■ Consider for all other patients. I (B) ■ Among lower-risk patients with normal left ventricular ejection fraction in whom cardiovascular risk factors are well controlled and revascularization has been performed, use of ACE inhibitors may be considered optional. IIa (B) Angiotensin receptor blockers: ■ Use in patients who are intolerant of ACE inhibitors and have heart failure or have had a myocardial infarction with left ventricular ejection fraction ≤40%. I (A) ■ Consider in other patients who are ACE inhibitor intolerant. I (B) ■ Consider use in combination with ACE inhibitors in systolic-dysfunction heart failure. IIb (B) Aldosterone blockade: ■ Use in postmyocardial infarction patients, without significant renal dysfunction[h] or hyperkalemia[i], who are already receiving therapeutic doses of an ACE inhibitor and β-blocker, have a left ventricular ejection fraction ≤40%, and have either diabetes or heart failure. I (A)

	Intervention Recommendations with Class of Recommendation and Level of Evidence
β-blockers:	■ Start and continue indefinitely in all patients who have had myocardial infarction, acute coronary syndrome, or left ventricular dysfunction with or without heart failure symptoms, unless contraindicated. I (A) Consider chronic therapy for all other patients with coronary or other vascular disease or diabetes unless contraindicated. IIa (C)
Influenza vaccination:	Patients with cardiovascular disease should have an influenza vaccination. I (B)

(Adapted from *Circulation.* 2006;113:2363–2372;).

[a]Patients covered by these guidelines include those with established coronary and other atherosclerotic vascular disease, including peripheral arterial disease, atherosclerotic aortic disease, and carotid artery disease. Treatment of patients whose only manifestation of cardiovascular risk is diabetes will be the topic of a separate American Health Association scientific statement. ACE, angiotensin-converting enzyme; HDL, high density lipoprotein.

[b]Non-HDL-C = total cholesterol minus HDL-C.

[c]Pregnant and lactating women should limit their intake of fish to minimize exposure to methylmercury.

[d]When LDL-lowering medications are used, obtain at least a 30% to 40% reduction in LDL-C levels. If LDL-C <70 mg/dL is the chosen target, consider drug titration to achieve this level to minimize side effects and cost. When LDL-C <70 mg/dL is not achievable because of high baseline LDL-C levels, it generally is possible to achieve reductions of >50% in LDL-C levels by either statins or LDL-C–lowering drug combinations.

[e]Standard dose of statin with ezetimibe, bile acid sequestrant, or niacin.

[f]The combination of high-dose statin + fibrate can increase risk for severe myopathy. Statin doses should be kept relatively low with this combination. Dietary supplement niacin must not be used as a substitute for prescription niacin.

[g]Patients with very high triglycerides should not consume alcohol. The use of bile acid sequestrant is relatively contraindicated when triglycerides are >200 mg/dL.

[h]Creatinine should be <2.5 mg/dL in men and <2.0 mg/dL in women.

[i]Potassium should be <5.0 m Eq/L.

guidelines state that lipid profiles should be obtained in all patients, preferably within 24 hours of an acute event. With mounting evidence suggesting that lower low-density lipoprotein-cholesterol (LDL-C) portends better outcomes, statins are still preferred in post-PCI patients even with LDL-C <100 mg per dL at baseline. Regular exercise should be encouraged, with a minimum of 30 to 60 minutes at least five times weekly. BMI should be calculated and documented, with the desirable approximate range of 18.5 to 24.9 kg per m². The above table summarizes the ACC/AHA recommendations regarding appropriate secondary prevention in these patients.

11 **Answer D.**   This patient probably should not have undergone coronary angiography in the first place, given her presentation, paucity of risk factors for CAD, and her otherwise low-risk stress test. Once the diagnostic images have been obtained, however, the interventionalist is faced with a dilemma—whether to proceed with an intervention, or to choose the primary medical management approach. Many factors are involved in this decision, but ultimately it is the interventionalist's job to integrate the entirety of the patient's presentation and make informed, conscientious decisions in the patient's best interest. PCI in this case may be a Class III recommendation according to the 2005 ACC/AHA/SCAI guidelines regarding PCI if the lesion is not hemodynamically significant (*Circulation.* 2006;113:2363–2372).

A Class III recommendation implies that based on the best available evidence, the intervention would extend more risk than benefit to the patient, and therefore should not be performed. This patient has CCS Class II angina on presentation, and there is no objective evidence of ischemia based on available information. Furthermore, the particular location of this lesion would place only a small area of myocardium at risk. Should the operator demonstrate a focal lesion in this patient that is well suited for PCI and that places a moderate or large-sized area of myocardium at risk, then proceeding with PCI would become a Class I recommendation. It is left to the discretion of the interventionalist to make these decisions with competence on behalf of each individual patient. One option would be doing FFR of the 50% stenosis to ascertain hemodynamic significance.

12 **Answer C.**   Routine periodic stress testing of patients who have undergone PCI with no high-risk features, and who are asymptomatic received a Class III recommendation from the ACC/AHA in 2002 (*J Am Coll Cardiol.* 2002;40:1531–1540). High-risk patients generally include those with decreased left ventricular function, multivessel CAD, proximal left anterior descending disease, previous sudden death, diabetes mellitus, hazardous occupations, and suboptimal percutaneous transluminal coronary angioplasty (PTCA) PCI results. In the presence of such high-risk features, exercise testing within 12 months of PCI to detect restenosis is a Class IIb recommendation, indicating additional studies are needed to confirm efficacy and safety of this approach. The only Class I recommendation for stress testing after revascularization is for recurrent symptoms that suggest ischemia. Another potential use for postrevascularization stress testing is to assist with activity counseling and to guide exercise training as part of a comprehensive cardiac rehabilitation program.

13 Answer E. Because this patient has undergone PCI within the last 6 months, she should be considered in the high-risk group, thereby making an early invasive strategy a Class I indication in managing her disease (*Available at:* http://www.acc.org/clinical/guidelines/unstable/unstable.pdf 2002). The ACC/AHA/SCAI 2005 Guideline Update for Percutaneous Coronary Intervention identifies nine such features that help identify patients as high risk and therefore more likely to benefit from an early invasive strategy when presenting with UA/NSTEMI (*Circulation.* 2006;113:e166–e286) and include:

- Recurrent ischemia despite intensive anti-ischemic therapy
- Elevated troponin level
- New ST-segment depression
- Heart failure (HF) symptoms or new or worsening MR
- Depressed LV systolic function
- Hemodynamic instability
- Sustained ventricular tachycardia
- PCI within 6 months
- Prior CABG

Many clinical trials (e.g., TIMI-IIIB, VANQWISH, and FRISC II) have evaluated different strategies for managing patients presenting with UA or NSTEMI, including both invasive and medical strategies to compare outcomes. More recent trials, such as RITA III, ISAR-COOL, and TACTICS-TIMI 18, suggest that patients who are treated with an early invasive strategy have reduced incidence of recurrent angina, and a combined endpoint of death and MI. On the basis of data compiled from these various trials, the most recent guidelines suggest that an early invasive approach is the preferred strategy in patients presenting with UA/NSTEMI with high-risk features.

14 Answer D. The latest ACC/AHA/SCAI guidelines for PCI state that elective PCI should not be performed at institutions without on-site cardiac surgery (*Circulation.* 2006;113:e166–e286). Under the guidelines, this would be a Class III recommendation (Level of Evidence: B), reflecting that such practice may carry increased risk and higher mortality in

patients undergoing elective PCI at such facilities. However, a compelling argument could be made for elective PCI in certain well-selected patients at institutions without on-site cardiac surgery if a plan for immediate transfer to such an institution is in place. For this patient, the closest facility with cardiac surgery is 120 miles away so immediate transfer would not be feasible. Therefore, arranging for elective PCI in the facility with on-site cardiac surgery is most appropriate. Although diagnostic angiography is also an option, the likelihood of this patient having hemodynamically significant CAD is high, making the option of diagnostic angiography immediately followed by PCI if needed the most attractive decision.

15 Answer A. In this scenario, you are faced with a patient with known CAD and a chest pain syndrome consistent with escalating angina. Diagnostic coronary angiography reveals a moderate lesion in the large diagonal branch, and no other potential "culprit" lesions. Appropriately, FFR is done to assess the hemodynamic significance of the lesion, but fails to demonstrate it. Using the technique of determining FFR to establish the hemodynamic significance of intermediate coronary lesions (30% to 70%) has been proved to be beneficial in many circumstances and carries a Class IIa indication in this patient group in the latest ACC/AHA PCI guidelines (*Circulation.* 2006;113:e166–e286). At this point, careful consideration must be given to the entirety of the patient's condition, and not just the angiographic appearance of the suspected culprit lesion. Most would agree that IVUS has no added benefit to the initial FFR determination in this situation. Although, depending on the interventionalist's interpretation of the significance of the angiographic appearance of the lesion, IVUS of the potential culprit lesion could be a Class IIa, IIb, or even Class III indication (if the angiographic appearance of the lesion is clear and no intervention is planned). It has been shown that deferring PCI for intermediate coronary lesions with normal physiology (i.e., normal FFR determination) produces similar results to intervening on such lesions with respect to event-free survival and freedom from anginal symptoms (*J Am Coll Cardiol.* 1998;31:841–847, *Circulation.* 2001;103:2928–2934, *J Am Coll Cardiol.* 1995;25:178–187). Proceeding with nuclear imaging once the FFR determination has been done is also unappealing, primarily because of the wealth of evidence, which correlates abnormal FFR determination with nuclear stress testing. In fact, an FFR of <0.75 has been consistently shown to identify physiologically significant stenosis associated with inducible myocardial ischemia with high sensitivity (88%), specificity (100%), positive predicted value (100%), and overall accuracy (93%). One must be impressed that the patient presented with poorly controlled BP and elevated resting pulse rate from the available information and physiologic data, would be the more beneficial target for the physician to focus.

16 **Answer D.** In the EPIC trial with abciximab, high-risk patients (including severe UA patients) had 35% lower incidence of ischemic complications (death, MI, revascularization) at 30 days compared with placebo (12.8% vs. 8.3%, $p = 0.0008$) (*N Engl J Med.* 1994;330:956–961). A 13% benefit was seen at 3 years, mainly attributable to decreased need for bypass surgery or repeat PCI in the group treated with abciximab (*JAMA.* 1997;278:479–484). Showing even greater benefit, patients with UA in the EPILOG trial demonstrated a 64% reduction (10.1% to 3.6%, $p = 0.001$) in the composite occurrence of death, MI, or urgent revascularization to 30 days with abciximab therapy compared with placebo (standard-dose weight-adjusted heparin) (*N Engl J Med.* 1997;336:1689–1696). Tirofiban was evaluated in the PRISM-PLUS trial, which included patients with UA and NSTEMI presenting within 12 hours of symptom onset (*N Engl J Med.* 1998;338:1488–1497). Here, the 30-day incidence of death, MI, refractory ischemia, or rehospitalization for UA was 15.3% in the group that received heparin alone compared with 8.8% in the tirofiban/heparin group. After PCI, death or nonfatal MI occurred in 10.2% of those receiving heparin versus 5.9% in those treated with tirofiban. Eptifibatide has been evaluated in two randomized clinical trials and has also demonstrated efficacy in reducing ischemic complications in patients with UA. In the PURSUIT trial such patients were randomized to receive placebo or eptifibatide in addition to standard therapy of aspirin with or without UFH. (*N Engl J Med.* 1998;339:436–443). In patients undergoing PCI within 72 hours of randomization, eptifibatide administration resulted in a 31% reduction in the combined endpoint of nonfatal MI or death at 30 days (17.7% vs. 11.6%, $p = 0.01$).

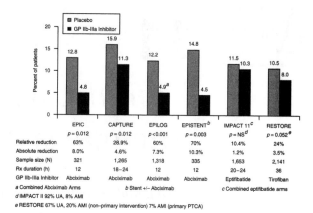

	EPIC	CAPTURE	EPILOG	EPISTENT[b]	IMPACT II[c]	RESTORE
	$p = 0.012$	$p = 0.012$	$p < 0.001$	$p = 0.003$	$p = $ NS[d]	$p = 0.052$[e]
Relative reduction	63%	28.9%	60%	70%	10.4%	24%
Absolute reduction	8.0%	4.6%	7.3%	10.3%	1.2%	3.5%
Sample size (N)	321	1,265	1,318	335	1,653	2,141
Rx duration (h)	12	18–24	12	12	20–24	36
GP IIb-IIIa Inhibitor	Abciximab	Abciximab	Abciximab	Abciximab	Eptifibatide	Tirofiban

a Combined Abciximab Arms   b Stent +/– Abciximab   c Combined eptifibatide arms
d IMPACT II 92% UA, 8% AMI
e RESTORE 67% UA, 20% AMI (non–primary intervention) 7% AMI (primary PTCA)

Death, MI, and Urgent Intervention at 30 days after PCI in patients with ACS: GPIIb/IIIa trials. (Adapted from the ACC/AHA 2002 Guideline for Management of Patients with Unstable Angina and Non–ST-Segment Elevation Myocardial Infarction.)

17 **Answer B.** In patients who present with UA or NSTEMI, statin therapy as well as diet should be instituted soon after admission in patients whose LDL exceeds 100 mg per dL (Class IIa indication, Level of Evidence: B). It is therefore recommended that fasting lipid profiles be drawn on all such patients and acted on accordingly. Ticlopidine is approved only for *combination* therapy with aspirin after PCI, and not alone. Clopidogrel 75 mg daily is a Class I indication in patients post-PCI who cannot tolerate aspirin because of hypersensitivity or gastrointestinal intolerance. According to the ACC/AHA 2002 Guideline Update for the Management of Patients with Unstable Angina and Non–ST-Segment Elevation Myocardial Infarction, ACE inhibitor therapy is advised for patients with CHF, LV dysfunction (EF <0.40), hypertension, or diabetes (Class I indication, Level of Evidence: A). (Available at: http://www.acc.org/clinical/guidelines/unstable/unstable.pdf 2002). The same guideline states that the target BP in such patients should be <130/85 mm Hg (not 120/80), though most feel that a side effect and symptomatic approach should be used in titrating antihypertensive medications to offer the patient maximal benefit.

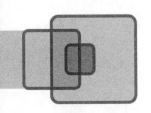

11
Primary, Rescue, and Facilitated Angioplasty

David J. Moliterno, Leslie Cho, and Debabrata Mukherjee

Questions

1 The currently accepted maximum medical contact-to-balloon or door-to-balloon time for patients with ST-segment elevation myocardial infarction (STEMI) is:

(A) 30 minutes
(B) 60 minutes
(C) 90 minutes
(D) 120 minutes
(E) 360 minutes

2 A 76-year-old man presents with an acute anterior wall myocardial infarction (MI). Emergent coronary angiography reveals a completely occluded left anterior descending (LAD) artery with thrombolysis in myocardial infarction (TIMI) 0 flow (see figure below) and a 70% to 80% stenosis of the right coronary artery (RCA) with TIMI

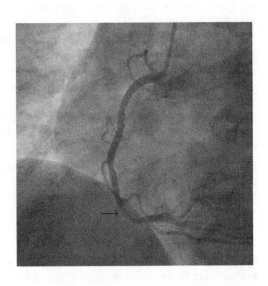

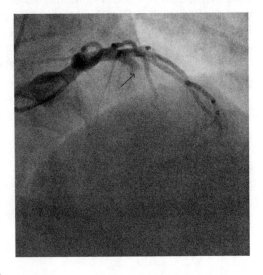

3 flow (see figure above). Left ventriculogram shows anterolateral hypokinesis. His heart rate is 88 and blood pressure (BP) is 127/78 with an oxygen saturation of 98% on room air. Optimal management of this patient will include:

(A) Bypass surgery because he has two-vessel disease involving the LAD artery
(B) Percutaneous coronary intervention (PCI) of the LAD artery only and consideration of PCI of the RCA at a later date (staged PCI) or noninvasive evaluation to assess RCA territory ischemia postdischarge, and PCI if indicated
(C) PCI of the LAD and the RCA
(D) PCI of the LAD and measurement of fractional flow reserve (FFR) of the RCA to assess

hemodymanic significance followed by PCI if indicated

3 A 69-year-old man presents to the emergency room of a community hospital without a PCI facility with an acute ST-segment elevation anterior wall MI. He is a tachycardiac and tachypneac with a heart rate of 112, BP of 76/43 and has rales in both the lung fields. Optimal management of this patient includes:

(A) Immediate administration of full-dose fibrinolysis

(B) Immediate administration of half-dose fibrinolysis with full-dose abciximab

(C) Immediate administration of half-dose abciximab with full-dose fibrinolysis

(D) Arrangement for transfer to the nearest hospital with PCI facility that is 70 minutes away

4 A 68-year-old woman presents to your office for evaluation of chest discomfort she had the previous evening. The discomfort lasted for approximately 30 to 40 minutes and subsequently resolved. Currently, she is pain free with a heart rate of 74 and a BP of 118/71. Her lungs are clear to auscultation and you do not hear any significant murmurs on cardiac exam. Electrocardiogram (EKG) reveals evolving STEMI. On further questioning she states discomfort started at approximately 7:00 PM last evening and lasted till 7:45 PM or so. It is now 10:00 AM the next morning. Appropriate management would include:

(A) Admission to the hospital and treatment with aspirin, heparin, clopidogrel, statins, and β-blockers

(B) Admission to the cardiac catheterization laboratory for emergent angiography with a goal of primary PCI

(C) Administration of full-dose fibrinolysis, admission to hospital, and treatment with aspirin, heparin, clopidogrel, statins, and β-blockers

(D) Administration of full-dose fibrinolytics and then admission to the catheterization laboratory for emergent angiography

5 Transfer of patients with STEMI to PCI-capable center rather than immediate fibrinolysis should be considered in all of the following situations, *except*:

(A) When fibrinolytic therapy is contraindicated or unsuccessful

(B) When cardiogenic shock ensues

(C) When the anticipated delay to PCI is 90 to 120 minutes

(D) When symptoms have been present for >2 to 3 hours

6 In patients with STEMI, compared with fibrinolysis, primary PCI lowers the odds of death by:

(A) 5%

(B) 10%

(C) 15%

(D) 20%

(E) 25%

7 The role of embolic protection devices in primary PCI is best characterized as being:

(A) Strongly recommended for all patients undergoing primary PCI (Class I recommendation)

(B) Strongly recommended for primary PCI only in patients with large thrombus burden (Class I recommendation)

(C) Currently not recommended for primary PCI

(D) Recommended for patients with no reflow after PCI

8 A 67-year-old man undergoes bypass surgery for severe three-vessel coronary disease. Approximately 12 hours after the surgery he becomes short of breath and has 3 mm ST elevation in the inferolateral leads. The best management strategy at this time is:

(A) Conservative management without coronary angiography

(B) Coronary angiography followed by catheter-based treatment strategy with subsequent PCI

(C) Coronary angiography followed by surgical-based treatment strategy readmitting patients to emergency redo-coronary artery bypass graft (CABG)

(D) Coronary angiography followed by conservative treatment

9 Predictors of 1-year mortality among 30-day survivors after primary PCI include all *except*:

(A) Age >70 years

(B) Any tachyarrhythmia during index hospitalization (defined as ventricular or supraventricular tachycardia that required treatment)

(C) Weight <80 kg

(D) Number of diseased coronary arteries

(E) Left ventricular ejection fraction (LVEF)

(F) Female gender

10 Among patients undergoing primary PCI, outcomes are best in those who are:

(A) Underweight or thin (body mass index [BMI] <18 kg/m^2)

(B) Normal weight (BMI <25 kg per m^2)

(C) Overweight (≥25 to <30 kg per m^2)

(D) Obese (≥30 kg per m^2)

11 A 44-year-old man presents with chest heaviness and 0.5 mm ST-segment elevation in EKG leads I and avL. Coronary angiogram is performed (see following figure). The most likely etiology of his chest pain is:

(A) Pericarditis
(B) Occluded coronary artery
(C) Anomalous coronary artery
(D) Kawasaki disease
(E) Congenital coronary artery fistula

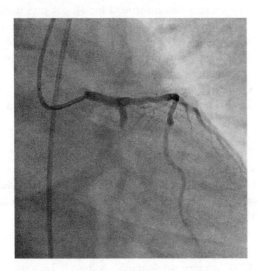

12 A 63-year-old woman presents with an acute STEMI. Emergent coronary angiography reveals completely occluded RCA with large thrombus burden (see following figure). Optimal management of this lesion includes:

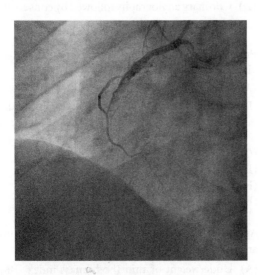

(A) Rheolytic thrombectomy
(B) Emboli protection device
(C) Balloon angioplasty followed by stenting
(D) Medical therapy

13 A 57-year-old man presents with an acute anterior wall MI. The patient is administered aspirin, clopidogrel, abciximab, and undergoes emergent coronary angiography (see following figure). The best management strategy in this individual is:

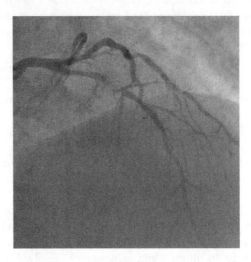

(A) Balloon angioplasty
(B) Fibrinolytic therapy followed by PCI in 3 to 4 days
(C) Bare-metal stent (BMS) implantation
(D) Drug-eluting stent (DES) implantation

14 A 34-year-old woman lawyer presents with chest discomfort after a particularly challenging tennis match. EKG reveals a 1 mm ST-segment elevation in leads II, III, and avF. An emergent coronary angiogram is performed (see following figure). The most likely etiology of her chest pain is:

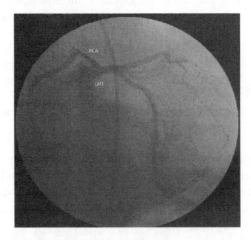

(A) Anomalous coronary artery
(B) Musculoskeletal chest pain
(C) Coronary artery dissection (CAD)
(D) Coronary embolus

15 You are asked to consult on an 83-year-old woman for possible PCI. Eight days ago she was admitted to the hospital with chest pain and ST elevation in leads V2–V4. She was diagnosed with acute anterior MI. However, she was not given thrombolytic therapy because of her history of stroke 4 months before admission and she refused cardiac catheterization. She was treated with aspirin, heparin, clopidogrel, simvastatin, metoprolol, and lisinopril. She responded well to the treatment, and her chest pain eventually resolved. Her EKG now has Q waves in the anterior leads. She has been free of chest pain since hospital day 1, and hemodynamically stable without any arrhythmias. Her echocardiogram on hospital day 4 was unremarkable except for anterior wall hypokinesis and LVEF of 35%. Her physician son has come in from out of town and wants her to undergo cardiac catheterization and possible PCI. Will catheterization and PCI decrease morbidity and mortality?

(A) Yes, rescue PCI results in improved VEF, greater freedom from adverse in-hospital clinical events, and decreases long-term MI and death from CAD

(B) Yes, rescue PCI results in improved LVEF and greater freedom from adverse in-hospital clinical events, but does not decrease long-term MI and death from CAD

(C) No, there is no convincing data to support the routine use of late adjuvant PCI days after MI in patients who did not receive reperfusion therapy

(D) No, there is no convincing data to support the routine use of late adjuvant PCI days after MI in patients who did not receive reperfusion therapy except to lower the rate of recurrent angina

16 A 61-year-old woman is brought to the emergency room by paramedics with chest pain for 2 hours. She is found to have ST elevation anteriorly. Her initial BP was 90/60 with heart rate of 100. She is given reteplase as the local hospital where she presents does not have a catheterization laboratory and is 2 hours drive from your large tertiary center. She is then immediately transferred to your hospital. Upon transfer she is without any chest pain; however, she still has ST elevation anteriorly. Is there any evidence of decreased mortality and morbidity from rescue PCI in this patient?

(A) Yes, rescue PCI in this patient would decrease chances of death and MI

(B) Yes, rescue PCI in this patient would decrease MI, but not chances of death

(C) No, rescue PCI in this patient would decrease neither MI nor chances of death

(D) No, rescue PCI in this patient would only decrease rates of arrhythmia

17 You are asked to examine a 58-year-old man with inferior wall MI by the hospital quality assessment board. The patient presented the previous night with chest pain and ST elevation inferiorly and was given tissue plasminogen activator (TPA). He had resolution of his chest pain and EKG abnormalities within 30 minutes. The next day another physician takes him to the catheterization laboratory and finds a large tortuous RCA with 95% stenosis with TIMI 3 flow, which he tries to open without success. He is unable to pass a balloon to the RCA because of extreme tortuosity. The procedure is aborted. The patient is doing well without any pain, arrhythmias or hemodynamic compromise. His EKG continues to be normal. It is now 24 hours after the attempted PCI. According to the current American College of Cardiology (ACC)/American Heart Association (AHA) guideline, what are the indications for rescue PCI?

(A) Persistent ischemia

(B) Hemodynamic compromise

(C) Heart failure

(D) Electrical instability

(E) All of the above

18 A 59-year-old nurse presents to the emergency room with lateral ST elevation and chest pain for 4 hours. She receives reteplase and has a resolution of her chest pain and ST elevation. She is discharged from the hospital on day 4 with aspirin (ASA), clopidogrel, vytorin, and metoprolol. She is doing well and has a stress echo that shows no evidence of ischemia and a small area of hypokinesis on her echo and her LVEF is 45%. However, she is still very concerned and feels that she should have undergone PCI. Would there have been any benefit to this patient undergoing routine PCI of the stenosis infarct-related artery immediately after fibrinolysis?

(A) There is no benefit with routine PCI in regard to salvage of jeopardized myocardium or prevention of reinfarction or death after successful fibrinolysis

(B) There is benefit with routine PCI in regard to salvage of jeopardized myocardium, but not with regard to prevention of reinfarction or death after successful fibrinolysis

(C) There is benefit with routine PCI in regard to death or MI, but no appreciable benefit to salvage of jeopardized myocardium after successful fibrinolysis

(D) There is benefit to salvage of myocardium, prevention of reinfarction, and death after successful fibrinolysis with routine PCI

19 A 71-year-old man is admitted to the hospital after promptly receiving a fibrinolytic agent, heparin, aspirin, and clopidogrel for an inferior wall MI. Primary angioplasty was not performed because the catheterization laboratory was not readily available at 2:00 AM when he presented. The patient's chest pain gradually resolved over several hours, and you see him later that morning when making rounds. He remains free of chest pain though he complains of dyspnea. His BP is 110/68, with a pulse rate of 92, and a respiratory rate of 20. On physical examination a third heart sound is faintly heard, and crackles are noted over the lower third of the posterior lung fields. Although he is free of chest pain, you decide to urgently send him for coronary angiography. In the catheterization laboratory the RCA is found to be completely occluded with faint left-to-right collateral. No other severe coronary artery disease is noted, and the LVEF is 40% to 45%. Which of the following would be the appropriate treatment?

(A) The MI is completed, therefore place a swan-ganz catheter and return the patient to the intensive care unit for diuretic therapy, and initiation of angiotensin-converting enzyme (ACE) inhibitors

(B) Perform rescue PCI and give a repeat loading dose of clopidogrel

(C) Begin intravenous IIb/IIIa inhibition and have the patient return tomorrow for follow-up angiography and possible PCI

(D) Consult cardiothoracic surgery for consideration of bypass grafting to the RCA

20 The Middlesbrough Early Revascularization to Limit INfarction (MERLIN) trial enrolled 307 patients with STEMI and failed thrombolytic therapy. They were randomized to an emergency coronary angiography with or without rescue PCI, or to conservative treatment. Thirty-day all-cause mortality was similar in the rescue and conservative groups. According to the subgroup analysis which group had the highest rate of 30-day all-cause mortality?

(A) Rescue PCI with resolution of ST elevation

(B) Rescue PCI without resolution of ST elevation

(C) Conservative therapy with resolution of ST elevation

(D) Conservative therapy without resolution of ST elevation

21 In the REACT trial patients presenting with failed pharmacologic reperfusion therapy were randomized to repeat thrombosis, conservative therapy, or rescue PCI. Which of the following best describes the findings of this study?

(A) No difference in all-cause mortality among the three groups

(B) A several-fold reduction in recurrent MI with rescue PCI versus repeat thrombolytic therapy

(C) More cerebrovascular accidents and major bleeding events in the rescue PCI group compared with the other groups

(D) Highest cost associated with PCI

(E) A and B

22 Nearly 20 years ago the TIMI 2 investigators randomized patients with STEMI receiving thrombolytic therapy to immediate versus delayed (18–48 hours) angiography and possible angioplasty (TIMI 2A phase, $n = 391$). They observed a similar rate of mortality between the two groups though a higher rate of bleeding among those randomized to early catheterization. Recently, the ASSENT-4 investigators performed a similar study whereby patients unable to promptly (1–3 hours) undergo primary PCI were randomized to standard PCI or to PCI preceded by full-dose tenecteplase. With 1,320 patients enrolled, what did the ASSENT-4 investigators find among patients randomized to the facilitated strategy of routine PCI urgently after thrombolytic therapy:

(A) Similar mortality and similar non–central nervous system (CNS) major bleeding rates

(B) Higher mortality and similar non-CNS major bleeding rates

(C) Similar mortality and higher non-CNS major bleeding rates

(D) Higher mortality and higher non-CNS major bleeding rates

23 In the 2005 ACC/AHA/Society for Cardiovascular Angiography and Intervention (SCAI) Practice Guidelines for PCI, what classification is given to facilitated PCI?

(A) I

(B) II

(C) III

(D) IV

Answers and Explanations

1 Answer C. The current ACC/AHA guidelines recommend that PCI for acute STEMI should be performed as quickly as possible, with a goal of a medical contact-to-balloon or door-to-balloon time within 90 minutes (*J Am Coll Cardiol.* 2006;47: 216–235). Time from symptom onset to reperfusion remains an important predictor of patient outcome even with PCI.

2 Answer B. The current ACC/AHA guidelines clearly state that elective PCI should not be performed in a noninfarct-related artery at the time of primary PCI of the infarct-related artery in patients without hemodynamic compromise, and is considered a contraindication (*J Am Coll Cardiol.* 2006;47: 216–235). The elective PCI of the noninfarct artery may actually worsen the outcomes in this setting. Although bypass surgery is an alternative in elective patients with severe multivessel disease particularly diabetes, waiting for bypass is not an option in this patient with an occluded LAD artery and a large amount of myocardium at jeopardy.

3 Answer D. Primary PCI should be performed for patients younger than 75 years old with ST elevation or presumably new left bundle-branch block who develop shock within 36 hours of MI, and are suitable for revascularization that can be performed within 18 hours of shock, unless further support is futile because of the patient's wishes or contraindications/unsuitability for further invasive care (*J Am Coll Cardiol.* 2006;47:216–235). PCI appears to have its greatest mortality benefit in high-risk patients. In patients with cardiogenic shock, an absolute 9% reduction in 30-day mortality with mechanical revascularization instead of immediate medical stabilization was reported in the SHOCK trial (*N Engl J Med.* 1999;341:625–634). Fibrinolysis is not very effective in patients with cardiogenic shock, and there is no data to support combination therapy in these patients. Consideration should be given to the placement of an intra-aortic balloon pump (IABP) before transfer if feasible.

4 Answer A. Current guidelines state that primary PCI should not be performed in asymptomatic patients, who are hemodynamically and electrically stable more than 12 hours after the onset of STEMI (*J Am Coll Cardiol.* 2006;47:216–235). Delayed revascularization after 12 hours is not supported by available clinical data although one ongoing trial, Open Artery Trial (OAT), is evaluating this.

5 Answer C. The time from symptom onset to reperfusion is an important predictor of patient outcome. After adjustment for baseline characteristics, the time from symptom onset to balloon inflation is significantly correlated with 1-year mortality in patients undergoing primary PCI for STEMI (relative risk equals 1.08 for each 30-minute delay from symptom onset to balloon inflation, $p = 0.04$) (*Circulation.* 2004;109:1223–1225). Delays in door-to-balloon time versus door-to-needle time of >60 minutes because of interhospital transfer might actually negate the potential mortality benefit of transfer for primary PCI over immediate intravenous fibrinolysis demonstrated in these trials (*Am J Cardiol.* 2003;92:824–826). Transfer of patients to PCI-capable centers should be considered when fibrinolytic therapy is contraindicated or unsuccessful, when cardiogenic shock ensues, when the anticipated delay is <60 minutes, or when the symptoms have been present for >2 to 3 hours.

6 Answer E. Primary PCI with stenting has been compared with fibrinolytic therapy in 12 randomized clinical trials. These investigations demonstrate that PCI-treated patients experience lower mortality rates (5.9% vs. 7.7%, OR 0.75, 95% CI 0.60 to 0.94, $p = 0.013$), fewer reinfarctions (1.6% vs. 5.1%, OR 0.31, 95% CI 0.21 to 0.44, $p = 0.0001$), and fewer hemorrhagic strokes than those treated by fibrinolysis (see following figure) (*Lancet.* 2003;361: 13–20). Compared with percutaneous transluminal coronary angioplasty (PTCA) alone, intracoronary stents achieve a better immediate angiographic result with a larger arterial lumen, less reclosure of the infarct-related artery, and fewer subsequent ischemic events.

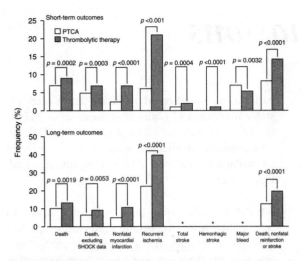

Short-term and Long-term Clinical Outcomes in Individuals Treated with Primary Percutaneous Coronary Interventions versus Fibrinolytic Therapy. (Adapted with permission from Killip et al. *Lancet.* **2003;361:13–20.)**

7   Answer C. Embolic protection devices have not shown any benefit in the setting of primary PCI for STEMI, as noted in the Enhanced Myocardial Efficacy and Recovery by Aspiration of Liberated Debris (EMERALD) trial (GuardWire), where distal protection did not convey significant benefit (*JAMA.* 2005;293:1063–1072). The subsequent trials such as the PCI Treatment of Myocardial Infarction for Salvage of Endangered Myocardium (PROMISE) study have also failed to show any benefit with these devices (*Circulation.* 2005;112:1462–1469). Embolic protection devices are not currently recommended for primary PCI.

8   Answer B. The best approach for the treatment of acute graft failure after CABG was unclear for a long time. A recent study compared primary PCI, emergency reoperation, and conservative therapy in a cohort of patients who developed an acute myocardial infarction (AMI) after bypass because of graft failure. The study reported that re-revascularization with emergency PCI may limit the extent of myocardial cellular damage compared with the surgical-based treatment strategy in patients with acute perioperative myocardial ischemia because of early graft failure following CABG (*Eur J Cardiothorac Surg.* 2006).

9   Answer F. An analysis from the CADILLAC trial using a multivariate logistic regression model identified age >70 years (OR 3.3, 95% CI 1.9 to 5.7), weight <80 kg (OR 1.9, 95% CI 1.1 to 3.6), any tachyarrhythmia during index hospitalization (defined as ventricular or supraventricular tachycardia that required treatment) (OR 2.4, 95% CI 1.2 to 4.8), number of diseased coronary arteries (OR 1.5, 95%

CI 1.1 to 2.1), and LVEF (each 10% decrease, OR 1.5, 95% CI 1.2 to 1.8) as factors independently associated with risk of death at 1 year among 30-day survivors. Female gender was not a multivariate predictor of outcomes (*Am J Cardiol.* 2006;97:817–822).

10   Answer C. A recent study analyzed the impact of BMI on the outcome of patients with AMI. Obese patients compared with normal-weight patients had lower in-hospital mortality (0.9% vs. 2.7%, p = 0.03) at 30 days (1.1% vs. 3.8%, p = 0.02) and 1 year (1.8% vs. 7.5%, p < 0.0001). Obese patients with AMI have an improved prognosis after primary PCI compared with normal-weight patients, a finding most likely related to AMI onset at younger age, with better renal function and less anterior infarction (*Am Heart J.* 2006;151:168–175).

11   Answer B. The coronary angiogram reveals acute occlusion of the left circumflex artery explaining his chest symptoms and lateral MI. Although pericarditis should be considered in the differential diagnosis of chest pain in a relatively young individual, the presence of an occluded coronary artery rules out this diagnosis. The angiogram does not reveal any coronary anomalies or arteriovenous fistula. Patients with Kawasaki disease are younger and typically have coronary artery aneurysms rather than occlusions. The EKG changes may often be subtle in patients with left circumflex artery disease.

12   Answer C. There is no evidence that either the thrombectomy devices or the emboli protection devices are useful in native coronary arteries with thrombus. A study conducted using AngioJet failed to reduce infarct size in patients with STEMI Angio-Jet Rheolytic Thrombectomy in Patients Undergoing Primary Angioplasty for (AiMI). In the treatment of X-TRACT randomized study, patients with saphenous vein graft (SVG) or thrombus-containing native coronary arteries were prospectively allocated to stent implantation with versus without prior thrombectomy with the X-Sizer device (*J Am Coll Cardiol.* 2003;42:2007–2013). Periprocedural MI at 30 days occurred in 15.8% of the patients assigned to the X-Sizer device compared with 16.6% of control patients (not significant). Early and late event-free survival was not improved by routine thrombectomy with this device. On the basis of the EMERALD and PROMISE trials, emboli protection devices are not effective in thrombus-containing native coronary arteries. Angioplasty followed by coronary stenting with adjunctive dual antiplatelet therapy and glycoprotein IIb/IIIa inhibitor is a reasonable alternative and will effectively restore normal flow in such patients. An attempt at revascularization is indicated in all patients with STEMI and medical therapy alone would not be appropriate in this situation.

13 Answer D. Available data suggest that compared with conventional BMS, DES implantations are not associated with increased risk when used for primary PCI in patients with STEMI. Postprocedure vessel patency, biomarker release, and the incidence of short-term adverse events were similar in patients receiving sirolimus-eluting stent (SES) or BMS. Thirty-day event rates of death, reinfarction, or revascularization were 7.5% versus 10.4%, respectively ($p = 0.4$) (*J Am Coll Cardiol.* 2004;43:704–708). Hofma et al. reported the safety and efficacy of currently available DES in patients with acute MI and demonstrated that there were no significant differences in major adverse cardiac outcomes (MACE)-free survival at 1 year between SES and paclitaxel-eluting stents for the treatment of AMI with very low rates of reintervention for restenosis with both (*Heart.* 2005;91:1176–1180). In this patient with a relatively proximal left anterior descending artery stenosis, a DES rather than BMS or balloon angioplasty is the best option. There is no reason to administer fibrinolytic therapy after performing coronary angiography in this patient.

14 Answer A. The angiogram reveals anomalous RCA. Subsequent CT angiogram revealed a course between the aorta and pulmonary artery. She developed ST-segment elevation on vigorous exercise with a treadmill. The following table lists the common congenital coronary anomalies and their clinical manifestations.

15 Answer C. No, there is no convincing data to support the routine use of late (days to weeks) adjuvant PCI days after MI in patients who did not receive reperfusion therapy. This patient had her event 8 days ago and is not stable without hemodynamic compromise or arrhythmia. The most recently conducted largest study, the DECOPI study, failed to find any difference in death, VT and MI at 6 months. However, this study was underpowered to detect differences. Currently, the Occluded Artery Trial is under way to study whether routine PCI days to weeks after MI improves long-term clinical outcome in asymptomatic high-risk patients with occluded infarct-related artery (*Am Heart J.* 2001;142: 411–421).

16 Answer B. The recently published Rescue Angioplasty versus Conservative Treatment or Repeat Thrombolysis (REACT) trial tested medical therapy, repeat fibrinolytic therapy, or PCI in patients with acute MI in whom thrombosis failed. They found that rescue PCI in this patient population reduced recurrent acute MI, but did not decrease death. The patients in whom reperfusion failed to occur (<50% ST-segment resolution) within 90 minutes of thrombolytic treatment were included in this study (*N Engl J Med.* 2005;353:2758–2768).

17 Answer E. In the 2006 ACC/AHA practice guideline for PCI, persistent ischemia, hemodynamic or electrical instability, and severe heart failure are all indications for rescue PCI. The patient had no indication for PCI.

Incidence of the most common coronary artery anomalies in the author's experience and their possible clinical manifestations

Coronary Artery Anomaly	Incidence (%)	Possible Clinical Manifestations
Separate origin of the LAD and LCx	0.31	—
Ectopic origin of the LCx from the RCA	0.25	—
Ectopic origin of the LCx from the right sinus	0.13	—
Myocardial bridge	0.11	UA, AMI, MA, SD
Ectopic origin of the LCA from right sinus	0.098	UA, AMI, MA, SD
Single coronary artery	0.098	SA, UA, SD
Atresic coronary artery	0.039	SI
Dual LAD type IV	0.039	—
Ectopic origin of the RCA from the left sinus	0.039	UA, AMI, MA, SD
Coronary artery fistula	0.039	HF, UA, AMI, SYC
Ectopic origin of the RCA from the PA	0.020	SD
Ectopic origin of the LCA from the PA	0.020	HF, SA, UA
Total	1.21	

LAD, left anterior descending coronary artery; LCx, left circumflex coronary artery; RCA, right coronary artery; UA, unstable angina; AMI, acute myocardial infarction; MA, malignant arrhythmias; SD, sudden death; LCA, left coronary artery; SA, stable angina; SI, silent ischemia; HF, heart failure; SYC, syncope; PA, pulmonary artery.

18 Answer A. Routine PCI in the absence of spontaneous or provocable ischemia does not improve LV function or survival. Some studies have shown increased incidence of bleeding, recurrent ischemia, emergency CABG, and death with routine PCI. However, most studies were done before stents, GPIIb/IIIa inhibitors, and improved anticoagulation therapy. This patient is different from the group studied in the DANAMI trial, which randomized patients with STEMI with spontaneous or inducible angina to catheterization or standard medical therapy (*Circulation.* 1992;85:533–542). The current ACC/AHA guidelines do not recommend routine PCI after fibrinolysis, but the 2005 European guidelines that were published before the reporting of the Assessment of Safety and Efficacy of a New Treatment Strategy for ASSENT-4 trial did recommend routine PCI as a Class I indication.

19 Answer B. According to the 2005 ACC/AHA/SCAI practice guidelines for PCI, there is a Class I indication for performing PCI after failed fibrinolytic therapy among patients, who have severe congestive heart failure within 12 hours of symptom onset. This patient fits within this scenario having a third heart sound, rales, and an occluded RCA within 12 hours of symptom onset.

20 Answer B. As has been reported in previous post hoc analyses of primary angioplasty studies, patients who undergo emergent PCI for AMI and who do achieve TIMI 3 flow or do not have resolution of their ST-segment elevation have a particularly poor outcome. Indeed, in the MERLIN trial patients undergoing rescue PCI, but who failed to have resolution of their ST-segment elevation had a 30-day all-cause mortality of 20% as compared with 6% for those who were treated conservatively, but who attained resolution of their ST-segment elevation, and compared with 3% for those who had rescue PCI and also attained resolution of their ST-segment elevation. It is not clear which pharmacologic adjuncts may best benefit patients at increased risk for failed reperfusion following rescue angioplasty. Several small trials have shown benefit from intracoronary VT such as nitroprusside, while others have shown improved reperfusion with the use of intravenous IIb/IIIa inhibitors. In the MERLIN trial only 3% of patients undergoing rescue angioplasty received a GPIIb/IIIa inhibitor, and 12% were treated with an IABP.

21 Answer E. Although the rescue PCI group did have a numerically lower rate of all-cause mortality compared with repeat thrombosis (6.2% vs. 12.7%) this did not reach statistical significance. On the other hand, there was a significantly lower rate of recurrent MI and a halving of the composite of death, repeat MI, stroke, and severe heart failure (15.3% vs. 31.0%) with PCI versus repeat thrombolytic therapy. There was no difference in the rate of stroke or major bleeding among the groups. The REACT study did not assess the financial implications of the treatment groups (*N Engl J Med.* 2005;353:2758–2768).

22 Answer B. Early and late follow-up in the TIMI 2 study (*JAMA.* 1988;260:2849–2858 and *J Am Coll Cardiol.* 1993;22:1763–1772) showed similar mortality between the treatment groups randomized to aggressive versus conservative strategies. The higher bleeding rates, particularly in TIMI 2A portion of the study, resulted from the close time pairing of the thrombolytic therapy, and the relatively large arterial access sheaths ($\geq$8 F). More recently, with the use of smaller access sheaths and newer thrombolytic regimens, it was hoped that bleeding and mortality would be improved with a contemporary facilitated PCI approach among patients unable to quickly undergo primary PCI. The ASSENT-4 study (*Lancet.* 2006;367:543–546) was discontinued well before the planned enrollment of 4,000 patients because of a higher mortality rate in the group undergoing facilitated PCI (6% vs. 3%). Several other adverse end points (e.g., reinfarctions, stroke, and repeat revascularization) were also higher in the facilitated PCI group though the rate of non-CNS major bleeding was similar in both the groups.

23 Answer B. The latest PCI guidelines were written before the data from ASSENT-4 were fully available, and some information suggests that high-risk patients may benefit from a facilitated PCI approach when primary PCI is not imminently available. Currently available guidelines give facilitated PCI a class IIb indication. There is no class IV indication.

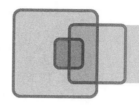

12

Periprocedural Myocardial Infarction and Emboli Protection

Telly A. Meadows and Deepak L. Bhatt

Questions

1 Which of the following is the most common cause of periprocedural myocardial infarction (MI)?

(A) Side branch closure
(B) Occlusive dissection
(C) Microvascular obstruction due to embolization
(D) Epicardial obstruction due to thrombus formation

2 In which of the following percutaneous coronary interventions (PCIs) is there no risk of embolization?

(A) Rotational atherectomy
(B) Directional coronary atherectomy (DCA)
(C) Balloon angioplasty
(D) Extraction atherectomy
(E) Angioplasty with stent deployment
(F) None of the above

3 Which of the following is *not* associated with an increased degree of embolization during percutaneous intervention?

(A) Large plaque burden
(B) Use of DCA
(C) Use of glycoprotein IIb/IIIa (GPIIb/IIIa) inhibitors
(D) Saphenous vein grafts (SVG) interventions
(E) Diffuse atherosclerosis

4 In the Enhanced Myocardial Efficacy and Recovery by Aspiration of Liberated Debris (EMERALD) trial, the use of a balloon occlusion and aspiration distal microcirculatory system during PCI for acute ST-segment elevation myocardial infarction was shown to improve, which of the following?

(A) Microvascular flow
(B) Success of reperfusion
(C) Infarct size
(D) ST-segment resolution
(E) None of the above

5 Which of the following treatments has been shown, in a reasonably powered randomized trial, to significantly reduce the risk of periprocedural MI?

(A) Pretreatment with atorvastatin before elective coronary intervention
(B) Pretreatment with intragraft verapamil before SVG intervention
(C) Thrombectomy before stent implantation in SVG intervention
(D) Rotational atherectomy
(E) Intracoronary urokinase

6 In which of the following interventions has the use of abciximab been shown to reduce the rate of periprocedural MI?

(A) Percutaneous transluminal angioplasty
(B) DCA
(C) Elective stenting
(D) Bailout stenting
(E) All of the above
(F) None of the above

7 Which of the following has been shown to decrease distal embolization during percutaneous intervention of SVGs?

(A) Aspiration thrombectomy with a transluminal extraction catheter

(B) Use of polytetrafluoroethylene (PTFE)-covered stent

(C) DCA

(D) Use of distal balloon occlusion and aspiration system

(E) None of the above

8 Which of the following is an advantage of a filter device as compared with a balloon occlusion device for embolic protection?

(A) Increased impedance of distal flow of cytokines and other vasoactive substances

(B) Better retrieval profile

(C) Better embolic protection

(D) Better visualization of vessel

(E) Better crossing profile

9 In the SVG Angioplasty Free of Emboli Randomized (SAFER) trial, the use of a balloon occlusion/aspiration system (PercuSurge GuardWire) was associated with which of the following outcomes?

(A) Statistically significant reduction in mortality

(B) Statistically significant increase in incidence of complications including distal dissection and perforation

(C) Statistically significant reduction in MI and "no reflow" phenomenon

(D) A and B

(E) A, B and C

10 What is the average rate of major adverse cardiovascular events (MACEs) at 30 days with the use of the currently approved emboli protection devices (EPDs) during PCI of SVGs?

(A) 0% to 15%

(B) 16% to 30%

(C) 31% to 45%

(D) 46% to 60%

(E) >60%

11 Which of the following patient characteristics does *not* increase the risk of periprocedural myonecrosis?

(A) Increased arterial inflammation

(B) Aspirin resistance

(C) Use of clopidogrel

(D) Genetic predisposition

(E) None of the above

12 What is the current rate of periprocedural myonecrosis, defined as any elevation above normal in total creatine kinase (CK) or CK-MB, associated with PCI?

(A) 0% to 15%

(B) 15% to 30%

(C) 31% to 45%

(D) 46% to 60%

(E) >60%

13 In the Evaluation of Platelet IIb/IIIa Inhibition for Prevention of Ischemic Complication (EPIC) trial, an increase in mortality was seen with which of the following magnitudes of periprocedural CK elevation?

(A) ≥10 times the normal CK level only

(B) ≥5 times the normal CK level only

(C) ≥3 times the normal CK level only

(D) ≥1 time the normal CK level only

(E) All of the above

(F) None of the above

14 Periprocedural myonecrosis (MI) has prognostic significance in association with which of the following outcomes?

(A) Immediate in-hospital mortality

(B) Short-term (<30 days) mortality

(C) Long-term (>1 year) mortality

(D) A and B

(E) A, B and C

15 Which of the following factors is *not* associated with a decreased risk of periprocedural MI?

(A) Clopidogrel therapy

(B) High-pressure stenting

(C) Aspirin therapy

(D) Statin therapy

(E) None of the above

16 Intravascular ultrasound (IVUS) has shown which of the following to be associated with higher periprocedural CK elevations?

(A) Plaque burden

(B) Lesion site calcification

(C) IVUS lumen dimension at the lesion site

(D) A and B

(E) A, B and C

17 How does carotid artery stenting with use of an emboli protection device compare with carotid endarterectomy in high risk patients with severe carotid artery stenosis?

(A) Carotid artery stenting with EPDs has been shown to be superior to endarterectomy

(B) Carotid artery stenting with EPDs has been shown to be inferior to endarterectomy

(C) Carotid artery stenting with EPDs has been shown be equivalent to endarterectomy

(D) Carotid artery stenting with EPDs has been shown to be noninferior to endarterectomy

18 Which of the following factors have been shown to be independent predictors of distal embolization during SVG interventions?

(A) Use of DCA
(B) Presence of thrombus
(C) Diffusely diseased vein grafts
(D) A and B
(E) A, B and C

19 During coronary angiography, a patient was discovered to have a total occlusion in the right coronary artery (RCA) (Panel A of the figure below). After percutaneous intervention is performed on the occlusion, the patient is discovered to have another abnormality in the RCA (Panel B of the figure below). What is the abnormality shown at the *arrow* in Panel B?

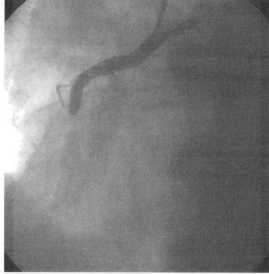

A

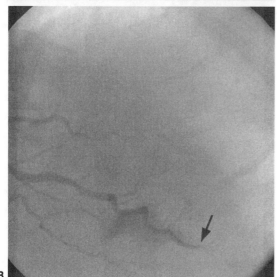

B

(A) Perforation
(B) Distal embolization and cutoff
(C) Vasospasm
(D) Dissection
(E) Stenosis

20 Match the following items listed with the appropriate image (as seen in Panels A–F in the following figure).

(A)

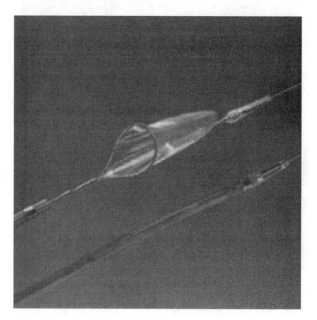

(B)

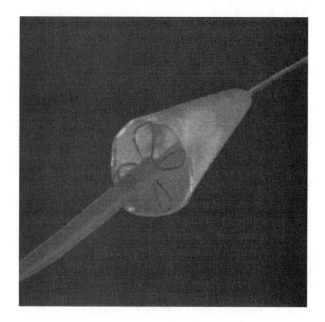

(C)

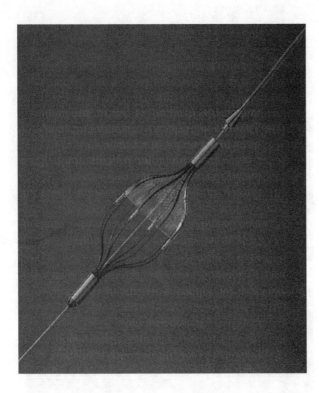

(D)

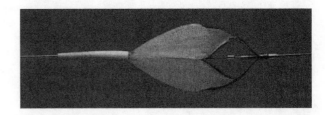

(E)

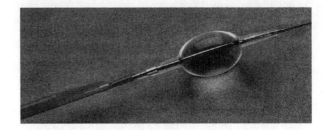

1.   PercuSurge GuardWire device
2.   AngioGuard device
3.   Boston Scientific FilterWire
4.   Guidant AccuNet
5.   IntraTherapeutics IntraGuard

Answers and Explanations

1 Answer C. Periprocedural MI may be caused by all of the answers provided, but the major mechanism is due to embolization of microscopic debris with subsequent platelet activation and inflammation leading to impairment in microvascular flow. The relationship between procedural MI and embolization was revealed through analysis of trials investigating DCA (*Textbook of interventional cardiology*. 2003;251–266). In the Coronary Angioplasty Versus Excisional Atherectomy Trial (CAVEAT) (*N Engl J Med*. 1993;329:221–227), patients undergoing DCA as compared with angioplasty had a significant increase in MI and mortality (8.6% vs. 4.6%; $p = 0.007$) at 6 months perhaps due to increased distal embolization.

2 Answer F. Embolization occurs in all of the PCI modalities listed. DCA and rotational atherectomy have been shown to cause more embolization than balloon angioplasty. In the CAVEAT trial (*N Engl J Med*. 1993;329:221–227), there was a significant increase in death and MI at 6 months associated with DCA when compared with balloon angioplasty, despite there being a significant increase in postprocedural lumen size with DCA. Patients with high-risk lesions in SVGs and native coronary arteries who underwent transluminal extraction atherectomy in the New Approaches to Coronary Interventions (NACI) registry had a high rate of distal embolization at 8.3%. Distal embolization was associated with an in-hospital mortality of 18.5% versus an in-hospital mortality of 3.0% in patients without distal embolization (*Catheter Cardiovasc Interv*. 1999;47:149–154). There is also a higher rate of embolization and periprocedural MI in angioplasty with stenting as compared with balloon angioplasty alone. This is likely due to the "cheese grater" effect that occurs with stent deployment.

3 Answer C. GPIIb/IIIa inhibitors have been shown to decrease the rate of death and MI associated with any percutaneous device (*Am J Cardiol*. 2000;85:1060–1064). This is likely due to the GPIIb/IIIa inhibitors ability to preserve microvascular flow by minimizing the response to distal embolization. Plaque burden and diffuse atherosclerosis have been shown to be associated with embolization and periprocedural MI. SVG interventions are associated with increased risk of embolization due to the large atheroma burden seen in SVGs. More invasive methods of revascularization, such as DCA, are associated with increased embolization (*Textbook of interventional cardiology*. 2003;251–266).

4 Answer E. The EMERALD trial (*JAMA*. 2005;293:1063–1072) randomized 501 patients presenting with ST-segment MI to receive PCI with a balloon occlusion and aspiration distal microcirculatory system versus angioplasty without any distal protection. There was no difference among the treatment groups with respect to either of the coprimary endpoints, which were ST-segment resolution measured 30 minutes after PCI by continuous Holter monitoring and infarct size measured by single photon emission computed tomography (SPECT) imaging between days 5 and 14. There was also no improvement in microvascular flow or success of reperfusion. The secondary endpoint for the trial included major adverse cardiac events related to left ventricular dysfunction (death, new-onset sustained hypotension, new-onset severe heart failure, and hospital readmission for left ventricular dysfunction) and major adverse cardiac events related to ischemia (death, reinfarction, ischemic target vessel revascularization, and disabling stroke). There was no difference in MACE related to either left ventricular dysfunction or ischemic complications at 30 days or 6 months between the two groups even though the device was successful at retrieving embolic debris.

5 Answer A. In the Atorvastatin for Reduction of Myocardial Damage During Angioplasty (ARMYDA) trial (*Circulation*. 2004;110:674–678), patients pretreated with atorvastatin (40 mg per day) 7 days before elective coronary intervention had a significant reduction in all markers for myocardial injury, including CK-MB, troponin I and myoglobin measured at 8 hours and 24 hours after the procedure when compared with patients who did not receive atorvastatin. Postprocedural MI measured by CK-MB occurred in 5% of patients who received atorvastatin versus 18% in patients in the placebo group ($p = 0.025$). Intragraft verapamil before PCI in SVGs was examined in a small study and verapamil was shown to decrease the rate of "no reflow" and improve flow rate in the vessel; however, there was no difference in postprocedural cardiac enzyme release (*J Invasive Cardiol*. 2002;14:303–304). In a study of 797 patients with diseased SVGs or thrombus-containing native coronary arteries, routine thrombectomy before stent implantation did not decrease the incidence of periprocedural MI when compared with stent implantation without thrombectomy (*J Am Coll Cardiol.* 2003;42:2007–2013). Many studies have shown the increased rates of distal embolization and periprocedural MI with directional and rotational atherectomy.

6 Answer E. Embolization is known to occur with all PCI modalities. Abciximab, a GPIIb/IIIa inhibitor, has been shown to be beneficial in reducing the rate of periprocedural infarction and death regardless of the interventional device used (*Am J Cardiol.* 2000;85:1060–1064). GPIIb/IIIa inhibitors, through their antiplatelet effect, have been shown to reduce microvascular occlusion and the subsequent left ventricular dysfunction that occurs with distal embolization. This may manifest clinically as an improvement in long-term mortality seen with the GPIIb/IIIa inhibitors.

7 Answer D. Percutaneous intervention of SVGs is associated with an increased risk of embolization due to the presence of the large atheroma burden. Accordingly, periprocedural MI rates are increased with PCI of vein grafts as compared with PCI of native coronary arteries. In the SAFER trial (*Circulation.* 2002;105:1285–1290), the use of the PercuSurge GuardWire system (a distal balloon occlusion and aspiration system) was associated with a 42% relative risk reduction in major cardiovascular events at 30 days, which included a significant reduction in MI and "no reflow" phenomenon. In the CAVEAT I trial (*Circulation.* 1995;91:1966–1974), DCA of *de novo* vein graft lesions was associated with increased rates of distal embolization when compared with angioplasty alone. The Symbiot trial (*J Invasive Cardiol.* 2005;17:609–612.) failed to show any decrease in the rate of distal embolization with the use of the Symbiot, a PTFE-covered stent as compared with bare-metal stents during PCI of SVGs. Routine thrombectomy before stent implantation in PCI of SVGs has also never been shown to decrease periprocedural myocardial ischemia.

8 Answer D. The two basic types of EPDs available are the filter and balloon occlusion devices. Each device carries its own advantages and disadvantages when compared with the other. Some of the advantages of the filter device are that it allows blood to flow through it while preventing flow of embolic debris greater than its pore size. The balloon occlusion devices currently have a better crossing profile than the filter devices. The balloon occlusion device prevents flow to the distal circulation and traps all embolic debris. The disadvantage of preventing all distal flow is that it prohibits visualization of the vessel beyond the device. However, one potential benefit of preventing distal flow is the prevention of the passage of cytokines and other vasoactive substances.

9 Answer C. In the SAFER trial (*Circulation.* 2002; 105:1285–1290.), 801 patients undergoing percutaneous intervention to stenotic SVGs were randomly assigned to stent placement over the shaft of the PercuSurge GuardWire balloon occlusion and aspiration system versus stent placement over a conventional angioplasty guidewire. Use of the distal protection device resulted in a 42% relative risk reduction in the primary endpoint, which was a composite of death, MI, emergency bypass, or target lesion revascularization by 30 days. Analysis of the individual components of the primary endpoint revealed a statistically significant reduction in MI and "no reflow." There was a 50% reduction in mortality (2.32% vs. 1.0%) with use of the emboli protection device, but this did not reach statistical significance. The reduction in the primary endpoint was really driven by the reduction in periprocedural MI.

10 Answer A. The MACE rate with use of the current EPDs (including distal filters, proximal devices, and distal balloon occlusion/aspiration systems) is 7–12% depending upon the device. The SAFER trial, which evaluated a distal balloon occlusion and aspiration system (PercuSurge GuardWire), had a 9.6% MACE rate at 30 days. In the FilterWire EX Randomized Evaluation (FIRE) trial (*J Am Coll Cardiol.* 2002;40:1882–1888), which assessed the utility of a distal filter device (FilterWire EX), there was a 30-day MACE rate of 11.3%. The Protection Devices in PCI Treatment of Myocardial Infarction for Salvage of Endangered Myocardium (PROMISE) trial (*unpublished, presented at TCT 2005 meeting*), examining the efficacy of a proximal balloon and occlusion system (Proxis), had a 9.2% MACE at 30 days. The Protection During Saphenous Vein Graft Intervention to Prevent Distal Embolization (PRIDE) trial (*J Am Coll Cardiol.* 2005;46: 1677–1683), which examined the use of a balloon-protection flush and extraction system (TriActiv System), found an 11.2% MACE at 30 days.

11 Answer C. The PCI-CURE trial (*Lancet.* 2001;358: 527–533) was the first to show a significant reduction in cardiovascular death or MI with clopidogrel pretreatment in patients with non–ST-elevation acute coronary syndrome undergoing PCI. The ARMYDA-2 trial (*Circulation.* 2005;111:2099–2106) randomized patients undergoing PCI to a high loading dose of clopidogrel (600 mg) versus the conventional loading dose of clopidogrel (300 mg). There was a 50% reduction in the risk of MI with the higher loading dose. Genetic predisposition, aspirin resistance, and increased arterial inflammation are factors believed to increase the risk of periprocedural myonecrosis (*Circulation.* 2005;111:906–912).

12 Answer B. Many studies have shown the rate of myonecrosis associated with PCI to be approximately 25%. The rate of myonecrosis is even higher, at least 50%, if the more sensitive troponin measurement is used (*Circulation.* 2005;111:906–912). An important distinction between using CK and CK-MB measurements to assess periprocedural MI versus using troponin measurements is that CK and CK-MB values have more prognostic significance in regard to future clinical outcomes including short-term and long-term mortality.

13 Answer E. The EPIC trial (*JAMA.* 1997;278:479–484) was one of the first trials to demonstrate the association between periprocedural MI and increased mortality in the intermediate period after percutaneous intervention. The study demonstrated a direct relationship between degree of CK elevation postprocedure and 3-year mortality. Patients with CK elevations 10X, 5X, and 3X the normal CK level had an estimated mortality rate at 3 years of 16.5%, 14.8%, and 13.1%, respectively. As compared with those with normal CK levels, patients with CK levels greater than once the upper limit of normal also had an increased mortality rate at 3 years (10.2% vs. 7.3%).

14 Answer E. Total CK and CK-MB elevations after percutaneous interventions are associated with adverse outcomes, including mortality, beginning in the immediate in-hospital period and extending up to 10 years after the procedure. This relationship between periprocedural MI and clinical outcomes has been validated by many large studies and metaanalyses. Although many of the studies have used various CK and CK-MB elevations as their cutoff in defining periprocedural MI, a statistically significant increase in mortality has been shown with any periprocedural CK elevation (*Circulation.* 2005;112:906–915; discussion 923).

15 Answer B. High-pressure stenting and stent overexpansion have been shown to increase periprocedural CK-MB elevation (*J Am Coll Cardiol.* 2003;

42:1900–1905). On the contrary, potent antiplatelet and antithrombotic therapies including aspirin, clopidogrel, and GPIIb/IIIa inhibitors have been shown to attenuate the impact of embolization during PCI leading to reductions in periprocedural MI. Baseline levels of hsCRP, a marker of inflammation, have been shown to predict the occurrence of periprocedural MI. Statins, which have potent anti-inflammatory effects, have been shown to significantly reduce the risk of periprocedural MI when given before PCI. Clopidogrel has also been shown to attenuate periprocedural levels of hsCRP (*Am J Cardiol.* 2004;94:358–360). It is possible that the benefit of clopidogrel pretreatment may in part be due to its anti-inflammatory effects in addition to its antiplatelet effects.

16 Answer D. In a study of 2,256 patients undergoing intervention of native coronaries, IVUS found many determinants of periprocedural MI. Plaque burden at the lesion, lesion site calcification, positive remodeling, cross-sectional narrowing at the lesion, and reference sites were all associated with CK-MB elevations. In the multivariate analysis, age, sex, diabetes mellitus, and lumen dimension at the lesion site before and after intervention were not predictive of CK-MB elevation (*Circulation.* 2000;101:604–610).

17 Answer D. In the Stenting and Angioplasty with Protection in Patients at High Risk for Endarterectomy (SAPPHIRE) trial, 334 patients with symptomatic carotid artery stenosis >50% or asymptomatic stenosis of >80% with comorbidities that made them high risk for endarterectomy were randomized to carotid stenting with use of a filter wire protection device (Angioguard or Angioguard XP) or carotid endarterectomy. The primary endpoint, which was the cumulative incidence of MACE at 1 year occurred in 12.2% of the patients assigned to carotid artery stenting versus 20.1% in the patients randomly assigned to carotid endarterectomy. The trial was a noninferior study by design, and the less invasive treatment of carotid artery stenting with the use of an EPD was shown to be noninferior to carotid endarterectomy (*N Engl J Med.* 2004;351:1493–1501).

18 Answer E. The CAVEAT-II was a prospective, multicenter trial comparing percutaneous transluminal coronary angioplasty versus DCA in patients with SVG lesions. From this study, the use of DCA and the presence of thrombus were both determined to be independent predictors of distal embolization (*Circulation.* 1995;92:734–740). In another study that examined the angiographic predictors of distal embolization after balloon angioplasty of SVGs, diffusely diseased vein grafts and large plaque volume were determined to be independent predictors of distal embolization (*Am J Cardiol.* 1993;72:514–517). Other studies have also found graft age to be a predictor of distal embolization.

19 **Answer B.** The angiogram shows distal embolization and cutoff in the distal posterior descending artery (PDA) after intervention was performed to the complete occlusion in the mid segment of the RCA.

20 **Answer A-5, B-3, C-1, D-4, E-2.**

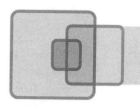

13

Chronic Total Occlusions

David E. Kandzari

Questions

1 Compared with percutaneous revascularization of nonocclusive coronary lesions, which statement best characterizes outcomes among patients with chronic total occlusions when using bare-metal stents (BMSs)?

(A) Chronic total occlusions have higher rates of restenosis and reocclusion

(B) Restenosis is higher with total occlusions, but reocclusion rates are similar

(C) Reocclusion is more frequent among total coronary occlusions, but restenosis rates are similar

(D) Rates of both restenosis and reocclusion are similar

2 Which variable best predicts improvement in left ventricular function following successful recanalization of a chronic total occlusion?

(A) History of prior myocardial infarction (MI)

(B) Baseline left ventricular dysfunction

(C) Angiographic presence of collateral flow

(D) Duration of occlusion

3 Compared with conventional BMSs, treatment with drug-eluting stents (DESs) following recanalization of chronic total occlusions is associated with all of the following, *except*:

(A) Reductions in restenosis

(B) Decrease in repeat target lesion revascularization

(C) Improved survival

(D) Decreased rates of reocclusion

4 Compared with procedural failure to recanalize chronic total occlusions, successful percutaneous revascularization of chronic total occlusions is associated with all of the following, *except*:

(A) Improved long-term survival

(B) Increased need for repeat revascularization procedures

(C) Reduced angina

(D) Improved left ventricular function

5 The most common reason for failure of percutaneous revascularization of chronic total occlusions is:

(A) Guidewire entry into a subintimal dissection plane

(B) Inability to cross the occluded segment

(C) Inability to deliver an angioplasty balloon

(D) Coronary artery perforation

6 Which of the following statements regarding coronary perforation in revascularization of total coronary occlusions is *true*?

(A) In-hospital mortality is similar among patients who do and do not experience cardiac tamponade

(B) Cardiac tamponade often develops hours following the interventional procedure

(C) Guidewire perforation most commonly occurs distal to the occluded segment

(D) Angiographic evidence of contrast extravasation excludes the diagnosis of cardiac tamponade

7   Which of the following statements regarding collateral flow in chronic total occlusions is *not* true?

(A) Collateral function is worse in patients with impaired regional wall motion

(B) The presence and extent of collateral flow predicts improvement in ventricular function following revascularization

(C) Collateral function regresses after recanalization of chronic total occlusions

(D) Growth factor expression is related to collateral function and the duration of occlusion

8   Which of the following technologies/strategies has demonstrated significantly higher procedural success over coronary guidewires in a randomized trial?

(A) Excimer laser guidewire
(B) Fibrinolytic infusion
(C) Optical coherence tomography guidewire
(D) None of the above

9   Advances in coronary guidewires for chronic total occlusions include all of the following, *except*:

(A) Tapered tip
(B) Hydrophilic coating
(C) Increased tip stiffness
(D) Absence of coiled tip

10   Which characteristic is *not* a predictor of procedural failure in chronic total coronary occlusion revascularization?

(A) Presence of sidebranch at site of occlusion

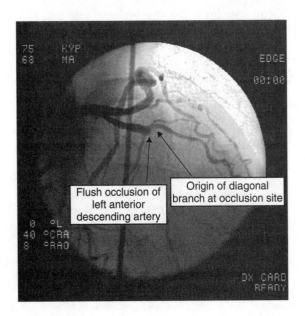

(B) Tapered stump of occlusion

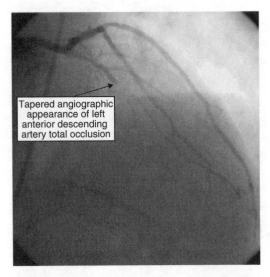

(C) Bridging collaterals

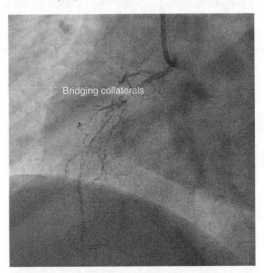

(D) Duration of total occlusion

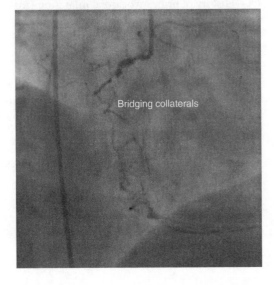

11 Compared with the treatment of nonocclusive lesions, percutaneous revascularization of chronic total occlusions is characterized by all of the following procedural characteristics, *except*:

(A) Increased use of iodinated contrast
(B) Increased exposure to ionizing radiation
(C) Increased stent length and number
(D) Increased risk of in-hospital death and myocardial infarction

12 Chronic total occlusions:

(A) Are present in approximately one-half of patients with other significant coronary disease
(B) Are identified in approximately one-third of all diagnostic coronary angiograms
(C) Account for approximately 10% of all percutaneous revascularization procedures
(D) All of the above

13 Chronic total coronary occlusions are most prevalent in which vessel?

(A) Left anterior descending artery
(B) Left circumflex artery
(C) Right coronary artery
(D) Left main artery

14 The pathophysiology of chronic total occlusions includes which of the following?

(A) Adventitial neovascularization
(B) Expression of collagen types I and III
(C) Organized thrombus
(D) All of the above

15 Angiographic collateral flow is a predictor of:

(A) Improvement in left ventricular function
(B) Restenosis
(C) Reocclusion
(D) None of the above

16 Before crossing a total coronary occlusion with a guidewire, appropriate adjunctive pharmacology includes treatment with which agent?

(A) Bivalirudin
(B) Unfractionated heparin
(C) Glycoprotein IIb/IIIa inhibitor
(D) Low-molecular-weight heparin

17 Which statement best characterizes the histology of chronic total coronary occlusions?

(A) Approximately one-half of chronic total occlusions are <99% stenotic despite their angiographic appearance
(B) The severity of lumen stenosis is related to lesion age
(C) Collagen-rich fibrous tissue is most dense in the midsegment of the total occlusion
(D) Inflammation is most prevalent in the adventitia

18 In patients with ST-segment elevation myocardial infarction who do not receive reperfusion therapy, a total occlusion is identified in approximately what percent of patients at 1 month?

(A) 10%
(B) 25%
(C) 50%
(D) 75%

19 In patients with chronic total occlusions who undergo attempted revascularization, which factor is most predictive of increased long-term mortality risk?

(A) Chronic kidney disease
(B) Diabetes mellitus
(C) Multivessel coronary disease
(D) Procedural failure

20 Technical maneuvers to confirm guidewire placement in the distal true lumen may include all of the following, *except*:

(A) Use of contralateral angiography
(B) Ability to deliver angioplasty balloon
(C) Use of intravascular ultrasound
(D) Contrast injection through end-hole catheter

Answers and Explanations

1 Answer A. Chronic total occlusion revascularization with BMSs is associated with considerably higher rates of restenosis and reocclusion compared with stenting of nonocclusive lesions. In the Total Occlusion Study of Canada (TOSCA)-1 (*Circulation.* 1999;100:236–242), the rates of restenosis and reocclusion at 6-month angiographic follow-up were 55% and 11%, respectively, among patients assigned to treatment with BMSs. In the Stenting in Chronic Coronary Occlusion (SICCO) trial (*J Am Coll Cardiol.* 1996;28:1444–14451), the reocclusion rate was 16% in the stent cohort.

2 Answer B. Compared with patients with normal or regional impairment of left ventricular function and chronic total occlusions, patients with global left ventricular dysfunction derive the greatest relative improvement in the percent ejection fraction (EF) and decrease in wall motion severity index following successful revascularization. In a recent study of patients with angiographic follow-up, baseline left ventricular dysfunction was an independent predictor of improvement in left ventricular function (*Am Heart J.* 2005;149:129–137). Variables including angiographic collateral flow, duration of occlusion or history of myocardial infarction were not predictive of improvement. Recent studies with cardiac magnetic resonance angiography have also identified dysfunctional but viable myocardium as the most significant predictor of improvement in the left ventricular EF and wall motion severity index (*Am Heart J.* 2005;96:165H). Finally, TOSCA examined the influence of successful revascularization on left ventricular EF and regional wall motion (*Am Heart J.* 2001;142:301–308). Although an occlusion duration ≤6 weeks was independently predictive of a significant increase in the percent EF, the greatest improvement was among patients with baseline EF <60%.

3 Answer C. Several recent studies have examined the safety and efficacy of DESs in chronic total occlusion revascularization. In most instances, nonrandomized observational studies have compared angiographic and clinical outcomes with historical controls of patients with total coronary occlusions treated with BMSs. A consistent finding among these trials is a significant reduction in angiographic binary restenosis, reocclusion, and the need for repeat target vessel revascularization. In the only randomized trial to date comparing sirolimus-eluting and BMSs, treatment with sirolimus-eluting stents was associated with an 81% relative reduction in in-stent restenosis at 6-month angiographic follow-up (36% vs. 7%, *p* <0.0001) (*Transcatheter therapeutics 2005 scientific sessions.* 2005). There were no differences in survival between patients treated with BMSs or DESs.

4 Answer B. Several observational studies examining the influence of attempted percutaneous revascularization of chronic total occlusions have demonstrated that compared with failed attempts, successful revascularization is associated with improved long-term survival, reduced angina, and improvements in left ventricular EF and regional wall motion (*J Am Coll Cardiol.* 2003;41:1672–1678, *Circulation.* 2001;104:2–415, *J Am Coll Cardiol.* 2001;38:409–414). Successful total occlusion revascularization is not associated with an increased need for repeat revascularization but instead a significant improvement in event-free survival from bypass surgery (*Circulation.* 2001;104:2–415).

5 Answer B. The most common mode of failure is inability to successfully pass a guidewire across the occluded segment into the distal true lumen of the vessel. Among 397 patients undergoing attempted total occlusion revascularization (*J Am Coll Cardiol.* 1995;26:409–415), the most common reasons for procedural failure were inability to cross the lesion with a guidewire (63% of cases), long intimal dissection with creation of a false lumen (24%), dye extravasation (11%), failure to cross with a balloon or dilate (2%), and thrombus formation (1.2%).

6 Answer B. In a series of patients who developed cardiac tamponade from complications related to percutaneous coronary intervention, cardiac tamponade was diagnosed on an average of 4.4 hours following completion of the procedure (*Am J Cardiol.* 2002;90:1183–1186). The occurrence of cardiac tamponade is associated with a high likelihood of in-hospital death and myocardial infarction. Guidewire perforation typically occurs at the site of the occluded segment; however, perforation may occur in the distal segment of the vessel, underscoring the need to exchange stiff, tapered, or hydrophilic guidewires for soft, less traumatic guidewires after successful crossing. Absence of contrast extravasation does not exclude the possibility of cardiac tamponade. Therefore, if perforation is suspected although not angiographically evident, important measures include serial echocardiography and hemodynamic monitoring.

7 **Answer B.**   Recovery of impaired left ventricular function after revascularization of a chronic total occlusion is not directly related to the extent of collateral function (*Am Heart J.* 2005;149:129–137). Growth factor expression, in particular, fibroblast growth factor, has been related to both the duration of occlusion and collateral function (*Circulation.* 2004;110:1940–1945). Collateral function is better in patients with a total coronary occlusion and normal regional wall motion than in patients with impaired regional function (*Circulation.* 2001;104:2784–2790). Collateral function also regresses during long-term follow-up after successful recanalization and may not be readily recruitable in the event of acute occlusion (*Circulation.* 2003;108:2877–2882).

8 **Answer D.**   Of the techniques listed, only the laser wire has been compared with conventional coronary guidewires in a randomized trial. In the Total Occlusion Trial with Angioplasty by using a Laser Wire (TOTAL) trial (*Eur Heart J.* 2000;21:1797–1805), 303 patients with chronic total occlusions were randomized to treatment with either the laser wire or conventional wire technique. Successful lesion crossing was achieved in 53% of the laser wire cohort versus 47% in the conventional wire group ($p = 0.33$).

9 **Answer D.**   Guidewires with a tapering tip diameter of 0.009 to 0.011 inches may facilitate wire engagement in microchannels of chronic total occlusions. Similarly, guidewires with incremental tip stiffness may penetrate the occluded segment more easily and provide greater shape retention. Hydrophilic wires typically advance with minimal resistance and are easily maneuverable in tortuous vessels, and are therefore used by some operators in chronic total occlusions. However, hydrophilic wires must also be used with caution because they are more likely to penetrate beneath the plaque and cause dissection and more frequently select small vessel branches, increasing the likelihood of perforation (*Catheter Cardiovasc Interv.* 2005;66:217–236).

10 **Answer B.**   Compared with a blunted appearance of the occlusion or side branch presence at site of occlusion, angiographic appearance of a tapered occlusion has been associated with an increased likelihood of procedural success (*Catheter Cardiovasc Interv.* 2000;49:258–264, *J Am Coll Cardiol.* 2003;41:1672–1678, *Catheter Cardiovasc Interv.* 2005;66:217–236, *Br Heart J.* 1993;70:126–131). Increasing duration of the occlusion and the presence of bridging collaterals are also associated with increased procedural failure (*Catheter Cardiovasc Interv.* 2000;49:258–264, *J Am Coll Cardiol.* 2003;41:1672–1678, *Catheter Cardiovasc Interv.* 2005;66:217–236, *Br Heart J.* 1993;70:126–131).

11 **Answer D.**   Attempted total occlusion revascularization is associated with increased use of iodinated contrast and exposure to ionizing radiation. Because significant disease distal to the occluded segment may not be readily visible on the initial angiogram, successful recanalization is often associated with considerably greater stent length and number compared with the treatment of nonocclusive disease.

Among 2,007 procedures for chronic total occlusion revascularization over a 20-year period, the annualized in-hospital major adverse event rate was 3.8%, which did not statistically differ from the major complication rate from a matched cohort of 2,007 patients undergoing treatment during the same period for nonoccluded vessels (*J Am Coll Cardiol.* 2001;38:409–414). However, compared with those patients in whom the procedure was successful, the in-hospital occurrence of major adverse cardiac events was significantly higher among patients with procedural failure (3.2% vs. 5.4%, $p = 0.02$).

12 **Answer D.**   Overall, a chronic total occlusion is identified in approximately one-third of all diagnostic coronary angiograms, yet attempted percutaneous revascularization of a total occlusion accounts for <10% of all percutaneous coronary interventions (*Am Heart J.* 1993;126:561–564, *Circulation.* 2002;106:1627–1633). However, in a summary of 8,004 patients presenting for diagnostic cardiac catheterization over a 10-year period, a chronic total occlusion was identified in 52% of patients with significant disease (≥70% stenosis) in another major epicardial vessel (*Am J Cardiol.* 2005;95:1088–1091).

13 **Answer C.**   According to the National Heart, Lung and Blood Dynamic Registry (*Circulation.* 2002;106:1627–1633), chronic total occlusions are most prevalent in the right coronary artery and least common in the left circumflex artery. The frequency of total occlusions also increases with advancing age. Total occlusion of the right coronary artery was identified in 18.2%, 21.3%, and 22.8% of patients <65 years, 65 to 79 years, and ≥80 years of age, respectively (*Am Heart J.* 2003;146:513–519).

14   **Answer D.**   Chronic total occlusions most commonly develop from thrombotic occlusion followed by thrombus organization and collagen deposition (in particular, types I and III) (*J Am Coll Cardiol.* 1993;21:604–611). Neovascularization is also prominent and begins within the adventitia. As total occlusions age, angiogenesis becomes more extensive, and the number and size of capillaries in the intima and adventitia become similar.

15   **Answer D.**   The presence and extent of angiographic collateral flow has been associated with the presence of viable and functional myocardium, but it does not predict the improvement in regional wall motion or occurrence of restenosis or reocclusion following successful revascularization (*Am Heart J.* 2005;149:129–137).

16   **Answer B.**   Attempted revascularization of chronic total occlusions is best performed using unfractionated heparin to achieve an activated clotting time of approximately 250 seconds (*Catheter Cardiovasc Interv.* 2005;66:217–236). If the lesion is successfully crossed, additional heparin and/or a glycoprotein IIb/IIIa antagonist may be administered. However, if a complication (e.g., coronary perforation) occurs, unfractionated heparin may be readily reversed with intravenous protamine sulfate. In contrast, antithrombin agents such as direct thrombin inhibitors (e.g., bivalirudin) and glycoprotein IIb/IIIa inhibitors are not readily reversible and therefore, present increased risk of bleeding complications if coronary perforation occurs.

17   **Answer A.**   By histology, approximately one-half of chronic total occlusions are <99% stenotic despite the angiographic appearance of thrombolysis in myocardial infarction (TIMI)-0 flow. Inflammation is most prevalent in the intima of chronic total occlusions, regardless of the lesion age (*J Am Coll Cardiol.* 1993;21:604–611). No relationship exists between the severity of stenosis and either plaque composition or lesion age. The concentration of collagen-rich fibrous tissue is particularly dense at the proximal and distal ends of the lesion with a midsegment characterized by soft lipid core and organized thrombus.

18   **Answer C.**   In patients with ST-segment elevation myocardial infarction not treated with reperfusion therapy, an occluded infarct-related artery has been identified in 87% of patients within 4 hours, 65% within 12 to 24 hours, 53% at 15 days, and 45% at 1 month (*Am Heart J.* 1979;97:61–69, *Circulation.* 1982;65:1099–1105, *N Engl J Med.* 1980;303:897–902).

19   **Answer D.**   Several observational studies have demonstrated increased long-term mortality among patients with failed attempts at total occlusion revascularization compared with successful revascularization (*Eur Heart J.* 2005;26:2630–2636, *J Am Coll Cardiol.* 2003;41:1672–1678, *Circulation.* 2001;104:2–415, *J Am Coll Cardiol.* 2001;38:409–414). In a multivariable model in 1,118 patients with chronic total occlusions in the British Columbia Cardiac Registry (*Circulation.* 2001;104:2–415), only the factors of end-stage renal disease and left ventricular dysfunction were more predictive of late mortality than procedural failure. The following table shows consistently higher mortality among patients undergoing failed versus successful percutaneous revascularization of chronic total occlusions.

Trial	Success (N)	Failure (N)	Follow-up Duration (years)	Mortality (%) Success	Failure	p value
British Columbia Cardiac Registry[a]	1,118	340	6	10.0	19.0	< 0.001
Suero et al.[b]	1,491	514	10	26.0	35.0	0.001
TOAST-GISE[c]	286	83	1	1.1	3.6	0.13
Aziz et al.[d]	377	166	2.4	2.5	7.3	0.049
Hoye et al.[e]	568	306	5	6.5	12.0	0.02

[a] *Am Heart J.* 1979;97:61–69.
[b] *Circulation.* 1982;65:1099–1105.
[c] *Circulation.* 1999;100:236–242.
[d] *Am J Cardiol.* 2005;95:1088–1091.
[e] *Am Heart J.* 2003;146:513–519.

20 **Answer B.** Use of contralateral angiography is essential to identify the distal true lumen through collateral vessels. Intravascular ultrasound may help distinguish a false passage into a subintimal dissection from the true lumen. Removal of the guidewire from an end-hole catheter placed distal to the occluded segment and contrast injection may help confirm placement into the true lumen if flow is observed without adventitial staining with contrast. Ability to deliver an angioplasty balloon past the occluded segment should not be interpreted as passage into the distal true lumen because the catheter may be easily advanced into a false lumen.

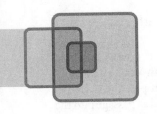

14

Ostial and Bifurcation Lesions

Antonio Colombo

Questions

1 The main difference between stent treatment of aorto-ostial and nonaorto-ostial stenosis is:

(A) There is no specific difference

(B) When treating a lesion located at the aorto-ostial location the stent should protrude a few millimeters into the aorta

(C) The need to have the stent protrude proximally a few millimeters applies also for nonaorto-ostial lesions

(D) Nonaorto-ostial lesions should be treated with the cutting balloon

2 Directional coronary atherectomy remains an important technique to be used for ostial lesions located in the left anterior descending (LAD) artery:

(A) Only registries and single-center experiences support this statement

(B) A study evaluating the outcome of directional atherectomy versus drug-eluting stents (DESs) confirmed the superiority of the second approach

(C) The combination of directional atherectomy and drug-eluting stenting is the most effective one

(D) None of the above

3 Which device among the ones listed has been proposed as a suitable device to treat ostial lesions?

(A) The cutting balloon as a stand-alone device in severely calcified lesions

(B) The Excimer laser in severe calcified lesions

(C) Rotational atherectomy

(D) None of the above

4 Regarding usage of bare-metal stents (BMSs) in bifurcation lesions:

(A) Elective implantation of two stents is an advisable approach provided final kissing balloon is performed

(B) The provisional side branch approach should always be considered first

(C) When feasible the side branch should be treated with cutting balloon dilatation before stenting

(D) Directional atherectomy performed before stenting will lower the risk of plaque shift toward the side branch

5 In a classic study by Al Suwaidi and others from Mayo Clinic (*J Am Coll Cardiol.* 2000;35:929–936) reporting results of bifurcational bare-metal stenting, the authors conclude:

(A) Acute procedural success was higher in the group treated with two stents

(B) There was a lower incidence of in-hospital major adverse cardiovascular event (MACE) (0% vs. 13%, $p < 0.05$) in patients treated with only one stent

(C) There was a significantly lower restenosis rate when only one stent was implanted on the main branch

(D) The authors conclude that selective implantation of two stents may be advantageous

6 The "stent pull-back technique" has been described as:

(A) An approach to treat aorto-ostial lesions

(B) An approach to treat nonaorto-ostial lesions

(C) A way to retrieve an embolized stent

(D) Demanding usage of a guide catheter, which is at least 7 French in size

7 The Atherectomy before MULTI-LINK Improves lumen Gain and clinical Outcomes (AMIGO) trial failed to demonstrate the primary endpoint (atherectomy and stenting reduces binary restenosis compared with stenting) but showed that in the subgroup of lesions with ostial location the benefit of atherectomy and stenting was significantly better compared with stenting alone:

(A) False
(B) True

8 The usage of DESs in bifurcational lesions is an approach evaluated in a randomized trial, which showed:

(A) No specific advantage compared with BMSs regarding restenosis at the ostium of the side branch
(B) No specific advantage of the Cypher stent versus the Taxus stent
(C) The provisional stent approach had a statistically significant advantage in terms of restenosis compared with the two-stent approach
(D) None of the above

9 The following classification of bifurcation lesion is:

Type A
Prebranch stenosis not involving the ostium of the side branch

Type B
Postbranch stenosis of the parent vessel not involving the ostium of the side branch

Type C
Stenosis of the parent vessel not involving the ostium of the side branch

Type D
Stenosis involving the parent vessel and the ostium of the side branch

Type E
Stenosis involving the ostium of the side branch only

Type F
Stenosis discretely involving the parent vessel and ostium of the side branch

(A) The Lefevre classification
(B) The Medina classification
(C) The Duke classification
(D) The Sanborn classification

10 When performing the crush technique with a sirolimus-eluting stent which of these is important?

(A) Always deploy stent using an 8 French guiding catheter
(B) Perform a final kissing balloon inflation
(C) Restenosis and thrombosis rates are influenced by the performance of final kissing balloon inflation
(D) The most frequent site for restenosis is the body of the side branch

11 For the lesion shown, which is the best treatment strategy?

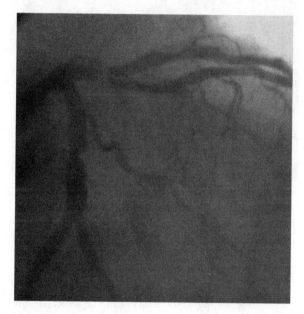

(A) Culottes stenting
(B) Crush stenting
(C) Provisional side branch stenting
(D) Any of the above

12 The best adjunctive pharmacologic approach when dealing with bifurcational lesions is:

(A) Elective administration of IIb/IIIa inhibitors
(B) Elective administration of bivalirudin
(C) Elective administration of bivalirudin and IIb/IIIa inhibitors in selected unstable patients
(D) No specific recommendations can be made at this time

13 Among the most likely causes of restenosis at the ostium of the side branch when two DESs are implanted on a bifurcation, the most likely explanation is:

(A) The stent was damaged while crossing the stent implanted on the main branch
(B) The operator left a gap between the main branch and the side branch stent

(C) The stent on the side branch has been underdilated

(D) All the above are true

14 If DES implantation is considered a clinically appropriate procedure in a patient with a lesion involving an unprotected left main artery shown below, the best approach is:

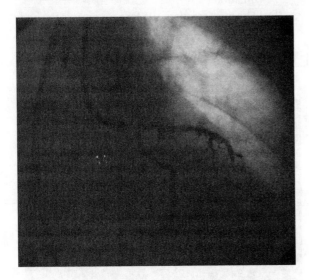

(A) Perform directional atherectomy and then implant two DESs

(B) Implanting a DES toward the LAD artery leaving the implantation of a second stent toward the circumflex a possible option

(C) Proceed with elective implantation of two stents: one in the LAD artery and the other in the circumflex

(D) B and C are correct

15 In a bench model evaluating flow dynamics in bifurcations, which of the following findings is *true*:

(A) The pattern of flow in the main branch was directly affected by alterations in the side branch alone

(B) Platelet activation but not leukocyte recruitment was directly influenced by changes in flow pattern

(C) Optimal side branch lumen will eliminate flow disturbances in the main branch

(D) All the above are true

16 The concept of "stent deformation" in the context of bifurcational stenting has been put forward to:

(A) Explain some insufficient results obtained with culottes stenting

(B) Explain the coverage of the ostium of the side branch and the importance of kissing balloon inflation

(C) Explain some cases of stent recoil in bifurcation located in tortuous segments

(D) Support the need for final kissing inflation when performing crush stenting

17 When performing culottes stenting, which of the following statements should be considered *invalid*:

(A) Implantation of two Cypher stents in a 3.5-mm bifurcation is appropriate

(B) Implantation of two Cypher stents in a 2.5-mm bifurcation is appropriate

(C) Implantation of two Cypher stents in a 3-mm bifurcation is appropriate

(D) Implantation of one 3.0-mm Cypher and one 2.5-mm Cypher in a bifurcation with the main branch 3 mm in diameter

18 Compared with nonbifurcation lesions, PCI with BMS implantation is associated with:

(A) Higher rates of myocardial infarction (MI) at 9 months

(B) Higher rates of death at 9 months

(C) Higher rates of target vessel revascularization (TVR) at 9 months

(D) Lower rates of TVR at 9 months

19 In bifurcational lesions, the measurement of fractional flow reserve (FFR) on side branches with >50% angiographic residual narrowing after stent implantation on the main branch provides the following findings:

(A) Most lesions have normal values of FFR (>0.75), indicating the absence of functional significance of the narrowing in all cases

(B) All the lesions have a normal value of FFR (<0.75), indicating the absence of functional significance of the narrowing in all cases

(C) All the lesions have a reduced value of FFR (<0.75), indicating the functional significance of the narrowing in all cases

(D) The measurement of FFR in this setting should be avoided due to the high rate of complications when recrossing through stent struts with the pressure guidewire

20 Which of the following statements is common to ostial and bifurcational lesions?

(A) They have never been evaluated in the context of randomized studies

(B) Both are ideally suitable for directional atherectomy

(C) The results following implantation of DESs are similar to the other lesion types

(D) None of the above is true

Answers and Explanations

1 Answer B. The most appropriate way to treat lesions located at the aorto-ostial location is to place a stent, which will slightly protrude into the aorta. This approach will guarantee optimal coverage of the ostium.

2 Answer A. Directional atherectomy can be used to treat ostial lesions located in the LAD artery and some centers still apply this technique with or without subsequent stenting (*Heart*. 2003;89:1050–1054, *Am J Cardiol*. 2002;90:1074–1078). Despite favorable results there are no data to support any specific advantage compared with stenting with a DES, an approach, which has given favorable results in a recently published registry (*J Am Coll Cardiol*. 2005;46:787–792).

3 Answer C. All the devices have been used and are suggested as appropriate to treat ostial lesions of the LAD artery. The cutting balloon as a stand-alone device is very likely not to cross the lesion. As general knowledge, a number of single-center studies (*J Invasive Cardiol*. 1999;11:231–232, *Heart*. 1997;77:350–352, *J Invasive Cardiol*. 1999;11:201–206) reported the beneficial combination of stenting preceded by cutting balloon dilatation. In bifurcation lesions, in which there is a large fibrotic plaque at the ostium of the side branch, use of the cutting balloon as a predilatation strategy before stenting seems reasonable. The Restenosis reduction by Cutting balloon Evaluation (REDUCE) III trial evaluated the role of cutting balloon predilatation before stenting versus standard balloon predilatation in a variety of lesions. This trial reported a lower restenosis rate when lesions were predilated with the cutting balloon. The Excimer laser is not effective in severely calcified lesions. Even if more specifically applied for calcific lesions, rotational atherectomy (rotablator) is the most appropriate answer (*Textbook of Interventional Cardiology*. 1999:345–366).

4 Answer B. When using BMSs one stent seems to give better results than two stents and this approach should be tried first (*Heart*. 2004;90:713–722).When using two BMSs the performance of kissing balloon is advisable but does not seem to improve the results to the extent of suggesting elective use of this technique (*J Am Coll Cardiol*. 2000;35:1145–1151). Some operators advise using cutting balloon dilatation to treat ostial side branch disease but this approach should not be considered standard (*J Invasive Cardiol*. 1999;11:201–206). Regarding the intuitive advantage of atherectomy in lowering the risk of plaque shifting, no specific study provided any demonstration of this property.

5 Answer B. This nonrandomized study receives a lot of citations in the literature dealing with stenting bifurcational lesions; therefore, the reader needs to be familiar with this study. In this report, the technique of implanting two stents was associated with more in-hospital MACE compared with the one-stent approach. All other comparisons favored the one-stent approach without reaching statistical significance. The difference in the acute MACE is most probably related to old stent delivery systems and it is unlikely to hold true with current stents, including DESs.

6 Answer B. The "stent pull-back technique" has been proposed as an approach to treat nonaorto-ostial lesions and demands usage of a balloon in the main vessel, which is inflated at low pressure while a stent is gently retrieved, before deployment toward the ostium of the side branch. This approach should increase the chance to obtain full coverage of the ostium of the side branch without making the stent protrude into the main branch (*Am J Cardiol*. 2005;96:1123–1128).

7 Answer A. No specific advantage has been shown in ostial lesions of atherectomy and stenting versus stenting alone in the AMIGO trial. The only subgroup showing a minor trend toward a possible benefit of prior atherectomy was bifurcational lesions; the binary restenosis rate was 9.8% after atherectomy and stenting and 20.9% after stenting alone ($p = 0.265$) (*Am J Cardiol*. 2004;93:953–958).

8 Answer D. So far, only two studies have been published that evaluate DESs in bifurcational lesions. The first study evaluated a provisional approach versus a two-stent approach with the two arms undergoing sirolimus-eluting stent implantation. The main findings of this study were: total restenosis rate at 6 months was 25.7%, and it was not significantly different between the double-stenting (28.0%) and the provisional side branch-stenting (18.7%) groups. Fourteen of the restenosis cases occurred at the ostium of the side branch and were focal. Target lesion revascularization was performed in 7 cases; target vessel failure occurred in 15 cases (17.6%) (*Circulation.* 2004;109:1244–1249). The second study showed numerically lower restenosis rates on the main and side branchs when one stent was implanted versus two stents but no comparison reached statistical significance (*Am Heart J.* 2004;148:857–864).

9   Answer C.   The classification shown is the Duke classification. Currently, five classifications for bifurcational lesions have been proposed (*J Am Coll Cardiol.* 2005;46:1446–1455).

10   Answer B.   When performing the crush technique it is important to perform final kissing inflation following recrossing into the side branch. This maneuver lowers the risk of restenosis at the ostium of the side branch but does not seem to affect the risk of thrombosis (*J Am Coll Cardiol.* 2005;46:613–620).

11   Answer D.   There is no recognized standard approach in the treatment of bifurcational lesions except for the preference of provisional side branch stenting with final kissing balloon when possible (*Heart.* 2004;90:713–722). In this specific example, there is significant stenosis involving both branches with a reasonable reference vessel diameter (3.0 mm or more). In such a lesion, the usage of two DESs as intention to treat appears a reasonable approach.

12   Answer D.   Each of the first three answers has some rationale and is somewhat correct. Nevertheless, we do not have at present any study to support why the Interventional Cardiologist should choose one versus another. The lack of any specific study on this topic makes the selection of D the most appropriate answer.

13   Answer D.   We do not know why, despite usage of DESs, we still see side branch restenosis in approximately 15% of the cases when two stents are implanted on a bifurcation. This finding is an improvement compared with results obtained following implantation of BMSs where the restenosis on the side branch was two times higher or more. All hypotheses presented as answers to the question are potentially correct. A recent study evaluating the results of implantation of two DESs (sirolimus) in bifurcational lesions proposed that the underexpansion or underdilatation of the side branch-stent is the main reason for a higher

incidence of restenosis at this site (*J Am Coll Cardiol.* 2005;46:599–605).

14   Answer D.   The lesion presented is a complex stenosis involving a left main coronary artery. Presently these lesions can be treated with stenting only in selected conditions such as the presence of a contraindication to the standard approach for left main stenosis, which is coronary artery bypass grafting (CABG). If the patient needs to be treated with a percutaneous technique, the two most accepted approaches are the ones given in B and C (*Circulation.* 2005;111:791–795, *J Am Coll Cardiol.* 2005;45:351–356). While some operators may perform directional atherectomy, this approach is not considered standard in most coronary lesions, in addition the stenosis presented here is likely to be calcific, a feature which makes directional atherectomy likely to fail.

15   Answer A.   Richter and others conducted a study with an in-vitro model and in an animal model of coronary bifurcations to evaluate the dynamics flow alterations and leukocyte adhesion as triggers for intimal hyperplasia. The main results of this study show that the flow dynamics in the side branch are a major determinant of the flow and patency of the main branch. The study evaluated leukocyte adhesion and not platelet activation. Contrary to the main findings of this study an optimal side branch lumen may disturb the flow pattern in the main branch (*J Clin Invest.* 2004;113:1607–1614).

16   Answer B.   The concept of stent deformation and side branch coverage is important when performing provisional side branch stenting. Some struts of the stent positioned in the main branch will slightly prolapse to partially stent the ostium of the side branch. If no final kissing balloon inflation is performed, the stent will be unfavorably deformed in the main branch (*Catheter Cardiovasc Interv.* 2000;49:274–283, *Heart.* 2004;90:713–722).

17   Answer A.   Cypher stents are made on the BxVelocity stent platform, which is a closed cell design with struts opening to 3 mm as maximal diameter; for this reason the main branch needs to be 3 mm or smaller in diameter. Implantation of Cypher stents in any branch larger than 3 mm will leave a relative narrowing due to the fact that the cell cannot be opened to a diameter larger than 3 mm. Usage of Taxus stents (Express platform) with an open cell design allows placement of these stents with the culottes technique in vessels larger than 3 mm.

18 **Answer C.** Higher rates of TVR is the only right answer. Data from the PRESTO trial indicate that, at 9 months, patients with bifurcational lesions had a higher incidence of TVR (17% vs. 14%; p <0.001), whereas death (1%), and MI (1%) were not different between the two groups (*J Am Coll Cardiol.* 2005;46:606–612).

19 **Answer A.** Many lesions at the ostium of a side branch do not demonstrate signs of ischemia. Among 97 bifurcation lesions evaluated with FFR on both branches, none of the 21 lesions with <75% stenosis had FFR <0.75, and among the 73 lesions with >75% stenosis, only 20 were functionally significant. Moreover, the FFR measurement in jailed side branch lesions is both safe and feasible (*J Am Coll Cardiol.* 2005;46:633–637).

20 **Answer B.** Both types of lesions had a very limited evaluation in the context of randomized trials. As a matter of fact, only bifurcational lesions were studied in two published randomized trials, while no specific trial has been published to evaluate ostial lesions. Despite the lack of specific evidence, directional atherectomy remains a very interesting option for ostial and bifurcational lesions. DESs give better results compared with BMSs when implanted on ostial and bifurcational lesions. Despite this improvement, the performance of DESs remains inferior in these lesions compared with other lesions.

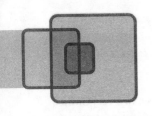

15

Long Lesions and Diffuse Disease

Joel A. Garcia and Ivan P. Casserly

Questions

1 According to the American College of Cardiology (ACC)/American Heart Association (AHA) lesions classification systems, what is the accepted lesion length that defines a "long" lesion?

(A) <5 mm of length
(B) >5 mm of length
(C) >10 mm of length
(D) >20 mm of length

2 Which of the following statements is *true* regarding the influence of lesion length on the AHA/ACC classification of lesion type?

(A) A lesion <10 mm in length represents an AHA/ACC Type A lesion
(B) A lesion >2 cm in length represents an AHA/ACC Type B1 lesion
(C) A lesion >2 cm in length represents an AHA/ACC Type B2 lesion
(D) A lesion 10 to 20 mm in length represents an AHA/ACC Type C lesion

3 The relationship between translesional flow across a lesion and lesion length is governed by Poiseuille law. Which of the following statements describes the relationship between these two variables?

(A) Flow is directly related to lesion length
(B) Flow is inversely related to lesion length
(C) Flow is directly related to the square of lesion length
(D) Flow is inversely related to the square of lesion length

4 Coronary vessel tapering is a significant issue in the interventional treatment of long lesions. Which of the following statements regarding coronary vessel tapering is *false*?

(A) Average coronary artery lumen tapering is 0.22 mm per 10 mm of arterial length
(B) Coronary artery lumen tapering is dependent on anatomic vessel tapering (i.e., tapering in EEM between proximal and distal vessel)
(C) In patients with documented coronary artery disease, coronary artery lumen tapering may be dependent on differential plaque accumulation (i.e., greater accumulation of plaque in distal compared with proximal segments)
(D) In patients with coronary artery disease, reverse coronary artery lumen tapering may occur in approximately 10% of coronary arteries
(E) Coronary artery lumen tapering is equal in the three major coronary arteries (left anterior descending [LAD], left circumflex [LCx], and right coronary artery [RCA])

5 Transplant vasculopathy is characterized by the diffuse concentric narrowing of the coronary arteries. Regarding its diagnosis, prognostic significance, and treatment, all of the following statements are true, *except*:

(A) Intravascular ultrasound (IVUS) offers earlier detection and better characterization of allograft vasculopathy when compared with routine angiography
(B) The presence of angiographic coronary disease posttransplantation is highly predictive of subsequent coronary disease-related events
(C) Flow-limiting lesions requiring intervention generally occur 5 years posttransplantation
(D) Primary procedural success for the interventional treatment of transplant vasculopathy lesions is less than for the treatment of native atherosclerosis

(E) Transplant vasculopathy is the second leading cause of death in cardiac transplant patients beyond 1 year from the time of transplantation

6 The angiogram below is consistent with which of the following diagnoses?

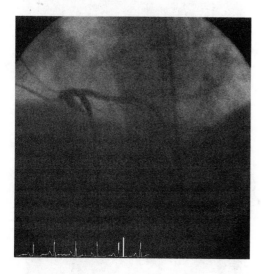

(A) Normal vessel tapering
(B) Allograft vasculopathy in LCx
(C) Allograft vasculopathy in LAD
(D) Diffuse coronary atherosclerosis
(E) None of the above

7 A 57-year-old woman presented with 2 hours of substernal chest pain, anterior ST elevation, and elevated cardiac biomarkers. On engagement of the left coronary artery (LCA), the following angiographic image was obtained. The angiographic appearance is most consistent with which of the following diagnoses?

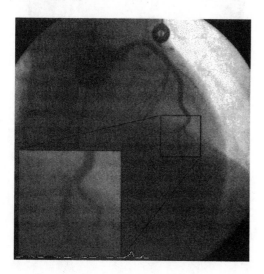

(A) Diffuse LAD atherosclerosis
(B) Unstable plaque in mid-LAD
(C) LAD dissection
(D) Nonocclusive thrombus in the LAD
(E) None of the above

8 In the present era, which of the following statements regarding the influence of lesion length on clinical outcomes with the use of balloon angioplasty was *true*?

(A) Lesion length was a predictor of acute procedural success
(B) Lesion length was a predictor of acute procedural complications
(C) Lesion length was a strong predictor of late lumen loss and restenosis
(D) All of the above

9 Comparing stand-alone angioplasty, rotational atherectomy, and Excimer laser angioplasty for the treatment of long coronary lesions, which of the following statements is *false*?

(A) Rotational atherectomy is associated with a higher rate of initial procedural success
(B) The incidence of periprocedural ischemic complications is equivalent for all treatment modalities
(C) Rotational atherectomy is associated with lower rates of restenosis compared with stand-alone angioplasty
(D) Excimer laser angioplasty is associated with higher rates of restenosis compared with stand-alone angioplasty

10 Which of the following statements regarding the use of bare-metal stents (BMS) for the treatment of long coronary lesions is *false*?

(A) The incidence of delivery failure is related to increased stent length
(B) Compared with stenting for treatment of focal lesions, stenting of long lesions is associated with significantly increased rates of lesion restenosis
(C) Compared with stenting for treatment of focal lesions, stenting of long lesions is associated with significantly increased rates of target lesion revascularization
(D) Restenosis following stenting of long coronary lesions has been correlated with both lesion length and total stent length
(E) Treatment of long lesions with a single long stent has been proven superior to treatment with multiple overlapping stents

11 Regarding the strategy of angioplasty with provisional Spot Stenting (SS) for the treatment of long lesions, which one of the following statements is *true*?

  (A) The rate of major procedural complications with SS is higher when compared with traditional stenting (TS) of long lesions

  (B) The rates of angiographic restenosis are less favorable with SS when compared with TS

  (C) The composite incidence of death, myocardial infarction (MI), or target lesion revascularization (TLR) at 6 months is lower with SS compared with TS

  (D) IVUS-guided SS has been proved to improve clinical outcomes over non–IVUS-guided SS

12 Comparing a strategy of angioplasty alone versus angioplasty and bare-metal stenting for the treatment of long coronary lesions, which of the following statements is *false*?

  (A) Bailout stenting is required in up to one third of patients treated with angioplasty alone

  (B) Both strategies have a similar acute angiographic result

  (C) Angiographic restenosis is lower with stents

  (D) Major adverse cardiovascular event (MACE) at 9 months favors the stented group

  (E) Bailout stenting led to a threefold increase in periprocedural infarction

13 The Taxus V trial randomized patients with complex coronary lesions to treatment with a paclitaxel-eluting stent versus a BMS. A subset of patients in this trial ($n = 379$) with a mean lesion length of approximately 25 mm required placement of multiple stents. Which of the following statements regarding clinical outcomes in this important subset is *false*?

  (A) In-stent restenosis rates were significantly reduced with the paclitaxel-eluting stent

  (B) The use of multiple stents was associated with a significantly increased risk of periprocedural MI

  (C) The use of multiple stents was associated with a significantly increased risk of significant side-branch stenosis

  (D) The incidence of stent thrombosis was significantly increased in patients receiving multiple stents

14 Match the following angiograms with the most likely clinical diagnoses:

(A)

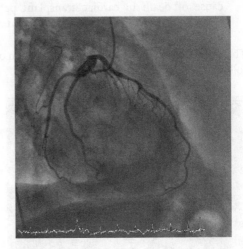

(B)

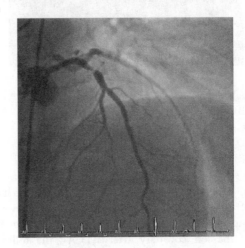

(C)

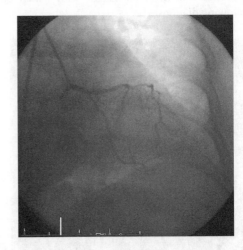

(D)

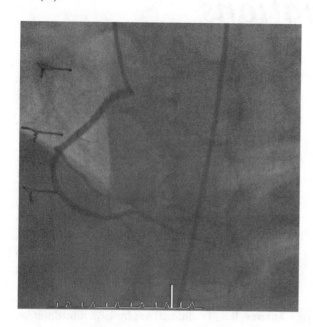

1. Normal coronary lumen tapering
2. Diabetic atherosclerosis
3. Transplant vasculopathy
4. Nondiabetic atherosclerosis

15 Regarding the relationship between the incidence of stent thrombosis and both stent length and lesion length, which of the following statements is *true*?

(A) With the use of BMSs, increased stent length is not predictive of an increased risk of stent thrombosis
(B) With the use of BMSs, increased lesion length is predictive of an increased risk of stent thrombosis
(C) With the use of drug-eluting stents (DESs), increased stent length is predictive of an increased risk of stent thrombosis
(D) With the use of DESs, increased lesion length is predictive of an increased risk of stent thrombosis

16 Which of the following statements regarding the use of adjunctive pharmacologic therapies during PCI for the treatment of long lesions is *true*?

(A) Preloading with a 300-mg dose of clopidogrel load is associated with decreased rate of periprocedural MI
(B) Preloading with a 600-mg dose of clopidogrel load is associated with decreased rate of periprocedural MI
(C) Bivalirudin is superior to unfractionated heparin in this cohort
(D) Adjunctive glycoprotein IIb/IIIa inhibition with abciximab decreases the risk of acute procedural complications in this cohort
(E) None of the above

Answers and Explanations

1 **Answer D.** According to the ACC/AHA and the Society for Coronary Angiography and Interventions lesion classifications systems, lesions <10 mm in length are discrete, lesions of 10 to 20 mm in length are referred to as tubular, and lesions >20 mm in length are long (*Am J Cardiol.* 2003;92:389–394).

2 **Answer A.** Type A lesions are considered discrete and are <10 mm in length. In terms of lesion length, both Type B1 and B2 lesions are 10 to 20 mm in length. Type B2 lesions have two or more Type B characteristics (e.g., eccentricity, moderate tortuosity, moderate angulation, moderate to heavy calcification, ovarial location, bifurcation lesions, presence of thrombus, total occlusion <3 months old). Finally, Type C lesions are considered diffuse and have a length of ≥2 cm (*Am J Cardiol.* 2003;92: 389–394).

3 **Answer B.** According to Poiseuille law,
$$\text{Flow} = \pi(\Delta P)(r^4)/8(\eta)(l)$$
where:

P = the pressure difference across the lesion

r = minimal lumen radius of the stenotic segment

η = blood viscosity

l = lesion length

The lesion length is inversely related to translesional flow. Therefore, for short, discrete lesions, length exerts relatively little impact on translesional flow, but for longer lesions (>20 mm), length can make a significant impact on translesional flow (*Textbook of interventional cardiology.* 2003;367–379).

4 **Answer E.** In two separate series (*Am J Cardiol.* 1992;69:188–193, *Am J Cardiol.* 1995;75:177–180) the mean coronary artery lumen tapering was found to be approximately 0.22 mm over a 10-mm length of coronary arterial length. In the series of patients with documented coronary artery disease reported by Javier and others there was a subset of coronary arteries (11%) that demonstrated reverse coronary artery lumen tapering (i.e., distal lumen CSA greater than proximal lumen CSA). In this same series, coronary artery lumen tapering was significantly greater in the LAD as compared with the LCx and RCA. Using IVUS, Javier examined the mechanism of coronary artery lumen tapering. It appears that in patients with coronary artery disease, lumen taping is dependent on both anatomic vessel tapering (i.e., decrease in EEM between proximal and distal segments) and differential plaque accumulation (i.e., greater accumulation of plaque in distal compared with proximal segments). Coronary artery lumen tapering is important in the treatment of long lesions because of the difference in vessel diameter at the proximal and distal margins of the lesion. Balloon and stent sizing to the vessel diameter at the proximal margin of the lesion may increase the risk of distal dissection. In contrast, sizing of balloon and stents to the vessel diameter at the distal margin of the lesion may result in inadequate lumen expansion and a suboptimal result.

5 **Answer D.** Traditional noninvasive modalities are insensitive in the detection of transplant vasculopathy. Although, conventional coronary angiography is the most commonly employed method for the detection of transplant vasculopathy, it is less sensitive than IVUS, which is the gold standard for the detection of this pathology (*Circulation.* 1998;98:2672–2678, *J Am Coll Cardiol.* 2005;45:1538–1542, *Circulation.* 1999;100:458–460). Significant flow-limiting lesions due to transplant vasculopathy are unusual in the first 5 years posttransplantation but show an exponential rise after this time-point. Interventional strategies including angioplasty and stenting have been reported for the treatment of these lesions, with similar primary procedural success compared with the treatment of native coronary atherosclerosis. There is a high rate of repeat procedures in this group, due to a combination of late restenosis at the treatment site and progression of transplant vasculopathy. Beyond 1 year from the time of cardiac transplantation, transplant vasculopathy is the second leading cause of death, with malignancy being the most common cause (*J Heart Lung Transplant.* 2005;24:945–955). In patients with end-stage transplant vasculopathy, the only treatment option currently is repeat transplantation.

6 **Answer C.** This is a left anterior oblique (LAO) cranial angiogram from the LCA approximately 6 years postcardiac transplantation. It demonstrates a decrease in the lumen caliber of the LAD that is significantly greater than one would expect due to normal vessel tapering. The circumflex is of normal caliber and shows normal vessel tapering. The angiographic findings are most consistent with the diagnosis of significant transplant vasculopathy in the LAD, which was confirmed by IVUS examination.

7 Answer C. This angiogram demonstrates a normal caliber proximal LAD with an abrupt decrease in caliber at the level of the third diagonal branch followed by diffuse narrowing of the distal LAD. Also note the prominent tortuosity of the distal LAD. This angiographic appearance is most consistent with a coronary dissection in the mid-LAD which propagated distally, resulting in diffuse luminal narrowing. The abrupt nature of the luminal diameter change differentiates this pathology from that of diffuse coronary atherosclerosis, and from normal vessel tapering. The presence of an unstable plaque alone would not be expected to be associated with diffuse narrowing distal to the lesion.

8 Answer D. In the present era, acute procedural success with short (<10 mm) lesions was 95%, with tubular lesions (10 to 20 mm) was 85%, and with long lesions (>20 mm) was 74%. Similarly, there was a significant increase in acute procedural complications such as abrupt vessel closure and dissection, and restenosis rates with increasing lesion length. The mechanism of these adverse outcomes with angioplasty alone is likely multifactorial, and is due to an association between increased lesion length and adverse morphologic characteristics (e.g., angulated segments, bifurcations points), and heterogeneity in composition of plaque resulting in uneven distribution of shear stresses during balloon dilatation and predisposition to dissection (*Textbook of interventional cardiology*. 2003;367–379).

9 Answer C. Two randomized studies performed in the present era provide comparative data regarding the treatment of long lesions with angioplasty, rotational atherectomy, and Excimer laser. The Excimer laser, Rotational Atherectomy, and Balloon Angioplasty Comparison (ERBAC) trial (*Circulation*. 1997;96:91–98) compared all three modalities for treatment of patients with complex lesion morphology (approximately 50% were >10 mm in length). This study showed a higher initial procedural success with rotational atherectomy (89% vs. 80% for angioplasty vs. 77% for Excimer laser). Periprocedural ischemic complications were equivalent for all treatment modalities. Despite the higher initial procedural success with rotational atherectomy, 6-month restenosis rates were significantly higher in the rotational atherectomy compared with angioplasty (42.4% vs. 31.9%). Similarly, restenosis rates with Excimer laser were significantly higher than with angioplasty (46% vs. 31.9%).

The AMRO trial randomized patients with lesions >10 mm in length and stable angina to treatment with Excimer laser or angioplasty. The findings mirrored those of the ERBAC trial, with similar initial angiographic success rates and incidence of periprocedural complications for the two treatment modalities, but a higher late lumen loss in the Excimer laser treated patients (*Lancet*. 1996;347:79–84).

10 Answer E. The use of BMSs for the treatment of long lesions is associated with significantly higher rates of restenosis and target lesion revascularization compared with the treatment of focal disease. In various series, restenosis rates for the treatment of long lesions varies from 20% to 40%, with target lesion revascularization rates of 15% to 25% (*Circulation*. 1997;96:1–472, *J Am Coll Cardiol*. 1995;25:156A, *Am Heart J*. 2001;141:971–976, *Catheter Cardiovasc Interv*. 1999;48:287–293 discussion 294–295, *Circulation*. 1996;94:I–685). This compares with a restenosis rate of 11.4% and TLR rate of 8% in the STRESS and BENESTENT trials of stenting of focal lesions (*N Engl J Med*. 1994;331:496–501, *N Engl J Med*. 1994;331:489–495). A large number of studies have examined the relationship between the rates of restenosis and both lesion length and total stent length. The data is conflicting, but in summary, there is evidence to suggest that both variables impact rates of restenosis. There are no randomized data demonstrating the superiority of a single long BMS versus multiple overlapping BMS for the treatment of long lesions. In practice, most operators prefer the approach of using a single long stent, since this reduces catheterization time, contrast load, and radiation exposure. However, in some cases, (e.g., because of difficulties with stent delivery, significant mismatch in the diameter between proximal and distal reference segments, lesion length greater than available stent lengths) multiple overlapping stents may be required to treat a long lesion.

11 Answer C. Colombo et al. showed that long-term outcomes with IVUS-guided SS (131 lesions in 101 patients), including angiographic restenosis and follow-up MACE, are superior to the outcomes achieved in a matched group of patients treated with TS. Although IVUS-guided SS has been associated with good outcomes for the treatment of long lesions, there are no comparative studies to determine the superiority of an IVUS guided versus non–IVUS-guided strategy (*J Am Coll Cardiol*. 2001;38:1427–1433).

12 Answer D. Serruys et al. reported a randomized comparison angioplasty with provisional stenting for suboptimal angiographic results versus angioplasty and elective stenting (using NIR stent) in 437 patients with long lesions (mean length 27 +/−9 mm). The strategy of angioplasty with provisional stenting resulted in bailout stenting in one third of patients (34%), with a threefold increase in periprocedural infarction. Angioplasty followed by elective stenting yielded a lower angiographic restenosis rate, but no reduction in MACE at 9 months (*J Am Coll Cardiol.* 2002;39:393–399).

13 Answer D. Taxus V represents the only randomized trial of DES versus BMS for the treatment of complex coronary lesions, including longer lesions (*JAMA.* 2005;294:1215–1223). A subset of patients in this trial received multiple stents (either planned for treatment of long lesions or as a bailout for treatment of complications or a suboptimal result). In this subset, although restenosis and target lesion revascularization rates were significantly reduced in the paclitaxel-eluting stent group, there was an excess of procedure related MIs in this group (8.3% vs. 3.3%, mainly non–Q wave MIs). The use of multiple stents was also associated with a significant increase in significant side-branch stenosis and occlusion (42.6% vs. 30.6%). The rate of stent thrombosis was not significantly different between the groups (1% in DES group vs. 0.5% in BMS group).

14 Answer A-1, B-4, C-2, D-3. Option A shows an angiographically normal LCA with normal vessel tapering. Option B represents focal nondiabetic atherosclerosis of the proximal LAD. Option C is an example of diabetic atherosclerosis. Note the severe diffuse vessel atherosclerotic narrowing evident in all vessel segments. Option D shows a case of severe transplant vasculopathy in the RCA. Note that there is concentric narrowing of the distal epicardial vessel with prominent involvement of the small side branches, which is the characteristic angiographic appearance of transplant vasculopathy.

15 Answer C. Increased stent length, both with BMS and DES, predicts an increased risk of stent thrombosis. In an analysis of 6 BMS trials, Cutlip et al. demonstrated a 30% increase in the risk of stent thrombosis per 10 mm of BMS (*Circulation.* 2001;103:1967–1971). In a large prospective observational series of patients receiving DES, Iakovou et al. demonstrated a similar magnitude of risk of increased stent thrombosis per 10 mm of DES length (*JAMA.* 2005;293:2126–2130). Lesion length does not appear to predict an increased risk of stent thrombosis (*J Am Coll Cardiol.* 2005;45:954–959).

16 Answer E. There is no randomized data regarding the use of antiplatelet or anticoagulant agents in the interventional management of long lesions. Despite the absence of such data, most operators are more aggressive with the use of antiplatelet and anticoagulant agents in the treatment of long lesions.

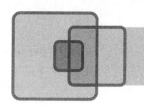

16

Restenosis and Percutaneous Options

Craig R. Narins

Questions

1 Which one of the following modifications to stent design has been associated with increased rates of in-stent restenosis?

(A) Thinner stent struts
(B) Use of a cobalt chromium platform instead of stainless steel
(C) Gold coating
(D) Heparin coating
(E) Use of a slotted tubular rather than a coil design

2 A 57-year-old man is referred for coronary angiography following a non–ST-elevation myocardial infarction (NSTEMI). The angiogram demonstrates a severe stenosis of the mid right coronary artery (RCA), and a 3.5 × 18 mm sirolimus-eluting stent is placed. Online quantitative coronary angiography (QCA) performed before and after stenting reveals the following measurements. Six months later the patient experienced two episodes of chest discomfort, and an exercise nuclear stress test suggested mild ischemia of the inferior wall. Angiography with QCA demonstrated a patent stent with measurements as described in the table. What is the in-stent late loss in this individual?

	Prestent	Poststent	6-month Follow-up
Vessel reference diameter (mm)	3.52	—	3.68
Minimum luminal diameter (mm)	1.03	3.28	2.95

(A) 0.33 mm
(B) 1.92 mm
(C) 0.16 mm
(D) 0.49 mm
(E) 0.73 mm

3 When a patient undergoes percutaneous coronary intervention (PCI) for the treatment of in-stent restenosis, which one of the following factors is *not* a predictor of recurrent restenosis?

(A) Diabetes mellitus
(B) Length of the initially placed stent
(C) Previous treatment for restenosis within the same stent
(D) Focal rather than diffuse pattern of restenosis
(E) Smaller final minimum luminal diameter following the repeat intervention

4 Randomized trial data confirms that thienopyridine therapy, for example, with clopidogrel, confers benefit for the prevention of subacute stent thrombosis after performing stand-alone balloon angioplasty for the treatment of in-stent restenosis.

(A) True
(B) False

5 Regarding the typical time course of restenosis within bare-metal stents (BMSs), which of the following statements is *true*?

(A) The degree of intimal hyperplasia within a stent usually reaches its peak within the first 6 months following stent implantation

(B) Between 6 months and 3 years following stent implantation, there is typically gradual but continued progressive narrowing within the stent on serial angiographic follow-up

(C) On serial intravascular ultrasound (IVUS) imaging, when compared with the immediate post-stent implantation results, late stent recoil at 6 months is a common phenomenon

(D) Patients presenting with in-stent restenosis <3 months following initial stent placement are more likely to have a favorable response to repeat PCI than patients presenting with restenosis at a later time

6 Intracoronary brachytherapy is an effective therapy for the treatment of in-stent restenosis. In comparing the properties of β versus γ-emitting isotopes, which of the following is *true*?

(A) β-emitters require longer intracoronary dwell times

(B) β-emitters have lower tissue penetration

(C) β-emitters have lower energy levels

(D) Shielding of cath lab personnel is more difficult with β-emitters

(E) When used in larger diameter vessels, catheter centering is not as critical with β-emitters as compared with γ-emitters

7 A 53-year-old woman underwent primary PCI involving placement of a 3.0×28 mm stent in the mid-RCA for treatment of an acute inferior myocardial infarction. She returned 5 months later with low-threshold angina despite medical therapy and the angiogram as shown below is obtained of the RCA in the right anterior oblique projection. Which one of the following potential therapies used for the treatment of in-stent restenosis would be associated with a reduced likelihood of recurrent restenosis when compared with conventional balloon angioplasty in this patient?

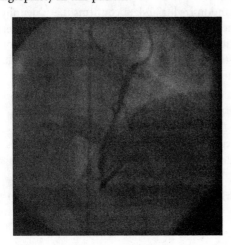

(A) Cutting balloon angioplasty

(B) Rotational atherectomy

(C) Excimer laser-assisted coronary angioplasty

(D) Directional coronary atherectomy

(E) BMS implantation ("stent within a stent")

(F) None of the above

8 Intracoronary brachytherapy is effective for reducing the likelihood of restenosis in all of the following lesion subsets, *except*:

(A) In-stent restenosis within a saphenous vein graft

(B) Diffuse (>30 mm in length) in-stent restenosis

(C) Recurrent in-stent restenosis (e.g., in-stent restenosis that has recurred after a previous attempt at percutaneous revascularization that did not involve brachytherapy)

(D) Prevention of restenosis when used following stent implantation for a *de novo* lesion

9 Which of the following is *not* true regarding the treatment of in-stent restenosis with vascular brachytherapy?

(A) Clopidogrel therapy should routinely be continued for at least 6 to 12 months following brachytherapy

(B) The placement of additional stents during the brachytherapy procedure reduces the risk of subsequent recurrent restenosis

(C) The presence of thrombus within a restenotic stent is considered a contraindication for the use of brachytherapy

(D) Recurrent angiographic restenosis 6 to 9 months following brachytherapy has occurred in >20% of patients treated with brachytherapy in most randomized clinical trials assessing this therapy

(E) The "edge effect," in which recurrent restenosis following brachytherapy occurs at the edge of the treated stent, is thought to occur when the radiation source fails to completely cover the length of the vessel segment injured by preradiation balloon dilation

10 Compared with balloon angioplasty, BMS implantation is associated with a lower likelihood of restenosis as a result of which one of the following biological mechanisms?

(A) Reduced degree of neointimal formation

(B) Reduced degree of negative remodeling

(C) Reduced vascular smooth muscle cell proliferation

(D) Increased collagen deposition

(E) All of the above

11 Rapamycin, used for the prevention of in-stent restenosis, is associated with which of the following biological characteristics?

(A) Inhibition of vascular smooth muscle cell migration

(B) Inhibition of vascular smooth muscle cell proliferation

(C) Immunosuppression

(D) Anti-inflammatory

(E) All of the above

12 Which of the following statements best describes the biological mechanism of action of paclitaxel?

(A) Stabilizes microtubule assembly

(B) Enhances microtubule breakdown

(C) Blocks cell cycle progression at the G1 to S phase transition in vascular smooth muscle cells

(D) Functions as a macrolide antibiotic

(E) All of the above

13 Various polymers can be used to affix pharmaceutical agents to stents. Some polymers themselves have been shown to increase the likelihood of restenosis.

(A) True

(B) False

14 The following figure shows a frequency distribution curve from a hypothetical trial comparing two stents, "Stent A" and "Stent B". On the basis of the figure, which one of the following statements is *true*?

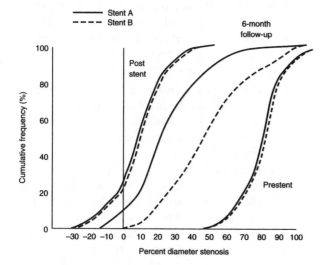

(A) The incidence of angiographic restenosis, defined as a stenosis severity of $\geq 50\%$ at 6-month follow-up, is greater for Stent A than for Stent B

(B) The differences in 6-month restenosis rates between the two stents can be attributed to better acute gain with Stent A

(C) Late loss is more pronounced for Stent B than for Stent A

(D) Angiographic restenosis is approximately 40% for Stent A

(E) All of the above

15 Which of the following pharmacologic agents has been associated with a significant reduction in subsequent restenosis compared with placebo when tested in the setting of a randomized controlled clinical trial?

(A) Pravastatin

(B) Valsartan

(C) Prednisone

(D) Troglitazone

(E) None of the above

(F) All of the above

16 Which one of the following statements regarding drug-eluting stent (DES) use in patients with diabetes mellitus is *true*?

(A) DESs have been shown to reduce the risk of angiographic restenosis and the need for repeat target lesion revascularization relative to BMSs among patients with diabetes

(B) Paclitaxel-coated stents are associated with significantly less late loss than Rapamycin-coated stents among patients with diabetes

(C) Patients with diabetes are at a greater risk of late stent thrombosis than patients without diabetes following DES placement

(D) When performing multivessel stenting in patients with diabetes, the use of DESs is associated with reduced late mortality compared with the use of BMSs

17 A 52-year-old man presented with low-threshold angina. During an exercise stress echocardiogram he developed typical angina at a moderate cardiac workload associated with 1.5 mm horizontal ST-segment depression in the inferolateral leads and transient hypokinesis of the inferior wall. Subsequent angiography demonstrated a lengthy 90% stenosis of the proximal-to-mid RCA, which was treated successfully with slightly overlapping 3.5×33 and 3.0×18 mm sirolimus-eluting stents. His angina resolved after the intervention, and he returns to your office for follow-up 1 year later. He continues to lead an active lifestyle and is free of angina. Which one of the following would constitute the most appropriate means to screen for stent patency at this time?

(A) Exercise stress echocardiogram

(B) Exercise treadmill test without adjunctive imaging

(C) Multislice computer tomography (CT) angiogram

(D) Coronary angiography

(E) No testing is indicated

18 Which one of the following features has *not* been identified as an independent predictor of angiographic in-stent restenosis following DES implantation?

(A) Longer stent length

(B) Diabetes mellitus

(C) Type B2 or C American College of Cardiology (ACC)/American Heart Association (AHA) lesion classification

(D) Smaller vessel reference diameter

(E) Ostial lesion location

19 A 74-year-old woman who underwent placement of a 2.5 × 15 mm BMS in her mid-left anterior descending (LAD) returned $4\frac{1}{2}$ months later with unstable angina and is found to have severe in-stent restenosis. Regarding the use of DESs for the treatment of in-stent restenosis in this patient, which one of the following statements is *true*?

(A) For the treatment of in-stent restenosis, DESs are more effective than balloon angioplasty in reducing recurrent angiographic but not clinical restenosis

(B) For the treatment of in-stent restenosis, DESs are more effective than balloon angioplasty in reducing both recurrent angiographic and clinical restenosis

(C) When used in the setting of in-stent restenosis, paclitaxel-eluting stents are associated with less subsequent late lumen loss than rapamycin-eluting stents

(D) DESs are associated with lower restenosis rates when used for the treatment of in-stent restenosis than when used for the treatment of *de novo* lesions

20 Which of the following patterns of in-stent restenosis is associated with the highest likelihood of recurrent restenosis following percutaneous intervention?

(A)

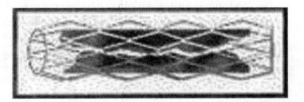

(B)

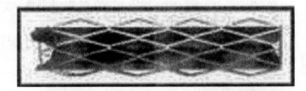

(C)

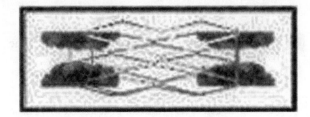

(D)

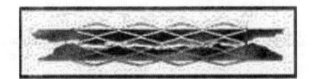

21 A 78-year-old otherwise healthy man underwent implantation of a 3.0 × 15 mm BMS at the ostium of his LAD coronary artery 6 months earlier for low threshold exertional angina. He is now referred for repeat angiography after experiencing two episodes of angina at rest. The angiogram demonstrates a concentric 70% stenosis involving the proximal portion of the ostial LAD stent and also involving the distal aspect of the left main trunk. The origin of the left circumflex (LCx) artery is widely patent. How is revascularization best approached?

(A) Place a single guidewire into the LAD and deploy a DES within the previous stent and distal left main. The LCx should be treated provisionally if there is significant plaque shift into the vessel origin

(B) Place guidewires in both the LAD and LCx and deploy "kissing" DESs in the LAD and LCx, allowing the proximal ends of the stents to cover the narrowing in the distal left main

(C) Place a guidewire in the LAD and perform cutting balloon angioplasty, with provisional stenting of the LAD and LCx only if the angioplasty result is inadequate

(D) Refer the patient for coronary artery bypass surgery, with placement of grafts to the LAD and LCx coronary arteries

22 Which one of the following statements regarding the use of intracoronary brachytherapy for the treatment of in-stent restenosis is *true*?

(A) The incidence of late aneurysm formation following brachytherapy is 6% to 8%

(B) γ-Emitting sources are associated with a lower incidence of recurrent restenosis than β-emitting sources

(C) Late recurrent restenosis, occurring from 6 months to 5 years following PCI for in-stent restenosis, is more common among patients treated with brachytherapy than placebo

(D) Among individuals who develop recurrent in-stent restenosis following brachytherapy, a repeat attempt at brachytherapy is contraindicated because of an unacceptably high risk of subsequent stent thrombosis

23 A 54-year-old man underwent placement of a 3.0 × 23 mm BMS in the mid-RCA. Eight months later he presented to the emergency room with chest pain. The electrocardiogram (EKG) showed no interval changes, and his serum troponin T concentration was within normal limits. Coronary angiography demonstrated diffuse restenosis within and proximal to the previously placed stent, and he underwent placement of a 3.0 × 32 mm paclitaxel eluting stent within and proximal to the original stent. Ten months later he again noted recurrent angina, and coronary angiography was repeated. Below is an image of the RCA in the right anterior oblique projection. Which one of the following statements is *true* regarding the use of DESs for the treatment of in-stent restenosis within a BMS?

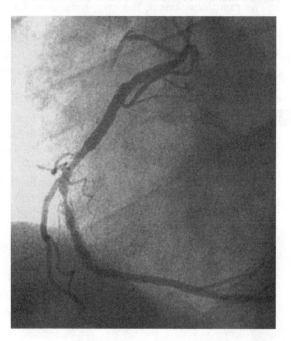

(A) Underexpansion of the DES used to treat in-stent restenosis is an important cause of recurrent restenosis

(B) The likelihood of restenosis is equivalent when DESs are used for the treatment of in-stent restenosis as with *de novo* lesions

(C) The immediate post-procedural minimal lumen diameter at the treatment site is typically greater following balloon angioplasty than following DES placement

(D) Negative vascular remodeling is a common contributor to recurrent restenosis following DES placement

24 Compared with the use of standard balloon angioplasty for the treatment of in-stent restenosis, which one of the following potential benefits is *not* associated with the use of cutting balloon angioplasty?

(A) Less recoil of the angioplasty site within the first 24 hours

(B) Lower likelihood of balloon slippage during inflation

(C) Less late luminal loss

(D) Lower number of balloons required during the intervention

25 Which of the following anticoagulant or antiplatelet agents, when used as an adjunct to balloon angioplasty during the treatment of in-stent restenosis, is associated with a lower rate of subsequent recurrent restenosis?

(A) Abciximab

(B) Clopidogrel

(C) Bivalirudin

(D) Aspirin

(E) None of the above

Answers and Explanations

1 Answer C. Two randomized studies have demonstrated that the use of stents with thinner struts is associated with a significant reduction of angiographic and clinical restenosis (*Circulation.* 2001;103: 2816–2821, *J Am Coll Cardiol.* 2003;41:1283–1288). Heparin coating has not been shown to affect the likelihood of subsequent in-stent restenosis, and likewise there is no evidence to suggest that the use of cobalt chromium stent platforms is related to higher rates of restenosis than stainless steel (*Am J Cardiol.* 2003;92:463–466). In fact, because the composition of cobalt chromium allows for thinner strut thickness, these stents may be associated with less risk of restenosis. Stents with a coil design, such as the Gianturco-Roubin stent, are associated with restenosis rates that are significantly greater than slotted tubular stents (*Am J Cardiol.* 2001;87:34–39, *Circulation.* 2000;102:1364–1368). Randomized studies have shown that gold coating is associated with higher rates of restenosis than implantation of identically designed stents that are not gold-coated (*Circulation.* 2000;101:2478–2483, *Am J Cardiol.* 2002;89:872–875, *Catheter Cardiovasc Interv.* 2004;62:18–25).

2 Answer A. Late loss is the key parameter used to quantitate the degree of intimal hyperplasia that has developed at the site of PCI between the time of the procedure and subsequent angiographic follow-up. Late loss within a stent is defined as the in-stent minimum lumen diameter immediately following stent placement minus the in-stent minimum lumen diameter on late follow-up angiography (*Circulation.* 1992;86:1827–1835, *J Am Coll Cardiol.* 1992;19:1493–1499).

3 Answer D. Diabetes, length of the initial stent, and smaller final minimum luminal diameter following the repeat intervention have all been associated with a higher likelihood of recurrent in-stent restenosis (*Textbook of Interventional Cardiology.* 2003;455–473). Long-term success is also less likely when in-stent restenosis presents in a diffuse or occlusive pattern rather than as a focal narrowing within the stent (*J Am Coll Cardiol.* 1998;32:980–984, *Circulation.* 1999;100:1872–1878).

4 Answer B. Although thienopyridine therapy is effective in reducing the incidence of stent thrombosis following implantation of BMSs or DESs and

following intracoronary brachytherapy, no prospective data have demonstrated the necessity of this therapy when stand-alone balloon angioplasty is used as a treatment for in-stent restenosis.

5 Answer A. In-stent restenosis typically occurs within the first 6 months of BMS implantation. After 6 months, serial angiographic follow-up studies have demonstrated a gradual spontaneous improvement in the degree of luminal narrowing within the stent (spontaneous regression) (*Am J Cardiol.* 1996;77:247–251, *N Engl J Med.* 1996;334:561–566). Late stent recoil, although occasionally noted, is an uncommon occurrence (*Am J Cardiol.* 1999;84:1247–1250, *Am J Cardiol.* 1998;81:9). Patients presenting with restenosis early (within the first 3 months of stent implantation) have an increased risk of recurrent restenosis following repeat PCI compared with patients who present later (*Am J Cardiol.* 2000;85:1427–1431).

6 Answer B. β-Emitters generate radiation in the form of electrons, whereas γ sources emit radiation in the form of photons. β-emitters demonstrate a rapid falloff in dose as distance from the source increases, which limits tissue penetration. Because of the rapid dose falloff, centering of the β-energy delivery source may be necessary in larger vessels to ensure adequate circumferential delivery of radiation to the vessel wall. The rapid dose falloff, however, reduces radiation exposure to cath lab personnel. Because β-emitters are associated with higher energy levels, shorter dwell times are required to achieve adequate tissue doses (*Internat J Cardiol.* 2004;93:1–5, *Cardiovasc Res.* 2004;63:22–30).

7 Answer F. Before the advent of vascular brachytherapy and, more recently, DESs to treat in-stent restenosis, several methods of tissue debulking were studied for the treatment of in-stent restenosis. Although data evaluating these techniques is limited, none appear to reduce the incidence of recurrent in-stent restenosis compared with stand-alone balloon angioplasty (*J Am Coll Cardiol.* 2004;43:936–942, *Eur Heart J.* 2003;24:266–273). In the randomized controlled angioplasty versus rotational atherectomy for the treatment of diffuse restenosis trial (ARTIST) study, rotational atherectomy used in the setting of in-stent restenosis was associated with an increased likelihood of recurrent clinical and angiographic restenosis compared with balloon angioplasty alone (*Circulation*. 2002;105:583–588). Anecdotal reports have described mixed results with the use of directional atherectomy and the excimer laser for the treatment of in-stent restenosis. The restenosis intrastent balloon versus stent trial (RIBS) trial, a randomized study of repeat BMS implantation versus balloon angioplasty for the treatment of in-stent restenosis, demonstrated no significant differences in angiographic or clinical outcomes between the two strategies (*J Am Coll Cardiol*. 2003;42:796–805). After encouraging registry studies examining the efficacy of cutting balloon angioplasty for treating in-stent restenosis, a more recent randomized trial failed to show a reduction in recurrent restenosis or major adverse cardiac events with the cutting balloon compared with conventional balloon angioplasty (*J Am Coll Cardiol*. 2004;43:943–949).

8 **Answer D.** Intravascular brachytherapy has been associated with a reduction in the likelihood of recurrent in-stent restenosis in all of the settings listed (*Catheter Cardiovasc Interv*. 2004;62:318–322, *N Engl J Med*. 2002;346:1194–1199, *Circulation*. 2000;101:1895–1898); however, brachytherapy has failed to reduce the likelihood of restenosis when used following stent implantation for a *de novo* lesion (*Am Heart J*. 2003;146:775–786).

9 **Answer B.** Because of delayed endothelialization of the stent following brachytherapy, which is associated with a propensity toward late stent thrombosis, clopidogrel therapy is advised for at least 12 months following brachytherapy (*Circulation*. 1999;100:789–792, *Circulation*. 2002;106:776–778). The presence of thrombus within a stent has been considered to represent a contraindication to brachytherapy (*Circulation*. 2003;107:1744–1749). The placement of additional stents during the brachytherapy procedure has been shown to *increase* the likelihood of subsequent recurrent restenosis, and may also increase the risk of stent thrombosis (*Am Heart J*. 2003;146:142–145). Although multiple randomized controlled trials of brachytherapy for in-stent restenosis using both β and γ-emitting isotopes have demonstrated significant reductions in recurrent restenosis compared with placebo, the incidence of recurrent angiographic restenosis following brachytherapy has remained >20% in nearly all of these trials (*ACC/AHA 2005 Guideline Update*. 2006). The "edge effect" is as defined in the question (*J Am Coll Cardiol*. 2001;37:1026–1030, *JAMA*. 2005;293:437–446).

10 **Answer B.** Compared with stand-alone balloon angioplasty, stent implantation is associated with an exaggerated vascular smooth muscle cell proliferative response and consequently, an increased degree of neointima formation (*Circulation*. 1999;99:44–52). Stent placement, however, essentially eliminates long-term negative remodeling of the vessel wall, which typically more than compensates for the exaggerated proliferative response and results in the reduced frequency of restenosis observed with stenting compared with balloon angioplasty (*Circulation*. 1997;95:363–370). Restenotic tissue obtained following balloon angioplasty demonstrates fewer smooth muscle cells and greater collagen deposition than tissue recovered from stents that have developed restenosis (*J Am Coll Cardiol*. 2000;35:157–163).

11 **Answer E.** Rapamycin (sirolimus) possesses all of the listed biological characteristics, which likely contribute to its antirestenosis effects (*Trends Cardiovasc Med*. 2003;13:142–148).

12 **Answer A.** Microtubules are a fundamental component of the mitotic spindle apparatus, and play essential roles in other cellular functions including migration and growth factor signaling. The assembly and disassembly of microtubules within a cell is maintained in a well-regulated equilibrium. Paclitaxel (Taxol) produces its antiproliferative effects by stabilizing microtubules, thus shifting the dynamic balance toward assembly, which consequently interrupts cellular division. Rapamycin (sirolimus) is a macrolide antibiotic that produces its cellular effects by blocking cell cycle progression at the G1 to S phase transition in vascular smooth muscle cells (*Ann Rev Med*. 2004;55:169–178).

13 **Answer A.** Polymer coatings are required for affixing most pharmaceutical agents to a stent platform for delivery. The coatings act as a reservoir for the drug, and can serve to regulate the rate of drug elution into surrounding tissues. A wide variety of potential coatings have been described, and the various polymers differ in terms of structure and biocompatibility (*Ann Pharmaco*. 2004;38:661–669). Some coatings, when affixed to a BMS, have been shown in animal models to elicit a more aggressive inflammatory and hyperplastic response than seen with nonpolymer-coated BMSs (*Circulation*. 1996;94:1690–1697).

14 **Answer C.** A great deal of information can be obtained from frequency distribution curves, which are typically used to display the immediate and late angiographic results of competing therapies in clinical trials of restenosis. The median acute luminal gain for each therapy can be determined by measuring the distance between the prestent and poststent curve for each stent on a horizontal line drawn at the 50% mark on the y(cumulative frequency)-axis. In the example, this distance is similar for Stents A and B. Late lumen loss can be determined by comparing the distance between the poststent and the 6-month follow-up curve for each stent, which in the example is greater for Stent B.

The angiographic restenosis rate for each therapy can be determined by drawing a vertical line upward from the 50% diameter stenosis point on the x-axis (percent diameter stenosis). The point on the y-axis that corresponds to where this vertical line intersects the 6-month follow-up curve for each stent reveals the percentage of individuals who had a $\leq$50% stenosis at 6-month follow-up. The frequency of angiographic restenosis for that particular stent is determined by subtracting this number from 100 (it is easier than it sounds!). In the example, the frequency of angiographic restenosis is approximately 10% for Stent A and 40% for Stent B.

15 Answer F. Small randomized trials have demonstrated significant reductions in angiographic restenosis for each of these agents. Oral prednisone therapy was examined in a study that included 83 patients with elevated serum C-reactive protein concentrations 72 hours following stenting (*J Am Coll Cardiol.* 2002;40:1935–1942). Patients were randomized to prednisone versus placebo for 45 days, and 6-month angiographic restenosis was significantly lower among patients treated with prednisone. In the 250-patient Valsartan for Prevention of Restenosis after Stenting (VAL-PREST) study, valsartan therapy was associated with a 50% reduction in angiographic restenosis compared with placebo (*J Invasive Cardiol.* 2001;13:93–97). Although 3-hydroxy-3 methyl-glutaryl (HMG)-CoA reductase inhibitor therapy has generally yielded disappointing results for restenosis prevention following PCI, pravastatin therapy was associated with a significant reduction in restenosis in the Regression Growth Evaluation Study (REGRESS) (*Eur Heart J.* 2001;22:1642–1681). A small trial examining the antidiabetic agent troglitazone also demonstrated a restenosis benefit (*J Am Coll Cardiol.* 2000;36:1529–1535). Although interesting, confirmation of these results in larger trials is necessary.

16 Answer A. Rapamycin and paclitaxel stents are both associated with a reduction in angiographic and clinical parameters of restenosis in patients with and without diabetes mellitus (*J Am Coll Cardiol.* 2005;

45:1172–1179, *Circulation.* 2004;109:2273–2278). In the intracoronary stenting and antithrombotic regimen (ISAR)-diabetes study, which randomized 250 patients with diabetes to implantation of rapamycin versus paclitaxel stents, the rapamycin-coated stent was associated with a significant reduction in late luminal loss at late angiographic follow-up (*New Engl J Med.* 2005;353:663–670). Diabetes has not heretofore been identified as a predictor of subacute or late stent thrombosis following DES placement. Although drug-coated stents significantly reduce the need for repeat revascularization compared with BMSs, they have not been shown to provide any relative mortality benefit.

17 Answer E. Routine stress testing (with or without adjunctive imaging) or other imaging studies to screen for stent patency have not been associated with improved prognosis, and in the absence of clinical symptoms are typically not indicated for screening purposes following successful PCI. As discussed in the ACC/AHA Practice Guidelines for Exercise Testing, routine periodic monitoring of asymptomatic patients after PCI or coronary artery bypass graft (CABG) without specific indications is considered not useful (Class III indication). The guidelines do suggest, however, that screening may be useful in patients considered to be at particularly high risk, for example, those with depressed left ventricular function, multivessel coronary disease, proximal LAD disease, multivessel disease, diabetes, hazardous occupations, or suboptimal PCI results (*J Am Coll Cardiol.* 2002;40:1531–1540). Routine follow-up coronary angiography is typically advised in patients who undergo stenting of an unprotected left main coronary artery.

18 Answer C. In a large registry of patients treated with a sirolimus-eluting stent, the following clinical, angiographic, and procedural variables were found to be independent predictors of subsequent in-stent restenosis: Treatment of in-stent restenosis odds ratio (OR) 4.16, 95% CI, 1.63 to 11.01; p <0.01), ostial location (OR 4.84, 95% CI, 1.81 to 12.07; p <0.01), diabetes (OR 2.63, 95% CI, 1.14 to 6.31; $p = 0.02$), total stented length (per 10-mm increase; OR 1.42, 95% CI, 1.21 to 1.68; p <0.01), reference diameter (per 1.0-mm increase; OR 0.46, 95% CI, 0.24 to 0.87; $p = 0.03$), and LAD artery (OR 0.30, 95% CI, 0.10 to 0.69; p <0.01)(*Circulation.* 2004;109:1366–1370).

19 Answer B. In a randomized trial of drug-eluting versus balloon angioplasty implantation for the treatment of in-stent restenosis, the use of either the sirolimus or paclitaxel-eluting stent was associated with significant reductions in both angiographic restenosis and the need for repeat target lesion revascularization. In this study, the sirolimus stent demonstrated an approximate threefold reduction in the incidence of recurrent angiographic restenosis compared with (BMS) (44.6 vs. 14.3%), and the paclitaxel-eluting stent was associated with a significant twofold reduction in angiographic restenosis (44.6 vs. 21.7%). Among patients receiving the sirolimus rather than the paclitaxel stent, there was a trend toward less late loss and a significant reduction in the need for repeat target vessel revascularization (8.0% in the sirolimus stent group versus 19.0% in the paclitaxel stent group, $p = 0.02$) (*JAMA.* 2005;293:165–171). Although effective as a means of therapy, DESs are associated with greater restenosis rates when used for the treatment of in-stent restenosis than when used for the treatment of *de novo* lesions (*Circulation.* 2004;109:1366–1370).

20 **Answer B.** Mehran et al. devised a classification system for restenosis based on the likelihood of late patency following repeat percutaneous intervention. In their analysis of 288 in-stent lesions treated with PCI, the focal pattern was associated with the lowest need for repeat revascularization (19%), followed by the diffuse intrastent (35%), diffuse proliferative (50%), and total occlusion (82%) patterns (*Circulation.* 1999;100:1872–1878).

ISR pattern I: Focal

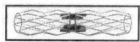

Type IA: Articulation or gap

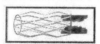

Type IB: Margin

Type IC: Focal body

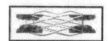

Type ID: Multifocal

ISR patterns II, III, IV: Diffuse

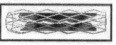

ISR pattern II: Intrastent

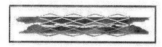

ISR pattern III: Proliferative

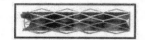

ISR pattern IV: Total occlusion

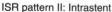

21 **Answer D.** This patient is best treated with bypass surgery. Although ongoing trials continue to assess the safety and efficacy of unprotected left main stenting, this scenario remains a contraindication to PCI (Class III) among individuals who are candidates for bypass surgery in the most recently published ACC/AHA/Society for Cardiovascular Angiography and Intervention (SCAI) PCI Guidelines (*ACC/AHA 2005 Guideline Update.* 2006).

22 **Answer C.** Following PCI for in-stent restenosis, adjunctive brachytherapy is associated with significant reductions in the incidence of clinical and angiographic restenosis at 6 months. Interestingly, late follow-up reports from both the Washington Radiation for In-Stent Restenosis Trial (WRIST) and Gamma-1 trials demonstrated an excess need for late target vessel revascularization between 6 months and 5 years among patients who received brachytherapy rather than placebo. Most restenosis events in the placebo arm occurred within the first 6 months. Although these findings suggest that in some individuals brachytherapy merely delays rather than prevents the development of recurrent in-stent restenosis, at 5 years the cumulative incidence of major adverse cardiac events remained significantly better among patients treated with brachytherapy versus placebo in both WRIST (46.2% vs. 69.2%, $p = 0.008$) and Gamma-1 (38.5% vs. 65.5%, $p = 0.02$) (*Catheter Cardiovasc Interv.* 2004;62:318–322, *Circulation.* 2002;105:2737–2740).

Late vascular wall aneurysm or pseudoaneurysm formation adjacent to the site of brachytherapy has been reported, but appears to be a rare event. Although there have been no prospective randomized trials comparing γ versus β radiation for the treatment of in-stent restenosis, observational data has not suggested that the two sources differ with respect to efficacy (*Am J Cardiol.* 2003;92:1409–1413). The use of repeat brachytherapy for recurrent in-stent restenosis that has failed a previous attempt at intracoronary radiation appears to represent a safe and potentially efficacious approach (*Circulation.* 2003;108:654–656).

23 **Answer A.** In the setting of in-stent restenosis, DES implantation is associated with improved acute luminal gain, less late loss, less negative remodeling, and fewer subsequent clinical events than balloon angioplasty (*JAMA.* 2005;293:165–171). Following DES placement for the treatment of in-stent restenosis, underexpansion of the newly placed DES has been found to represent a significant cause of late stent failure due to recurrent restenosis (*Circulation.* 2004;109:1085–1088).

24 **Answer C.** Although cutting balloon angioplasty for in-stent restenosis is associated with less early recoil at the treatment site than conventional angioplasty, (*Italian Heart J.* 2004;5:271–279) the cutting balloon technique does not appear to reduce the likelihood of recurrent restenosis. In the randomized Restenosis Cutting Balloon Evaluation Trial (RESCUT), 428 patients with in-stent restenosis were randomized to treatment with either conventional or cutting balloon angioplasty. The cutting balloon was associated with less balloon slippage and a lower number of balloons used during the intervention; however, there was no significant difference in angiographic restenosis between the conventional and cutting balloons at 7-month follow-up (*J Am Coll Cardiol.* 2004;43:943–949).

25 **Answer E.** None of the antiplatelet or anticoagulant agents listed have been associated with reductions in neointimal hyperplasia formation or clinical restenosis when administered in conjunction with the treatment of either *de novo* or restenotic lesions. In the Evaluation of ReoPro And Stenting to Eliminate Restenosis (ERASER) study, for example, abciximab therapy at the time of stent implantation was not associated with significant reductions in either IVUS or angiographic measures of restenosis compared with placebo at 6-month follow-up (*Circulation.* 1999;100:799–806).

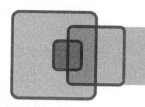

17

Atherectomy, Rotablation, and Laser

Robert J. Applegate

Questions

1 Which of the following best describes results from directional coronary atherectomy (DCA)?

(A) "Optimal" atherectomy with use of intravascular ultrasound to guide the extent of atherectomy does not result in lower restenosis rates compared with historical controls
(B) The mechanism of lumen enlargement following directional atherectomy occurs both by tissue extraction and by vessel stretching
(C) Recovery of deep wall elements (media and adventitia) correlates with the incidence of restenosis
(D) Restenosis following directional atherectomy occurs because of positive remodeling and intimal proliferation

2 Which of the following patients would be most likely to have a complication during directional atherectomy?

(A) A 50-year-old woman with a focal mid right coronary artery (RCA) lesion with a reference vessel size of 3.5 mm
(B) An 80-year-old man with tortuous calcified iliac arteries and a calcified mid circumflex lesion with reference vessel size of 2.5 mm
(C) A 70-year-old man with prior coronary artery bypass grafting and an ostial lesion of the saphenous vein graft (SVG) to a diagonal vessel with a reference diameter of 3.5 mm
(D) A 60-year-old man with restenosis of the mid left anterior descending (LAD) coronary artery with a reference segment of 3.5 mm

3 Randomized clinical trials of directional atherectomy versus balloon angioplasty for *de novo* lesions in native coronary arteries found which of the following comparing atherectomy with angioplasty?

(A) Lower complication rates, lower restenosis
(B) Lower complications rates, higher restenosis
(C) Higher complication rates, lower restenosis
(D) Higher complication rates, higher restenosis

4 Which of the following is most likely to cause a complication during directional atherectomy?

(A) Use of a 0.014-in. guidewire with polytetrafluoroethylene (PTFE) coating the distal portion of the wire
(B) Clockwise rotation and deep seating of a guide catheter to achieve a stable working platform
(C) Limiting device balloon inflation pressures to 40 psi or less
(D) Placing the guidewire tip 3 to 5 cm distal to device in the straight portion of target artery

5 A 64-year-old man is referred for DCA of the lesion shown (left figure). After the initial pass, the cutter could not be backed out over the guidewire (right figure). The angiogram following removal of the DCA device and guidewire is shown (middle figure).

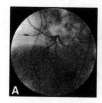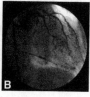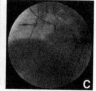

Which of the following is most likely responsible for this finding?

(A) Overaggressive wire manipulation during initial wiring of the lesion
(B) Use of a nitinol wire
(C) Distal migration of the guidewire with guidewire tip rotation
(D) Limiting DCA to four to six passes before removing device

6 Which one of the following is best treated with rotational atherectomy?

(A) Presence of visible thrombus
(B) Lesions >20 mm in length
(C) Recent angioplasty with evidence of localized dissection
(D) Severely angulated lesion

7 Which of the following is *true* with respect to rotational atherectomy and restenosis?

(A) When compared with balloon angioplasty in randomized clinical trials, restenosis is lower with rotational atherectomy
(B) Restenosis is lower with rotational atherectomy in small vessels compared with balloon angioplasty
(C) Adjunctive use of rotational atherectomy before coronary stenting is associated with lower restenosis rates compared with use of stenting alone
(D) No randomized clinical trial has shown reduced restenosis rates with rotational atherectomy

8 Which of the following is most likely to be associated with "slow flow" or "no reflow" during rotational atherectomy?

(A) Burr runs ≤1 minute in duration
(B) Burr speeds of 140,000 to 160,000 rpm
(C) Multiple burr runs <1 minute apart
(D) "Deceleration" <5,000 rpm

9 Which of the following is most likely to lead to potential complications during rotational atherectomy?

(A) Differential cutting
(B) Orthogonal displacement of friction
(C) Wire bias
(D) Microparticulate debris <12 μm

10 The following factor is most likely to result in burr stalling:

(A) Lightly tightened hemostatic valve
(B) Spasm of the coronary vessel

(C) Saline flush in the drive shaft
(D) Deceleration <5,000 rpm

11 Which of the following is most likely to result in a complication during rotational atherectomy?

(A) Initial burr-to-artery ratio of 0.5 to 0.6
(B) Continuation of burring until lesion is crossed for short, calcific lesions
(C) Platforming of the burr in a segment proximal to the stenosis
(D) Use of Rotaglide
(E) Use of vasodilators and frequent contrast injections

12 Rotational atherectomy of a mid circumflex coronary artery lesion (left figure) is performed in a stepped fashion with 1.5 mm and 2.0 mm burrs. The result is shown (right figure). The most likely cause of this result after rotational atherectomy is:

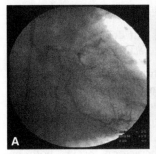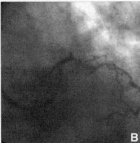

(A) Coronary vasospasm
(B) Wire bias
(C) Guide catheter dissection
(D) Centrifugal displacement of friction

13 Rotational atherectomy of a proximal RCA lesion (left figure) was performed using a 1.25-mm burr. Some difficulty was encountered in advancing a 1.75-mm burr into the left main coronary artery. During platforming of the burr, the patient complained of chest pain and the angiogram (on the right) was obtained. Which of the following is the best option for treatment of this patient at this time?

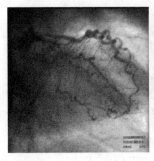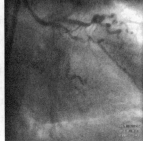

(A) Perform balloon angioplasty and stenting of the proximal ramus

(B) Upsize to a 2.25-mm burr and repeat atherectomy

(C) Perform immediate pericardiocentesis and prepare the patient for emergency cardiac surgery

(D) Inject RCA to determine if there is collateral flow to the ramus vessel

14 A 78-year-old man presented with unstable angina. Coronary angiography revealed diffuse, calcific disease of the LAD coronary artery as shown (left figure). Rotational atherectomy of the LAD coronary artery was performed with a 1.25-mm burr, followed by a 1.75-mm burr. The patient complained of chest pain and the following angiogram (right figure) was obtained. Which of the following is the best treatment for this patient?

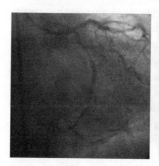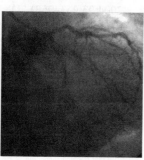

(A) Intracoronary thrombolytics

(B) Extraction atherectomy

(C) Stenting of the LAD

(D) Low-pressure balloon angioplasty with administration of intracoronary vasodilator

15 A calcific lesion in the mid LAD coronary artery is treated with initial rotational atherectomy followed by placement of a drug-eluting stent. Which of the following best describes the evidence base supporting this approach?

(A) Debulking before use of drug-eluting stent reduces restenosis rates

(B) There are no randomized trials of rotational atherectomy followed by use of drug-eluting stent

(C) "Facilitated stenting" with use of rotational atherectomy before use of drug-eluting stent

is reasonable with target burr-to-artery ratios of 0.7 to 0.8

(D) Minimizing the area of injury before use of drug-eluting stent reduces edge effects

16 Which of the following is least likely to explain lumen enlargement during laser atherectomy?

(A) Photothermal effects

(B) Dottering

(C) Photochemical dissociation

(D) Photoacoustic effects

17 Which of the following is most likely to be associated with increased risk of dissection during laser atherectomy?

(A) Saline flushes

(B) Restenotic lesions

(C) Contrast flushes

(D) Small-diameter laser catheters

18 Compared with balloon angioplasty, with which of the following is laser atheroblation associated:

(A) Decreased complications, decreased restenosis

(B) Decreased complications, increased restenosis

(C) Increased complications, decreased restenosis

(D) Increased complications, increased restenosis

19 Which of the following best describes the appropriate technique during laser ablation?

(A) Use of a 2.0-mm catheter for total occlusion crossed with a guidewire

(B) Use of 40 mJ per mm fluence, frequency of 20 Hz, and pulse sequence for 2.5 seconds

(C) Use of low osmolar contrast agent during laser ablation to minimize thrombus formation

(D) A power guide position is more important than coaxial guide positioning

20 Which of the following is a relative contraindication to the use of laser ablation?

(A) Ostial stenosis of the RCA

(B) In-stent restenosis of the body of SVG to OM1

(C) Chronic occlusion of 15 mm of the mid LAD

(D) Heavily calcified lesion of the mid circumflex involving OM2

Answers and Explanations

1 **Answer B.** Intravascular ultrasound studies have indicated that the mechanism of lumen enlargement is both by tissue extraction and by vessel stretching from the centering balloon. "Optimal atherectomy" was evaluated in the OARS trial (*Circulation.* 1998;97:332–339). In this registry trial, use of intravascular ultrasound guided the extent of atherectomy, with a target of <20% residual stenosis angiographically. Intravascular ultrasound led to greater luminal gain and decreased restenosis rates at the time of follow-up compared with historical controls. Although one might postulate that the presence of elements of the arterial wall in DCA tissue such as adventitia should correlate with the extent of restenosis, there is no correlation between recovery of deep wall elements from the media and adventitia and the rate of restenosis following DCA. In the late follow-up period (≥6 months), negative remodeling (not positive remodeling) and intimal proliferation are observed.

2 **Answer B.** Use of DCA in severely calcified lesions is relatively contraindicated because of poor calcium-cutting capabilities of DCA cutters. Moreover, the circumflex coronary artery is the least amenable to directional atherectomy. Finally, the presence of tortuous iliac arteries makes the use of larger guiding catheters that are necessary to perform atherectomy problematic. All of these factors and the small size of the target vessel make it most likely that this patient will have a complication compared with the other patients. Although there are no randomized trials evaluating the use of DCA in specific lesion types, clinical experience and observational studies indicate that bifurcation lesions and aorto-ostial lesions are both well treated by DCA. However, no reduction in restenosis has been observed when DCA is compared with simple balloon angioplasty. In the CAVEAT-II Trial comparing directional atherectomy with balloon angioplasty in SVG lesions, use of DCA was associated with similar acute benefit and similar restenosis rates (*Circulation.* 1995;91: 1966–1974).

3 **Answer C.** The CAVEAT and BOAT trials randomized directional atherectomy versus balloon angioplasty for *de novo* lesions in native coronary arteries (*Circulation.* 1998;97:322–331, *N Engl J Med.* 1993;329:221–227). In these trials, directional

atherectomy was associated with an increase in creatine phosphokinase (CPK)-MB elevations, which were ≥3 times normal, and periprocedural myocardial infarction (MI) compared with balloon angioplasty, and therefore had higher acute complication rates. By contrast, at the time of the angiographic follow-up, there was a statistically lower incidence of restenosis following directional atherectomy compared with balloon angioplasty in the BOAT trial, with a lower rate also observed in the CAVEAT trial (*p* < 0.06). The AMIGO trial was a randomized comparison of "optimal atherectomy" (<20% residual after DCA) followed by bare metal stenting compared with bare metal stenting alone (*Am J Cardiol.* 2004;93:953–958). Despite favorable early reports that debulking and stenting was associated with lower restenosis rates than stenting alone, the randomized trial results indicated equivalent acute gain, similar early complication rates, and no difference in major adverse cardiac events at 8-month follow-up including angiographic restenosis. The benefit of DCA followed by use of drug-eluting stent has not been evaluated in clinical trials.

4 **Answer B.** The optimal technique of directional atherectomy starts with coaxial positioning of the guide catheter. Deep seating of a guide catheter to achieve a "power position" is not necessary, and is associated with a higher incidence of guide catheter–induced coronary dissection. A 0.014-in. guidewire with PTFE coating the distal portion is recommended for use with a directional atherectomy device to facilitate rotation of the cutter on the guidewire. Limiting device balloon inflation pressures to 40 psi or less minimizes potential balloon trauma to the vessel. Finally, placing the guidewire tip 3 to 5 cm distal to the device in a straight portion of the vessel reduces the likelihood of developing guidewire tip dissection due to the spinning of the wire as the cutter spins within the atherectomy device.

5 **Answer C.** This sequence of angiograms depicts fracture of the guidewire tip with perforation of the apical portion of the LAD coronary artery. This may occur as a result of failure to secure the wire during atherectomy, with rotation of the tip as a consequence of rotation of the cutter and shaft over the guidewire. If the tip is anchored in a distal vessel, the wire may be fractured, usually at the junction of the tip and shaft of the wire as has occurred here. Use of a nitinol wire *per se* is not associated with this complication. Limiting DCA to four to six passes minimizes the likelihood that the cutter will be packed tightly with atherectomous material, and subsequently trapping the device on the guidewire.

6 **Answer B.** Although treating of lesions >20 mm in length may take longer than treating shorter lesions, clinical evidence suggests that longer lesions can be treated as effectively as shorter lesions with rotational atherectomy without an increase in complication rates. The presence of visible thrombus or the presence of a localized dissection after a recent balloon angioplasty are both associated with increased complications from use of rotational atherectomy. Severely angulated lesions are associated with increased perforation rates and should not be treated with rotational atherectomy.

7 **Answer D.** Although rotational atherectomy has been used extensively in the past to debulk lesions, the STRATAS trial, (*Am J Cardiol.* 2001;87:699–705) and the DART trial (*Am Heart J.* 2003;145:847–854) examined restenosis rates in randomized fashion comparing rotational atherectomy with balloon angioplasty. Neither study found a lower incidence of restenosis with rotational atherectomy.

8 **Answer B.** Burr speeds of 140,000 to 160,000 rpm have been examined in the experimental setting and have been found to be associated with less increase in local temperature during atherectomy compared with other burr speeds (*Cathet Cardiovasc Diagn.* 1998;45:208–214). This technique has been translated into clinical practice and is believed to be the optimal speed for larger burrs. For burr sizes <2 mm, speeds of approximately 160,000 rpm are currently recommended. Burr runs >1 minute in duration and multiple burr runs with inadequate time to allow for washout of microparticulate debris are believed to be associated with an increase in slow flow or no flow. Decelerations of >5,000 rpm have also been shown, in clinical studies, to be associated with a higher incidence of local complications including slow flow, CPK rises, and restenosis (*Am J Cardiol.* 2001;87:699–705).

9 **Answer C.** Wire bias refers to the position of the rotational atherectomy wire in an eccentric position within the coronary vessel. In spite of the relatively floppy nature of the rotational atherectomy wire, the physical strength of the wire in an eccentric position leads to atherectomy that follows the position of the wire. If the wire is eccentrically lying against

the lesion, this may facilitate the effectiveness of rotational atherectomy. However, if it is against the normal vessel, this may create a track outside of the normal vessel lumen, and may lead to local complications including perforation. Both differential cutting and orthogonal displacement of friction are believed to represent principles that contribute to effective use of rotational atherectomy. The small size of microparticulate debris allows the debris to pass through the distal coronary vasculature and minimizes plugging and vessel obstruction, although inadequate flushing of the vessel during atherectomy may still result in microvascular plugging.

10 **Answer D.** Burr stalling is a potential catastrophic complication associated with rotational atherectomy. Spasm of the coronary vessel may trap the burr and cause stalling. For this reason, use of vasodilators to prevent spasm is strongly encouraged. In the worst-case scenario, the burr may become wrapped and then trapped by the intima of the vessel, with ensuing vessel occlusion. Unless the burr can be removed by counterclockwise rotation of the drive shaft, emergency surgery may be required to deal with this situation. Lightly tightening the hemostatic valve prevents the drive shaft from stalling. Saline flush in the drive shaft will cool the motor drive unit, preventing burnout and stalling of the motor drive. Decelerations of <5,000 rpm frequently occur during rotational atherectomy and have not been found to be associated with slow flow, no reflow, or burr stalling (*Am J Cardiol.* 2001;87:699–705).

11 **Answer B.** The optimal technique of rotational atherectomy has been developed on the basis of extensive clinical experience and a consensus of expert operators. Although short calcific lesions are excellent targets for rotational atherectomy, they may require multiple passes with the atherectomy device before they can be crossed with the device. Continuation of burring until a lesion is crossed may increase local temperatures, causing local spasm and potentially perforation, as well as filling the distal vasculature with excessive microparticulate debris, leading to slow flow or no flow. Use of an initial burr-to-artery ratio of 0.5 to 0.6 provides a safe starting point for rotational atherectomy. Some experts believe that a final burr-to-artery ratio of 0.7 to 0.8 constitutes an optimal technique of rotational atherectomy as well, although in the era of drug-eluting stents the optimal ratio may be in the 0.5 to 0.6 range. Platforming the burr in a segment proximal to the stenosis is important so that the optimal burr speed can be used in the lesion, and sudden forward movement of the burr into the lesion during activation of the device can be prevented. Rotaglide is a lubricant composed of olive oil and egg yolk phospholipids, which facilitates rotation of the drive shaft, movement of the device over the wire, and movement of the burr within the vessel. Vasodilators are used to prevent spasm and minimize burr deceleration or stalling. Frequent contrast injections are used to maximize flushing of microparticulate debris through the distal vasculature, as well as to allow careful monitoring for perforations.

12 **Answer B.** In this case, wire bias resulted in rotational atherectomy of the "inner curve" of the bend in the mid circumflex, with a subintimal channel outside of the original coronary lumen. Wire bias represents the phenomenon of eccentric position of a guidewire "cutting the corner" of a tortuous vessel, with subsequent atherectomy within the vessel along this eccentrically positioned guidewire. Although coronary spasm and guide catheters may result in injury to the coronary circulation during rotational atherectomy, they are not likely to have caused this result. Centrifugal displacement of friction is one of the principles that allows movement of the burr over the guidewire with the minimal tolerances between burr lumen and guidewire size.

13 **Answer C.** This patient has developed a Type III, free-flowing perforation at the junction of the left main and ramus vessels. This may have occurred as a result of unrecognized wire bias and atherectomy of the carina of the left main and ramus vessels. Additionally, this may have been a result of formation of an unrecognized loop in the guidewire at the tip of the guide catheter during advancement of the burr up the guide catheter. In this situation, platforming of the burr may not have been in a path coaxial with the left main and ramus vessels, resulting in inadvertent atherectomy of the left main. It is unlikely that attempts at balloon tamponade of the perforation would be successful given the location of the perforation. Moreover, prolonged balloon inflation would likely be followed by hemodynamic collapse because of LAD and left circumflex flow obstruction from the inflated balloon. Reversal of anticoagulation and stopping glycoprotein (GP)IIb/IIIa inhibitors with platelet transfusion would also be reasonable but are unlikely to adequately treat the perforation without accompanying surgery.

14 **Answer D.** This patient has developed slow flow/no reflow, most likely secondary to excessive microparticulate debris embolization of the distal vasculature. Intracoronary thrombolytics are unlikely to be

of benefit because this complication is not thrombus mediated. Similarly, extraction atherectomy would not be useful, and may also have limited feasibility given the small caliber of the lumen and the presence of diffuse calcific disease. Stenting of the LAD without adequate visualization of the landing zone proximally and distally would be problematic, and would not address the microvascular plugging. Low-pressure balloon angioplasty is a reasonable choice to relieve local spasm, and also provides a means to deliver vasodilators to the distal vascular bed of the LAD. Use of an intra-aortic balloon pump (IABP) to augment coronary perfusion pressures may also be necessary if significant hypotension develops.

15 **Answer B.** There are no randomized studies evaluating debulking by rotational atherectomy before use of drug-eluting stent. Therefore, the statement that rotational atherectomy reduces restenosis rates before use of drug-eluting stents is incorrect. Most experts agree that the optimal technique of using rotational atherectomy before drug-eluting stent placement is to perform "facilitated" stenting with low burr-to-artery ratios, and minimizing the area of injury to reduce the likelihood of edge effects. However, there are few clinical trials that confirm the effectiveness of these strategies.

16 **Answer B.** The mechanism of tissue ablation during use of laser occurs as a result of vaporization of tissue, or the photothermal effect, correct breakdown of molecules, or photochemical dissociation, and ejection of debris, or the photoacoustic effect. It is not clear that there is one predominant mechanism of tissue ablation, although in an animal model photochemical dissociation would appear to be the predominant mechanism. Dottering of the vessel by the device itself is unlikely to occur in most circumstances and is not believed to contribute to lumen enlargement during laser atherectomy.

17 **Answer C.** A coronary artery dissection is increased during use of laser atheroblation compared with balloon angioplasty or other techniques in general. The use of contrast flushes or injections during laser runs is felt to increase local vessel disruption because of dispersion of laser energy. The use of saline flushes during laser runs has been shown to decrease the incidence of dissections, presumably because blood and contrast increase the photoacoustic effects of laser, resulting in greater tissue disruption. Clinical studies have identified bifurcation lesions, diabetes mellitus, and oversized laser atherectomy catheters as being associated with increased dissection rates.

18 **Answer D.** In the Excimer laser, rotational atherectomy and Balloon Angioplasty Comparison (ERBAC) trial, excimer laser angioplasty was associated with both an increase in coronary complications as well as higher restenosis rate compared with balloon angioplasty (*Circulation.* 1997;96:91–98). In this study, saline flushes were not used and may have been in part responsible for this higher rate of local complications.

19 **Answer B.** It is recommended that the fluence (laser power) start at 40 mJ per mm at a frequency of 20 Hz, using pulse sequences of 1 to 5 seconds as the initial laser strategy. If further lasing is indicated, the fluence rate is increased followed by an increase in the frequency rates. Use of a 2.0-mm catheter for total occlusion initially is likely to be unsuccessful. Use of any contrast agent, whether low or high osmolar, is felt to be associated with increased tissue disruption because of deflection of laser energy, and is therefore associated with increased risk of dissection. Finally, coaxial, not power, guide catheter alignment minimizes complications during laser atherectomy.

20 **Answer D.** Although it was initially hoped that laser atheroblation would be useful in heavily calcified lesions, the clinical evidence suggests that laser atherectomy is less efficient than rotational atherectomy in heavily calcified lesions, and is associated with a modest increase in clinical event rates at 6 months compared with simple balloon angioplasty. Although in-stent restenosis may be preferentially treated with drug-eluting stents, laser atherectomy was shown to be effective in in-stent restenosis including vein grafts. Chronic occlusions of coronary vessels are well suited for laser atherectomy as initial debulking strategy, as long as intraluminal position of the wire is confirmed before the use of laser.

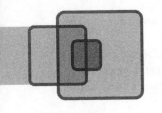

18
Stents

Stephen G. Ellis

Questions

1 With bare-metal stents (BMSs), direct stenting compared with stenting after predilatation results in:

(A) Less target lesion revascularization (TLR) at 6 months
(B) Shorter procedure times
(C) Less target vessel revascularization (TVR) at 6 months
(D) A and C
(E) All of the above

2 Angiographic correlates of stent thrombosis within 30 days of bare metal stenting include:

(A) Dissection remaining after stenting
(B) Stent length
(C) Final minimal lumen diameter (MLD)
(D) A and C
(E) All of the above

3 A 53-year-old man undergoes left anterior descending (LAD) artery stent for exertional angina. After stent deployment, there is intraluminal linear dissection. Is it safe to leave this alone after bare metal stenting?

(A) It is safe to leave mild luminal haziness alone but not intraluminal linear dissection
(B) Yes, it is safe to leave mild luminal haziness and intraluminal linear dissection alone
(C) Yes, it is safe to leave mild luminal haziness and intraluminal linear dissection alone, provided the patient is on glycoprotein IIb/IIIa antagonists
(D) No, it is not safe to leave any dissection behind

4 Correlates of stent thrombosis occurring 1 to 6 months after bare metal stenting include:

(A) Extensive plaque prolapse
(B) Radiation therapy
(C) Disruption of adjacent vulnerable plaques
(D) Stenting across side branches
(E) A, B, and C
(F) All of the above

5 Recognized complications of balloon rupture during stent implantation occurring in at least 10% of ruptures include:

(A) Coronary spasm
(B) Coronary perforation
(C) Coronary dissection
(D) A and C
(E) None of the above

6 Before implantation, coronary stents should not be touched by the operator because:

(A) There is greater risk of restenosis
(B) Glove talc may induce coronary spasm
(C) There is risk of infection
(D) Touching stents gently really does not matter
(E) A and C

7 A 36-year-old female smoker presents to you for evaluation. For the last 12 months, she has experienced morning chest pain, which does not get worse with exercise. She had an extensive workup with her primary cardiologist and was found to have variant angina. She is continuing to have chest pain on Norvasc, aspirin (ASA), and extended release nitroglycerin. She searched on the Internet and found that stenting might help. Expected outcomes of bare metal stenting for variant angina include:

(A) Improved but not total angina control
(B) Little, if any, improvement in symptoms
(C) Higher than usual risk of restenosis
(D) A and C

8 Which of the following is *not* a correlate of diffuse in-stent restenosis (ISR) with BMSs?

(A) Small reference vessel diameter (RVD)
(B) Coil stents
(C) Female gender
(D) High balloon inflation pressure
(E) None of the above

9 What is the relationship between intimal hyperplasia measured by intravascular ultrasound (IVUS) and stent size or BMSs?

(A) Intimal hyperplasia is independent of stent size
(B) Intimal hyperplasia is greater for large stents
(C) Intimal hyperplasia is greater for small stents

10 The best IVUS cross-sectional area (CSA) cutoff correlating restenosis in BMSs is:

(A) 7 mm^2
(B) 8 mm^2
(C) 9 mm^2
(D) 10 mm^2
(E) Once you factor in RVD, final CSA does not matter

11 The expected rate of TLR for proliferative pattern of bare metal stent-in-stent restenosis treated with either balloon angioplasty or bare metal stenting is:

(A) 25%
(B) 35%
(C) 50%
(D) 70%

12 The expected rate of TLR for focal pattern of bare metal stent-in-stent restenosis treated with either balloon angioplasty or bare metal stenting is:

(A) 10%
(B) 15%
(C) 20%
(D) 25%
(E) 30%

13 The absolute TVR benefit for BMSs compared with balloon angioplasty for lesions in vessels with RVD <3.0 mm is:

(A) 3%
(B) 5%
(C) 7%
(D) 10%

14 When limited to BMSs, when feasible, the best approach in treating a type 2 bifurcation lesion is:

(A) Stent across the side branch and finish with kissing balloon for side branch compromise
(B) Predilatate the side branch, stent across, and finish with kissing balloon
(C) Use cutting balloon for the side branch, stent across, and finish with kissing balloon
(D) T-stenting
(E) Culotte stenting

15 The likelihood of important side branch narrowing after high-pressure stent implantation across a side branch in a side branch with a >50% ostial narrowing is:

(A) 20%
(B) 30%
(C) 40%
(D) 50% or higher

16 The likelihood of important side branch narrowing after high-pressure stent implantation across a side branch in a branch *without* ostial narrowing is:

(A) 7%
(B) 15%
(C) 20%
(D) 25%

17 For BMSs, which characteristic has been convincingly shown to influence restenosis rate?

(A) Coil versus tubular design
(B) Strut thickness
(C) Longitudinal flexibility
(D) A and C
(E) All of the above

18 The expected TLR rate at 9 months for a contemporary BMS placed into a 3.5-mm vessel requiring a 15-mm length stent in a nondiabetic is:

(A) 3%
(B) 5%
(C) 8%
(D) 10%
(E) 12%

19 In evaluating the results of randomized trials with mandated 6- to 8-month angiography in some patients, by how much (relatively speaking) does angiography increase TLR rates compared with patients without mandated angiography?

(A) 30%

(B) 50%

(C) 70%

(D) The results between studies are too inconsistent to provide an answer

20 In the BMS era does bypass surgery or coronary stenting appear to provide better long-term (2-year) all-cause survival for dialysis patients, and does the availability of drug-eluting stents (DESs) appear to have changed this?

(A) Surgery is better

(B) Stenting is better

(C) DES has improved survival compared with BMS

(D) DES does not appear to have improved survival compared with BMS

(E) A and C

(F) A and D

21 In an attempt to stent a calcified mid-right coronary stenosis while advancing the stent, unfortunately, your guide catheter wire and balloon abruptly fall out of the vessel. You note that the stent seems to be left behind, halfway pushed into the lesion and the patient becomes ischemic. Your best option at this point is:

(A) Send the patient for emergency surgery

(B) Attempt to place a wire through the stent followed by a low-profile balloon and retrieve the stent by inflating the balloon and pulling back

(C) Attempt to snare the stent

(D) Pass a wire adjacent to the stent and compress the stent against the sidewall of the vessel

22 The most common IVUS correlate of subacute stent thrombosis is:

(A) Residual haziness suggested with thrombosis

(B) Residual haziness suggested of tissue protrusion

(C) Residual dissection

(D) Inadequate stent expansion

23 High-dose statin therapy has been chosen to reduce the risk of non-QA myocardial infarction (MI) complicating coronary stent implantation.

(A) True

(B) False

24 What are contraindications to stenting?

(A) Postdistal runoff

(B) Thrombus

(C) There are no true contraindications to stenting

(D) Heavily calcified lesion

25 A 53-year-old physician presents to your office for a second opinion. She underwent BMS to LAD percutaneous coronary intervention (PCI) because of her concern about stent thrombosis and came back 9 months later with restenosis for which she received a DES. Since then she is doing well; however, she was researching on the Internet and found that she should have had debulking before stent implantation to reduce the risk of restenosis. She would like your opinion.

(A) You agree with her because there are randomized studies that support reduction of restenosis if debulking occurs before stent implantation

(B) You disagree with her as there are studies that show no improvement in restenosis rate if debulking occurs before stent implantation

(C) You agree with her but there is no randomized data to date that supports this; there is only registry information

(D) You disagree with her but there is no randomized data to date that supports this

26 The patient in Question 25 is also insisting that she should have had adjunctive IVUS during her first PCI to reduce the risk of restenosis. Do you agree?

(A) Yes, the AVID study supports the use of adjunctive IVUS in all PCI patients

(B) No, because of conflicting results from the two studies: the AVID study only supports the use of adjunctive IVUS in complex lesions, but the optimization with intracoronary ultrasound to reduce stent restenosis (OPTICUS) study supports the use in all PCI patients

(C) No, the AVID study only supported the use of adjunctive IVUS in complex lesions, but the OPTICUS study showed no difference between the IVUS or routine angiography group

(D) Yes, both AVID and OPTICUS supported the use of adjunctive IVUS in LAD lesions

27 A 58-year-old man undergoes a stress test for new chest pain. He is found to have lateral wall ischemia and undergoes cardiac computed tomography (CT) scanning. He is found to have significant stenosis. He is referred by his internist. The patient wants to talk to you about the risk of PCI. He wants you to list the potential complications of stenting. In the current era, what is the rate of emergent coronary artery bypass grafting (CABG) and in-hospital mortality?

(A) 0.1% to 1.0% CABG and 0.1% in-hospital mortality rate

(B) 1% to 2% CABG and 0.7% to 1.5% in-hospital mortality rate

(C) 3% to 5% CABG and 1% to 3% in-hospital mortality rate

(D) 3% to 5% CABG and 0.7% to 1.5% in-hospital mortality rate

28 In the published trials and selected registries of unprotected left main trunk PCI with BMS, what is the long-term mortality rate?

(A) 1% to 3%

(B) 3% to 10%

(C) 3% to 15%

(D) 3% to 25%

29 A 78-year-old retired executive presents to you for a second opinion. He had CABG 10 years ago and has been having increasing chest pain. He underwent a stress test, which showed inferior ischemia and then underwent an angiogram. He had patent left internal mammary artery (LIMA) to LAD and saphenous vein grafts (SVG) to obtuse marginal 1 (OM1) and OM2. However, his SVG to right coronary artery (RCA) was found to have severe 85% diffuse stenosis in the graft. He read that covered stents might be helpful.

He would like you to use covered stent for SVG to RCA PCI. Do you agree?

(A) No, covered stents have not been studied in SVG PCI

(B) No, covered stents reduce embolization risk but not restenosis risk in SVG PCI

(C) No, covered stents do not reduce restenosis or embolization risk in SVG PCI.

(D) No, covered stents reduce restenosis but not embolization risk in SVG PCI

30 A 63-year-old patient underwent PCI to OM1 2 days ago. She had an uneventful procedure and was discharged home the next day. The following day, she noticed numbness and weakness of her right arm and legs and came back to the hospital. She underwent emergent CT, which showed no intracranial bleeding. The neurologist would like to do a magnetic resonance imaging (MRI). However, the radiologists are scared because of her recent PCI. What is your recommendation?

(A) MRI can be safely done 6 to 8 weeks after PCI

(B) MRI can be safely done 4 to 6 weeks after PCI

(C) MRI can be safely done 1 week after PCI

(D) MRI can be safely done 1 to 3 days after PCI

Answers and Explanations

1 **Answer B.** Overall, direct stenting was associated with a decrease in procedural time with lower fluoroscopic time, reduction in contrast volume, and a cost reduction. However, at 6 months, there was no reduction in death, MI, TLR, or TVR (*Am J Cardiol.* 2003;91:790–796).

2 **Answer E.** The variables most significantly associated with the probability of stent thrombosis in a pooled analysis were persistent dissection National Heart, Lung and Blood Institute (NHLBI) grade B or higher after stenting, total stent length, and final MLD within the stent (*Circulation.* 2001;103:1967–1971).

3 **Answer A.** It is safe to leave mild luminal haziness alone but not intraluminal linear dissection. Intraluminal linear dissection increases the risk of acute closure (*Circulation.* 2001;103:1967–1971).

National Heart, Lung and Blood Institute's Classification System of Coronary Dissection

Type	Description	Rate of Acute Closure (%)
A	Mild luminal haziness	0
B	Intraluminal linear dissection	3
C	Extraluminal contrast dye staining or extraluminal cap (with persistence of dye after dye clearance)	10
D	Spiral dissection	30
E	Dissection with filling defects	9
F	Dissection with limited or no flow	69

4 **Answer F.** Late stent thrombosis was defined as an acute thrombus within a stent that had been in place for >30 days. The pathologic mechanisms of late stent thrombosis were stenting across ostia of major arterial branches, exposure to radiation therapy, plaque disruption in the nonstented arterial segment within 2 mm of the stent margin, and stenting of markedly necrotic, lipid-rich plaques with extensive plaque prolapse and diffuse ISR (*Circulation.* 2003;108:1701–1706).

5 **Answer D.** Balloon rupture is a rare complication during stent implantation, which can usually be managed with stents (*Am J Cardiol.* 1997;80:1077–1080).

6 **Answer A.** In vivo analysis of rinsed versus non-rinsed stents demonstrated a reduced neointimal thickness, neointimal area, and vessel percent stenosis in rinsed, compared with nonrinsed, stents. A significant reduction in the inflammatory infiltrate around struts was also observed in untouched stents (*J Am Coll Cardiol.* 2001;38:562–568).

7 **Answer A.** Twenty percent of patients with variant angina are resistant to medical therapy. For these patients, stenting has improved angina control. However, in a small study, 33% of the patients continued to have angina after stent implantation (*J Am Coll Cardiol.* 1999;34:216–222).

8 **Answer E.** Diffuse restenosis was associated with a smaller RVD, longer lesion length, female gender, longer stent length, and the use of coil stents. Aggressive forms of ISR occur earlier and with more symptoms, including MI (*J Am Coll Cardiol.* 2001;37: 1019–1025).

9 **Answer A.** Intimal hyperplasia CSA and thickness at follow-up were calculated and compared with stent CSA and circumference. There was a weak, but significant correlation between mean and maximum intimal hyperplasia CSA versus stent CSA. However, there was no correlation between mean or maximum intimal hyperplasia thickness versus stent CSA or stent circumference. Intimal hyperplasia thickness was found to be independent of the stent size (*Am J Cardiol.* 1998;82:1168–1172).

10 **Answer C.** Patients with restenosis have a significantly longer total stent length, smaller reference lumen diameter, smaller final MLD by angiography, and smaller stent lumen CSA by IVUS. In lesions without restenosis, patients had 9.4 ± 3.4 mm CSA versus 8.1 ± 2.7 mm ($p <0.0001$) in patients with restenosis. IVUS guidance, IVUS stent lumen CSA was a better independent predictor than the angiographic measurements (*J Am Coll Cardiol.* 1998;32:1630–1635).

11 **Answer C.** Mehran et al. (*Circulation.* 1999;100: 1872–1878) developed an angiographic classification of ISR according to the geographic distribution of intimal hyperplasia in reference to the implanted stent: Pattern I includes focal lesions ($\leq$10 mm in length), pattern II is ISR >10 mm within the stent, pattern III includes ISR >10 mm extending outside the stent, and pattern IV is totally occluded ISR. TLR increased with increasing ISR class; it was 19%, 35%, 50%, and 83% in classes I to IV, respectively.

12 **Answer C.** See explanation for Question 11 (*Circulation.* 1999;100:1872–1878).

13 **Answer B.** Moreno et al. (*J Am Coll Cardiol.* 2004;43:1964–1972) performed a meta-analysis of 11 randomized trials comparing coronary stenting versus balloon angioplasty in small coronary vessels. The pooled rates of restenosis were 25.8% and 34.2% in stent versus balloon patients, respectively ($p = 0.003$). Stented patients had lower rates of major adverse cardiac events (15.0% vs. 21.8%, $p = 0.002$; RR 0.70; 95% CI, 0.57 to 0.87) and new TVRs (12.5% vs. 17.0%, $p = 0.004$; RR 0.75, 95% CI, 0.61 to 0.91).

14 **Answer A.** Balloon angioplasty of coronary bifurcation lesions is associated with a lower success and higher complication rate. Suwaidi et al. (*J Am Coll Cardiol.* 2000;35:929–936) performed a study where they treated 131 patients with bifurcation lesions. Patients were divided into two groups: Group 1 where a stent was deployed in one branch and percutaneous transluminal coronary angioplasty (PTCA) in the side branch, and Group 2 where stent deployment occurred in both branches. Group 2 was then divided into two subgroups depending on the technique of stent deployment. The Gp2a subgroup underwent Y-stenting, and the Gp2b subgroup underwent T-stenting. After 1-year follow-up, no significant differences were seen in the frequency of major adverse events (death, MI, or repeat revascularization) between Gp2a and Gp2b. Adverse cardiac events were higher with Y-stenting compared with T-stenting (86.3% vs. 30.4%, $p = 0.004$). Stenting of both branches offers no advantage over stenting one branch and performing balloon angioplasty of the other branch (*J Am Coll Cardiol.* 2000;35:929–936, *J Am Coll Cardiol.* 2000;35:1145–1151).

15 **Answer D.** Aliabadi et al. (*Am J Cardiol.* 1997;80:994–997) evaluated the incidence, angiographic predictors, and clinical outcome of side branch occlusion following stenting in 175 patients. By multivariate analysis, the presence of side branches with >50% ostial narrowing that arose from within or just beyond the diseased portion of the parent vessel was an angiographic predictor of side branch occlusion. At 9-month follow-up there was no difference in combined clinical events between those patients with and without side branch occlusion.

16 **Answer A.** See explanation for Question 15 (*Am J Cardiol.* 1997;80:994–997).

17 **Answer A.** Early coil stents had poor radial strength, allowing considerable tissue prolapse and higher restenosis rate. Thicker struts result in more intense formation of neointimal hyperplasia, which may result in higher restenosis rate. Longitudinal flexibility is associated with deliverability (*Textbook of interventional cardiology*, Vol. 4. 2003:591–630).

18 **Answer B.** In the recent DES trials such as SIRIUS (Sirolimus-Eluting Stent in *de novo* Native Coronary Lesions), TAXUS IV, and TAXUS V, TLR rate for BMS in 3.5 to 4.0 mm was only 5% at 9 months.

19 **Answer C.** Serruys et al. (*Lancet.* 1998;352:673–681) randomized patients to either clinical and angiographic follow-up or clinical follow-up alone in stent versus balloon angioplasty trial. At 6 months, a primary clinical endpoint had occurred in 12.8% of the stent group and in 19.3% of the angioplasty group ($p = 0.013$). This significant difference in clinical outcome was maintained at 12 months. In the subgroup assigned angiographic follow-up, restenosis rates occurred in 16% of the stent group and in 31% of the balloon angioplasty group ($p = 0.0008$). In the group assigned clinical follow-up alone, event-free survival rate at 12 months was higher in the stent group than in the balloon angioplasty group (0.89 vs. 0.79, $p = 0.004$).

20 **Answer F.** Herzog et al. (*Circulation.* 2002;106:2207–2211) analyzed dialysis patients in the United States hospitalized from 1995 to 1998 for first coronary revascularization procedures. The in-hospital mortality was 8.6% for CABG patients, 6.4% for PTCA patients, and 4.1% for stent patients. The 2-year all-cause survival was highest for CABG patients and lowest for stent patients.

21 **Answer D.** Passing a wire adjacent to the stent and compressing the stent against the sidewall of the vessel is probably the safest and easiest method in this situation. To pass a snare device into a calcified mid-RCA would be difficult and sending the patient to surgery without attempting stent compression is not prudent. It may be quite difficult to pass a wire through an undeployed stent.

22 **Answer D.**   Cheneau et al. (*Circulation*. 2003;108: 43–47) analyzed 7,484 consecutive patients without acute MI who were treated with PCI and stenting and who underwent IVUS imaging during the intervention. Of these, 0.4% had angiographically documented subacute closure <1 week after PCI. Subacute closure lesions were compared with a control group. In 48% of the patients with subacute stent thrombosis there were multiple causes. They included dissection (17%), thrombus (4%), and tissue protrusion within the stent struts leading to lumen compromise (4%), and reduced lumen dimension post-PCI (final lumen <80% RLD) (83%). Inadequate postprocedure lumen dimensions, alone or in combination with other procedurally related abnormal lesion morphologies (dissection, thrombus, or tissue prolapse), was the most common correlate of subacute thrombosis.

23 **Answer A.**   The Atorvastatin for Reduction of Myocardial Dysrhythmia After Cardiac Surgery (ARMYDA) trial randomized 153 patients with chronic stable angina without previous statin treatment to coronary PCI with pretreated statin versus placebo. There was less myocardial injury as measured by creatinase kinase-MB (CK-MB) and troponin in the statin group after PCI. Pretreatment with statin therapy 7 days before PCI significantly reduces procedural myocardial injury in elective coronary intervention (*Circulation*. 2004;110:674–678).

24 **Answer A.**   Poor distal runoff is a contraindication to stenting due to increased risk of stent thrombosis due to slow flow. Lesions that cannot be dilated are also not suitable for stent due to stent thrombosis. Lesions with extensive thrombus should undergo some type of thrombectomy before stent insertion.

25 **Answer B.**   The Atherectomy and Multilink Stenting Improves Gain and Outcome (AMIGO) and the Stenting Post Rotational Atherectomy Trial (SPORT) studies both failed to showed reduction in restenosis with debulking before stent implantation.

26 **Answer C.**   Angiography versus IVUS directed coronary stent placement (AVID) and OPTICUS demonstrated that IVUS did not improve the outcome. However, AVID did show improvement in high-risk lesions such as SVG, small vessel, and vessels with severe stenosis.

27 **Answer B.**   According to the American College of Cardiology National Cardiovascular Data Registry (ACC-NCDR) (1998–2000) and the NHLBI registry (1997–1998), emergent CABG rate is 1.9% and mortality rate is 0.7% to 1.4%.

28 **Answer D.**   In the registries presented by Park et al. the death rate at 25 months was 3.1% and at 31 months was 7.4%. In Takagi et al. the death rate at 31 months was 16% and in the unprotected left main trunk intervention multicenter assessment (ULTIMA) registry death rate at 1 year was 24.2%.

29 **Answer C.**   Treatment of lesions located in SVGs is associated with increased procedural risk and a high rate of restenosis. A randomized trial of a polytetrafluoroethylene (PTFE)-covered stent compared with a bare stainless steel stent for prevention of restenosis and major adverse cardiac events in patients undergoing SVG treatment was done. There was no difference in restenosis rate and 6-month clinical outcome between the PTFE-covered stent and the BMS for treatment of SVG lesions. However, a higher incidence of nonfatal MIs was found in patients treated with the PTFE-covered stent.

30 **Answer D.**   Despite emerging evidence that MRI is safe within 8 weeks of bare metal coronary stenting, there are limited data on the safety of MRI very early (1 to 3 days) after stent implantation. Porto et al. found that it was safe to undergo MRI 1 to 3 days after stent implantation without increase in major adverse cardiac events. There were no cases of acute stent thrombosis and at 9-month clinical follow-up only two patients (4%) developed adverse events (1 target vessel restenosis and 1 nontarget vessel revascularization) (*Am J Cardiol*. 2005;96:366–368).

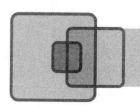

19

Drug-Eluting Stents and Local Drug Delivery for the Prevention of Restenosis

Peter Wenaweser and Bernhard Meier

Questions

1 Stents coated with drugs like sirolimus and paclitaxel reduce the incidence of in-stent restenosis. The main effect of the drugs is on:

(A) Elastic recoil
(B) Arterial remodeling
(C) Smooth muscle cell proliferation/migration
(D) Extracellular matrix production

2 Which of the following is *true* regarding sirolimus?

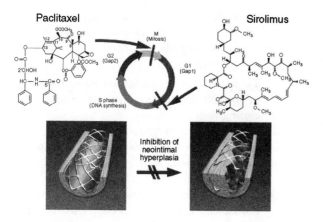

(A) Sirolimus is a macrolide
(B) Sirolimus is the metabolic substrate of the fungus *Streptomyces hygroscopicus*
(C) Sirolimus was at an early stage targeted as rapamycin for use in renal transplantation

(D) Sirolimus influences regulator genes that control the cell cycle
(E) A, B, C, and D are correct

3 Which of the following statements concerning paclitaxel (*Taxus*) is *wrong*?

(A) Paclitaxel induces disassembly of microtubules
(B) Paclitaxel was discovered in a crude extract from the bark of a Pacific yew
(C) Paclitaxel is an antimicrotubule drug
(D) Paclitaxel was first evaluated as an antitumor drug

4 Which of the following statements regarding drug-eluting stent platforms is *not* correct?

(A) The sirolimus-eluting (Cypher) stent is composed of a stainless steel stent coated with a nonerodable polymer
(B) Paclitaxel can only be used in combination with a polymer-based stent platform
(C) Polymers are long-chain molecules, which form a reservoir, and facilitate controlled and prolonged drug delivery
(D) A conceptually ideal drug-eluting stent should have a large surface area, minimal gaps between cells, and no strut deformation after deployment

5 Polymeric materials coated on stents:

(A) Allow a controlled and sustained release of agents

(B) Minimize the potential of underdosing or overdosing of drug levels

(C) Serve as drug reservoir

(D) Are potentially toxic

(E) A to D are true

6 The first randomized comparison of a sirolimus-eluting stent with a standard bare-metal stent reduced the rate of in-stent restenosis after 6 months to:

(A) 20%

(B) 15%

(C) 10%

(D) <5%

7 Which of the following treatments is suitable for a patient with in-stent restenosis following bare-metal stent implantation?

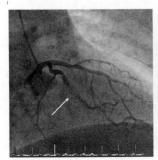 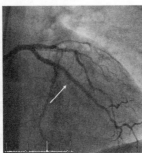

(A) Balloon angioplasty is always the treatment of choice

(B) A treatment with a sirolimus- or paclitaxel-eluting stent appears to be superior to balloon angioplasty

(C) A treatment with β-radiation has shown to be inferior to balloon angioplasty

(D) Paclitaxel-eluting stent implantation appears to be superior to sirolimus-eluting stent implantation

8 Experimental models of stent implantation in human coronary arteries show:

(A) A complete healing after bare-metal stent implantation within 2 to 4 months

(B) That the deployment of sirolimus-eluting or paclitaxel-eluting stents is associated with an increase in neointimal thickness at 28 days in comparison with bare-metal stents

(C) A delayed healing with persistence of fibrin and incomplete endothelialization after drug-eluting stent implantation

(D) Always a greater inflammatory reaction after drug-eluting stent implantation in comparison with bare-metal stent within 28 days

9 Which of the following statements is *wrong*? Very late (>1 year) stent thrombosis after drug-eluting stent implantation:

(A) May be associated with chronic inflammation of the arterial wall

(B) May be due to a hypersensitivity reaction to the polymer

(C) Can be avoided by prescribing prolonged dual antiplatelet therapy

(D) Carries a high morbidity and mortality

10 Which of the following antiproliferative agents is under clinical investigation as new drug-eluting stent systems?

(A) Tacrolimus

(B) Everolimus

(C) Biolimus

(D) Zotarolimus

(E) All of the above

11 The SIRTAX trial, a randomized, controlled, single-blind study comparing sirolimus-eluting stents with paclitaxel-eluting stents in approximately 1,000 all-comer patients favors a treatment with a sirolimus-eluting stent because of:

(A) Lower incidence of cardiac death

(B) Lower incidence of stent thrombosis

(C) Fewer major adverse cardiac events, primarily by decreasing rates of clinical and angiographic restenosis

(D) Better acute gain and higher success of stent implantation

(E) B and C

12 A meta-analysis of randomized trials by Kastrati et al. comparing sirolimus-eluting with paclitaxel-eluting stents in patients with coronary artery disease reported all *except*:

(A) Target lesion revascularization is less frequently performed in patients treated with a sirolimus-eluting stent

(B) Rate of death is comparable

(C) Angiographic restenosis is more frequently observed in patients treated with a paclitaxel-eluting stent

(D) Rates of myocardial infarction and stent thrombosis are lower in sirolimus-eluting stent treated patients

13 A 58-year-old man underwent coronary angiography due to angina pectoris CCS 3. The invasive evaluation showed a subtotal proximal left anterior descending (LAD) lesion. The result after balloon dilatation and stent implantation is good (see the figure on the left). Six months later the patient suffered from acute, ongoing chest pain with anterior ST-segment elevation in the electrocardiogram (EKG). The coronary angiography at this point of time is depicted in the figure on the right. What is your diagnosis and treatment?

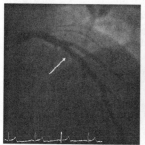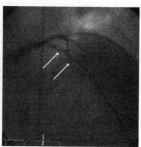

(A) Complete in-stent restenosis with plaque rupture
(B) Late stent thrombosis with a large amount of visible thrombus
(C) Balloon angioplasty and additional stent implantation
(D) Balloon angioplasty, possible thrombus aspiration/removal, and use of abciximab
(E) A and C
(F) B and D

14 Evaluation of the cost-effectiveness of drug-eluting stents in an unselected patient population in the year 2003 to 2004 (*Lancet.* 2005;366:921–929) shows that:

(A) The use of drug-eluting stents in all patients is less effective than in studies with selected patients
(B) A restriction to patients in high-risk groups should be evaluated in further trials
(C) With respect to the current prices of drug-eluting stent, an unrestricted use of these stents is not justified
(D) A to C are correct

15 A large prospective observational cohort study evaluated the incidence and predictors for stent thrombosis following drug-eluting stent implantation. The overall incidence amounted to 1.3% in a 9-month follow-up. Which of the following parameters was the strongest predictor?

(A) Premature antiplatelet therapy discontinuation
(B) Renal failure
(C) Bifurcation lesions
(D) Diabetes
(E) Low ejection fraction

16 The assessment of coronary endothelial function 6 months after comparing sirolimus-eluting stent implantation with bare-metal stent implantation, assessed with bicycle exercise as a physiologic stimulus (see following figure), revealed that:

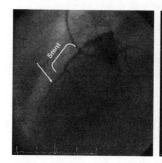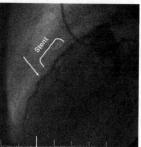

(A) Implantation of a bare-metal stent does effect physiologic response to exercise proximal and distal to the stent
(B) Implantation of a bare-metal stent does not effect physiologic response to exercise proximal and distal to the stent
(C) Implantation of a sirolimus-eluting stent does not effect physiologic response to exercise proximal and distal to the stent
(D) Implantation of a sirolimus-eluting stent does effect physiologic response to exercise proximal and distal to the stent
(E) B and D
(F) B and C

17 What are possible pitfalls of drug-eluting stents?

(A) Prolonged dual antiplatelet treatment after stent implantation
(B) Severe allergic reactions
(C) Hypersensitivity reactions caused by polymer-based stent platforms
(D) Loss of radial force of the stent after complete drug-release
(E) A, B, and C
(F) A and C

18 For the treatment of patients with multivessel disease:

(A) Coronary artery bypass grafting (CABG) is obsolete and inferior to multivessel stenting with drug-eluting stents
(B) CABG is still superior to multivessel percutaneous coronary intervention (PCI)
(C) Drug-eluting stents may provide a comparable long-term outcome to CABG, but there is a lack of conclusive data

(D) Not more than three stents or 50 mm total drug-eluting stent length should be implanted in the same patient

19 The sirolimus-eluting (Cypher) and paclitaxel-eluting (Taxus) stent platform share the following characteristics, *except*:

(A) Stainless steel stent
(B) Nonbiodegradable polymer
(C) Strut thickness 130 to 140 μm
(D) Equal release rate of the drug (sirolimus or paclitaxel)

20 A meta-analysis of all published, randomized trials comparing the clinical outcome of drug-eluting stents (sirolimus and paclitaxel) with bare-metal stents until 2004 favors the use of drug-eluting stents because of:

(A) Significant reduction of myocardial infarction
(B) Significant reduction of mortality
(C) Significant reduction of restenosis and major adverse cardiac events
(D) Significant reduction of stent thrombosis

Answers and Explanations

1   **Answer C.**   The stent accounts for arterial remodeling; the drugs for smooth muscle cell proliferation/migration; and extracellular matrix production does not occur.

2   **Answer E.**   Although developed as an antibiotic, it was found more useful as an immunosuppressant.

3   **Answer A.**   Paclitaxel promotes the polymerization of tubulin and does not induce the disassembly of microtubules like other antimicrotubule agents such as vinca alkaloids (*N Engl J Med.* 1995;332:1004–1014).

4   **Answer B.**   Some drugs can be loaded directly onto metallic surfaces (e.g., prostacyclin, paclitaxel) (*Circulation.* 2003;107:2274–2279).

5   **Answer E.**   (*Pharmacol Ther.* 2004;102:1–15).

6   **Answer D.**   None of the patients in the sirolimus-stent group, as compared with 26.6% of those in the standard stent group, had restenosis of 50% or more of the luminal diameter ($p < 0.001$) (*N Engl J Med.* 2002;346:1773–1780).

7   **Answer B.**   A direct comparison of balloon angioplasty with a treatment with sirolimus-eluting (Cypher) and paclitaxel-eluting (Taxus) stent showed a significantly lower restenosis rate with either stent. Sirolimus-eluting stent implantation may be superior to paclitaxel-eluting stent implantation. β-radiation significantly reduced in-stent restenosis in comparison with balloon angioplasty (right-hand panel in the figure after percutaneous transluminal coronary angioplasty (PTCA) and drug-eluting stent implantation) (*JAMA.* 2005;293:165–171, *Circulation.* 2000;101:1895–1898).

8   **Answer C.**   (*Coron Artery Dis.* 2004;15:313–318).

9   **Answer C.**   Even under dual antiplatelet treatment with acetylsalicylic acid and clopidogrel very late stent thrombosis has been reported (*J Am Coll Cardiol.* 2005;45:2088–2092).

10   **Answer E.**

11   **Answer C.**   (*N Engl J Med.* 2005;353:653–662).

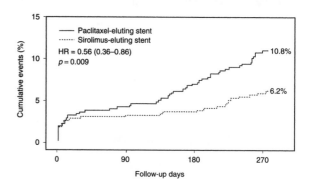

12   **Answer D.**   (*JAMA.* 2005;294:819–825).

13   **Answer F.**   Stent thrombosis is angiographically defined as reduced thrombolysis in myocardial infarction (TIMI) flow and visible thrombus. Clinically, stent thrombosis can be suspected if the patient presents with acute chest pain and dynamic ST changes in the leads of the previously treated target vessel.

14   **Answer D.**

15   **Answer A.**   All of the mentioned variables were associated with stent thrombosis. In this specific multivariate analysis, the premature discontinuation of antiplatelet therapy emerged as strongest predictor for stent thrombosis and emphasizes the importance of dual antiplatelet treatment following coronary stenting with a drug-eluting stent. (*JAMA.* 2005;293:2126–2130).

16   **Answer E.**   Studies evaluating the coronary vasomotion have shown that bare-metal stents do not interfere with the physiologic response of coronary endothelial function proximal and distal to the stented segment. However, drug-eluting stents appear to have an influence on the non-stented segments proximal and distal to the stent. (*J Am Coll Cardiol.* 2005;46:231–236).

17   **Answer F.**   Severe allergic reactions to drug-eluting stents have been rarely reported. Apart from other pitfalls being discussed like late malapposition and "black holes," a prolonged dual antiplatelet therapy might negatively influence the outcome of patients, despite the protection against stent thrombosis, mainly due to higher bleeding complications.

18 Answer C.   Head-to-head comparisons of CABG versus multivessel stenting with drug-eluting stents are under way. The results of these studies might provide specific information for a better management of patients with multivessel disease.

19 Answer D.   Paclitaxel is released more slowly than sirolimus.

20 Answer C.   (*Lancet*. 2004;364:583–591).

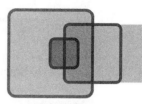

20

Percutaneous Interventions in Aortocoronary Saphenous Vein Grafts

Christophe A. Wyss and Marco Roffi

1 Which of the following statements about the historical background of surgical revascularization is *true*?

(A) Coronary artery bypass grafting (CABG) using venous conduits was first performed in humans in the 1960s
(B) The first conduit used was the left internal mammary artery (LIMA)
(C) The first aortocoronary saphenous vein graft (SVG) was implanted in humans in the 1950s
(D) SVGs were used as bypass grafts in humans earlier than LIMA
(E) A and B are true

2 Which of the following statements concerning patency rate of aortocoronary SVGs is true?

(A) Less than 5% of vein grafts are occluded at 1 year
(B) 20% of vein grafts are occluded at 10 years
(C) 40% of vein grafts are occluded at 10 years
(D) 80% of vein grafts are occluded at 10 years
(E) A and C are true

3 Which of the following statements best describes the need for further revascularization (redo-CABG or percutaneous coronary intervention [PCI]) among patients who had undergone bypass surgery using SVGs?

(A) Further revascularization is required in approximately 60% of cases at 10 years
(B) Further revascularization is required in approximately 40% of cases at 10 years
(C) Further revascularization is required in approximately 20% of cases at 10 years

(D) Further revascularization is required in approximately 5% of cases at 10 years

4 Which of the following statements about redo-CABG among patients who had undergone bypass surgery previously is *not* correct?

(A) Redo surgery carries a higher mortality rate than the first CABG
(B) Redo surgery carries a higher morbidity rate than the first CABG
(C) Redo surgery conveys the same degree of relief from angina as the first CABG
(D) Redo surgery conveys less relief from angina than the first CABG
(E) Redo surgery is associated with reduction in SVG patency as compared with initial surgery

5 A 74-year-old gentleman presents with angina Canadian Cardiovascular Society (CCS) III 15 years following CABG. Before coronary angiography, he wants to know which potential therapeutic options may be applicable for him:

(A) PCI, if the lesions are suitable
(B) Owing to the nature of graft atherosclerosis, medical management is the only strategy with acceptable risk
(C) Redo-CABG is the default approach in these cases
(D) In patients with advanced SVG-disease, redo-CABG should be considered, particularly if no internal mammary artery (IMA) grafting has been previously performed
(E) A and D are correct

6 Which of the following morphologic features is the least characteristic for vein graft atherosclerosis?

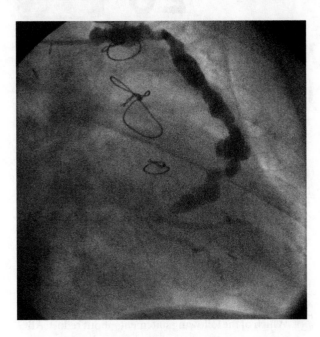

(A) Extensive calcification
(B) Atherosclerotic plaque with poorly developed fibrous cap
(C) Thrombosis
(D) Neointimal hyperplasia
(E) Diffuse involvement

7 A 75-year-old woman presents with acute coronary syndrome (ACS) and dynamic ST-segment depression in the lateral leads. She had undergone CABG 4 months earlier (LIMA to left anterior descending artery [LAD], right internal mammary artery [RIMA] to right carotid artery [RCA], SVG to the first diagonal branch, and jump-graft to the first marginal branch of the left circumflex artery [LCX]) and her preoperative ejection fraction (EF) was 30%. Coronary angiography demonstrated an occlusion of the SVG to the diagonal branch. Which of the following statements about early SVG occlusion (i.e., within the first 6 months of surgery) is *true*?

(A) A postoperative high graft flow damages the endothelium and therefore predisposes to early SVG occlusion
(B) Preoperative congestive heart failure is a significant predictor of early SVG occlusion
(C) Grafting to diagonal branches carries a higher early SVG occlusion rate compared with other territories
(D) Female gender is a significant predictor of early SVG graft occlusion
(E) B and C are correct

8 Which of the following statements about vein graft thrombosis is *not* correct?

(A) Vein graft thrombosis is the principal underlying mechanism of early vein graft occlusion
(B) Bypass surgery is characterized by a prothrombotic state
(C) Even when performed under optimal conditions, harvesting of venous conduits is associated with focal endothelial cell loss or damage
(D) Reduction of graft flow due to anastomosis proximal to an atherosclerotic segment or to a stricture at the anastomosis site predisposes to graft thrombotic occlusions
(E) Oral anticoagulants are superior to aspirin in preventing SVG thrombosis

9 A 68-year-old man with diabetes presented with ACS and dynamic ST depression in the leads V_4 through V_6. Eight months earlier, he had undergone CABG (LIMA to LAD, vein to diagonal branch, and jump-graft to LCX, vein to RCA). In this patient, the likely cause for ischemia between 1 month and 1 year following CABG is:

(A) A stenosis at the distal anastomosis site
(B) A subacute thrombotic graft occlusion
(C) A mid-graft stenosis due to neointimal hyperplasia
(D) A stenosis at the proximal anastomosis due to aorto-ostial disease
(E) A, B, and C are true

10 Which of the following statements about SVG atherosclerosis is *not* correct?

(A) Lipid handling of SVG endothelium is characterized by fast lipolysis, less active lipid synthesis, and low lipid uptake
(B) Late thrombotic occlusion occurs frequently in old degenerated SVG with advanced atherosclerotic plaque formation
(C) SVG atherosclerosis tends to be diffuse and friable with a poorly developed fibrous cap and little evidence of calcification
(D) Compared with the native vessel atherosclerotic process, SVG atherosclerosis is more rapidly progressive
(E) From a histologic perspective, SVG atherosclerosis has more foam cells and inflammatory cells than the native coronary one

11 Which of the following factors influence long-term SVG patency?

(A) Native vessel diameter
(B) Cigarette smoking
(C) Hyperlipidemia

(D) Severity of native vessel atherosclerosis proximal to the anastomotic site

(E) All of the above

12 One of your referring general practitioners wonders which strategy leads to an improvement in outcomes among patients following CABG. What is *not* your answer?

(A) Antiplatelet therapy
(B) Smoking cessation
(C) Lipid-lowering therapy
(D) The use of arterial grafts
(E) Yearly coronary angiograms

13 The same general practitioner wants to know more about antithrombotic therapy in the CABG setting. Which of the following statements is *not* correct?

(A) Dipyridamole in addition to aspirin therapy is more effective than aspirin alone for SVG patency
(B) Clopidogrel 300 mg as a loading dose 6 hours after surgery followed by 75 mg per day PO is a safe alternative for patients undergoing CABG who are aspirin intolerant
(C) In patients who undergo CABG for non–ST-segment elevation ACS, clopidogrel 75 mg per day for 9 to 12 months following the procedure in addition to aspirin is recommended
(D) For patients undergoing CABG and mechanical valve replacement, aspirin is recommended in addition to warfarin (Coumadin).

14 You are starting an elective PCI of an aorto-ostial long-segment stenosis in a 7-year-old vein graft (see following figure). Which of the following complications should be of *least* concern in this setting?

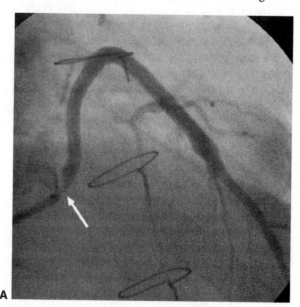

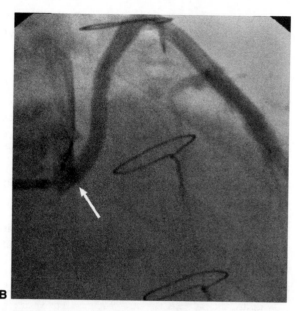

An aorto-ostial saphenous vein graft lesion (*arrow*) is demonstrated in panel A. Panel B shows the result following stenting.

(A) Proximal anastomosis rupture
(B) Distal embolization
(C) No reflow
(D) Abrupt closure
(E) Dissection

15 Percutaneous interventions of SVG have been associated with worse outcomes compared with endovascular treatment of the native circulation. Reasons may include:

(A) Percutaneous treatment of SVG disease is inappropriate. Instead, these patients should be managed conservatively
(B) Patients with SVG disease have a worse risk profile at baseline
(C) Owing to the nature of the disease, SVG interventions carry a higher risk of complication, such as periprocedural myocardial infarction (MI)
(D) The paucity of data on SVG interventions does not allow the conclusion that patients undergoing SVG interventions have a worse outcome compared with those undergoing native vessel revascularization
(E) B and C are correct

16 Platelet glycoprotein (GP) IIb/IIIa receptor antagonists:

(A) Should be used routinely in SVG interventions
(B) Are not recommended in SVG interventions
(C) Are equivalent to mechanical emboli protection devices in preventing complications during SVG interventions

(D) Are superior to mechanical emboli protection devices in preventing complications during SVG interventions

(E) A and C are true

17 Stenting in SVG:

(A) Should never be performed, because of exacerbation of distal embolization at the time of deployment

(B) Is associated with a low restenosis rate

(C) Improves outcome when a polytetrafluoroethylene (PTFE)-covered stent is used

(D) Is only recommended in ostial lesions

(E) Appears to improve outcomes compared with balloon angioplasty; however, randomized data is limited

18 A major breakthrough in SVG interventions has been:

(A) GPIIb/IIIa receptor antagonists

(B) Mechanical distal emboli protection

(C) Atherectomy

(D) Ultrasound thrombosis

(E) All of the above

19 A 77-year-old man underwent unprotected stent-based PCI of a 15-year-old vein graft and suffered a periprocedural MI following prolonged no-reflow poststenting of a long segment involving the proximal portion and the proximal anastomosis of the graft. What could have been done differently?

(A) The use of a mechanical emboli protection device may have reduced the risk of periprocedural MI

(B) In this case, a filter device may have been a safer option than a distal balloon occlusion system

(C) A distal balloon occlusion device should have been used because it has been demonstrated to be superior to filter devices in SVG PCI

(D) It was correct to not use mechanical emboli protection devices because safety and efficacy data are insufficient

(E) A and B are true

20 A 65-year-old man presents with diffuse in-stent restenosis following PCI of a vein graft 6 months earlier. His cardiovascular risk factors include diabetes, hypertension, and hyperlipidemia. His left ventricular function is moderately impaired. What are your therapeutic options in this setting?

(A) You may consider endovascular radiation (brachytherapy) if you have this option in your facility

(B) You may consider drug-eluting stents, although the current data in SVG PCI are sparse

(C) You proceed to ultrasound thrombosis

(D) You perform rotablation, because this technology has proven to be effective in this setting

(E) A and B are true

21 The most promising future strategy to improve outcomes of SVG interventions is:

(A) Drug-eluting stents

(B) Low-molecular-weight heparin

(C) Covered stents

(D) Atherectomy devices

(E) None of the above

22 A 65-year-old man comes to your office for a checkup. He had had CABG 10 years earlier. His cardiovascular risk factors include diabetes, hypertension, and hypercholesterolemia. Despite being asymptomatic, he is very concerned since he has read in the news that bypass grafts may occlude 10 years after surgery. The thallium stress test is negative and the left ventricular function normal. Nevertheless, he pushes for coronary angiography. At this point you:

(A) Agree for a coronary angiography because in SVG percutaneous plaque sealing by stenting even angiographic nonsignificant lesions has proved to efficaciously prevent further cardiovascular events

(B) Tell him that the only meaningful thing you can suggest at this point in time is an aggressive risk-factor management

(C) Perform a multislice computed tomography (CT) angiography to address SVG patency

(D) Agree for coronary angiography to perform intravascular ultrasound (IVUS) as baseline information before high-dose statin therapy. You then plan to repeat IVUS at 1 year to assess the response to lipid-lowering therapy

(E) Do not suggest any of the above

Answers and Explanations

1   **Answer E.** The first aortocoronary SVG was implanted by Garrett et al. in May 1967 (*JAMA.* 1973;223:792–794) and the technique was subsequently refined and successfully implemented by René Favaloro, an Argentinean cardiac surgeon working at the Cleveland Clinic Foundation. The LIMA was the first conduit used as a coronary bypass graft in humans. A sutured end-to-end anastomosis between the LIMA and a marginal branch of the left circumflex coronary artery was first performed in February 1964 in Leningrad (*J Thorac Cardiovasc Surg.* 1967;54:535–544).

2   **Answer C.** A major limitation of SVG as a conduit for CABG is the atherothrombosis and accelerated atherosclerosis of the vein grafts. During the first year after surgery, up to 15% of venous conduits occlude. At 10 years, 40% of vein grafts are occluded and only 50% are free of significant stenosis (see following figure) (*J Am Coll Cardiol.* 1996;28:616–626).

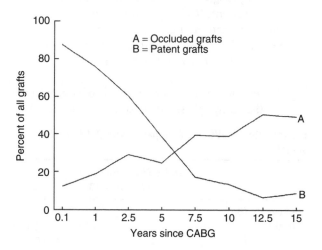

3   **Answer C.** Additional revascularization (redo-CABG or PCI) is required in approximately 5% of patients at 5 years, 20% at 10 years, and 30% at 12 years after surgery (*Am J Cardiol.* 1994;73:103–112).

4   **Answer C.** As compared with the first surgery, redo-CABG is associated with higher mortality rate (3% to 7%) and higher rate of perioperative MI (4% to 11.5%). In addition, redo surgery is less efficacious in relieving angina and the patency rate of venous conduits is decreased (*Circulation.* 1998;97:916–931).

5   **Answer E.** SVG PCI is a viable option if the lesions are suitable. In patients with advanced SVG disease, redo-CABG should be considered, particularly if no IMA grafting has been previously performed. Accordingly, the use of LIMA has been associated with long-term graft patency and survival.

6   **Answer A.** Three pathophysiologically distinct and temporally separated processes are observed in SVG disease: Subacute thrombosis (usually occurring within 1 month of surgery), neointimal hyperplasia (between 1 month and 1 year post-CABG), and vein graft atherosclerosis (usually clinically significant >3 years after surgery). Morphologically, vein graft lesions tend to be diffuse, concentric, and friable with a poorly developed or absent fibrous cap and little evidence of calcification (*Circulation.* 1998;97:916–931).

7   **Answer E.** Optimal graft flow as assessed at the end of surgery has a protective effect against graft occlusion. Good flow conditions are observed in patients with larger target vessels, lack of significant disease distally to the anastomosis, and several runoff branches. Significant predictors of SVG occlusion or disease at 6 months after surgery include congestive heart failure, grafting to diagonal arteries, larger vein graft size, and poor runoff. Traditional cardiovascular risk factors, such as hypertension, sex, diabetes mellitus, and previous MI, do not seem to affect early graft patency (*J Thorac Cardiovasc Surg.* 2005;129: 496–503).

8   **Answer E.** Vein graft thrombosis is the principal underlying mechanism of early vein graft occlusion. Vein graft thrombosis is caused by alterations in the vessel wall, altered flow dynamics, or changes in blood rheology (Virchow's Triad). Bypass surgery has a systemic effect on circulating levels of factors influencing hemostasis, creating a prothrombotic state. Focal endothelial cell loss and damage is associated with high-pressure distension of the venous conduits due to harvesting. Reduction of graft flow due to implantation proximal to an atherosclerotic segment or a stricture at the anastomosis is a predisposing factor for occlusion by thrombosis. Several comparative antithrombotic trials have shown that oral anticoagulants are equivalent to aspirin in terms of 1-year vein graft patency rates (*Circulation.* 1998;97:916–931).

9 **Answer E.** Although within the first month of surgery thrombosis is the main mechanism of vein graft disease, from 1 month to 1 year, ischemia in territory supplied by an SVG is most often due to lesions at the distal perianastomotic site or midgraft stenosis caused by neointimal hyperplasia. Neointimal hyperplasia, defined as the proliferation of smooth muscle cells and accumulation of extracellular matrix in the intimal compartment, is the characteristic adaptive mechanism of venous conduits to systemic blood pressures. This process represents the foundation for later development of graft atherosclerosis. Graft occlusion due to subacute thrombosis is a more rare cause of ischemia between 1 month and 1 year after CABG.

10 **Answer A.** Although the fundamental processes of atherosclerosis in native coronary vessels and in vein grafts are similar, there are several temporal, histologic, and metabolic differences. Lipid handling of SVG endothelium is characterized by slow lipolysis, more active lipid synthesis, and high lipid uptake than in the native coronary arteries. In addition, SVG atherosclerosis is more rapidly progressive. From a histologic point of view, SVG atherosclerosis is characterized by more foam and inflammatory cells. SVG atherosclerotic involvement is diffuse and lesions are friable with a poorly developed fibrous cap and little evidence of calcification (*Circulation.* 1998;97:916–931).

11 **Answer E.** A number of morphologic factors have been associated with reduced vein graft patency. It has been observed that 1-year vein graft patency was significantly lower if the grafted vessel was <1.5 mm compared with grafted vessels with a diameter >1.5 mm (*Ann Thorac Surg.* 1979;28:176–183). Severity of native vessel atherosclerosis proximal to the anastomotic site influences the flow in the vein graft. Sustained competitive flow through mild stenotic native vessels has been described as a predisposing factor for vein graft occlusion. However, this mechanistic view remains a source of debate because the available data is conflicting (*J Thorac Cardiovasc Surg.* 1981;82:520–530, *Ann Thorac Surg.* 1979;28:176–183). Cigarette smoking is an important predictor of recurrent angina during the first year after surgery and of poor long-term clinical outcome. The evidence implicating hyperlipidemia as a key risk factor in the development of vein graft atherosclerosis is as consistent and strong as it is for native coronary disease.

12 **Answer E.** Aspirin has been shown to increase short- and midterm vein graft patency. Cessation of smoking is a highly effective strategy in preventing atherosclerosis. Accordingly, it has been shown that persistent smokers had more than twice the risk of suffering MI or required redo surgery at 1 year following CABG compared with patients who quit smoking at the time of surgery (*Circulation.* 1996;93:42–47). Several trials have shown a clear-cut benefit for aggressive lipid-lowering therapy in the post-CABG setting. Similarly, the use of arterial grafts has been a major breakthrough in bypass surgery owing to the better long-term patency compared with SVG.

13 **Answer A.** For patients undergoing CABG, addition of dipyridamole to aspirin therapy is not recommended (*BMJ.* 1994;308:159–168). According to the American College of Chest Physicians (ACCP) guidelines, for patients intolerant to aspirin, an oral loading dose of 300 mg clopidogrel 6 hours after surgery followed by 75 mg per day is recommended. Patients undergoing CABG who require oral anticoagulation at the same time (e.g., for atrial fibrillation or mechanical valve replacement) also qualify for aspirin (*Chest.* 2004;126:600S–608S). In patients who undergo CABG for non–ST-segment elevation ACS, the Clopidogrel in Unstable Angina to Prevent Recurrent Events (CURE) study has demonstrated that the combination of aspirin and clopidogrel, 75 mg per day for 9 to 12 months, is superior to aspirin alone (*N Engl J Med.* 2001;345:494–502).

14 **Answer A.** Suture line rupture is of concern only in the early phase after surgery. Characteristic

Event's rates in SVG-PCI (compared with PCI in native vessels)

	Grafts PCI $n = 627$	Native PCI $n = 13,158$	p
30-d events (%)			
Death	2.1	1.0	0.006
MI	13.1	7.7	<0.001
Urgent revascularization	2.6	3.6	0.15
Death/MI	14.0	8.2	<0.001
Death/MI/urgent revascularization	15.2	10.0	<0.001
6-mo events (%)			
Death	4.7	2.0	<0.001
MI	18.3	9.4	<0.001
Revascularization	24.5	19.1	0.003
Death/MI	20.4	10.6	<0.001
Death/MI/ revascularization	37.1	25.4	<0.001

SVG, saphenous vein graft; PCI, percutaneous coronary intervention; MI, myocardial infarction.

complications of PCI in degenerated SVG include distal embolization, no-reflow, dissection, and abrupt closure. Overall, SVG PCI are associated with significantly worse outcomes compared with interventions in native circulation (see preceding table) (*Circulation*. 2002;106:3063–3067).

15 Answer E. Patients with SVG disease requiring revascularization have a more pronounced risk profile than their counterparts undergoing native coronary artery intervention. The former are usually older and have more comorbidities such as prior MI, diabetes, hyperlipidemia, hypertension, stroke, heart failure, and peripheral vascular disease. Patients undergoing PCI of a bypass graft have higher death rates and more nonfatal cardiac events than patients undergoing native coronary intervention. Although partially explained by the increased prevalence of high-risk characteristics among the patients undergoing graft intervention, it has been demonstrated that SVG PCI *per se* is associated with worse outcomes compared with interventions of the native circulation (*Circulation*. 2002;106:3063–3067).

16 Answer B. GPIIb/IIIa receptor inhibitors are potent antiplatelet agents shown to be highly effective in reducing adverse events following PCI across a wide variety of coronary lesions. Overall, the greater the baseline risk profile of the patient or the complexity of the intervention, the greater the benefit derived from therapy. The one exception to that rule has been the use of these agents in SVG interventions. Accordingly, a pooled analysis of five large-scale randomized GPIIb/IIIa inhibitor trials including over 600 patients undergoing bypass graft intervention detected no benefit from active treatment compared

with placebo (*Circulation*. 2002;106:3063–3067). The likely explanation for this failure is that the amount and/or composition of the material embolized during the procedure overwhelms the capacity of these agents to protect the distal vasculature. Therefore, routine use of GPIIb/IIIa inhibitors for SVG PCI is not recommended.

17 Answer E. Randomized data on the safety and efficacy of stenting in vein graft intervention is scarce. The only trial randomizing patients undergoing SVG interventions to balloon angioplasty or stenting failed to demonstrate a reduction in binary restenosis (37% in the stent group and 46% in the angioplasty group; $p = 0.24$) among 220 patients (*N Engl J Med*. 1997;337:740–747). Nevertheless, a benefit in terms of freedom from death, MI, or repeat revascularization was observed (73% vs. 58%, respectively; $p = 0.03$) (see following figure). Despite the paucity of data, stenting is frequently used

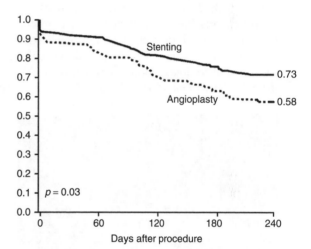

Efficacy of different treatment strategies in percutaneous intervention of vein grafts

Therapy	Efficacy	Comments
Stents	Likely	Not prospectively addressed in large-scale randomized trials
		Most SVG PCIs performed are stent-based
Covered stents	Failed	Lack of efficacy demonstrated in a randomized trial
		Preliminary data on new generation covered stents promising
Drug-eluting stents	Promising	Current safety/efficacy data in SVG PCI insufficient
GPIIb/IIIa inhibitors	Failed	Not recommended
Emboli protection devices	Highly effective	Efficacy demonstrated in randomized trials
		Distal balloon occlusion and filter devices equally effective
Ultrasound thrombosis	Failed	Tested in a randomized trial
Atherectomy devices	Unknown	Insufficient safety and/or efficacy data
Brachytherapy	Highly effective for in-stent restenosis	Efficacy demonstrated in randomized trials
		Therapy cumbersome and logistically challenging

SVG, saphenous vein graft; PCI, percutaneous coronary intervention.
Modified from Roffi M. Percutaneous intervention of saphenous vein grafts. *ACC Curr Jour Rev*. 2004;14:45–48.

as the default approach in SVG PCI. Even though the idea that a covered stent may be able to entrap friable degenerated material, and therefore decrease the probability of distal embolization, is appealing, clinical trials showed no improvement in outcomes associated with the use of covered stents in SVG PCI (*Circulation.* 2003;108:37–42).

18 Answer B. As discussed in Question 15, GPIIb/IIIa inhibitors showed no benefit in SVG interventions. Mechanical emboli protection is based on the concept of interposing a device between the lesion treated and the distal vasculature supplied by the graft as a prevention of distal embolization. The use of mechanical emboli protection devices has been a major breakthrough in SVG PCI (see table in preceding text). A randomized trial enrolling over 800 patients using distal balloon occlusion demonstrated a 42% relative risk reduction of major adverse cardiac events (MACE) at 1 month among patients allocated to emboli protection (see following figures) (*Circulation.* 2002;105:1285–1290). Most of the benefit was due to a reduction in periprocedural MI. The hypothesis that ultrasound thrombosis may be beneficial in patients with ACSs and SVG culprit lesion was tested in a randomized trial involving 181 patients (*Circulation.* 2003;107:2331–2336).

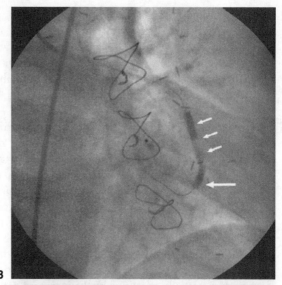

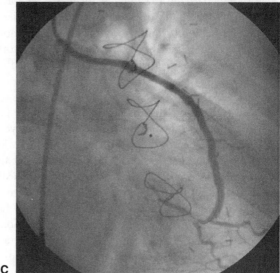

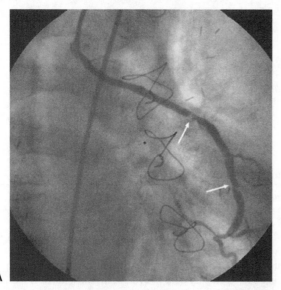

The use of a distal balloon occlusive emboli protection system (PercuSurge GuardWire, Boston Scientific, Natick, MA) is demonstrated. Panel A shows two significant lesions (*arrows*) in the mid-to-distal portion of a saphenous vein graft to the marginal branch of the left circumflex artery. In panel B, the distal balloon is inflated (*large arrow*) and the graft occluded. The no-flow state is documented by the stagnant column of contrast media (*small arrows*). Panel C demonstrates the final result following stent and retrieval of the distal protection.

However, use of this device was associated with more cardiac adverse events and, in particular, more MIs. Few thrombectomy devices have undergone preliminary testing in the setting of SVG disease, but none of them has yet delivered sufficient safety and efficacy data (*ACC Curr J Rev.* 2004;14:45–48).

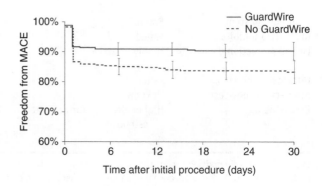

19 **Answer E.** Mechanical emboli protection is based on the concept of interposing a device between the lesion treated and the distal vasculature supplied by the graft as a prevention of distal embolization. This can be achieved by placing either a filter or an occlusive distal balloon. Filter-based emboli protection allows blood flow throughout the procedure, but particles smaller than the pore size (usually 100 μm) may reach the distal vasculature. In addition, these devices are currently stiffer and bulkier than distal balloon occlusion. The latter is low profile and allows for a more complete retrieval of small particles suspended in the blood column at the time of intervention. The disadvantage of distal balloon occlusion is the potential for ischemia and the poor visualization of the lesion. Use of a filter device was proved to be equivalent to distal balloon occlusion for reducing periprocedural MI in a randomized trial involving 651 patients (see following figure) (*Circulation*. 2003;108:548–553). Distal balloon occlusive devices should not be used during intervention of aorto-ostial vein graft lesions as, owing to the lack of antegrade flow during distal occlusion, debris from the intervention may embolize into the ascending aorta.

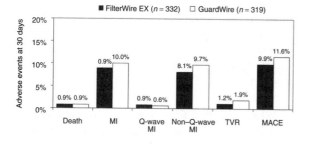

20 **Answer E.** Venous conduits are prone to neointimal hyperplasia in the setting of PCI, translating into restenosis rates as high as 40% to 60%. For patients with in-stent restenosis of a bypass graft, endovascular radiation (brachytherapy) may be considered, particularly for long or recurrent lesions (*N Engl J Med*. 2002;346:1194–1199). Preliminary data suggests that drug-eluting stents are a promising technology for SVG intervention to impact the high restenosis rate. Finally, there is no evidence for the use of ultrasound thrombosis, rotablator, or atherectomy devices (see also Question 17).

21 **Answer A.** Drug-eluting stents are a promising technology particularly for SVG interventions because of the associated high restenosis rate (see preceding table). However, the data available are preliminary and no randomized comparisons have so far been published. Despite the rationale that a covered stent may enable entrapment of friable degenerated material, and may therefore decrease the probability of distal embolization, clinical application of these devices showed no reduction in restenosis and an increase in MI. Few thrombectomy devices have undergone testing in the setting of SVG disease, but none of them has delivered sufficient safety and efficacy data.

22 **Answer B.** The most efficacious strategy for this patient is aggressive cardiovascular risk-factor control. In case of recurrent ischemia, the different therapeutic options (i.e., PCI, redo-CABG, medical management) will be evaluated on the basis of coronary anatomy.

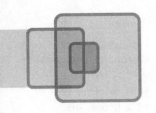

21
Closure Devices

Leslie Cho and Debabrata Mukherjee

Questions

1 The potential benefits of vascular closure devices include all of the following, *except*:

(A) Reduction in time to hemostasis
(B) Earlier ambulation of patients
(C) Lower incidence of hematoma and pseudoaneurysm
(D) Increased patient comfort
(E) Earlier discharge for some patients

2 Which of the following is a patented product that enhances the natural method of achieving hemostasis by delivering collagen extravascularly to the surface of the femoral artery?

(A) Angio-Seal
(B) Duett
(C) FemoStop
(D) Perclose
(E) Syvek
(F) VasoSeal

3 Which of the following is an arch with a pneumatic pressure dome, connection tubing, and a two-way stopcock, a belt, and a pump for inflation?

(A) Angio-Seal
(B) Duett
(C) FemoStop
(D) Perclose
(E) Syvek
(F) VasoSeal

4 Which of the following is a device that creates a mechanical seal by sandwiching the arteriotomy between a bioabsorbable anchor and the collagen sponge, which dissolves within 8 to 12 weeks?

(A) Angio-Seal
(B) Duett

(C) FemoStop
(D) Perclose
(E) Syvek
(F) VasoSeal

5 Which of the following is a suture-mediated closure device that can be used in anticoagulant patients?

(A) Angio-Seal
(B) Duett
(C) FemoStop
(D) Perclose
(E) Syvek
(F) VasoSeal

6 Which of the following is a balloon catheter that initiates hemostasis and ensures the precise placement of procoagulant (a flowable mixture of thrombin, collagen, and diluent) at the puncture site in the entire tissue tract?

(A) Angio-Seal
(B) Duett
(C) FemoStop
(D) Perclose
(E) Syvek
(F) VasoSeal

7 Which of the following is made of a soft, white, sterile, nonwoven pad of cellulosic polymer, and poly-*N*-acetyl glucosamine isolated from a microalgae?

(A) Angio-Seal
(B) Duett
(C) FemoStop
(D) Perclose
(E) Syvek
(F) VasoSeal

8 Clinical studies have suggested increased vascular complications with which of the following devices?

(A) Angio-Seal
(B) Duett
(C) FemoStop
(D) Perclose
(E) Syvek
(F) VasoSeal

9 The incidence of which complication is higher with vascular closure devices than with concomitant use of glycoprotein (GP) IIb/IIIa inhibitors:

(A) Local hematoma
(B) Arteriovenous fistula
(C) Pseudoaneurysm
(D) Retroperitoneal hematoma
(E) Femoral vein thrombosis

10 The most common infectious complication associated with percutaneous vascular closure devices is:

(A) Generalized sepsis
(B) Infective endocarditis
(C) Mycotic pseudoaneurysm
(D) Carbuncle
(E) Femoral endarteritis

11 A 45-year-old woman undergoes a diagnostic catheterization after having a positive stress test for atypical chest pain. She is found to have mild luminal irregularities, and the cardiologist decides to use an Angio-Seal device to close her groin. She responds well and is sent to the recovery room with instructions to return home in 2 hours. An hour after the procedure, she is found to be pulseless and have pain, pallor, and paresthesia of her right leg. What should you do next?

(A) Give pain pills for relief
(B) IV heparin and GPIIb/IIIa inhibitor
(C) IV fibrinolytic therapy
(D) Urgent surgery consult or urgent percutaneous peripheral vascular intervention

12 The patient mentioned in the preceding text responds well to the treatment and is discharged after 2 weeks in the hospital. She returns to your office demanding to know what had happened. She is convinced that the closure device is unsafe and should have never been used on her. She wants to know whether manual pressure would have been safer to use. Is she correct?

(A) Yes, in a large analysis, manual pressure was safer compared with vascular closure devices regardless of the type of case

(B) No, in a large analysis, manual pressure was safer only in diagnostic cases, but not in percutaneous coronary intervention (PCI) cases
(C) No, in a large analysis, both manual pressure and vascular closure devices had similar major complication rates
(D) No, in a large analysis, manual pressure was safer only in PCI cases, but not in diagnostic cases

13 The same patient wants to know why she had femoral artery thrombosis. All of the following are risk factors for femoral artery thrombosis, *except*:

(A) Small femoral artery size
(B) Peripheral vascular disease
(C) Diabetes
(D) Female gender
(E) Obesity

14 A 67-year-old woman presents to your office for a second opinion. She underwent PCI 3 months ago and did well. On a routine physical examination she was found to have a pulsatile mass in her right groin. She then has a duplex ultrasound, which shows a 3.8 cm pseudoaneurysm. She was seen by a vascular surgeon and was given thrombin injection. However, her pseudoaneurysm is unchanged. She has been told that she will need surgery. She is convinced that this is because her groin was sealed with vascular closure device. Is the incidence of pseudoaneurysm higher with vascular closure devices?

(A) No, it is the same with manual and vascular closure devices
(B) Yes, it is higher with vascular closure devices
(C) No, it is higher with manual pressure

15 The patient mentioned in the previous question would like your opinion regarding treatment options. What are her other options?

(A) Surgery is the only option because she has failed thrombin injection
(B) Manual compression is another option and if that fails, then surgery
(C) Another round of thrombin injection should be tried
(D) Conservative management should be tried with blood pressure control
(E) Surgery is not needed at this time because she is asymptomatic

16 What are the distinguishing features on the physical examination of a groin hematoma from femoral artery pseudoaneurysm?

(A) Groin mass
(B) Pain and audible bruit

(C) Continuous groin pain and neuralgia

(D) Pulsatile groin mass and bruit

17 Your hospital administrator contacts you regarding the catheterization laboratory revenue. He states that with drug-eluting stent usage, the margin for profit has decreased significantly. He is convinced that you can save money by not using vascular closure devices. He asks you about the disadvantages of *not* using vascular closure devices. You reply:

(A) There will be more hematoma with manual pressure

(B) Prolong bed rest with manual pressure

(C) There will be more atrioventricular (AV) fistulas

18 An 81-year-old patient undergoes an urgent catheterization for acute myocardial infarction (MI). She is found on angiogram to have 100% occlusion of left anterior descending (LAD) artery. She has a successful PCI to LAD with 3.0/33 drug-eluting stent and 3.0/28 drug-eluting stent with heparin and GPIIb/IIIa inhibitor, abciximab. She is allergic to latex. She is unable to keep her leg still. Can you use Angio-Seal?

(A) Yes, Angio-Seal can be used in patients with latex allergy

(B) No, Angio-Seal cannot be used in patients with latex allergy

(C) Only manual pressure should be applied to patients with latex allergy

(D) No, only Perclose can be used in patients with latex allergy

19 A 78-year-old man undergoes PCI to the right coronary artery (RCA) with bivalirudin. He responds well and is sealed with Perclose without any complication. He is discharged home. He returns to your office within a month, complaining of severe right leg pain with minimal exertion. You examine him, and he is found to have slightly decreased right lower extremity pulse, but otherwise unremarkable. He undergoes duplex and is found to have Perclose-induced right femoral artery stenosis. What are the treatment options?

(A) No treatment is required; it will go away within 2 to 3 weeks

(B) There is no such thing as subacute limb ischemia from vascular closure device; therefore, he has peripheral arterial diseases (PAD)

(C) Access from contralateral femoral artery and balloon angioplasty of the affected side

(D) Surgical intervention

20 An 80-year-old woman undergoes an elective PCI to dominant circumflex (CX). Her right femoral artery is sealed with new generation Angio-Seal. Three days later she presents with chest pain, ST elevation, and hypotension in the emergency room (ER). She is taken back to catheterization laboratory. Can you reaccess the same site?

(A) Yes, as long as it is 1 cm proximal to the previously accessed site

(B) No, right femoral artery cannot be accessed for 90 days

(C) No, the same site cannot be accessed for 30 days

(D) No, the same site cannot be accessed for 7 days

Answers and Explanations

1 Answer C. Vascular closure devices have some obvious advantages. The time spent by catheterization laboratory staff in manually compressing the puncture site is reduced, which in turn improves the patient flow throughput in busy catheterization laboratories. Other potential benefits include the reduction in time to hemostasis, earlier ambulation of patients, increased patient comfort and earlier discharge for some patients. A rigorously performed systematic review and meta-analysis suggested that vascular closure devices may actually increase the risk of hematoma and pseudoaneurysm (*JAMA*. 2004;291:350–357).

2 Answer F. VasoSeal (see following figure) enhances the body's natural method of achieving hemostasis by delivering collagen extravascularly to the surface of the femoral artery. Type 1 collagen produced from bovine tendons activates platelets in the arterial puncture, forming a clot on the surface of the artery, resulting in a seal at the arterial puncture site for immediate sheath removal after angioplasty and stent procedures. VasoSeal devices do not require leaving a foreign body inside the artery, do not increase the size of the arterial puncture, and do not require the user to leave a clip on the patient or surgical suturing after the procedure. In addition, the collagen reabsorbs over a 6-week period and no fluoroscopy is needed before use.

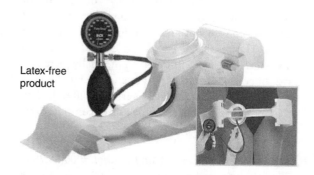

Latex-free product

3 Answer C. The FemoStop Femoral Compression System (see following figure) provides an alternative to manual pressure and other methods of manually achieving femoral artery hemostasis. The FemoStop dome applies a focused, controlled pressure to the puncture site, minimizing the pain and discomfort associated with excessive pressure. Although the dome is made of a soft latex-free material occupying the smallest area necessary to achieve hemostasis, it minimizes the risk of venous congestion or pain associated with ligament and nerve compression. Its inflatable transparent dome facilitates accurate placement of pressure and allows clear visibility of the puncture site. The other advantages over manual compression are that FemoStop allows hands-free operation and compression, potentially less discomfort and more freedom of movement for patients, accurate manometer-controlled pressure, and less contact with blood.

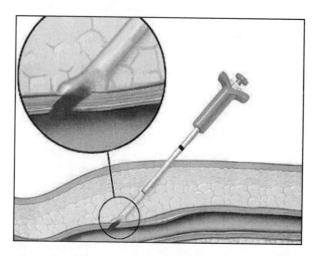

4 Answer A. The Angio-Seal Vascular Closure Device quickly seals femoral artery punctures following catheterization procedures, allowing for early ambulation and hospital discharge. The device creates a mechanical seal by sandwiching the arteriotomy between a bioabsorbable anchor and collagen sponge, which dissolve within 60 to 90 days (see following figure). The Angio-Seal STS PLUS platform is composed of an absorbable collagen sponge and a specially designed absorbable polymer anchor connected by an absorbable self-tightening suture. The device seals and sandwiches the arteriotomy between its two primary components, the anchor and the collagen sponge. Hemostasis is achieved primarily through mechanical means and is supplemented by the platelet-inducing properties of the collagen.

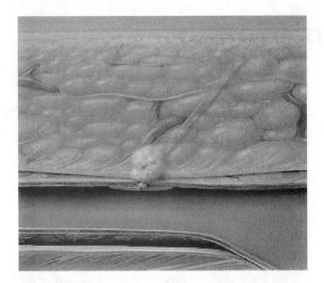

5 **Answer D.** The Perclose system (see following figure) uses percutaneous delivery of suture for closing the common femoral artery access site of patients who have undergone diagnostic or interventional catheterization procedures using 5 to 8 F sheaths. The modified Perclose A-T (Auto-Tie) is intended to simplify the complex knot-tying step that many physicians consider the most difficult step of the procedure. This innovation adds convenience, increases ease of use, and reduces the vessel closure procedure time.

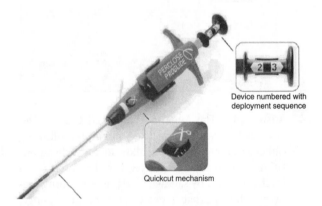

Device numbered with deployment sequence

Quickcut mechanism

6 **Answer B.** The Duett sealing device (see following figure) is used to seal the arterial puncture site following percutaneous procedures such as angiography, angioplasty, and stent placement. Using a dual approach (a balloon catheter and procoagulant), the Duett sealing device is designed to rapidly and safely stop bleeding. The Duett sealing device can quickly seal the entire puncture site with a one-size-fits-all device that leaves nothing rigid behind that could interfere with reaccess or potentiate an infection.

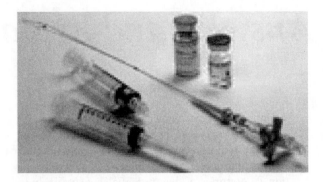

7 **Answer E.** The Syvek patch (see following figure) is made of a soft, white, sterile, nonwoven pad of cellulosic polymer and poly-*N*-acetyl glucosamine isolated from a microalgae. It leaves no subcutaneous foreign matter, is nonallergenic, and does not restrict immediate same site reentry. Although there are no known contraindications, it does not eliminate manual compression, but may shorten the duration of compression needed.

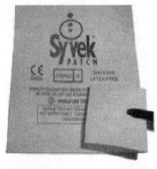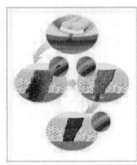

8 **Answer B.** The pooled analyses by Vaitkus et al. (*J Invasive Cardiol.* 2004;16:243–246) demonstrated that the Angio-Seal and Perclose devices might be superior to or at least equivalent to manual compression for both interventional and diagnostic cases. The results of controlled clinical trials with VasoSeal, however, indicated a potentially increased risk of complications. Another analysis by Nikolsky et al. (*J Am Coll Cardiol.* 2004;44:1200–1209) showed that in interventional cases the rate of complications was also higher with VasoSeal.

9 **Answer D.** Cura et al. (*Am J Cardiol.* 2000;86:780–782, A9) analyzed approximately 3,000 consecutive patients who underwent PCI and demonstrated that the use of femoral closure devices in a broad spectrum of patients was associated with an overall risk similar to manual compression. Even in patients treated with GPIIb/IIIa platelet inhibition, the incidence of access-site events between those receiving manual compression and those treated with closure devices was quite comparable. However, in this cohort, the incidence of retroperitoneal hemorrhage was significantly increased among patients treated with closure devices compared with manual compression (0.9% vs. 0.1%, $p = 0.01$).

10 **Answer C.** Sohail MR et al. reviewed all cases of closure device–related infection seen in their institution and searched the English language medical literature for all previously published reports (*Mayo Clin Proc.* 2005;80:1011–1015). They identified 46 cases from the medical literature and 6 cases from their institutional database. Diabetes mellitus and obesity were the most common comorbidities. The median incubation period from device insertion to presentation with access-site infection was 8 days (with a range of 2 to 29 days). The most common presenting symptoms were pain, erythema, fever, swelling, and purulent drainage at the access site. Mycotic pseudoaneurysm was the most common complication (22 cases). *Staphylococcus aureus* was responsible for most of the infections (75%). The mortality rate was 6% (3 patients). This suggests that infection associated with closure device placement is uncommon, but is an extremely serious complication. Morbidity is high, and aggressive medical and surgical interventions are required to achieve cure.

11 **Answer D.** She has acute femoral artery thrombosis. There is approximately 1% to 2% risk of major complication from vascular closure device. Acute femoral artery thrombosis requires urgent intervention (*JAMA.* 2004;291:350–357).

12 **Answer C.** In a large propensity score analysis of 24,000 patients from a single-center retrospective study, the risk-adjusted occurrence of vascular complications was similar for manual pressure when compared with vascular closure devices (*Catheter Cardiovasc Interv.* 2006;67:556–562). However, in a meta-analysis by Koreny et al. (*JAMA.* 2004;291:350–357) using only randomized studies, there appeared to be slightly higher hematoma and pseudoaneurysm incidence with vascular closure devices.

13 **Answer E.** Obesity is not a risk factor for femoral artery thrombosis (*UpToDate.* 1997).

14 **Answer C.** In a large meta-analysis by Koreny et al. (*JAMA.* 2004;291:350–357) using only randomized studies of 4,000 patients, there appeared to be slightly higher hematoma and pseudoaneurysm incidence with vascular closure devices.

15 **Answer A.** She has a large pseudoaneurysm with failed injection. Her option is surgery (*J Am Coll Cardiol.* 2006;47:1239–1312).

16 **Answer D.** Pseudoaneurysm can be diagnosed on physical examination by pulsatile mass and audible bruit. Most are asymptomatic.

17 **Answer B.** The use of vascular closure devices reduces the time to hemostasis and the duration of bed rest (*JAMA.* 2004;291:350–357).

18 **Answer A.** Angio-Seal can be used in patients with latex allergy.

19 **Answer C.** Subacute limb ischemia has been reported from vascular closure devices. This may be treated with balloon angioplasty (*Catheter Cardiovasc Interv.* 2002;57:12–23).

20 **Answer A.** Applegate RJ et al. studied the restick issue with Angio-Seal and found that restick can occur safely within 1 to 7 days of Angio-Seal (*Catheter Cardiovasc Interv.* 2003;58:181–184).

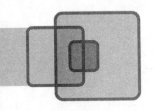

22

Management of Intraprocedural and Postprocedural Complications

Ferdinand Leya

Questions

1 A 69-year-old man with hypertension (HTN) and renal insufficiency (glomerular filtration rate [GFR] 65) presents to your office for consult from an Internist. He has been experiencing chest pain with exertion and underwent stress thallium which showed anterior defect. He then had cardiac catheterization that showed severe three-vessel disease with ejection fraction (EF) of 45%. He refused coronary artery bypass grafting (CABG) and presents to your office for multivessel percutaneous coronary intervention (PCI). He is concerned about his risk. What is his risk of emergent CABG with percutaneous revascularization?

(A) 0.4%
(B) 1.5%
(C) 3.7%
(D) 5.0%

2 During the selective cannulation of the left main coronary ostium, the blood pressure (BP) waveform, as seen in the figure, was recorded. Which of the following is the most likely explanation for the waveform?

(A) The pressure waveform indicates that the catheter tip prolapsed into the left ventricle
(B) The pressure transducer contains air
(C) There is catheter kink
(D) The catheter is up against the wall
(E) The catheter is engaged into a diseased left main artery

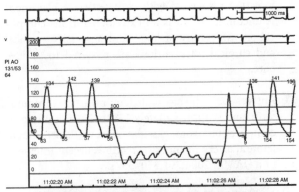

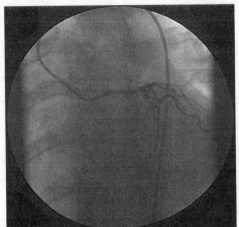

3 A 67-year-old retired lawyer with diabetes mellitus (DM), hyperlipidemia, and HTN presents to you for a second opinion. He underwent cardiac catheterization for increasing exertional chest pain and was found to have chronically occluded moderate-size right coronary artery (RCA) and 50% left anterior descending (LAD) artery, and circumflex (CX) lesions. He underwent PCI to RCA and had 2.5/28, 2.5/33, and 2.25/28 bare-metal stent. Drug-eluting stents were not used because of the patient's history of ulcers. Immediately after the intervention, the patient started complaining of chest pain and had inferior ST elevation. He underwent immediate catheterization and was found to have occluded RCA. However, the artery could not be successfully opened. In the stent era, all factors have been correlated with abrupt vessel closure, *except*:

(A) Stent length
(B) Small vessel diameter
(C) Poor distal run off
(D) Excessive tortuosity
(E) Unstable angina

4 A 51-year-old woman presents to you for second opinion. She underwent successful elective PCI to CX for exertional chest pain. Her hospitalization was uneventful until the time of discharge when she was told that her creatine kinase-MB (CK-MB) isoform was three times the normal limit. She was discharged home and has been doing well but cannot stop worrying. Which of the following statements is *true* regarding procedure-related enzyme release?

(A) CK-MB elevation does not occur after angiographically successful uncomplicated coronary interventions
(B) Routine monitoring of cardiac enzymes is not necessary to detect patients who suffer from myocardial injury after coronary intervention
(C) The incidence of CK-MB enzyme elevation after angiographically successful percutaneous intervention is >50%
(D) Elevation of CK-MB after PCI predicts increased long-term cardiac mortality and morbidity

5 A 45-year-old patient with diabetes who was hypercholesterolemic, hypertensive, and a heavy (two-packs-a-day) smoker underwent a successful angioplasty and stent placement to mid-LAD lesion. Before angioplasty, the patient received acetylsalicylic acid (ASA) 325, and glycoprotein (GP) IIb/IIIa inhibitor treatment. The angioplasty procedure was uneventful. The Cypher 3.0 × 28-mm stent was deployed at 16 atm. The final angiogram showed a well-expanded vessel with thrombolysis in

myocardial infarction (TIMI) 3 flow. The following morning, a routine troponin was 1.5 ng/mL. The patient remained asymptomatic and his cardiac examination was normal. His electrocardiogram (EKG) showed nonspecific ST–T-wave changes, which were unchanged from the admitting EKG. The best course of action for this patient now is as follows:

(A) Discharge the patient immediately with β-blockers, nitrates, statin, ASA, Plavix, and an angiotensin-converting enzyme (ACE) inhibitor
(B) Bring the patient back to the catheterization laboratory for a repeat angiogram
(C) Transfer the patient to a coronary care unit (CCU)
(D) Continue to monitor the patient in telemetry for 48 hours
(E) Check another set of troponin in 8 hours. If the trend is down then discharge him on Plavix, ASA, β-blockers, statins, and an ACE inhibitor

6 A 75-year-old patient traveled 4 hours by car to get to the hospital for a 7:00 AM, first case, elective, complex, multilesion, multivessel coronary intervention. Although the angioplasty procedure was difficult to perform because of lack of adequate guide support, finally after trying several guide catheters, an Amplatz no. 3 guide catheter was found to give a good guide support to deliver three long Taxus stents. At the end of the procedure, the operator informed the patient that he was successful in opening all the blockages. The catheterization laboratory staff moved the patient to the recovery room. The patient was asymptomatic without any complaint and had normal vital signs. Later, the recovery room registered nurse (RN) noticed that the patient became progressively lethargic and less responsive to her. The physician in charge was notified. After obtaining the vital signs, which were noted to be unchanged, the most appropriate action at this time should be:

(A) Have the RN check the patient's EKG and his vital signs again
(B) Give him naloxone (Narcan)
(C) Perform a screening neurologic examination or obtain an urgent neurology consult
(D) Check the patient's complete blood count (CBC), blood sugar, blood urea nitrogen (BUN), and creatinine level

7 The patient mentioned in the preceding text recovers and is discharged without any residual deficits. He has filed a formal complaint against you to the hospital. The Chief of Staff's office would like to know about periprocedural stroke during coronary interventions. Which of the following statements is correct?

(A) Periprocedural stroke occurs approximately 0.5%
(B) Patients who suffer a stroke have an increased in-hospital mortality of 37%
(C) Patients who suffer a stroke have an increased 1-year mortality of 56%
(D) It is mostly embolic and not hemorrhagic stroke
(E) A, B, and C are true
(F) B, C, and D are true
(G) C and D are true
(H) A, B, C, and D are true

8 You are asked to examine a 65-year-old heavy smoker with a strong family history of coronary artery disease (CAD), status post (s/p) multivessel PCI in the past with left-sided stroke for cardiology evaluation. His past medical history is notable for PCI to heavily calcified ostial LAD and mid-CX 8 months ago. Recently, he has been under treatment for methicillin-resistant *Staphylococcus aureus* (MRSA) bacteremia following his right below-knee amputation for gangrene. At baseline, he has an abnormal EKG with nonspecific ST changes in the precordial leads. The two-dimensional (2D) echo demonstrated moderate aortic insufficiency (AI) with multiple large vegetations on the aortic valve. He is examined by the cardiothoracic surgeons who would like to operate on him. They would like to visualize his coronary anatomy first and then ask for your opinion. The most appropriate action at this time is:

(A) Because of high risk of embolization with left heart catheterization, he should undergo cardiac computed tomography (CT) to assess patency of ostial LAD and mid-CX stents
(B) Send the patient for emergency heart surgery without cardiac angiogram
(C) Perform left-sided cardiac catheterization to visualize coronary anatomy
(D) Transfer the patient to neuro intensive care unit (ICU) for stroke management and treat endocarditis medically

9 A 75-year-old morbidly obese patient (378 pounds, 5 ft. 5 in. tall) is referred from an outside hospital for angioplasty and stenting of a large proximal dominant RCA lesion. The patient has an infected skin lesion in the right groin beneath a large abdominal pannus. The operator decides to cannulate the left groin instead, and after multiple sticks he is finally able to cannulate the left leg artery and to place a 7 F arterial introducer. The angioplasty

procedure is successful using a 3.5/33 mm Cypher stent to RCA with heparin and GPIIb/IIIa inhibitor eptifibatide (Integrilin). Following the angioplasty procedure, all equipment is removed from the patient's heart. At the end of the procedure the activated clotting time (ACT) is measured at 287 seconds. The operator decides to close the left groin artery entry site with an 8 F Angio-Seal device. Before doing so, he performs a peripheral angiogram using the introducing sheath to inject dye. The angiogram shows that the introducer was placed in the proximal profunda femoris artery too close to its bifurcation. The operator elects to place the Fem Stop instead. The Fem Stop is successfully applied and the patient is moved to the recovery room. In the recovery room, the RN notices that the patient's BP has dropped from 130/90 to 96/70, and her pulse has increased from 68 to 78 bpm. The physician is notified, and he orders an increase in intravenous fluids to 200 mL/hour for 1 hour. The patient's BP normalizes, but an hour later it drops again. This time it measures 90/68, with a pulse of 90 bpm. Soon after that, the patient starts to complain that the Fem Stop causes her to have left groin pain. The physician comes and adjusts the Fem Stop. He examines the groin and it appears normal. The intravenous fluids are increased and the systolic BP returns to 102/70 mm Hg. After a while, the patient again starts complaining of being uncomfortable in bed with the Fem Stop compressing her groin, and she becomes diaphoretic, her BP drops to 75/50, and her heart rate (HR) slows down to 45 bpm. The physician is notified. The most appropriate initial response at this time should be:

(A) Loosen or reposition the Fem Stop and give the patient a pain medication with sedation for comfort
(B) Send the patient for CT scan
(C) Send the patient to vascular laboratory for ultrasound
(D) Order patient's CBC, and type and cross
(E) Remove Fem Stop and apply direct manual pressure on the artery entry site
(F) Continue rapid fluid infusion to expand the volume
(G) Stop GPIIb/IIIa inhibitors
(H) Consult a vascular surgeon to consider surgery
(I) A, B, and C are correct
(J) D, E, F, and G are correct
(K) A–H are correct

10 The patient mentioned in the preceding text does well with manual pressure and goes upstairs to the telemetry floor. In 3 hours, you are called to see the patient because she has developed pulselessness, pain, pallor, and paresthesia of her left leg. What is the best way to treat this patient at this time?

(A) Start intravenous heparin and careful clinical monitoring

(B) Start intravenous heparin, GPIIb/IIIa inhibitor, and careful monitoring

(C) Intravenous fibrinolytic therapy

(D) Urgent peripheral vascular (PV) surgery consultation or urgent percutaneous PV intervention

11 Complication of groin hematoma may lead to sensory or motor neurologic deficit by compressing the surrounding nerves. Which nerves are most commonly affected by groin hematoma?

(A) Femoral and sciatic nerves

(B) Sciatic, femoral, and lateral cutaneous nerves

(C) Femoral and lateral cutaneous nerves

12 The most common cause of procedurally related retroperitoneal hematoma includes:

(A) Spontaneous retroperitoneal venous bleeding triggered by aggressive anticoagulant therapy

(B) Arterial bleed caused by a back wall puncture of the femoral artery distal to the origin of the superficial CX iliac artery

(C) Arterial bleeding caused by a back wall puncture of the femoral artery proximal to the origin of the deep CX iliac artery

13 A 54-year-old woman is transferred to the medical center from an outside hospital for an elective angioplasty of the RCA artery lesion. Three days before admission, the patient suffered an acute inferior wall myocardial infarction (MI), which was successfully treated with IV tPA. On the day of the procedure, the patient was asymptomatic, but she was quite anxious about the upcoming coronary angioplasty. The 80% lesion in the proximal RCA was opened with a 3.5 × 23 mm Cypher stent. The final angiogram showed a widely patent RCA, normal left coronary system, and EF of 50% with moderate inferior wall hypokinesis. The right groin entry site was successfully closed with a Perclose device after angiogram was taken (see following figure).

The patient was transferred to the recovery unit, and within 45 minutes she began to complain of right groin and right flank pain, which improved when she adjusted her position. Thirty minutes later, her BP and pulse, which previously read 130/70 and 70 respectively, measured 100/60 and 80. Fluids were administered, and her BP improved, but she continued to complain about the right lower abdominal quadrant pain. The physician was called. He examined the groin and found no evidence of bleeding and hematoma. Bowel sounds were weak but present. He reassured the patient and returned to the catheterization laboratory. Fifteen minutes later, her BP dropped again to 76 mm Hg with a pulse of 60 bpm. The patient became slightly diaphoretic and restless, complaining of increasing abdominal discomfort. Soon thereafter, her BP dropped to 60/40, HR was 45 bpm, the patient began to retch, but could not vomit. The most likely diagnostic explanation of this patient's problem is:

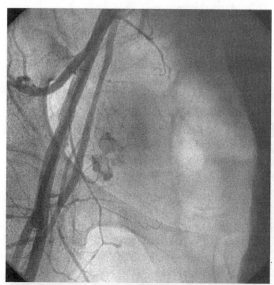

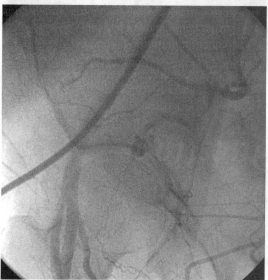

(A) Patient is allergic to intravenous pyelogram (IVP) dye

(B) Patient has femoral artery dissection

(C) Patient has spontaneous RP bleed

(D) Patient has adverse reaction to midazolam (Versed) and fentanyl

(E) Patient has arterial external iliac artery perforation with retroperitoneal dye extravasation

14 The best treatment for a patient who, during the percutaneous intervention, suffers an accidental large right iliac artery laceration is:

(A) Aggressive fluid and blood replacement therapy
(B) Emergency consult to PV surgery
(C) Immediate percutaneous intervention using contralateral approach to block bleeding from the iliac artery by inflating properly sized angioplasty balloon followed by placing covered stent to seal the vessel wall
(D) Manual pressure

15 Match each of the following figures to a diagnosis:

(A)

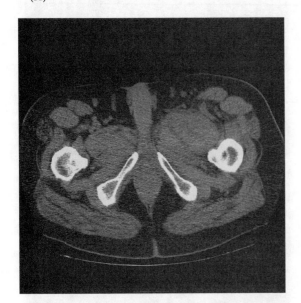

(B)

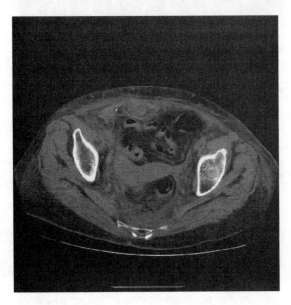

(C)

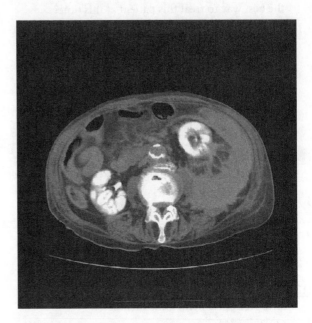

(D)

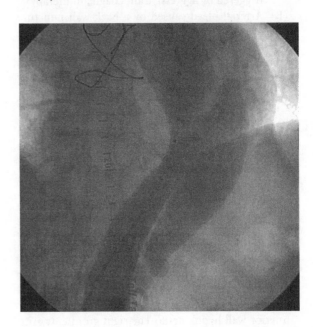

(E)

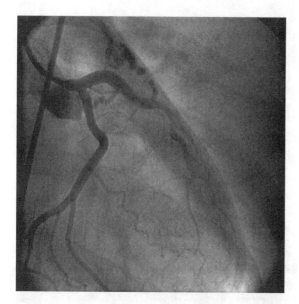

(F)

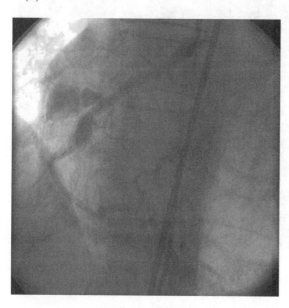

1. Retroperitoneal hematoma
2. Thigh hematoma
3. Rectus muscle hematoma
4. Aortic dissection
5. Coronary atrioventricular (AV) malformation
6. Coronary perforation

16 A 63-year-old morbidly obese woman presents to your office for follow-up. She underwent successful uneventful PCI to RCA, which was complicated by the development of pseudoaneurysm. On initial duplex, it was measured at 2.5 cm. It was treated with ultrasound-guided thrombin injection. She underwent repeat duplex 2 months later, and the aneurysm has remained unchanged. However, she is asymptomatic. What are the appropriate therapeutic options at this time?

(A) Ultrasound-guided compression of the neck of the pseudoaneurysm
(B) Injection of the cavity of the pseudoaneurysm with procoagulant or embolization coils
(C) Surgery
(D) Conservative management with good BP control and repeat ultrasound in 2 months

17 The angiogram in the following figure demonstrates which of the following abnormalities?

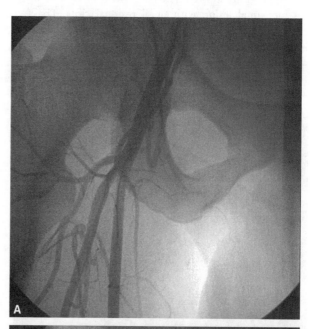

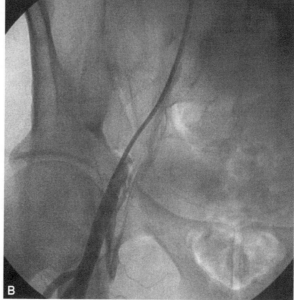

(A) Iliac artery lesion
(B) Femoral artery dissection
(C) Postprocedural AV fistula
(D) Right groin mass
(E) Congenital AV malformation

18 A 75-year-old woman with HTN and hyperlipidemia was admitted to an outside hospital for an anterior wall MI 4 days ago. She was given thrombolytic therapy and was doing well until this morning when she developed shortness of breath (SOB). She has been transferred to your hospital, and a diagnostic angiogram was performed. The coronary angiogram showed TIMI 3 flow in LAD with 85% proximal lesion with small residual clots. The LV angiogram was performed, demonstrating an EF of 65% and no mitral regurgitation (MR) (see following figure). The best course of action for the patient is to have:

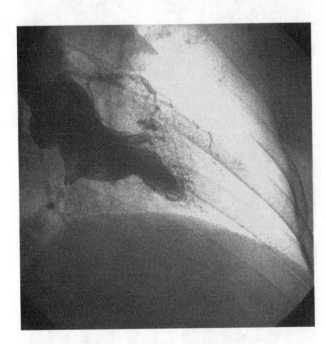

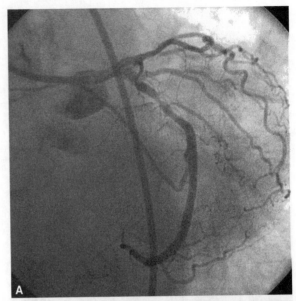

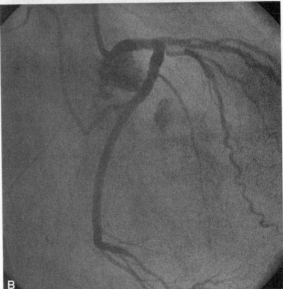

(A) PTCA + stent of the residual LAD lesion
(B) Intracoronary thrombolysis, followed by PTCA + stent of the LAD lesion
(C) AngioJet procedure, followed by PTCA + stent of the LAD lesion
(D) Immediate Doppler echocardiogram and open heart surgery

19 The incidence of coronary perforation during coronary intervention is low. These pre- and postprocedural angiograms demonstrate:

(A) Type I coronary perforation
(B) Type II coronary perforation
(C) Type III coronary perforation

20 Which of the following options is *not* a correct choice to treat coronary perforation?

(A) Prolonged inflation of the balloon across the perforation
(B) Reverse anticoagulation, giving protamine 1 mg for each 1,000 units of heparin
(C) Reverse anticoagulation, giving protamine 0.1 mg for each 1,000 units of heparin
(D) Use of covered stent
(E) Use of coils to embolize leaking branch
(F) Pericardiocentesis

21 If a severe reaction to dye occurs, with which of the initial concentration of IV epinephrine can it be reversed before it is diluted further?

(A) 1 mL of 1:1,000 epinephrine
(B) 1 mL of 1:100,000 epinephrine
(C) 1 mL of 1:10,000 epinephrine

22 A 68-year-old man with s/p CABG 10 years ago presents with chest pain. He is noted to have nonspecific ST changes, but his initial troponin is 2.0 ng per mL. He is brought to the cardiac catheterization laboratory. His angiograms are given in the following figure. He undergoes PCI to a diseased saphenous vein graft (SVG) with embolic protection device. During the procedure after stent deployment, he has severe chest pain with ST elevation. An angiogram at that time is shown in the following figure. What would you do next?

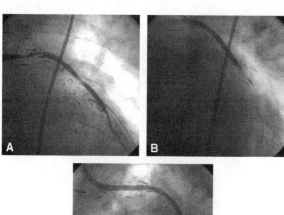

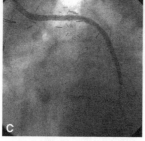

(A) Capture and remove the filter device because it did not adequately capture the debris
(B) Capture and remove the filter device because it is full of debris
(C) Give intracoronary nitroglycerin (IC NTG)
(D) Intravascular ultrasound (IVUS) of the stent site because there might be a dissection

23 What is the most common cause of no reflow and CK elevation during SVG PCI?

(A) No reflow is primarily caused by intense vasospasm
(B) No reflow is caused by acute platelet aggregation
(C) No reflow is caused by particulate matter embolization from friable plaque and thrombus

(D) No reflow is completely preventable by using emboli protection device

24 A 24-year-old patient was admitted to the emergency room (ER) with severe chest pain and anterior wall ST elevation. The patient was partying and drinking alcohol, and using cocaine all night long. The patient was taken to the catheterization laboratory, and the selective coronary angiogram showed severe mid-LAD lesion (see following figure). What would you do next?

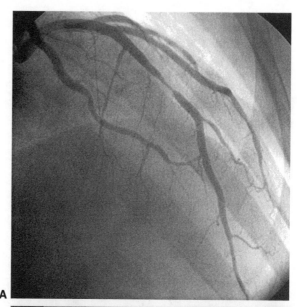

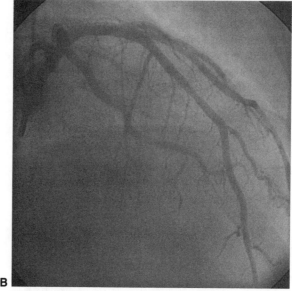

(A) Heparin and GPIIb/IIIa inhibitor
(B) Angioplasty and stent
(C) IC NTG and repeat angiogram
(D) IV β-blockers

25 A 51-year-old man comes to your ER with severe chest pain for 2 hours. His past medical history is unremarkable except for hyperlipidemia. He is found to have ST elevation in the anterior leads and is taken to the catheterization laboratory, where he undergoes successful PCI to mid/distal LAD with 3.0/28 drug-eluting stent, heparin, and abciximab (ReoPro). His EF is 50%. He does well, and is transferred to CCU. Two hours later, he becomes very short of breath and hypoxemic. He has hemoptysis, goes into respiratory distress, and is intubated. His chest x-ray shows alveolar infiltrates. What is the most likely cause of his SOB?

(A) Pulmonary hemorrhage from ReoPro
(B) Congestive heart failure
(C) LV rupture
(D) Papillary muscle rupture
(E) Aortic dissection

Answers and Explanations

1 **Answer C.** Typically, CABG is performed as a rescue revascularization procedure to treat acute ischemia or infarction resulting from PCI-induced acute coronary occlusion. In the balloon angioplasty era, the rate of emergent CABG was 3.7%. However, in the stent era, the reported rate has been 0.45% (*Circulation.* 2000;102:2945–2951).

2 **Answer E.** There is ostial left main coronary trunk (LMT) stenosis with no reflux of dye.

3 **Answer D.** In the stent era, unstable angina, bailout stenting, small vessel diameter, long lesions, large plaque volume, residual uncovered dissection, slow flow or poor distal runoff, and suboptimal final procedural lumen have all been associated with abrupt vessel closure. Excessive tortuosity is a risk factor for abrupt vessel closure during balloon angioplasty but not stent thrombosis (*Textbook of interventional cardiology* Chapter 13).

4 **Answer D.** Elevation of CK-MB over five times the normal baseline carries the same adverse impact on long-term prognosis as a Q-wave infarction (*Circulation.* 1996;94:3369–3375, *Catheter Cardiovasc Interv.* 2004;63:31–41, *J Am Coll Cardiol.* 1999;34:672–673).

5 **Answer E.** The long-term prognostic significance of smaller postprocedural troponin T elevations is unknown. Therefore, there is no need to prolong hospitalization beyond what is necessary to document that troponin has peaked and has begun to fall. It is of note that one study suggests a postprocedural increase in troponin T of five times normal is predictive for adverse events at 6 years (*ACC/AHA 2005 Guideline Update.* 2006).

6 **Answer C.** Strokes are rare but devastating complications of cardiac interventions. The interventionalist should be familiar with potential etiologies, preventive strategies, and treatments for catheterization-related stroke, and should develop the routine habit of speaking with the patient directly at the end of the procedure. If the patient is less alert, has slurred speech, and has visual, sensory, or motor symptoms, there should be a low threshold for performing a screening neurologic examination or obtaining an urgent stroke neurology consult. For most hemispheric events, an urgent carotid angiogram and neurovascular rescue should be considered (*Cathet Cardiovasc Diagn.* 1998;44:412–414).

7 **Answer C.** Stroke related to contemporary PCI is associated with substantial increased mortality. Patients who suffer procedural stroke tend to be older, have lower left ventricular EF and more diabetes, and experience a higher rate of intraprocedural complications necessitating emergency use of intra-aortic balloon pump. The in-hospital mortality and 1-year mortality are substantially higher in patients with stroke (*Circulation.* 2002;106:86–91).

8 **Answer C.** The question of central nervous system (CNS) embolic risk arises when it is necessary to perform catheterization on a patient with endocarditis of left-sided (aortic or mitral) heart valves. Although echo appearance of these vegetations looks friable and they can embolize spontaneously, left heart catheterization can be done safely in these patients. In a series of 35 patients with active endocarditis who had left heart catheterization, none had catheterization-induced embolic events. Patency is difficult to visualize with heavily calcified arteries with cardiac CT (*Am J Cardiol.* 1979;44:1306–1310).

9 **Answer C.** Occult bleeding at the arterial entry site is the cause of this patient's hypotension. The patient needs to be stabilized first before being sent to CT scan or vascular laboratory (*J Am Coll Cardiol.* 2005;45:363–368).

10 **Answer D.** This patient has acute femoral artery thrombosis. This is an emergency case that needs immediate surgery or PV intervention.

11 **Answer C.** Nerve complications following cardiac catheterization through the femoral route are rare. Although femoral nerve is most likely to be affected, lateral cutaneous nerve can also be affected (*Catheter Cardiovasc Interv.* 2002;56:69–71).

12 **Answer C.** Arterial back wall puncture is the most common cause of retroperitoneal hematoma (*Eur J Vasc Endovasc Surg.* 1999;18:364–365).

13 **Answer E.** The angiogram shows external iliac artery perforation with dye extravasation.

14 **Answer C.** Bleeding from lacerated iliac artery could be fatal within a matter of minutes without catheter-based control of large bleeding. Therefore, immediate posterior tibial artery (PTA) using contralateral approach is appropriate.

15 **Answer .** A-2, B-3, C-1, D-4, E-5, F-6.

16 **Answer C.** This aneurysm has been treated in the past, and still persists after 2 months. Therefore, it should be operated (*J Vasc Surg.* 1993;17:125–131, discussion 131–133, *Catheter Cardiovasc Interv.* 2001; 53:259–263, *J Vasc Surg.* 1999;30:1052–1059).

17 **Answer C.** AV fistula is noted in the preceding figure. Small AV fistulas are often monitored with ultrasound imaging. Indications for intervention are lack of spontaneous closure, increase in fistula size, and/or the development of symptoms.

18 **Answer E.** The LV angiogram demonstrates impending LV rupture (high anterior wall) with dye staining the fistula track in the LV wall. Echo showed moderate pericardial effusion. The patient had an emergency surgery.

19 **Answer B.** The angiographic appearance of coronary perforations could be classified as: Type I— Extraluminal crater without extravasation, Type II— Pericardial and myocardial blush, and Type III—Dye extravasation (*Circulation.* 1994;90:2725–2730).

20 **Answer C.** The current dose of protamine is 1 mg for each 1,000 units of heparin (*Am J Cardiol.* 2002; 90:1183–1186).

21 **Answer C.** Epinephrine of 0.5 to 1.0 mL of 1:10,000 administered intravenously over several minutes should be considered. This may be repeated at intervals of 5 to 10 minutes, preferably with cardiac monitoring because adverse effects of intravenous epinephrine may occur. In the setting of profound hypotension, a continuous infusion of epinephrine (5 to 15 µg per minute) titrated to effect may be administered. If intravenous access cannot be obtained immediately, epinephrine (3 to 5 mL of 1:10,000 dilution of epinephrine) can be delivered through the endotracheal tube.

22 **Answer B.** The filter device is full of debris. Although it is possible that distal embolization occurred, if there was good apposition of the filter to the vessel wall throughout the case, it is less likely. Therefore, at this point, you can wire with another wire and capture and remove the emboli filter device. After the removal of filter wire, the angiogram shown in the preceding figure was taken.

23 **Answer C.** The Saphenous Vein Graft Angioplasty Free of Emboli Randomized (SAFER) trial compared emboli protection device versus conventional therapy in SVG PCI. The primary endpoint (a composite of death, MI, emergency bypass, or target lesion revascularization by 30 days) was observed in 16.5% assigned to the control group and 9.6% assigned to the embolic protection device ($p = 0.004$). This 42% relative reduction in major adverse cardiac events was driven by lower MI and no-reflow phenomenon in the emboli filter arm. This study demonstrated the importance of distal embolization in causing major adverse cardiac events and the value of embolic protection devices in preventing such complications (*Circulation.* 2002;105:1285–1290, *J Am Coll Cardiol.* 2002;40:1882–1888).

24 **Answer C.** The follow-up angiogram demonstrates the normal LAD lumen size, indicating the presence of cocaine-induced coronary spasm. An IV β-blocker would not be appropriate and may cause more spasm. Calcium channel blockers would be more appropriate.

25 **Answer A.** Pulmonary alveolar hemorrhage has been rarely reported during use of abciximab. This can present with any or all of the following in close association with ReoPro administration: Hypoxemia, alveolar infiltrates on chest x-ray, hemoptysis, or an unexplained drop in hemoglobin.

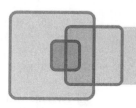

23

Qualitative and Quantitative Angiography

Sorin J. Brener

Questions

1 Which of the following characteristics of a lesion predicts a lower rate of procedural success in the stent era?

(A) Total occlusion <3 months old
(B) Excessive tortuosity of proximal segment
(C) Ostial location
(D) Segment angulation >45 and <90 degrees

2 Which of the following lesion characteristics is associated with both increased early procedural failure and late restenosis?

(A) Irregular contour
(B) Moderate calcification
(C) Length >20 mm
(D) Angulation >45 degrees

3 Of the bifurcation lesions, which are related to higher rates of procedural complications during parent vessel percutaneous coronary intervention (PCI)?

(A) Parent vessel stenosis and ostium of branch vessel has >50% stenosis
(B) Normal branch originating from diseased parent vessel
(C) Branch not involved by parent vessel lesion but in jeopardy during balloon inflation
(D) All of the above

4 The thrombolysis in myocardial infarction (TIMI) flow classification scheme was derived from:

(A) Patients undergoing elective PCI
(B) Patients undergoing primary PCI for acute myocardial infarction (MI)

(C) Patients receiving IV fibrinolysis for acute MI
(D) Patients receiving intracoronary (IC) fibrinolysis for acute MI

5 Correlation between the assessment of coronary flow by clinical centers and angiographic core laboratory is best for:

(A) TIMI 0–1 flow
(B) TIMI 2 flow
(C) TIMI 3 flow
(D) All of the above

6 As compared with TIMI 0–2 flow, TIMI 3 flow after reperfusion therapy is associated with:

(A) Improved 30-day survival
(B) Improved 1-year survival
(C) Improved left ventricular ejection fraction
(D) All of the above

7 The distal landmark for the right coronary artery (RCA) TIMI frame count (TFC) is as follows:

(A) The bifurcation of RCA
(B) The first branch of the posterolateral artery off RCA
(C) The end of posterior descending coronary artery (PDA)
(D) The first septal perforator off PDA

8 Ninety minutes after fibrinolysis-based reperfusion therapy, a TFC of 40 in left anterior descending (LAD) artery is likely to be graded as:

(A) TIMI 3 flow
(B) TIMI 2 flow

(C) TIMI 1 flow

(D) TIMI 0 flow

9 Patients with TFC <14 after reperfusion for acute MI have:

(A) "TIMI 4" flow and the best prognosis at 30 days

(B) An error in measurement

(C) Similar outcome as patients with TFC of 23

(D) Worse outcome than patients with TFC of 23

10 The following pair of values is typical of TFC in noninfarct arteries after reperfusion and in arteries examined during elective angiography:

(A) 45 and 28

(B) 35 and 28

(C) 21 and 21

(D) 31 and 21

11 The Myocardial Perfusion Grade (MPG) evaluates the quality of:

(A) Epicardial flow

(B) Myocardial flow

(C) Epicardial and myocardial flow

(D) Neither

12 The relation between maximal ST-segment elevation resolution (STR), optimal MPG after reperfusion, and recovery of function of the infarcted zone is that:

(A) STR correlates better with early (before hospital discharge) recovery and MPG correlates better with late (within 6 months) recovery

(B) STR correlates better with late (within 6 months) recovery and MPG correlates better with early (before hospital discharge) recovery

(C) STR and MPG correlate with early (before hospital discharge) recovery

(D) STR and MPG correlate with late (within 6 months) recovery

13 As compared with quantitative methods, visual estimation of diameter stenosis before PCI is:

(A) Greater

(B) Similar

(C) Lower

(D) Unpredictable

14 Computerized algorithms for detection of vessel contour use a mixture of first and second derivative extremes of density to identify vessel margins. An algorithm weighted more toward the first derivative than toward the second derivative will systematically result in:

(A) Larger diameters

(B) Similar diameters

(C) Smaller diameters

(D) Unpredictable results

15 Repeated quantitative angiographic measurements of the same angiographic frame are likely to result in intraobserver variability in minimal lumen diameter (MLD) of:

(A) 1.0 to 2.0 mm

(B) 0.5 to 1.0 mm

(C) 0.1 to 0.5 mm

(D) 0.05 to 0.1 mm

16 The determination of the reference diameter (RD) is based on:

(A) The 10-mm segment proximal to lesion

(B) Two 10-mm segments without irregularities proximal and distal to lesion

(C) The 10-mm segment distal to lesion

(D) The diameter of the proximal "shoulder" of the lesion

17 The loss index is:

(A) The late loss in MLD divided by the acute gain

(B) The late loss in MLD divided by the RD

(C) The difference between balloon size and MLD at end of procedure

(D) The net gain divided by the RD

18 Which of the following determinants is the least critical in predicting late loss?

(A) Diabetes mellitus

(B) Lesion length

(C) Lesion location (which coronary artery is involved)

(D) Postprocedural MLD

19 As compared with balloon angioplasty, stenting results in:

(A) Smaller late loss

(B) Larger late loss

(C) Similar late loss

(D) Unpredictable late loss

20 All the following definitions describe restenosis after PCI, *except*:

(A) Late loss ≥0.72 mm

(B) Loss of >50% acute gain at follow-up

(C) Diameter of stenosis >50% at follow-up

(D) Diameter of stenosis >70% at follow-up

Answers and Explanations

1 **Answer B.** In general, stents have overcome many of the limitations of balloon-only coronary revascularization. Nevertheless, the presence of excessive tortuosity of the segment proximal to lesion impedes passage of stents and is more prone to dissection while attempting to advance devices (*J Am Coll Cardiol*. 2006;47:216–235).

2 **Answer C.** Many lesion characteristics have been studied for their predictive value with respect to early and late failures. Stents have eliminated the adverse prognostic effect of many lesion characteristics. Longer lesions remain associated even in the current era with higher rates of procedural failure and restenosis. In fact, longer lesion length is one of the major high-risk features in the new classification offered by the American College of Cardiology/Society for Cardiovascular Angiography and Interventions (ACC/SCAI) in the latest guideline update (*J Am Coll Cardiol*. 2006;47:216–235, *J Am Coll Cardiol*. 1992;19:1641–1652, *J Am Coll Cardiol*. 1991;17:22–28).

3 **Answer A.** The optimal management of bifurcation lesions has remained elusive because of the absence of stents dedicated to this type of lesion. Many techniques were empirically adopted for treatment of bifurcation lesions and classification systems were derived to predict immediate and long-term success. The key finding in these classifications is the presence of plaque at the ostium of the branch and the extent to which it obstructs the lumen (*Catheter Cardiovasc Interv*. 2000;49:274–283, *J Am Coll Cardiol*. 1992;19:1641–1652).

4 **Answer C.** The first (and still) most applied method of reperfusion for ST-segment elevation myocardial infarction (STEMI) is fibrinolytic therapy. Initially, it was administered through the IC route, and subsequently, it became available for IV use. The seminal observation that the extent, durability, and completeness of flow restoration correlates with mortality has led to efforts to standardize the evaluation of flow after reperfusion therapy. This classification has been widely accepted for results of angioplasty and for patients who are not suffering STEMI at the time of presentation (*N Engl J Med*. 1985;312:932–936).

5 **Answer A.** The best correlation between site investigators and independent reviewers at a core laboratory for the assessment of flow quality exists for occluded arteries (TIMI 0-1 flow) (*Circulation*. 1996;93:879–888).

6 **Answer D.** In Global Utilization of Streptokinase and tPA for Occluded coronary arteries I (GUSTO I), the patients who attained TIMI 3 flow 90 minutes after lysis had improved survival and myocardial function, as compared with those with less complete reperfusion. At 30 days, patients with TIMI 3 flow at 90 minutes after lytics had a mortality rate of 4.6% as compared with 8% for those with TIMI 0–2 flow. At 2 years, this benefit persisted: 7.9% versus 15.7%, respectively (*N Engl J Med*. 1993;329:1615–1622).

7 **Answer B.** The measurement of TFC requires visualization of the artery at intermediate or low magnification (to prevent the need for panning) and the identification of the frames when contrast enters the artery and when it reaches prespecified, easily identifiable, and reproducible landmarks (*Circulation*. 1996;93:879–888).

8 **Answer A.** The LAD TFC needs correction because of its length—therefore, the corrected TIMI frame count (cTFC) is 40:1.7 or 23.5, which is typically reflective of TIMI 3 flow (*Circulation*. 1998;98:2805–2814, *J Am Coll Cardiol*. 1994;24:1602–1610, *Circulation*. 1997;95:351–356, *J Am Coll Cardiol*. 2005;45:351–356).

9 **Answer A.** Patients treated with reperfusion therapy soon after onset of symptoms and who achieve complete reperfusion can manifest flow that is more rapid than those with noninfarct arteries. It is presumed that profound vasodilatation in the infarct bed, without significant damage to the microcirculation, is responsible for this phenomenon. When it occurs, excellent prognosis can be anticipated (*Circulation*. 1999;99:1945–1950).

10 **Answer D.** During the analysis of infarct-artery flow in reperfusion studies with fibrinolytic agents, it was observed that the flow in noninfarct arteries is slower (higher TFC) than the flow observed in patients undergoing elective angiography. This important observation strengthens the current paradigm claiming that, during an acute coronary syndrome, systemic activation of platelets occurs, and marked secretion of vasoactive substances leads to diffuse slowing of coronary flow (*Circulation*. 1996;93:879–888, *J Am Coll Cardiol*. 1999;34: 974–982).

11 **Answer B.** There are two important methods for the determination of MPG: The densitometric method (evaluates maximal density of contrast in region of interest) (*Circulation*. 1998;97:2302–2306) and the kinetic method (evaluates the speed of entry and exit of contrast in the area of interest) (*Circulation*. 2002;105:1909–1913). Although epicardial flow is necessary for myocardial perfusion, it is not sufficient. Patients may experience TIMI 3 flow in the infarct-artery with poor myocardial perfusion due to destruction of the microcirculation or distal embolization of plaque and thrombus after reperfusion. Conversely, patients may have suboptimal TIMI flow (usually TIMI 2) in the infarct-artery with excellent myocardial perfusion. Rarely, even collateral flow may be sufficient to provide adequate myocardial perfusion (MPG 2 or 3) (*Circulation*. 1996;93:223–228, *Circulation*. 1998;97:2302–2306).

12 **Answer A.** Although immediate restoration of epicardial and myocardial perfusion with resolution of ST-segment changes and symptoms is desirable, these events may occur at various intervals after successful reperfusion. In a study of patients undergoing primary PCI, recovery (at least one grade by echocardiography) of regional myocardial function before hospital discharge occurred in 62% of those with >50% ST-deviation resolution and 55% of those with MPG 2–3. It was noted in only 23% of those without significant ST-deviation resolution before hospital discharge, but 86% of those with MPG 2–3 still showed improved function at 6 months (*Circulation*. 2002;106:313–318).

13 **Answer A.** Visual estimation of lesion severity remains crucial in the delivery of care in routine clinical practice. Nevertheless, lesion severity measured by quantitative coronary angiography (QCA) is typically lower than the visual estimate before PCI and greater than the visual estimate after PCI (*J Am Coll Cardiol*. 1991;18:945–951).

14 **Answer C.** Smoothing algorithms used to detect arterial contour mathematically extrapolate differences in contrast densities between arterial lumen and its surroundings. If a first-order derivative is used predominantly (CMS, CAAS-II), the resulting lumen is smaller than if additional derivatives are weighted

in (ArTrek). These factors are important when comparing results of angiographic studies analyzed with different software (*Circulation*. 1995;91:2174–2183).

15 **Answer D.** Overall, the differences in arterial measurements in repeated evaluations by the same observer are extremely small. This bodes well for the reliability and reproducibility of QCA parameters (*J Am Coll Cardiol*. 1993;22:1068–1074).

16 **Answer B.** There are two methods to estimate RD at the point of maximal stenosis. The interpolation method uses a second-order polynomial equation to estimate the RD by tracking the arterial contour proximal and distal to the lesion. A second method uses an arithmetic average of the diameter of two 10-mm segments without obvious irregularities located equidistantly from the maximal stenosis (*Cathet Cardiovasc Diagn*. 1992;25:110–131, *Cathet Cardiovasc Diagn*. 1997;40:343–347).

17 **Answer A.** By convention, the loss index is the ratio between the late loss and acute gain. This calculation uses the concept that larger acute gains are typically associated with larger losses, yet the remaining lumen is still larger. In other words, every millimeter gained loses only a fraction during arterial healing, analogous to income taxation (*J Am Coll Cardiol*. 1993;21:15–25).

18 **Answer C.** Many clinical and angiographic parameters influence late loss. Diabetes and lesion length are the most important, whereas lesion location is the least important, particularly with stenting (*Am J Cardiol*. 1997;80:77K–88K, *Circulation*. 1992;86:1827–1835).

19 **Answer B.** As mentioned above, larger acute gains are typically associated with larger late loss due to arterial injury. Stenting, as compared with balloon angioplasty, clearly demonstrated this phenomenon (*J Am Coll Cardiol*. 1992;19:258–266, *J Am Coll Cardiol*. 1999;34:1067–1074).

20 **Answer D.** Numerous definitions have been used to describe the response to arterial injury during PCI. Classically, binary restenosis has been defined as >50% stenosis at follow-up. The 0.72-mm cutoff point is derived from doubling the expected variability in serial angiographic studies. The 70% cutoff is better associated with recurrent angina, positive stress tests, or ischemia-driven revascularization (*J Am Coll Cardiol*. 1992;19:258–266, *Circulation*. 1985;71:280–288, *J Am Coll Cardiol*. 1992;19: 939–945).

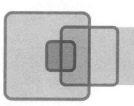

24

Interventional Coronary Physiology

Morton J. Kern

Questions

1 Myocardial oxygen demand is balanced by oxygen supply. Which of the following is *not* involved in increasing myocardial oxygen demand?

(A) Myocardial contractility
(B) R-R interval
(C) Left ventricular (LV) end diastolic dimension
(D) Diastolic relaxation
(E) Systolic pressure

2 Coronary reserve is the ratio of maximal flow to basal (resting) coronary blood flow. Which of the following is most likely associated with a normal increase in coronary flow reserve (CFR)?

(A) A 75-year-old man with left ventricular hypertrophy (LVH) and hypertension
(B) A 62-year-old woman with three-vessel coronary artery disease (CAD)
(C) A 59-year-old man with 80% proximal left anterior descending artery (LAD)
(D) A 39-year-old woman with insulin-dependant diabetes mellitus since high school
(E) A 48-year-old man with 60% mid-LAD

3 Which of the following best states the rationale for use of in-laboratory coronary physiology to assess stenoses?

(A) The use of stress testing has a low specificity and sensitivity
(B) The angiogram cannot provide enough information to determine flow for lesions 40% to 70% narrowed
(C) Chest pain syndromes are unreliable

(D) CAD is diffuse, obscuring the degree of atherosclerosis
(E) Intravascular ultrasound (IVUS) imaging shows plaque distribution and flow limitations

4 Coronary flow velocity reserve using a Doppler-tipped guidewire can measure coronary vascular resistance (CVR) accurately. In addition to mean velocity, which of the following is required to measure volumetric coronary flow?

(A) Peak instantaneous velocity
(B) Phasic systolic/diastolic flow ratio
(C) Mean vessel cross-sectional area
(D) Percent diameter narrowing
(E) Lesion length

5 CFR by Doppler is no longer used as a reliable indicator of lesion significance. Which of the following explains this?

(A) Doppler was too difficult to use by the average interventionalist
(B) The wire was too stiff
(C) An abnormal CVR did not necessarily mean that the lesion was flow limiting
(D) The Doppler signal did not reflect volumetric flow
(E) Pharmacologic hyperemia was unreliable compared to exercise

6 A 55-year-old man has atypical chest pain and undergoes cardiac catheterization and coronary angiography. His examination shows the following angiogram of the LAD. What is the best way to determine lesion significance?

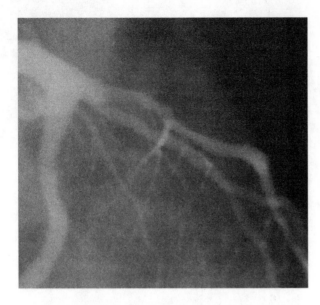

(A) Additional angiographic views with left anterior oblique (LAO), steep cranial

(B) IVUS

(C) CFR

(D) Fractional flow reserve (FFR)

(E) Single photon emission computed tomography (SPECT) myocardial perfusion imaging, next day

7 After stenting a proximal LAD (see following figure) in a 67-year-old woman with diabetes, the distal FFR is still abnormal (FFR is 0.41). What is the best way to assess the final result of stenting in this patient?

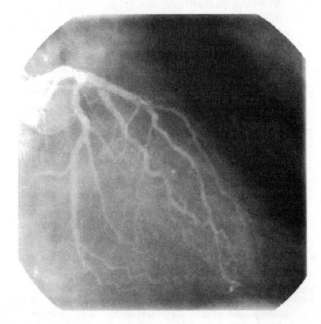

(A) IVUS

(B) CFR

(C) FFR during pullback

(D) SPECT scanning

(E) Relative coronary flow reserve (RCFR)

8 A 42-year-old man returns to your laboratory for follow-up 3 years after cardiac transplantation. He is asymptomatic. Routine angiography is normal. The attending physician wants to evaluate his microcirculatory responses to a new antirejection drug. What is the best method to evaluate this agent?

(A) FFR

(B) RCFR

(C) CFR

(D) IVUS

(E) Magnetic resonance imaging (MRI)

9 A 60-year-old woman with diabetes mellitus has atypical chest pain and an equivocal stress echocardiographic examination. She smokes one pack of cigarettes per day. Her electrocardiogram (EKG) is normal. Her weight is 285 pounds. She is 5 ft 2 in. tall. On angiography, she has an intermediate stenosis as shown below. Which is the best way to treat this lesion?

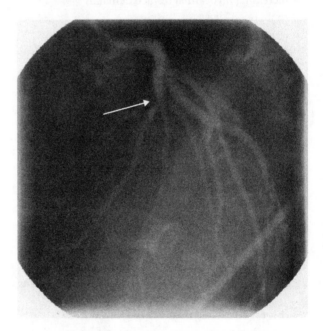

(A) Rotablator

(B) Crush stenting

(C) Plain old balloon angioplasty

(D) Determine CFR for individual branches

(E) Determine FFR for individual branches

(F) Coronary artery bypass grafting (CABG)

10 You have performed both FFR and CFR on an intermediate 60% diameter narrowing in the LAD in a patient with hyperlipidemia. CFR was 1.7 and FFR was 0.88. What is the most likely explanation?

(A) The FFR overestimated lesion severity
(B) The FFR underestimated lesion severity
(C) There is an inadequate response to pharmacologic hyperemia
(D) There is an impairment of the microcirculation
(E) The lesion is physiologically significant

11 In assessing the physiology of a coronary artery narrowing, in which of the following relationships is the flow related to the pressure?

(A) Directly and linearly
(B) Directly and exponentially
(C) Indirectly and linearly
(D) Indirectly and exponentially
(E) Inversely and linearly

12 Which of the following is the correct calculation of FFR?

(A) Aortic pressure/coronary pressure distal to the lesion at hyperemia
(B) Coronary pressure/aortic pressure proximal to the lesion at hyperemia
(C) Coronary pressure/aortic pressure distal to the lesion at rest
(D) Coronary pressure/aortic pressure distal to the lesion at hyperemia
(E) Aortic pressure/coronary pressure distal to the lesion at rest

13 A 65-year-old woman has a right carotid artery (RCA) stent placed for acute inferior ST-elevation myocardial infarction (STEMI). She has a LAD lesion of 65% on angiography. She returns 4 weeks later for evaluation of the LAD and on stress testing demonstrates hypertension (200/105), dyspnea, nonsustained ventricular tachycardia (NSVT) (4 to 6 beats) and 2-mm ST-segment depression (LVH on EKG at rest). The referring physician sends the patient to the catheterization laboratory before the radionuclide perfusion study result is available. Angiography shows the RCA stent to be patent, normal LV function, and a 60% LAD lesion in only one view. The radionuclide perfusion images are normal. What is the best way to approach this patient?

(A) Place LAD stent
(B) IVUS and place LAD stent if cross-section area (CSA) <4 mm^2
(C) Stop procedure and repeat stress test
(D) FFR and place stent if abnormal
(E) Obtain true lateral image of LAD lesion then stent

14 A 75-year-old man with progressive angina and positive stress testing undergoes catheterization and is found to have multivessel CAD: LAD 60%, circumflex (CFX) 80%, and RCA 90% with normal LV systolic function. Which of the following correctly states the case for the use of coronary physiology in this setting?

(A) FFR of all vessels is unnecessary, proceed to CABG
(B) FFR of all vessels provides information useful to the surgeon alone
(C) FFR of the LAD alone is sufficient to assist in revascularization by percutaneous coronary intervention (PCI) or CABG
(D) FFR of the LAD is not reliable in 3V CAD
(E) IVUS is preferable to FFR in patients with 3V CAD

15 An 81-year-old woman has an acute STEMI and comes to the emergency room (ER). She has blood pressure (BP) of 80/60, heart rate (HR) of 95 bpm, clear lungs, elevated neck veins, and distant heart sounds. The EKG shows 2-mm ST-segment elevation in leads II, III, and AVF. The patient develops a brief run of nonsustained VT, and the chest pain abates and the ST segments are substantially reduced. In the catheterization laboratory, the LAD has a 65% narrowing, the CFX is nondominant and unobstructed, and the RCA has a 50% hazy-appearing lesion. Which of the following is an appropriate use of FFR?

(A) FFR of the RCA to determine necessity to stent
(B) FFR of the LAD only to determine necessity to stent at this time
(C) FFR of both the RCA and LAD to determine necessity to stent both in this sitting
(D) FFR of the LAD only to determine necessity to stent at another time
(E) FFR of both the RCA and LAD to determine necessity to stent both at another time

16 A 69-year-old man had a STEMI 2 weeks ago and now comes to the catheterization laboratory with atypical chest pain. No risk stratification testing has been performed. The EKG shows evolutionary changes with small inferior Q-waves and no dynamic or acute EKG changes. His physical examination is unremarkable with normal and stable BP and HR. In the catheterization laboratory, the LAD has a 65% narrowing; the CFX is nondominant and unobstructed; and the RCA has a 50% hazy-appearing lesion. Which of the following is an appropriate use of FFR?

(A) FFR of the RCA to determine necessity to stent
(B) FFR of the LAD only to determine necessity to stent at this sitting

(C) FFR of both the RCA and LAD to determine necessity to stent both in this sitting

(D) FFR of the LAD only to determine necessity to stent at another time

(E) FFR of both the RCA and LAD to determine necessity to stent both at another time

17 A 42-year-old man with multiple CAD risk factors has a positive exercise Cardiolite perfusion imaging study with reversible anterior perfusion. He has had minor atypical chest pain. The EKG shows LVH without repolarization abnormalities. At coronary angiography, the RCA is normal. The CFX has minimal lumen irregularities. The LAD has two narrowings: Lesion 1 (55%) is proximal to the first septal and lesion 2 (60%) is 25 mm more distal at the second diagonal branch. What is the best use of FFR to treat this patient?

(A) FFR across lesion 1 only, then treat if FFR abnormal, defer treatment of lesion 2

(B) FFR across both lesions 1 and 2, treat both lesions 1 and 2

(C) FFR across both lesions 1 and 2, treat only the lesion with the biggest gradient

(D) FFR across only lesion 2, treat Lesion 2 and defer treatment of lesion 1

(E) FFR across both lesions 1 and 2, treat the lesion with the greatest gradient and then repeat FFR across the remaining lesion

(F) Do not use FFR for serial lesions

18 A 59-year-old man presents with chest pain at rest and LVH with nonspecific STT wave changes. Troponins are negative. Coronary angiography demonstrates a 50% to 60% narrowing of the LAD. What is the role of FFR/CVR in this setting?

(A) FFR will indicate whether to proceed with intervention

(B) CVR is better than FFR to assess a lesion in the acute coronary syndrome (ACS)

(C) Neither FFR nor CVR is indicated in ACS

(D) IVUS will better define the need to intervene

(E) FFR with pullback is most accurate to define the lesion

19 A 49-year-old woman who received radiation therapy to the chest for Hodgkin's lymphoma >15 years ago complains of atypical chest pain. Her EKG shows normal sinus rhythm with nonspecific STT changes. The physical examination is normal; laboratory work is normal; and echocardiogram is normal. An exercise stress test shows equivocal small area of reperfusion. Coronary angiography shows a 40% to 50% left main in one projection only. Catheter damping is inconsistent during several angiograms. What is the preferred method of using FFR to assess the ostial LM lesion?

(A) Intracoronary (IC) bolus adenosine through the engaged guide catheter

(B) IV infusion adenosine, guide catheter engaged, with side holes

(C) IV infusion adenosine, guide catheter engaged, no side holes

(D) IV infusion adenosine, guide catheter disengaged

(E) IV bolus adenosine, guide catheter disengaged

20 A 79-year-old man has atypical chest pain with exertional dyspnea. He has no CAD risk factors. No other medical problems or significant past surgical or medical history exists. A maximal exercise Cardiolite perfusion study is negative. Because of persistent chest pain at rest without EKG abnormalities, coronary angiography was performed and demonstrated a 50% LAD lesion and no other evidence of CAD. FFR is 0.88. Treatment with PCI is deferred. ASA, β-blockers, ACE, and statins are prescribed. What is the expected major adverse cardiovascular event (MACE) rate for this patient over the next 2 years?

(A) Greater than 15% at 1 year

(B) 4% the same as any patient with CAD

(C) 10% twice the rate as patients with CAD

(D) Unpredictable because CAD is highly variable

(E) Acute myocardial infarction (MI) can be expected because this is an intermediate lesion

Answers and Explanations

1 **Answer D.** Myocardial oxygen consumption (MVO_2) is directly related to contractility, LV wall stress, and frequency of contraction (HR or RR interval). LV wall stress is related to LV diameter and generated systolic pressure. Although diastolic function is energy consuming, it is not one of the major determinants of MVO_2. Myocardial ischemia results from an imbalance between the myocardial oxygen supply and demand. Coronary blood flow provides the needed oxygen supply for any given myocardial oxygen demand, and normally increases automatically from a resting level to a maximum level in response to increases in myocardial oxygen demand from exercise, neurohumoral, or pharmacologic hyperemic stimuli.

2 **Answer E.** Hypertension, diabetes, severe CAD, and >75% diameter narrowing of target vessel are all associated with impaired coronary reserve for different reasons. The one patient who likely has a normal coronary reserve is the patient with an intermediate angiographic lesion. Angiography alone cannot completely characterize the clinical significance of a coronary artery stenosis. This well-recognized limitation has been repeatedly documented by IVUS imaging and ischemia stress testing. Coronary angiography produces a silhouette image and can neither identify intraluminal detail nor provide the angiographer with information about the characteristics of the vessel wall.

3 **Answer B.** While it is true that stress testing has a highly variable sensitivity and specificity depending on the test, the study population, and incidence of CAD, the rationale for in-laboratory physiology is that the angiogram for intermediate lesions cannot predict which lesions will or will not produce ischemia by whatever measures are used for testing. It is also true that chest pain syndromes are not specific but the patient still has to have a coronary narrowing to require further testing. IVUS shows diffuse disease and its distribution but does not directly give a picture of flow responses in a single cross-sectional image. Coronary angiography produces a silhouette image and can neither identify intraluminal detail nor provide the angiographer with information about the characteristics of the vessel wall. Furthermore, the accurate identification of both the normal and diseased vessel segments is complicated by diffuse disease as well as angiographic artifacts of contrast streaming, image foreshortening, or calcification. Bifurcation or ostial lesion locations may be obscured by overlapping branch segments. Even with numerous angiographic angulations to reveal the lesion in its best view, the physiologic significance of a coronary stenosis, especially for an intermediately severe luminal narrowing (approximately 40% to 70% diameter narrowing), cannot be accurately determined.

4 **Answer C.** Volume flow (cm^3 per second) equals mean velocity (cm per second) times CSA (cm^2).

5 **Answer C.** CVR, although difficult at times to some operators and laboratories, was only useful if normal. If abnormal, CVR did not differentiate between flow impairment due to a stenosis or abnormal microvascular circulation. The technical aspects of the Doppler wire could easily be overcome and pharmacologic hyperemia is as reliable as exercise for ischemic induction. CFR is a combined measure of the capacity of the major resistance components (the epicardial coronary artery and supplied vascular bed), to achieve maximal blood flow in response to hyperemic stimulation (see following figure). A normal CFR implies that both the epicardial and minimally achievable microvascular bed resistances are low and normal. However, when abnormal, CFR does not indicate which component is affected, a fact limiting the clinical applicability of this measurement.

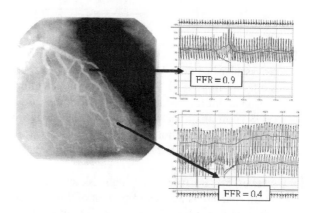

6 **Answer D.** FFR is lesion specific and, unlike CFR, is unaffected by the microcirculation. IVUS may suggest an abnormal FFR when CSA is <4.0 mm^2.

Additional angiographic views are of limited value for this type of lesion. SPECT myocardial perfusion imaging performed on the next day is not cost-effective. A nonischemic threshold value range of 0.75 to 0.80 has been prospectively confirmed and was compared with noninvasive stress testing. An FFR <0.75 was associated with inducible ischemia (specificity, 100%), whereas a value >0.80 indicates absence of inducible ischemia in most patients (sensitivity, 90%). In summary, for the assessment of an epicardial stenosis, the beyond-lesion to aortic pressure ratio at maximal hyperemia (FFR) is a measurement of lesion significance that, unlike CFR, has low variability, high reproducibility, and is relatively unaffected by changes in hemodynamics.

7 **Answer C.** FFR during pullback will show the physiologic impact of the entire artery and any focal lesions as well as the effect of flow immediately distal to stent. CFR will be abnormal in diffuse disease and in patients with diabetes and microvascular impairment. IVUS will show diffuse disease but not specific lesions in a diffuse disease vessel. SPECT scanning will likely be abnormal but not helpful in diffuse disease. RCFR may be helpful, but not for diffuse disease.

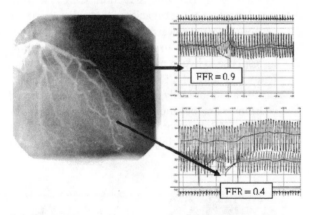

8 **Answer C.** CFR measures both conduit and microvascular bed flow. FFR is only useful when there is a lesion in a vessel. RCFR would also give information about the bed but only relative comparison. IVUS is an anatomic tool without physiologic information. MRI is not yet widely available to test coronary flow and reserve.

9 **Answer E.** Because of the high risk and complex lesion characteristics, determination of the ischemic potential is needed. No percutaneous intervention is optimal for trifurcation lesions. CFR is not lesion specific. FFR for each branch will identify which, if any, narrowing needs to be treated. FFR for each

branch in this patient was 0.90, 0.91, and 0.90. No intervention was performed. Gastroesophageal reflux disease (GERD) was treated successfully.

10 **Answer D.** Assuming that the technique of FFR and CFR was correctly performed, the FFR accurately reflects the ischemic potential of the narrowing. The CFR reflects the status of both the conduit and the microvascular bed. Therefore, the CFR is not lesion specific and in the presence of a near-normal FFR, microvascular disease is likely the explanation.

11 **Answer A.** Flow is related to pressure directly in relationship to viscous friction and exponentially in terms of the separation coefficient. Overall the pressure–flow relationship is curvilinear and approximately exponential.

12 **Answer D.** Coronary pressure/aortic pressure distal to the lesion at hyperemia.

13 **Answer D.** FFR and stent if abnormal. The FFR turned out to be 0.89×2 with 50, 60 µg IC adenosine. The correspondence between radionuclide stress and FFR is good. ST-segment changes on exercise tolerance test (ETT) with an abnormal resting EKG are unreliable. VT is not specific in this setting and symptoms of dyspnea with uncontrolled hypertension are likewise not specific for ischemia.

14 **Answer C.** FFR is useful to identify which vessels have hemodynamically significant lesions. If FFR of the LAD is abnormal, CABG > PCI for revascularization strategies is suggested, whereas if FFR of the LAD is normal, PCI of the CFX and RCA is preferred. FFR can be used in multivessel disease, and it is superior to IVUS for physiologic decisions. IVUS is mainly indicated for anatomic information.

15 **Answer D.** The FFR of the RCA is unnecessary and may be misleading. The RCA lesion is hazy and recently had spontaneous reperfusion as shown by the VT- and ST-segment reductions after STEMI. This lesion should be treated. More importantly, acute FFR physiology data are neither available nor validated in the dynamic environment of ACS. As for the LAD, FFR would be helpful to see whether PCI of the 65% lesion is needed at another time when the patient stabilizes from the acute right ventricular (RV) infarction. Few operators perform nontarget artery PCI in the setting of a complicated STEMI, and it is a class III indication (i.e., contraindicated).

16 **Answer C.** This patient is stable after his infarction and several weeks away from the acute event. DeBruyne et al. found that the correlation between FFR and SPECT 2-methoxyisobutylisonitrile (MIBI) scanning for ischemia was high with a threshold value of approximately 0.80. In this patient, FFR can be used for both the RCA and LAD to identify the correlation to ischemia and for selection of revascularization on that basis. One might also stage the procedure and do only one of the two lesions but at this time after the acute event, most operators would intervene on both lesions in one setting.

17 **Answer E.** The achievement of the exact FFR of each individual lesion is difficult in most clinical settings and can be obtained only with a coronary occlusion wedge pressure. For clinical purposes, FFR across both lesions, use the biggest hyperemic gradient to identify lesion to treat first, then repeat FFR across the remaining lesion and treat according to FFR thresholds. Deferring treatment when the FFR can confirm the lesion significance is inappropriate.

18 **Answer C.** Neither FFR nor CVR is indicated in ACS. The dynamic and rapidly changing status of the artery, microcirculation, and the patient precludes accurate use of FFR/CVR. This dynamic variability holds for the acute MI as well. No data exists for the ACS within the first 24 hours or for the acute MI before 6 days of the event.

19 **Answer D.** IV infusion adenosine, guide catheter disengaged. Obstruction of the presumed ostial lesion by the guide catheter will give a false high-pressure gradient and low FFR. Disengaging the guide is a key maneuver. Side holes may produce some relief of the obstruction but may create a stenosis of lesser magnitude. IC bolus and quick withdrawal of the guide catheter have been used but are more difficult and less reliable than an IV adenosine infusion of 140 µg/kg/min. IV bolus adenosine is not used for FFR.

20 **Answer B.** Deferring PCI in patients with stable angina or atypical chest pain with normal FFR yields an excellent, low 2-year MACE. Patients with stable CAD have an event rate of 4% per year. MI has not been demonstrated in stable lesions undergoing FFR and being followed up. CAD is highly variable but should be controllable with treatment and is associated with a low event rate.

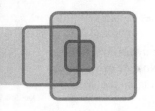

25

Intravascular Ultrasound

Hussam Hamdalla and Khaled M. Ziada

Questions

1 Following an intravascular ultrasound (IVUS) imaging of a moderately diseased coronary artery (see left figure), offline measurements are performed (see right figure). All of the following statements about these measurements are true, *except*:

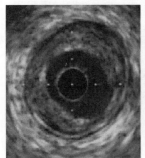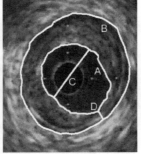

(A) Line A traces the leading edge of the intima, defining the lumen area
(B) Line B traces the leading edge of the media, defining the vessel area
(C) Line C is the minimal luminal diameter in this cross section
(D) The difference between areas A and B represents the atheroma area
(E) Line D represents the minimal atheroma thickness

2 The Reversal of Atherosclerosis with Aggressive Lipid Lowering (REVERSAL) trial examined the effect of intensive versus moderate lipid- lowering therapies on coronary disease progression. All of the following statements are true, *except*:

(A) The primary end point of the study was the percentage change in the total atheroma volume (TAV)

(B) The change in TAV was proportionate to the change in the low density lipoprotein (LDL) cholesterol level
(C) There was a significant reduction in the percent TAV with intensive lipid lowering
(D) There was a significant progression in the percent TAV in the moderate lipid-lowering arm
(E) There was no reported difference in the clinical endpoints between the two arms of the study

3 A physically active 66-year-old hypertensive patient is referred for coronary angiography because of typical angina precipitated by moderate exertion. In the catheterization laboratory, there is fluoroscopic evidence of calcification in the left main trunk. Right coronary angiography showed a severe focal lesion in the mid segment. Left coronary angiography revealed not only moderate disease in a marginal branch of the circumflex artery, but more importantly it also revealed, ostial left main disease (see left figure). An IVUS imaging is then performed to better define the left main trunk disease. The minimal lumen area in the left main trunk was measured to be 7.4 mm^2 (see right figure). What is the most appropriate next step?

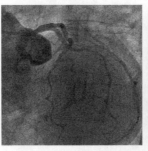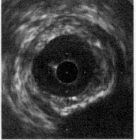

(A) Measure fractional flow reserve (FFR) distal to the left main stenosis

(B) Place an intra-aortic balloon pump and arrange for three-vessel bypass surgery

(C) Consider right coronary angioplasty for symptom relief

(D) Reevaluate the patient with a pharmacologic nuclear stress test

4 The OPTICUS study compared an ultrasound-guided stent implantation strategy with an angiography-guided stent implantation strategy. Which of the following statements regarding this trial is *true*?

(A) There was no significant difference between both groups in the restenosis rate at 6-month follow-up

(B) The significantly higher acute gain seen in the ultrasound-guided stent implantation group translated into a significantly lower acute loss compared with the angiography-guided group

(C) An angiography-guided approach to stenting was associated with an increased number of balloons used per case

(D) Myocardial reinfarction was significantly reduced with the use of an ultrasound-guided approach for stent implantation

(E) At 6 months, percent diameter stenosis was significantly larger in the angiography-guided arm

5 A 70-year-old male patient with hypertension and hyperlipidemia presents with recurrent episodes of chest burning for several days. His electrocardiogram reveals T-wave inversion in leads V_3 through V_6 that resolve with the resolution of chest pain. His troponin I is 3.0, but the creatine kinase-MB (CK-MB) is not elevated. Coronary angiography is performed: The right coronary angiogram is unremarkable, and the left coronary angiogram is seen here (figure below). An IVUS imaging was then performed to better define the mid left anterior descending

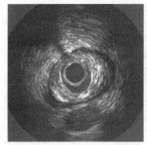 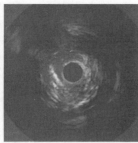

(LAD) segment. The (above) right and left figures demonstrate the representative images from the LAD at the level of the diagonal bifurcation and just proximal to the bifurcation, respectively. On a review of the angiograms and the IVUS images, which of the following statements would be considered as correct?

(A) The haziness of the mid LAD is caused by heavy calcification

(B) An IVUS imaging did not provide an explanation for the angiographic haziness in the mid LAD

(C) The clinical management of the patient will be influenced by the IVUS findings

(D) FFR in the distal LAD will be ≥0.85

(E) The patient is unlikely to develop more chest pain

6 Following a difficult engagement of a large and mildly diseased right coronary artery (RCA), a subsequent angiogram reveals an extensive dissection (see following figure). Emergent bailout stenting is planned, and a guiding catheter is advanced to engage the RCA. The angioplasty wire is passed to the distal vessel with some difficulty.

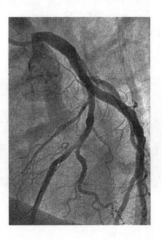

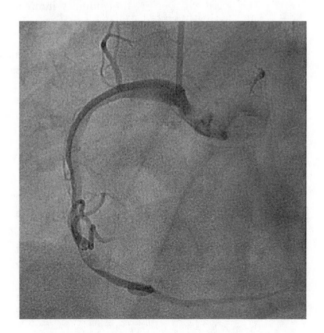

An IVUS catheter is then advanced over the wire to confirm its position. The following figures are obtained from the mid and proximal RCA. The next best course of action is as follows:

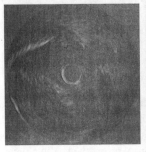 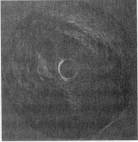

(A) The wire should be removed and the procedure terminated

(B) The wire should remain in place; percutaneous transluminal coronary angioplasty (PTCA) and/or stenting should follow

(C) The wire should be removed, and another attempt at passing it in the true lumen should be performed

(D) The wire should remain in place, but another wire should be used to access the true lumen

7 Serial IVUS imaging of coronary lesions following the balloon angioplasty and atherectomy improved our understanding of the mechanisms of acute lumen gain and subsequent restenosis. Regarding these mechanisms, the following statement is *true*:

(A) At 6 months, the change in lumen area correlates more strongly with the change in the plaque area than with the change in the vessel area

(B) The serial changes in the minimal luminal diameter seen by angiography correlate with the changes seen by IVUS imaging

(C) At 1 month, the increase in vessel area is more significant in the nonrestenotic lesions compared with the restenotic lesions

(D) Between 24 hours and 1 month after balloon angioplasty, there is significant adaptive remodeling

(E) Between 1 month and 6 months, constrictive remodeling was less significant in restenotic lesions than in nonrestenotic lesions

8 All of the following applications of IVUS imaging are appropriate, *except*:

(A) Assessment of an angiographically hazy segment in the marginal branch of the circumflex artery after PTCA

(B) Measurement of the minimum lumen area and the adequacy of strut apposition after stenting the mid RCA

(C) Evaluation of an ostial LAD lesion considered for directional atherectomy

(D) Confirmation of the presence of atherosclerotic coronary disease in a patient with atypical symptoms whose angiograms reveal minimal disease

(E) Evaluation of a 40% to 50% ostial left main coronary artery lesion in a patient with class 2 to 3 angina

9 The following figure represents a longitudinal section of a severe focal coronary stenosis. Which of the following measurements are needed to calculate the remodeling index?

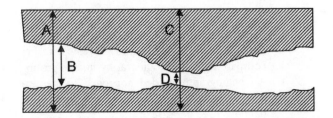

(A) A and B
(B) C and D
(C) A and C
(D) B and D
(E) A to D

10 A 52-year-old patient presented with angina on moderate exertion. On the treadmill, he stopped after 5.5 minutes because of chest pressure and 2-mm ST depression. A diagnostic angiogram of the left coronary system (lower left figure) revealed a tight lesion in the major obtuse marginal branch of the circumflex artery. After deciding to proceed with percutaneous coronary intervention (PCI), a 6 F extra backup guiding catheter was selected. The catheter engagement was difficult, and the patient developed chest discomfort. Another angiogram was obtained just before passing the angioplasty wire (lower right figure). IVUS imaging of the left main trunk was performed (figure on next page). What is the most appropriate next step?

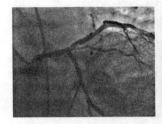 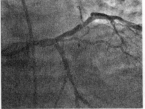

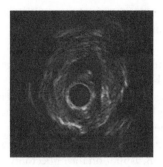

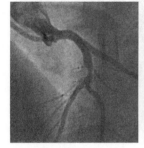

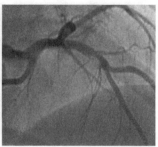

(A) Abort the planned PCI, and schedule the patient to see a cardiac surgeon

(B) Abort the planned PCI, and consult with the cardiac surgeon in the laboratory

(C) Proceed with the planned PCI of the left circumflex artery

(D) Proceed with the planned PCI after inserting an intra-aortic balloon pump

11 Which of the following images is obtained from the saphenous vein graft of a patient presenting with chest pain for the first time, 5 years after his bypass surgery?

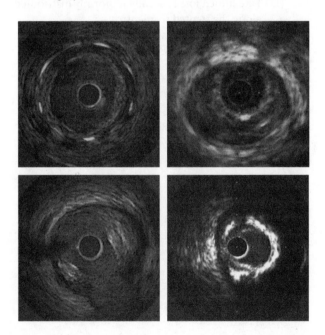

12 A patient with typical angina is referred for coronary angiography after a nuclear stress test reveals an anterior reversible perfusion defect. The LAD angiograms reveal a 50% to 60% diameter stenosis in the mid segment (see following figures), though the other vessels contain only mild irregularities.

An IVUS examination of the LAD is performed. The following figure on the left shows the section with the narrowest lumen. Representative images from the more proximal LAD (middle and right figures) are shown. Which of the following conclusions about this patient is *true*?

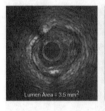 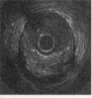 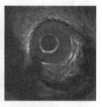

(A) IVUS imaging did not explain the discrepancy between the angiogram and the result of the stress test

(B) The IVUS images explain why the stress test result was false positive

(C) An FFR of 0.70 would confirm the findings of the IVUS images

(D) The IVUS images are inconclusive because of the proximity of the diagonal branch

13 IVUS imaging is frequently used to assess the results of high-pressure stent deployment. Which of the following images of coronary stents is the *least* likely to need the use of a larger balloon and/or higher inflation pressure?

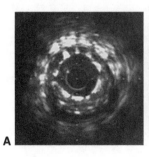 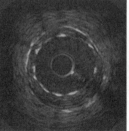

A   B

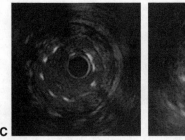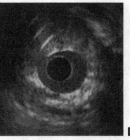

14 A patient is referred for PCI to a severe proximal LAD lesion. IVUS imaging is performed to evaluate the lesion and plan the intervention. A representative image from the diseased segment is shown in the following figure.

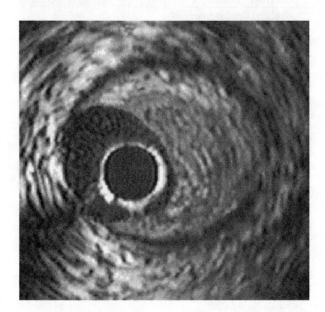

On evaluating this lesion, which of the following statements would be considered *true*?

(A) Directional atherectomy before stenting will result in greater acute lumen gain compared with direct stenting

(B) Adequate stent expansion cannot be achieved in this lesion without pretreatment with rotational atherectomy

(C) Because of the thrombotic nature of this lesion, aspiration thrombectomy is a reasonable alternate strategy

(D) In these lesions, ultrasound-guided debulking using directional or rotational atherectomy will reduce late lumen loss

15 All of the following statements regarding in-stent restenosis are correct, *except*:

(A) Late lumen loss correlates strongly with tissue growth inside the stent

(B) Late lumen loss measured by IVUS correlates with angiographic late loss

(C) Negative remodeling is a major determinant of in-stent restenosis

(D) Late lumen loss is usually uniformly distributed along the stented segment

(E) Late lumen loss distal to the edge of the stent is most likely because of negative remodeling

Answers and Explanations

1 **Answer B.** As a general rule, the measurements on ultrasound images are performed from the leading edge of an echo-dense layer to the leading edge of another echo-dense layer. The lumen area is defined as the area bound by the leading edge of the intima, or the interface between the echo-dense intima and the echo-lucent blood elements in the lumen. The vessel area is the area bound by the external elastic membrane (EEM) that can be identified as the interface between the leading edge of the echo-dense adventitia and the echo-lucent medial layer (Line B on the right figure). The difference between the lumen and EEM areas is the atheroma area. In fact, this area includes the atheroma and the thickness of the media. This has traditionally been accepted to avoid the inaccurate tracing around the trailing edge of the atheroma. In addition, the thickness of the medial layer is relatively unchanged by the presence or severity of disease. The minimum diameter between the lumen and EEM tracings is measured to define the presence or the absence of disease (Line D on the right figure). Several definitions have been used but, in general, a minimum diameter of 0.5 mm is considered abnormal. The minimum lumen diameter is the shortest line through the center point of the lumen (Line C on the right figure) (*J Am Coll Cardiol.* 2001;37: 1478–1492, *Curr Probl Cardiol.* 1999;24:541–566).

2 **Answer C.** In the REVERSAL trial, patients were randomly assigned to receive a moderate lipid-lowering therapy of pravastatin 40 mg per day versus a more intensive regimen of atorvastatin 80 mg per day. An IVUS assessment of a mildly diseased coronary segment was performed upon enrollment and after 18 months. The primary end point of the study was the percentage change in TAV, which was computed as:

$$\frac{TAV \text{ (follow-up)} - TAV \text{ (baseline)} \times 100}{TAV \text{ (baseline)}}$$

The TAV was calculated as the sum of differences between EEM and lumen areas across all evaluable slices in the target segment. In the moderate lipid-lowering arm, there was a positive change in the TAV (2.7%; 95% CI 0.24 to 4.67), indicating net progression ($p = 0.001$) compared with baseline. In the intensive lipid-lowering arm, there was no evidence of progression in TAV compared with baseline (-0.04%; 95% CI -2.35 to 1.49, $p = 0.98$). These findings suggested that intensive lipid lowering could result in arrest of progression of disease in mildly narrowed coronary arteries. As expected, the reduction in LDL cholesterol was significantly larger in magnitude in the atorvastatin arm. The change in TAV was directly proportional to the change in LDL cholesterol. In addition, there was a direct relationship between change in percent TAV and change in C-reactive protein (CRP) levels, which were significantly lower with atorvastatin therapy, suggesting a potential non–lipid-lowering role for statins. The study was powered on the basis of the expected change in atheroma volume and did not enroll enough patients to detect differences in clinical outcomes (*JAMA.* 2004;291:1071–1080).

3 **Answer C.** In the absence of a reference segment to compare with, defining stenosis severity can be difficult. This is true for all ostial lesions, particularly in cases of ostial left main disease. In addition to the angiographic appearance, the absence of backflow of contrast into the aortic cusp when the catheter is engaged is a worrisome sign that needs to be identified immediately. An additional clue is the pressure waveform, which is "ventricularized" or shows "dampening" if the catheter is obstructing flow into the ostial left main trunk. However, pressure dampening can occur in the absence of a severe obstruction if the catheter tip is directed toward and makes contact with the arterial wall. In most cases of suspicious left main lesions, an adjunctive modality is utilized to assess stenosis severity. This can be achieved by using a pressure wire and calculating the FFR or by an IVUS imaging. Several studies have demonstrated the predictive value of the measurements obtained through either modality. An FFR ≥ 0.75 predicts a low risk of death or cardiac events in the ensuing 2 to 3 years on medical therapy alone. Similarly, an IVUS left main lumen area ≥ 5.9 mm^2 correlated with an FFR ≥ 0.75, both measures strongly predicting an event-free survival over a 3-year period. Given the stable clinical presentation and the lumen area exceeding 7 mm^2, placing a balloon pump and sending the patient to surgery would not provide any clinical benefit compared with medical therapy alone. FFR measurement in equivocal left main stenosis is appropriate, and very useful in guiding therapy, but it would be redundant to perform both IVUS imaging and FFR measurement. With the availability of adjunctive modalities such as the pressure wire and

IVUS imaging, the decision about hemodynamic significance of such lesions can be made in the catheterization laboratory (*Heart.* 2001;86:547–552, *Circulation.* 2004;110:2831–2836).

4 **Answer A.** The OPTICUS study investigators randomized 550 patients to ultrasound-guided versus angiography-guided stent implantation strategy. The primary endpoints were the incidence of angiographic restenosis (>50% lumen diameter reduction), minimal lumen diameter, and percent diameter stenosis at 6-month follow-up. The ultrasound-guided approach was associated with increased utilization of balloons, contrast, fluoroscopy, and procedural time. This resulted in a significantly larger acute lumen gain and less residual diameter stenosis than in the angiography-guided arm. Despite the larger acute gain, there was no significant difference in the angiographic restenosis (24.5% vs. 22.8%, $p = 0.68$) or minimal lumen diameter (1.95 vs. 1.91 mm, $p = 0.52$) at 6 months. Similar findings have been reported by Schiele et al. (*J Am Coll Cardiol.* 1998;32:320–328) and others (*Circulation.* 2001;104:1343–1349, *Circulation.* 2003;107:62–67). In a smaller study on stenting of long lesions transurethral laser incision of the prostrate (TULIP), the increase in the acute luminal gain did translate into a reduction in angiographic restenosis, although these data have not been validated in larger trials.

5 **Answer C.** On the basis of clinical and laboratory evidence, it is seen that this patient had sustained a myocardial infarction, probably a few days before presentation. The angiograms reveal an area of haziness in the mid LAD at the level of a diagonal bifurcation, although diameter reduction compared with the adjacent segments is not significant. Haziness could be the result of calcification of the arterial wall, but a more important differential diagnosis for haziness in this context would be plaque rupture and/or overlying intraluminal thrombosis (see following figures). Another possibility is an eccentric lesion that is more severe than what the angiogram reveals in this projection. In these situations, an IVUS can be very helpful in making the diagnosis.

An IVUS imaging of the mid-LAD segment revealed a large plaque burden with minimal calcification at the level of the diagonal bifurcation, but with a minimal lumen area of 3.4 mm², indicating a hemodynamically severe stenosis. Just proximal to the diagonal bifurcation (right figure), there is evidence of plaque rupture, with flow communication between the true LAD lumen (surrounding the IVUS catheter artifact) and the ulcerated plaque "underneath" the fibro-calcific cap (*arrow*). On the basis of these findings, percutaneous or surgical revascularization would be more appropriate than medical therapy. In acute myocardial infarction patients, the utility of FFR is not well studied, and with an area of 3.4 mm², one would expect the FFR to be <0.75. Given the severity of disease and the measured lumen area, it is likely that this patient will have postinfarction angina if the lesion in not treated (*Circulation.* 1999;100: 250–255, *Curr Probl Cardiol.* 1999;24:541–566).

6 **Answer B.** In extensive coronary artery dissections, it is challenging to distinguish between the true and the false lumens. Usually this is the first most important step in bailout stenting, which is intended to restore flow in the true lumen and obliterate the false channel. Passage of the angioplasty wire in a side branch and injecting contrast through the distal tip of a balloon are some of the maneuvers used to confirm the position of the wire. However, this does not exclude the possibility of "fenestration" (i.e., that the wire passed from the false to the true lumens). An IVUS can assist in confirming the position of the wire before stenting. The two important features of the true lumen are the trilaminar appearance of the wall and the presence of side branches. The left figure (below) shows a side branch (*arrow*) in continuity with the vessel lumen that is surrounding the IVUS catheter, confirming the fact that the catheter is in a true lumen. The right figure (below) reveals the characteristic trilaminar appearance (*arrows*) of the true lumen with an intra-arterial wall hematoma (*asterisk*) seen in the false lumen. These findings confirm the true lumen position of the wire, and proceeding with PTCA/stenting would be the appropriate next step.

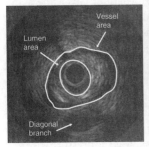
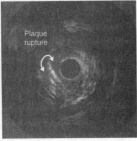
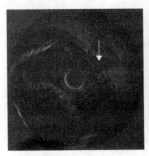
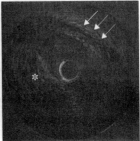

7 **Answer D.** The serial ultrasound restenosis (SURE) study assessed the patients who underwent coronary balloon angioplasty or atherectomy by serial angiographic and ultrasound examinations performed at preintervention, postintervention, 24-hour, 1-month and 6-month follow-up. The serial examination of the treated lesion sites provided great insight into the remodeling responses and the mechanisms of late lumen loss or restenosis. Typically, lesions treated with PTCA or atherectomy undergo a biphasic remodeling response: A significant increase in vessel area between 24 hours and 1 month (adaptive remodeling) followed by a significant decrease (constrictive remodeling) between 1 and 6 months. At any point of time, the change in the vessel area (remodeling) was the most important determinant of the resultant lumen area. This correlation was much stronger than the correlation between changes in lumen area and those in plaque area. As for the mechanism of restenosis, the early adaptive remodeling response of the vessel was not different between lesions that did and did not develop restenosis, which meant that there was no apparent difference in vessel area at the 1-month time point. However, the constrictive remodeling response (between 1 and 6 months) was more significant in lesions that eventually developed restenosis compared with those that ended with a favorable outcome. In this study, IVUS imaging revealed a significant increase in lumen diameter between 24 hours and 1 month, which could not be identified by quantitative angiography (*Circulation.* 1997;96:475–483).

8 **Answer D.** IVUS imaging provides a detailed tomographic perspective of both the lumen and the wall of the artery. The IVUS findings frequently clarify and/or complement our understanding of the luminal silhouettes provided by contrast angiography. The American College of Cardiology (ACC)/American Heart Association (AHA) guidelines outline the clinical situations in which there is reasonable evidence for the benefit of IVUS imaging. These include assessment of the adequacy of stent deployment (measurement of the minimal in-stent lumen area and evaluating strut apposition), assessment of a suboptimal angiographic result after PTCA, determination of the mechanism of restenosis to enable appropriate management, evaluation of coronary anatomy at a location difficult to image angiographically, and the preinterventional assessment of the coronary calcium extent and distribution in which use of an atherectomy device is contemplated. IVUS imaging may also be considered in the assessment of coronary atherosclerosis in patients with both characteristic angina and positive functional study without a clear angiographic lesion. IVUS is also the golden standard for the accurate identification and quantification of cardiac allograft vasculopathy or transplant coronary disease. There is no role for IVUS when an angiographic diagnosis is clear and there is no planned intervention (*Circulation.* 2006;113:156–175).

9 **Answer C.** As initially described by Glagov et al. in a necropsy study, arterial remodeling is the expansion of the EEM of the arterial wall at sites of atherosclerosis to accommodate atheroma volume and preserve lumen size. Stenoses develop when the ability of the artery to remodel is overcome by the progressive enlargement of the atheroma. This is known as *positive or adaptive remodeling.* Another form of arterial remodeling known as *negative (or constrictive) remodeling* is the local shrinkage of the vessel size at the site of disease, which has been implicated in the stenotic atherosclerotic lesions and restenosis after balloon angioplasty. The IVUS investigators examining the phenomenon of remodeling compare the lesion of interest with a proximal reference segment free of disease and express a "remodeling index," which is calculated as the ratio of the EEM area at the lesion site to the EEM area at the proximal reference site. A remodeling index of >1.05 is consistent with positive remodeling, <0.95 is consistent with negative remodeling, and 0.95 to 1.05 is consistent with absence of remodeling. A positively remodeled atheroma is usually larger in size and more likely to present with unstable coronary syndromes (*Circulation.* 2000;101:598–603, *J Am Coll Cardiol.* 2001;38:297–306).

10 **Answer B.** This is a case of left main trunk dissection on engagement with an extra backup guiding catheter. The clue to the diagnosis was the change in the angiographic appearance of the left main trunk after the difficult engagement, although the projection was identical. IVUS imaging was used to confirm the diagnosis. There are two false channels in the following figure (*arrows*), with the IVUS catheter artifact occupying the true lumen of the vessel. The false channels in cases of dissection and/or plaque rupture can be better visualized with saline or contrast injection while imaging, as this accentuates the difference in echo-density between the lumen and the arterial wall structures. In addition, the injected fluid can be seen traveling from the true to the false lumen in real time.

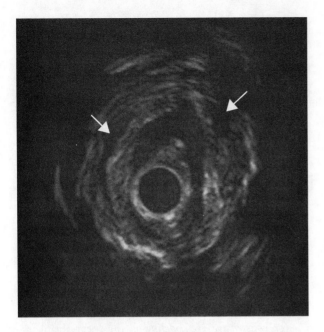

The left main coronary dissection requires urgent management. If the patient is hemodynamically stable or can be stabilized with the help of an intra-aortic balloon pump, then urgent coronary bypass surgery is probably the treatment of choice. If the patient is considered too unstable (e.g., severe on-going ischemia, hypotension, and/or life-threatening ventricular arrhythmia), emergent stenting of the left main may be an acceptable alternative. In either situation, the cardiac surgeon needs to be notified as soon as the diagnosis is made in the catheterization laboratory. Any elective PCI should be aborted and the situation should be managed immediately. A balloon pump would be helpful to support the patient's hemodynamics on the way to the surgery suite or if stenting of the left main trunk is considered, but not to support PCI of the circumflex artery.

11 **Answer B.** The upper left figure shows the struts of a slotted-tube stent, which are seen as bright ultrasound reflections around the circumference of the artery. The presence of a layer of echo-lucent tissue (distinct from the speckle of blood elements in lumen) is evidence of intimal hyperplasia within the boundaries of the stent, thereby indicating that this stent has been implanted in this artery in a prior procedure. In this section, the intimal hyperplasia appears nonobstructive. The upper right figure is obtained from a tight stenosis in the middle of a 5-year-old vein graft. The atheroma is heterogeneous in density, but mostly echo-lucent. Vein graft lesions are typically echo-lucent in appearance, and represent mixtures of lipid pools, collagen, and thrombotic material. In these lesions, heavy

calcification is rare. The minimum lumen diameter is <2 mm. The lower left figure is obtained from a native coronary artery at a bifurcation point. There is mild-to-moderate degree of atherosclerosis. The branch arising from the imaged vessel can be identified by following the continuity of the speckle of the blood elements around the IVUS catheter into the branch with an interruption of the layers of the wall (in the 5 o'clock direction). In this image, the wire artifact and its shadow are very apparent (in the 9 o'clock direction). The lower right figure is obtained from a heavily calcified segment of a coronary artery. The arc of calcification occupies approximately three quadrants of the section, and is seen as a bright echo with a shadow caused by the inability of the ultrasound beams to penetrate the tissue. Although this is not uncommon to see in native coronary arteries with advanced atherosclerosis, this degree of calcification does not develop in vein graft lesions (*Circulation.* 1998;97:916–931).

12 **Answer C.** This is a case of a diffusely diseased LAD, in which the more severe segmental stenosis (shown in the upper left figure) is superimposed on a moderate and diffuse disease (shown in the upper middle and right figures). Coronary angiograms are traditionally interpreted in a segmental fashion, where the least stenosed segment is assumed to be the "normal" reference to which the other segments are compared. In the presence of diffuse disease, this segmental approach to interpretation results in underestimation of stenosis severity. Another problem with angiographic interpretation is the projection of usually complex lumen shapes within stenosed segments onto a two-dimensional screen. Angiographers compensate by obtaining orthogonal views, but the choice of those projections is still arbitrary. Therefore, it is conceivable that the projection that would be perfectly perpendicular to the minimum lumen diameter may not be obtained. In this case, IVUS imaging did demonstrate a severe stenosis in the mid vessel with a minimum lumen diameter of <2 mm and an area of <4 mm^2. These measurements indicate a hemodynamically significant stenosis that is likely to cause ischemia on a stress test. This minimum lumen area by IVUS has a good correlation with an FFR of <0.75, which explains why the stress test was positive, despite the apparently "moderate" narrowing on angiography. The degree of narrowing in a bifurcation lesion can be difficult to angiographically assess, but that does not apply to a tomographic imaging modality such as IVUS. The branching point of the diagonal branch is not seen in any of the images shown here. In all the three images, the interruption of the circumference of the arterial wall is caused by the shadow of the wire artifact (*Circulation.* 1999;100:250–255, *Curr Probl Cardiol.* 1999;24:541–566).

13 **Answer B.** Following high-pressure stenting, a small postprocedure minimum in-stent lumen area is the most important predictor of target vessel revascularization. The various proposed IVUS criteria for optimal stent deployment emphasize achieving the largest possible in-stent lumen area. Increasing the in-stent lumen area usually requires larger balloons and/or higher inflation pressures; however, that would be limited by the reference vessel size. Panels A and B of the figure depict stents with relatively small lumen areas, which predisposes a high risk of restenosis. Panels C and D depict a stent with gross malapposition of struts. Historically, such degrees with malapposition were commonly observed before routine use of high-pressure inflations and are considered a precipitating factor for stent thrombosis. In all three situations, operators typically resort to higher inflation pressures and/or balloon oversizing. The upper right figure depicts a well-expanded and well-opposed stent with a minimum area exceeding 7 mm^2. Even with bare-metal stents, such lumen areas are associated with target vessel revascularization rates in the single digits (*Eur Heart J.* 1998;19:1214–1223, *J Am Coll Cardiol.* 1994;24:996–1003, *Am Heart J.* 2001;141:823–831).

14 **Answer A.** The IVUS image shows a heterogeneous plaque with areas of echo-lucency suggesting a mixture of fibrous and fibro-fatty tissues. These lesions, when located in proximal vessels, are ideal for directional atherectomy. Aggressive atherectomy guided by repeated ultrasound imaging will result in significant debulking and improved acute lumen gain; however, there has been no evidence of reduction in restenosis with this approach. Pretreatment with rotational atherectomy has not been shown to improve acute or late outcomes. It remains useful in heavily calcified lesions where stents cannot be delivered or adequately expanded. IVUS imaging is not a reliable tool for identification of intracoronary thrombus. The echogenic characteristics of thrombus are similar to heterogeneous plaque. In certain situations, a thrombus can be identified in the context of an acute myocardial infarction and when it is located within the lumen (*Am Heart J.* 2004;148:663–669, *Am J Cardiol.* 2004;93:953–958).

15 **Answer C.** In-stent restenosis is a result of neointimal tissue growth in the stent. Neointimal growth is uniformly distributed throughout the stent. In articulated stents (Palmaz-Schatz), immediate postprocedure tissue prolapse and subsequent neointimal hyperplasia tended to be worse at the central articulation point. Late lumen loss within the stented segments is directly proportional to the degree of neointimal hyperplasia. Slotted-tube stents abolish the negative remodeling response that is the primary driver of restenosis following balloon angioplasty. Therefore, the correlation between late loss and negative remodeling (shrinkage of the vessel area) is very weak in the stented segment. However, negative remodeling is more apparent in the few millimeters of the artery just distal to the edge of the stent and is the primary mechanism of late loss in this region of the artery. These changes are seen equally in native coronaries and saphenous vein grafts as well as in lesions treated with one or two stents. IVUS late lumen loss was found to correlate with, but was consistently smaller than, angiographic late lumen loss (*Circulation.* 1996;94:1247–1254).

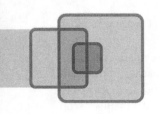

26

Approach to Patients with Hemodynamic Compromise

Zoran S. Nedeljkovic and Alice K. Jacobs

Questions

1 A 68-year-old woman with a past history of well-controlled hypertension presents to the hospital with several days of intermittent substernal chest pressure and shortness of breath. On arrival to the emergency room, her blood pressure is 90/70 mm Hg, her heart rate is 105 beats per minute, and her respiratory rate is 26 breaths per minute. She is diaphoretic and in visible respiratory distress. Cardiovascular examination is notable for a jugular venous pressure of 8 cm, bibasilar rales at the bases, and a 3/6 harsh systolic murmur at the left sternal border. Her extremities are cool. Her electrocardiogram reveals sinus tachycardia with 2 mm ST-segment elevation in V_1 through V_4 and 1 mm ST-segment depression in II, III, and aVF. Her baseline complete blood count (CBC), serum electrolytes, and renal function are normal.

She is given aspirin and heparin and undergoes endotracheal intubation for airway support. She is taken to the cardiac catheterization laboratory for emergent angiography. Single-frame cineangiogram in the left anterior oblique (LAO)-cranial projection of her left coronary and left ventricular angiogram are shown in the following figures. The next most appropriate course of action would be:

(A) Administration of abciximab followed by primary percutaneous coronary intervention (PCI) of the left anterior descending (LAD) artery
(B) Insertion of an intra-aortic balloon pump (IABP) followed by primary PCI of the LAD
(C) Primary PCI of the LAD and referral for emergency coronary artery bypass surgery
(D) Insertion of IABP and referral for emergent coronary artery bypass surgery

2 A 36-year-old man undergoes diagnostic coronary and left ventricular angiography for evaluation of chest pain. His cardiac examination is notable for the presence of a mid-peaking systolic ejection murmur, heard best at the left sternal border without radiation. His lungs are clear to auscultation. His electrocardiogram shows left ventricular hypertrophy with secondary repolarization abnormalities. His coronary angiogram demonstrates normal left and right coronary arteries, and left ventricular angiography reveals normal systolic function. A simultaneous left ventricular and femoral arterial pressure tracing is shown in the following figure.

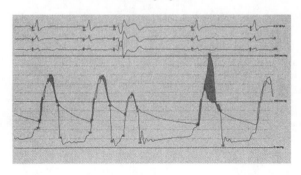

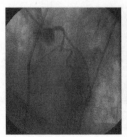 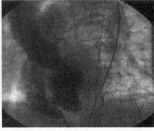

The procedure was uneventful, but during recovery, the patient complains of chest pain and lightheadedness. On physical examination, his blood pressure is 70/50 mm Hg with a heart rate of 88 beats per minute. He appears diaphoretic and the extremities are cool. In addition to administration of intravenous fluids, which of the following should be administered?

(A) Dobutamine
(B) Dopamine
(C) Phenylephrine
(D) Atropine

3 An 80-year-old woman presents to a community hospital with unstable angina associated with transient inferolateral ST-segment depression. She is treated with aspirin, clopidogrel, enoxaparin, and eptifibatide, in addition to metoprolol and atorvastatin. She is stabilized and subsequently "rules in" for a myocardial infarction (MI) with a cardiac troponin I of 2.1 ng per mL. Her CBC, serum electrolytes, and renal function are normal. She undergoes diagnostic coronary and left ventricular angiography, which reveal normal left ventricular systolic function and single vessel coronary artery disease with a 90% stenosis in the mid right coronary artery. She is transferred to a tertiary hospital where she undergoes placement of a drug-eluting stent with an excellent angiographic result. The femoral arteriotomy site is closed using a collagen plug closure device.

Two hours later, she complains of nausea, abdominal pain, and vague chest discomfort. Her blood pressure is 90/60 mm Hg and heart rate is 44 beats per minute. She appears pale and diaphoretic. Her lungs are clear to auscultation and her cardiac examination is without murmurs, rubs, or gallops. Her abdomen is soft with no reproducible tenderness. Her right groin has a small hematoma with no evidence of bleeding. Her electrocardiogram shows nonspecific findings.

Following administration of 0.5-mg atropine intravenously and normal saline, her blood pressure and heart rate rise to 108/68 mm Hg and 70 beats per minute, respectively. Which of the following should be done next?

(A) Continued observation
(B) Urgent coronary angiography to exclude acute stent thrombosis
(C) Discontinue eptifibatide and obtain stat CBC and type and crossmatch
(D) Computed tomography (CT) of the abdomen

4 Which of the following is *not* a contraindication to IABP insertion?

(A) Severe peripheral arterial disease
(B) Aortic insufficiency
(C) Recent fibrinolytic therapy
(D) Abdominal aortic aneurysm

5 A 66-year-old woman with a history of hypertension and hyperlipidemia undergoes diagnostic coronary angiography for an abnormal exercise stress test. The patient receives standard premedication for the procedure, including midazolam and fentanyl. The catheter is advanced smoothly around the aortic arch and the left main coronary is engaged. A sample of her initial left coronary angiogram is shown in the following figure.

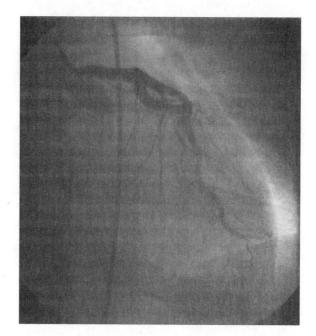

The patient suddenly complains of shortness of breath and chest pain. Physical examination is notable for a blood pressure of 82/50 mm Hg, heart rate of 94 beats per minute, respiratory rate of 24 breaths per minute, and oxygen saturation of 92%. Cardiac examination reveals no murmurs or gallops and her lungs demonstrate diffuse inspiratory and expiratory wheezing. Which of the following should be done next?

(A) Switch to a lower osmolar iodinated contrast agent
(B) Repeat left coronary angiography to exclude dissection of the left main coronary artery
(C) Administer diphenhydramine, antihistamines, and epinephrine
(D) Administer flumazenil to reverse the effects of the benzodiazepine

6 A 63-year-old man is admitted to the hospital for evaluation of exertional shortness of breath and chest pain. His risk factors for ischemic heart disease include hypertension, hyperlipidemia, and obesity. His initial treatment includes aspirin and unfractionated heparin. Cardiac enzymes are negative for MI, and the remainder of his laboratory values is normal. A pharmacologic nuclear study is performed and demonstrates a medium-sized moderately severe perfusion defect in the inferolateral wall with near-complete reperfusion on the resting images. He presents to the cardiac catheterization laboratory for diagnostic right and left heart catheterization through the transfemoral approach. Using a balloon-tipped flotation catheter, right-sided pressures are recorded as follows: Right atrial (RA) pressure (mean, mm Hg) 11; right ventricular (RV) pressure (systolic, end diastolic, mm Hg) 52/10; and pulmonary arterial (PA) pressure (systolic, diastolic, mean, mm Hg) 54/20, 31.

The catheter is advanced into the left-sided pulmonary wedge position and the mean pressure is 18 mm Hg. Following deflation of the balloon, an appropriate rise in the mean pressure is seen, confirming that the catheter was in the wedge position. The patient suddenly develops hemoptysis with rapid oxygen desaturation. The most appropriate immediate management includes:

(A) Placement of the patient in the left lateral decubitus position and emergency thoracic surgical consultation for presumed rupture of the pulmonary artery
(B) Reinflation of the balloon-tipped catheter in the pulmonary artery for presumed rupture of the pulmonary artery
(C) Administration of protamine
(D) Surgical consultation for emergency chest tube insertion

7 A 53-year-old man presents to the hospital with 3 hours of nearly constant substernal chest discomfort. He has no significant past medical history, but his risk factors for cardiovascular disease include current tobacco use and a family history of premature coronary artery disease. On physical examination, his blood pressure is 100/70 mm Hg and heart rate is 84 beats per minute. His lung fields are clear to auscultation and percussion and cardiovascular examination is notable for normal heart sounds and no audible murmurs. His electrocardiogram shows 2 to 3 mm of ST-segment elevation in leads II, III, and aVF, with 1 mm ST depression in V_1 through

V_3. He is taken to the cardiac catheterization laboratory for emergency percutaneous revascularization. Angiography of the left coronary artery was normal. A single-frame cineangiogram of the right coronary artery before and after dilation of the stenosis with a 2.5-mm balloon is shown in the following figures.

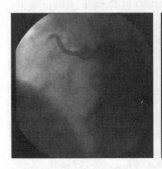 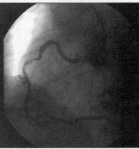

The patient subsequently complains of nausea and vomits. The hemodynamic tracing from the monitor is shown in the following figure.

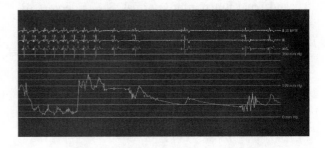

Which of the following would you do next?
(A) Insert a temporary transvenous pacemaker
(B) Administer dopamine
(C) Administer atropine and intravenous fluids
(D) Reinflate the angioplasty balloon in the proximal segment of the coronary artery and prepare for emergency pericardiocentesis

8 Which of the following is *not* responsible for the hemodynamic disturbances seen with RV infarction?

(A) Reduction in left ventricular preload
(B) Increase in left ventricular afterload
(C) Pericardial constraint
(D) RV dysfunction

9 Which of the following hemodynamic profiles is most consistent with cardiogenic shock secondary to inferior wall MI with RV involvement?

The following table contains the answer choices.

				Pressure (mm Hg)			
	RA	RV	PA	PCW	Ao	CO L/min	SVR dyne S/cm⁵
A	3	20/3	20/8	7	88/56	3.2	1,590
B	15	35/14	36/15	15	85/60	3.5	1,220
C	2	22/3	24/8	8	82/40	7.2	600
D	15	50/18	52/28	30	90/62	2.9	1,550

RA, RV, PA, PCW, and Ao denote right atrial, right ventricular, pulmonary arterial, pulmonary capillary wedge, and aortic pressure measured in mm Hg, respectively; CO denotes cardiac output expressed in liters/minute; SVR denotes systemic vascular resistance in dyne-sec-cm⁻⁵

10 Which of the following agents is *least* likely to be of benefit in a patient with cardiogenic shock demonstrating persistent hypotension despite IABP counterpulsation?

(A) Dobutamine
(B) Dopamine
(C) Norepinephrine
(D) N^G-monomethyl L-arginine (L-NMMA)

11 In which of the following patients would percutaneous cardiopulmonary support (CPS) offer the greatest benefit?

(A) A 33-year-old woman with fulminant myocarditis and hypotension despite high-dose inotropic support
(B) An 82-year-old male with cardiogenic shock treated with an intra-aortic balloon undergoing primary PCI
(C) A 64-year-old woman with ovarian cancer and a normal ejection fraction undergoing unprotected left main PCI
(D) A 46-year-old male with a recent anterior MI and mildly reduced left ventricular function (40% with anterior wall severe hypokinesis) undergoing PCI of a proximal LAD/diagonal artery bifurcation lesion

12 A 74-year-old woman presents to the emergency room with a history of substernal chest pain and shortness of breath starting 4 hours ago. She has a history of longstanding hypertension and known coronary artery disease with a prior MI 6 years ago. At that time, an implantable cardiac defibrillator (ICD) was implanted. On physical examination, her blood pressure is 100/40 mm Hg with a heart rate of 88 beats per minute and a respiratory rate of 16 breaths per minute. The lung fields are clear to auscultation and the heart sounds are regular with a systolic flow murmur heard in the second right intercostal space.

The electrocardiogram shows an acute infero-posterior wall ST-segment elevation MI. The chest x-ray is shown in the following figure.

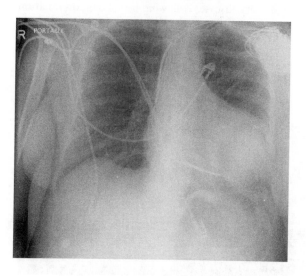

She is treated with aspirin, heparin, and a single intravenous dose of metoprolol and taken to the cardiac catheterization laboratory for emergency PCI. Angiography of the left coronary artery revealed moderate disease in the mid LAD and diffuse mild disease in the left circumflex artery. The right coronary artery was occluded in the mid portion with thrombus. The mid right coronary artery was successfully treated with a single drug-eluting stent and there was no residual stenosis. However, following stent deployment, there was grade 2 thrombolysis in myocardial infarction (TIMI) flow in the distal bed of the right coronary artery, which did not improve despite multiple doses of intracoronary nitroprusside. Right heart catheterization was performed and revealed a PA pressure of 44/16 mm Hg and a mean pulmonary capillary wedge (PCW) pressure of 16 mm Hg. An IABP was placed and there was appropriate diastolic augmentation and systolic unloading. Upon arrival to the coronary care unit, the patient rapidly develops severe shortness of breath with a blood pressure of 100/50 mm Hg and a heart rate of 110 beats per minute. The electrocardiogram shows nonspecific changes. She is emergently intubated for pulmonary edema.

Which of the following is likely contributing to the patient's sudden decompensation?

(A) Acute stent thrombosis
(B) Acute ventricular septal rupture
(C) Acute severe aortic insufficiency
(D) Acute severe mitral insufficiency

13 A 54-year-old man undergoes rescue angioplasty following unsuccessful reperfusion with fibrinolytic therapy for an acute anterior wall MI. Coronary angiography revealed thrombotic occlusion of the proximal LAD with no other significant epicardial coronary disease. Following initial balloon inflation across the stenosis in the proximal LAD, there is restoration of antegrade flow. The electrocardiogram and arterial pressure from the guiding catheter are shown in the following figure. Which of the following should be done next?

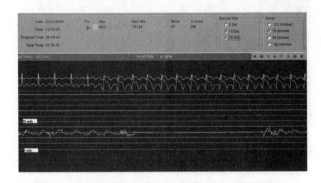

- (A) Administration of bolus and infusion of amiodarone
- (B) Administration of bolus and infusion of lidocaine
- (C) Electrical cardioversion
- (D) Observation

14 In which of the following situations is coronary perforation most likely to occur during PCI?

- (A) Rotational atherectomy of a stenosis in the mid portion of a tortuous right coronary artery
- (B) Balloon angioplasty of a densely calcified proximal LAD stenosis using a high-pressure balloon
- (C) Stent placement in a stenosis in the proximal right coronary artery following failed fibrinolysis for an acute inferior wall MI
- (D) Stent placement in a stenosis in the mid portion of a saphenous vein graft to the obtuse marginal branch

15 In which of the following clinical situations would prophylactic IABP counterpulsation likely be the most beneficial?

- (A) A 62-year-old male undergoing PCI of the mid LAD and mid right coronary artery with an LVEF of 40%, blood pressure of 110/70 mm Hg, and PCW pressure of 16 mm Hg
- (B) A 54-year-old woman with a history of coronary artery bypass grafting (CABG) undergoing PCI of the distal left main coronary artery with a patent left internal mammary graft to the LAD, and an occluded saphenous vein graft to an obtuse marginal branch of the left circumflex artery in addition to an LVEF of 30%, blood pressure of 100/70 mm Hg, and PCW pressure of 6 mm Hg
- (C) An 82-year-old woman undergoing PCI of a calcified proximal LAD with an LVEF of 60%, blood pressure of 140/60 mm Hg, and PCW pressure of 22 mm Hg
- (D) A 78-year-old woman undergoing PCI of the proximal LAD with an LVEF of 20%, blood pressure of 95/50 mm Hg, and PCW pressure of 26 mm Hg

16 A 68-year-old woman is undergoing rotational atherectomy of an angulated lesion in the mid right coronary artery with a 1.5 mm burr. Her blood pressure suddenly drops to 70/30 mm Hg and angiography demonstrates contrast extravasation into the pericardial space. In preparation for emergency pericardiocentesis for cardiac tamponade, protamine sulfate should be given if which of the following antithrombotic agents had been given before PCI?

- (A) Heparin
- (B) Enoxaparin
- (C) Heparin or bivalirudin
- (D) Bivalirudin

17 A 50-year-old woman with a long history of cigarette smoking and hypertension undergoes coronary angiography for Class III stable angina and an exercise echocardiogram notable only for anterolateral ischemia and normal left ventricular function. Left coronary angiography reveals a 90% stenosis in the mid LAD and insignificant disease in the left circumflex artery. Following catheter placement in the right coronary ostium, the patient complains of severe angina. Blood pressure falls from 150/80 to 100/70 mm Hg and the heart rate increases to 90 beats per minute. Angiography reveals a 95% stenosis of the proximal right coronary artery without signs of dissection. The patient continues to complain of severe chest pain and the monitor reveals ST-segment elevation in leads II and III. Which of the following would you do next?

- (A) Administer atropine 0.6 mg IV and IV fluids
- (B) Replace the diagnostic catheter with a guiding one and prepare for emergency PCI of the right coronary artery
- (C) Insert an IABP in preparation for emergency PCI of the right coronary artery
- (D) Administer 100 μg of intracoronary nitroglycerin in the right coronary artery

18 An 82-year-old man with a history of hypertension, type 2 diabetes, and dyslipidemia is brought in by his family to the emergency room after being noted to be lethargic with difficulty in breathing. On examination, he is diaphoretic with a blood pressure of 85/50 mm Hg and a heart rate of 110 beats per minute. His heart sounds are normal without any murmurs, and rales are present over the lower third of the lung bases. His electrocardiogram shows evidence of an evolving anteroseptal MI with Q waves in V_1 through V_3 and 2 to 3 mm ST-segment elevation. What class of recommendation do the 2004 American College of Cardiology/American Heart Association (ACC/AHA) Guidelines for the Management of Patients with ST-Elevation Myocardial Infarction assign to primary percutaneous intervention for this clinical situation?

(A) Class I
(B) Class IIa
(C) Class IIb
(D) Class III

19 An 82-year-old woman with peripheral vascular disease is admitted to the catheterization laboratory for diagnostic catheterization for an acute coronary syndrome. She is given 1.0 mg of midazolam and 25 μg of fentanyl, both intravenously for conscious sedation. Following insertion of a sheath into the right femoral artery, a left diagnostic catheter is positioned over a wire into the ascending aorta. Before angiography of the left coronary artery, the patient is noted to be confused with incoherent speech. Her blood pressure is 108/80 mm Hg and heart rate is 78 beats per minute. Which of the following would be the next most appropriate course of action?

(A) Administration of flumazenil and naloxone
(B) Emergent neurologic evaluation
(C) Administration of an additional 0.5 mg of intravenous midazolam
(D) Administration of 0.5 mg of intravenous halo-peridol

20 A 59-year-old man presents to the hospital with chest pain and is found to have anterior T-wave inversions and an elevated cardiac troponin. He is treated with aspirin, clopidogrel, and unfractionated heparin. He is taken to the cardiac catheterization laboratory and following angiography of the left coronary artery, he complains of severe chest pain with evidence of ST-segment elevation on the monitor. His blood pressure is 80/40 mm Hg with a heart rate of 90 beats per minute. A single frame cineangiogram of the left coronary artery in the right anterior oblique (RAO) projection with caudal angulation is shown in the following figure. Which of the following should be done next?

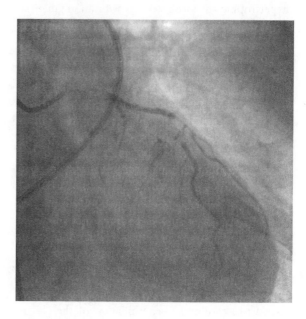

(A) Insertion of an IABP
(B) Emergent coronary artery bypass surgery for dissection of the left main coronary artery
(C) Administration of 100% oxygen
(D) Administration of abciximab and preparation for emergency PCI of the left main and LADs

Answers and Explanations

1 Answer D. The patient is presenting with an acute anterior wall MI caused by thrombotic occlusion of the mid-LAD, complicated by rupture of the ventricular septum and cardiogenic shock. Percutaneous revascularization of the LAD should not be performed. This patient appears to be a surgical candidate and should have an IABP inserted, followed by emergency cardiac surgery and repair of the ventricular septum.

2 Answer C. The patient has evidence of probable hypertrophic subaortic stenosis with an augmentation of the left ventricular and aortic gradient and a fall (narrowing) of the pulse pressure following a premature ventricular beat (Brockenbrough-Braunwald sign). Following the procedure, he develops signs and symptoms of acute left ventricular outflow obstruction that should initially be managed by bed rest and administration of intravenous fluids to augment preload. Refractory hypotension should be managed with intravenous phenylephrine (a pure α-agonist, vasoconstrictor). Dopamine should not be given because any inotropic agent may worsen the outflow tract obstruction and exacerbate hypotension. Atropine can be used for situations associated with increased vagal tone, but would not be appropriate in the acute management in this setting.

3 Answer C. The patient has likely had an acute retroperitoneal bleed and should be treated with supportive care and discontinuation of the glycoprotein (GP) IIb/IIIa platelet receptor antagonist. Compression of the femoral arteriotomy site may be helpful and blood transfusion should be performed for ongoing bleeding, which is causing hemodynamic instability or results in unacceptably low hemoglobin. Femoral arterial puncture above the inguinal ligament (particularly with puncture of the back wall) may predispose the patient to bleeding in the retroperitoneal space. This patient's diagnostic angiogram was performed in another hospital and, therefore, the information regarding the arterial access may not have been available. Continued administration of eptifibatide may have aggravated any ongoing bleeding. *The diagnosis of retroperitoneal bleeding should be suspected in any patient who develops an unexplained vagal reaction or transient hypotension following transfemoral catheterization.* The diagnosis can be confirmed with CT scanning, but the diagnosis is usually made on clinical grounds and the treatment is generally supportive with surgical exploration and repair seldom being required.

4 Answer C. Contraindications to IABP insertion include severe peripheral arterial disease or prior peripheral arterial bypass surgery, moderate or severe aortic insufficiency, or an abdominal aortic aneurysm. Recent fibrinolytic therapy is not a contraindication to an IABP.

5 Answer C. Reactions to iodinated contrast media occur in <1% of patients but may occur in 17% to 35% of patients with a prior contrast reaction (*Ann Intern Med.* 2003;139:123–136). Common clinical manifestations can range from mild (pruritus and urticaria) to serious (bronchospasm and angioedema) to life-threatening (shock). These manifestations are due to release of histamine from direct degranulation of tissue mast cells and circulating basophils and are anaphylactoid reactions in contrast to immunoglobulin E (IgE)-mediated true allergic reactions. Acute management of anaphylactoid contrast reactions in the catheterization laboratory includes administration of intravenous antihistamines (both anti-H_1 and anti-H_2) and corticosteroids (although these do not work immediately). Severe reactions that lead to respiratory and hemodynamic compromise should be treated with epinephrine (*Cathet Cardiovasc Diagn.* 1995;34:99–104).

6 Answer A. Pulmonary artery rupture is a rare, but often lethal, complication of Swan-Ganz catheterization. Risk factors include older age, pulmonary hypertension, improper balloon inflation or positioning, manipulation of an inflated balloon-tipped catheter in the wedge position, and possibly anticoagulation (*Chest.* 1995;108:1349–1352). Patients universally develop acute hemoptysis, which can be massive. Hemothorax can develop rapidly and the patient should initially be turned to the side of the hemothorax to protect the unaffected lung. Immediate thoracotomy is likely the only life-saving therapy for patients who develop hemothorax. Reversal of anticoagulation is also reasonable once initial stabilizing measures have been performed. A chest tube can be inserted as a temporizing measure, but is not a substitute for prompt surgical correction.

7 **Answer C.** Nausea and vomiting, often associated with hypotension and bradycardia, are common with MI, particularly when it involves the inferior wall of the left ventricle. This constellation of findings is often attributed to direct activation of parasympathetic/vagal reflex pathways or left ventricular stretch receptors (Bezold-Jarisch reflex) that lead to bradycardia and peripheral vasodilation. The Bezold-Jarisch reflex most commonly occurs after acute reperfusion of the infarct artery in a patient with an inferior MI.

8 **Answer B.** RV ischemia and infarction almost exclusively occur in the setting of infarction of the inferior wall of the left ventricle. This is most often seen with occlusion of the right coronary artery, proximal to the origin of the acute marginal branches. The characteristic triad of hypotension, clear lung fields, and elevation of the jugular venous pressure in the setting of an acute MI are classic features of RV infarction. Acute ischemia of the right ventricle causes the chamber to dilate, and in the presence of an intact pericardium, causes the interventricular septum to shift toward the left ventricle. This leads to RV systolic dysfunction and a decrease in LV preload, both of which can lead to hypotension. Initial management strategies should include optimization of LV preload with volume loading. Prompt revascularization is beneficial in relieving RV and LV ischemia. Other important features of the management of RV infarction include avoiding agents that may reduce preload, including nitroglycerin and diuretics. Inotropic agents (dobutamine) and IABP counterpulsation are sometimes needed to augment the cardiac output (CO) and improve hemodynamics (*N Engl J Med.* 1994;330: 1211–1217).

9 **Answer B.** RA pressure is elevated with a mildly elevated PCW and systemic vascular resistance (SVR) and with a normal CO. In **A**, filling pressures are all low and SVR is elevated, consistent with hypovolemic shock. In **C**, filling pressures are also low, but CO is elevated and SVR is low, consistent with sepsis. In **D**, PCW is elevated, CO is relatively low, and SVR is elevated, consistent with cardiogenic shock.

10 **Answer A.** Dopamine, at doses >10 μg/kg/min, acts predominantly as an α-adrenergic agonist and potent vasoconstrictor. At doses <10 μg/kg/min but >3 μg/kg/min, it acts as a β-adrenergic agonist and positive inotrope. Dopamine is often used as a first-line agent for the treatment of persistent hypotension in cardiogenic shock. However, because of its β-agonist effects, it can also lead to tachycardia. Norepinephrine (Levophed) is a potent adrenergic ($\alpha > \beta$) agent that is used for refractory hypotension. Dobutamine is a positive inotropic agent that also causes systemic vasodilation, and is not a preferred agent for the treatment of persistent hypotension in cardiogenic shock. There is literature suggesting that inappropriately high levels of nitric oxide (NO), a potent vasodilator, are produced in states of systemic inflammation, including cardiogenic shock. A preliminary investigation on the use of L-NMMA, an inhibitor of nitric oxide synthase (NOS), in 11 consecutive patients with refractory cardiogenic shock despite percutaneous revascularization and IABP demonstrated a 64% survival rate at 30 days (*Circulation.* 2000;101: 1358–1361). An international phase III study in cardiogenic shock, Tilarginine Acetate for Injection in a Randomized International Study in Unstable AMI Patients with Cardiogenic Shock (TRIUMPH), is ongoing to determine the benefit of NOS inhibition in patients with cardiogenic shock.

11 **Answer A.** Percutaneous CPS involves insertion of large catheters into the systemic venous and arterial circulations and active aspiration of blood from the venous circulation and passage through an extracorporeal system that oxygenates the blood and pumps it back into the arterial circulation. Possible indications include fulminant myocarditis (as a bridge to cardiac transplantation) or as an adjunct to high-risk PCI in the setting of severely reduced left ventricular function, or dilation of the artery serving the only viable myocardium.

12 **Answer C.** Moderate or severe aortic insufficiency is a contraindication to an IABP. Inflation of the balloon during diastole raises the aortic pressure and increases coronary blood flow. Clues that this patient may have had chronic underlying aortic insufficiency are the presence of a wide pulse pressure, presence of a systolic murmur (due to overall increased blood flow across the aortic valve), and cardiomegaly on the chest x-ray. Placement of an IABP in this patient caused more acute, severe aortic insufficiency and pulmonary edema. An IABP would not be expected to cause clinical deterioration in the presence of an acute ventricular septal defect or acute severe mitral insufficiency. Acute stent thrombosis would not necessarily cause acute pulmonary edema, and is usually associated with chest pain and ST-segment elevation on the electrocardiogram.

13 **Answer D.** The initial portion of the electrocardiogram demonstrates sinus tachycardia with a rate of approximately 100 beats per minute. The arterial pressure is 78/44 mm Hg. The wide-complex rhythm that develops is an accelerated idioventricular rhythm (AIVR) that is often seen following successful reperfusion in acute MI, either by pharmacologic or mechanical means and is usually transient. The blood pressure seen toward the end of the screen remained stable. Antiarrhythmic therapy is not indicated for AIVR. Likewise, electrical cardioversion is also usually not needed.

14 **Answer A.** Coronary artery perforation is an infrequent occurrence following PCI. Perforations during PCI can occur as a result of guidewire manipulation ("wire exit") or improper sizing of the balloon. Elderly patients and women appear to be at increased risk. However, PCI following fibrinolytic therapy and PCI of a saphenous vein graft are not associated with increased risk of perforation. In a prospective study of the incidence of coronary artery perforation in the early 1990s, use of newer devices to treat coronary lesions by cutting or ablating tissue (atherectomy, laser) were associated with an increased incidence of perforation compared with balloon angioplasty alone (*Circulation*. 1994;90:2725–2730). These investigators defined a scheme for classifying coronary artery perforations into one of three groups: Extraluminal crater without extravasation (Type 1), pericardial or myocardial blush without contrast extravasation (Type 2), or extravasation through frank (≥1 mm) perforation (Type 3). Type 1 and Type 2 perforations can usually be managed with prolonged balloon inflations and reversal of anticoagulation. Type 3 perforations are usually associated with a higher incidence of adverse events (death, MI, tamponade, or emergency cardiac surgery).

Prolonged balloon inflations may not be well tolerated, and perfusion balloons have been used in this setting to seal off the perforation and maintain adequate distal perfusion. Heparin anticoagulation is usually reversed with protamine, and pericardial tamponade is treated with pericardiocentesis. If these measures fail, emergency surgery is needed. In recent years, polytetrafluoroethylene (PTFE)-covered stents have emerged as an attractive alternative to the nonsurgical management of coronary artery perforations, with promising results (*Circulation*. 2000;102: 3028–3031).

15 **Answer D.** Prophylactic IABP placement should be considered before PCI in patients who demonstrate hemodynamic compromise and/or have impaired hemodynamic reserve. One should consider a prophylactic IABP in a patient undergoing high-risk PCI, in the face of a severely reduced left ventricular function or markedly elevated filling pressures. Although an IABP is often used in PCI of an unprotected left main coronary stenosis, it is not necessarily needed when PCI is performed in the setting of a patent bypass graft to the LAD or left circumflex artery ("protected left main" PCI).

16 **Answer A.** Protamine sulfate is given intravenously to neutralize the anticoagulant effect of heparin. The usual dose is 1 mg of protamine sulfate for each 100 units of unfractionated heparin. Protamine is not as effective in neutralizing the effect of low-molecular-weight heparins (enoxaparin). Neither direct thrombin inhibitors (bivalirudin) nor GP IIb/IIIa inhibitors are affected by protamine.

17 **Answer D.** Catheter-induced coronary spasm, most common in the right coronary artery, should be considered in this patient on the basis of the timing of the onset of symptoms. Although the chest pain could precipitate a vagal reaction, the increase in heart rate makes this less likely. In addition, the absence of inferior ischemia on the previous stress test makes the diagnosis of coronary spasm more likely. Intravenous or intracoronary nitrates should be given before PCI whenever this diagnosis is suspected. Coronary spasm should be considered in the presence of a proximal stenosis in the right coronary artery that is smooth and concentric, particularly if catheter engagement occurs too quickly.

18 **Answer B.** According to the ACC/AHA Guidelines for the Management of Patients with ST-Elevation Myocardial Infarction, emergency revascularization is given a Class I recommendation (conditions for which there is evidence and/or general agreement that a given procedure or treatment is beneficial, useful, and effective) for suitable patients <75 years of age who develop cardiogenic shock within 36 hours of MI, in whom revascularization can be performed within 18 hours of the onset of shock (*J Am Coll Cardiol*. 2004;44:671–719). The SHOCK trial was a multicenter, randomized trial comparing emergency revascularization (either PCI or CABG) with initial medical stabilization (including an IABP) for patients with ST elevation or new left bundle branch block (LBBB) MI and cardiogenic shock. Although the 30-day mortality (primary endpoint) between the two groups was not statistically different, at 6 months and 1 year, mortality was better in the group assigned to emergency revascularization, compared with the group treated with initial medical stabilization (*N Engl J Med*. 1999;341:625–634, *JAMA*. 2001;285:190–192). A prespecified subgroup of patients <75 years of age similarly showed an overall benefit with emergency revascularization, with respect to 30-day mortality; however, of those >75 years ($n = 56$), there was no difference in mortality between the two treatment strategies. This might have been explained by the unexpectedly low mortality rate among elderly patients assigned to the initial medical stabilization arm, as their survival was similar to younger patients assigned to medical stabilization. Therefore, for patients >75 years of age, the ACC/AHA guidelines assign primary PCI a Class IIa (conditions for which there is conflicting evidence and/or divergence of opinion about the usefulness/efficacy of a procedure or treatment, but for which the weight of the evidence is in favor of such a procedure or treatment).

19 **Answer A.** Elderly patients are at increased risk for idiosyncratic reactions to benzodiazepines and narcotics. In the outlined scenario, one would be concerned about an acute cerebrovascular event (particularly because there has been manipulation of a guidewire and catheter in the ascending aorta and aortic arch); however, the initial management should include reversal of the benzodiazepine and narcotic. Additional sedatives or psychoactive medications should be avoided until the patient's neurologic status is clarified.

20 **Answer C.** Coronary air embolus is a preventable complication of cardiac catheterization. When it does occur, treatment is usually supportive with administration of 100% inhaled oxygen. If the chest pain or ischemia persists despite oxygen, an IABP and pressor support may be necessary; however, coronary artery bypass surgery is not indicated.

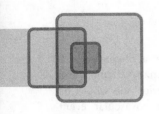

27

Peripheral Interventional Procedures

Matthew C. Becker and Samir Kapadia

Questions

1 Which of the following patients is *not* an appropriate candidate for carotid artery stenting (CAS) according to the SAPPHIRE trial criteria?

(A) An 82-year-old woman with a recent history of transient ischemic attack (TIA), poorly controlled hypertension, and 60% stenosis of the internal carotid

(B) A 72-year-old man with a history of myocardial infarction (MI) 3 weeks ago and an 80% stenosis of the right internal carotid artery (ICA)

(C) A 60-year-old diabetic man with a history of cerebrovascular accident (CVA) 6 weeks ago resulting in residual left upper extremity paresis with 90% left internal carotid stenosis

(D) An asymptomatic 85-year-old man with severe emphysematous lung disease, NYHA (New York Heart Association) class III congestive heart failure (CHF) and bilateral 80% stenosis of the internal carotid arteries

2 All of the following are complications of CAS, *except*:

(A) Stroke
(B) Hypotension/Bradycardia
(C) MI
(D) Hyperperfusion Syndrome
(E) All of the above

3 The following angiogram was performed on a 74-year-old man, a diabetic patient with a recent history of hospitalization for transient left upper extremity paresis. On the basis of the data reported by

large, randomized trials evaluating the efficacy of traditional carotid endarterectomy (CEA), which of the following statements is *true*?

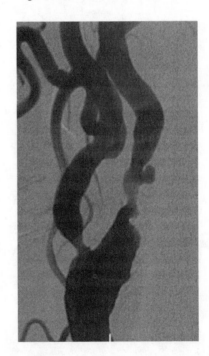

(A) This patient is *not* an appropriate candidate for CEA because of his recent transient left upper extremity paresis, and should be considered for CAS for an optimum outcome

(B) The patient *would be* appropriate for CEA, and can expect a lower risk of any major or fatal ipsilateral stroke in the 2 years following the procedure at the expense of an initial increase in the 30-day risk of death and stroke as compared with medical therapy

(C) The patient *is* a candidate for CEA, and can expect a lower risk of stroke or death immediately following the procedure but the benefit becomes insignificant at 2 years as compared with medical therapy

(D) The patient *is* a candidate for CEA, and can expect a lower risk of any ipsilateral or contralateral stroke in the 2 years following the procedure

4 As a part of an executive physical, a healthy 65-year-old man with a history of hypertension and tobacco use, but no history of stroke or TIA, was referred for a carotid ultrasound that revealed 70% and 40% stenoses of the left and right common carotids, respectively. On the basis of the information provided by the multiple, randomized trials evaluating the efficacy of CEA in patients with asymptomatic carotid disease, which of the following statements is *true*?

(A) Performing CEA on the left carotid artery at this time would likely expose the patient to a perioperative risk of stroke, death, and MI around 3% to 7%, and would not likely result in a lower risk of subsequent stroke

(B) Performing CEA on the left carotid artery would likely result in an elevated risk of perioperative stroke, death, or MI around 3%, but would result in a reduced incidence of *ipsilateral* stroke by 2 years postoperatively

(C) U.S. Food and Drug Administration (FDA) does not approve carotid stenting for asymptomatic patients at this time

(D) There is no randomized data suggesting a long-term benefit of performing CEA in asymptomatic patients with carotid stenosis <80%

(E) Both B and C

5 Periprocedural stroke during carotid stenting is most commonly attributable to distal embolization. During which portion of the procedure are distal embolic events most likely to occur?

(A) Wiring
(B) Predilatation
(C) Stenting
(D) Postdilatation
(E) Guide placement

6 Which of the following types of procedure has the least detectable amount of embolization by transcranial Doppler?

(A) Carotid stenting with filter on a wire emboli protection device

(B) Carotid stenting with distal occlusion emboli protection device

(C) Carotid stenting with proximal occlusion emboli protection device

(D) CEA

7 Which of the following statements regarding symptomatic peripheral arterial disease (PAD) is *incorrect*?

(A) Most patients participating in formal exercise rehabilitation programs have been shown to double their symptom-free walking period

(B) Because of their high rate of comorbid cardiovascular disease (CVD) and vascular events, all patients with PAD should be considered to have coronary artery disease (CAD) until proved otherwise, and initiated on drug therapy until their low-density lipoprotein C (LDL-C) levels are reduced to <100 mg per dL

(C) The presence of low ankle-brachial indices (ABIs) in hypertensive patients is a predictor of increased mortality

(D) The FDA has approved both pentoxiphylline and clopidogrel for the treatment of intermittent claudication

8 All of the following are acceptable indications for endovascular intervention to the superficial femoral arterial lesion shown in the following figure, *except*:

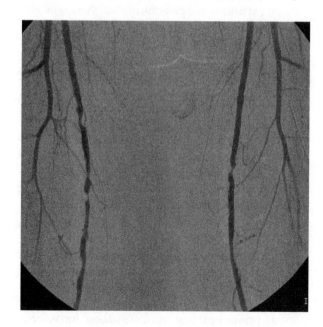

(A) Incapacitating, intermittent claudication
(B) Rest pain
(C) Development of nonhealing ulcerations or wounds of the lower extremity

(D) Presence of a 5-cm eccentric 80% lesion of the proximal superficial femoral artery (SFA) in a patient with mild, intermittent claudication

9 The following angiogram is that of a 65-year-old man who has a history of poorly controlled diabetes, hypertension as well as tobacco abuse, and complains of claudication symptoms after walking approximately 100 feet. His symptoms have been stable for older than 3 years, and he denies rest pain or chronic, nonhealing wound infections. Which of the following statements regarding this patient's future management is *incorrect*?

(A) The patient should be counseled on risk factor modification including smoking cessation and should be referred to a formal exercise rehabilitation program

(B) Because of the high rate of complications during infrapopliteal interventions, including thrombosis and perforation, angioplasty of these lesions is contraindicated

(C) The indications for endovascular intervention of these lesions include critical limb ischemia, rest pain, nonhealing wounds, or limb salvage

(D) Long-term patency rates for infrapopliteal interventions are not as favorable as those for iliac or femoral procedures

(E) After aggressively controlling this patient's hypertension and diabetes, medical therapy including antiplatelet agents and cilostazol should be the first line intervention

10 A 75-year-old woman with an ongoing history of hypertension, hypercholesterolemia, tobacco abuse, and moderately severe, intermittent claudication presents with a complaint of sudden onset, unbearable pain in the right lower extremity for the past 3 hours. An examination reveals a cool and mottled extremity with no popliteal arterial pulsation detected. Which of the following statements regarding this condition is *incorrect*?

(A) The most common etiologies of this condition are *in situ* thrombosis and embolism; however, the differential diagnosis must also include dissection, trauma, vasculitis, or abdominal aortic aneurysm (AAA) thrombosis or dissection

(B) Treatment options for this condition include primary surgical revascularization, intravenous thrombolysis, or percutaneous mechanical thrombectomy

(C) Primary surgical therapy is the traditional approach for this situation but carries a mortality rate approaching 30% in some cases

(D) Without rapid diagnosis and treatment, this patient is at high risk for amputation and/or mortality under any circumstance

11 Which of the following is *not* an indication for renal arteriography?

(A) Onset of hypertension in an individual younger than 30 or older than 55 years or rapidly accelerating hypertension in a previously well-controlled patient

(B) Azotemia after the initiation of an angiotensin-converting enzyme inhibitor (ACEI)

(C) Asymmetric kidney size as documented by non-invasive imaging in association with an unexplained elevation in creatinine (>1.5 mg per dL)

(D) The finding of an abdominal bruit on physical examination

(E) Following the completion of a diagnostic left-heart catheterization in a patient with severe coronary atherosclerosis with normal renal function

12 Which of the following is *not* an indication for percutaneous revascularization of the lesion seen in the following figure?

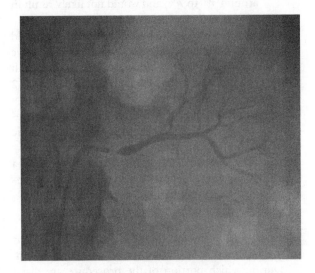

(A) Recurrent admission for decompensated heart failure or flash pulmonary edema in a medically compliant 72-year-old patient

(B) Hypertension refractory to >3, maximally dosed, antihypertensive medications

(C) Subacute renal failure (creatinine <3.0 mg per dL) in normal-sized kidneys (>9 cm) on noninvasive imaging

(D) Chronic kidney disease in a 65-year-old nondiabetic requiring renal replacement therapy (i.e., dialysis) instead of an alternative etiology

(E) Severe coronary atherosclerotic disease without associated chronic kidney disease in a male, diabetic patient

13 Which of the following statements regarding the treatment of renal artery stenosis (RAS) is *true*?

(A) Trials evaluating percutaneous revascularization of significant RAS (>70% lesion) in patients with renovascular hypertension have consistently demonstrated a significantly greater reduction in blood pressure as compared with patients treated with medical therapy alone

(B) Angioplasty with stent placement is superior to angioplasty alone in patients with fibromuscular dysplasia (FMD)

(C) Especially in patients with aorto-ostial or proximal RASs, angioplasty with stenting is superior to angioplasty alone

(D) ACEIs should not be used in patients with a significant unilateral RAS, secondary to a high risk of azotemia from the accentuated transglomerular pressure gradient

14 A 65-year-old diabetic man with a history of hypertension, hypercholesterolemia, and heavy tobacco abuse presents to his local emergency department complaining of increasing lower abdominal pain over the past 3 weeks. During his physical examination, a tender, pulsatile mass is detected in the lower abdomen with an associated systolic murmur. High-resolution computed tomography (CT) scan reveals an infrarenal AAA with a maximal diameter of 6 cm without evidence of rupture or leak. Which of the following statements regarding the management of this patient's condition is *true*?

(A) Current data regarding the long-term efficacy of endovascular aneurysm repair (EVAR) indicates that this patient would likely have a significantly reduced all-cause mortality if he underwent EVAR as opposed to open surgical repair

(B) If the preceding CT scan revealed extensive calcification and intramural thrombus involving >90 degrees the circumference of the proximal neck of the AAA, EVAR would offer technical advantages over open surgical repair

(C) If the length of the proximal neck of the AAA is noted to be <10 mm, surgical repair should be recommended

(D) If the preceding CT scan revealed a significant aortic tortuosity resulting in aneurysmal neck angulation >60 degrees, EVAR would be preferable to open repair due to the reduced risk of graft leak

(E) If records from the patient's primary care physician revealed that the AAA was actually discovered the previous year and was 5.0 cm in maximal diameter at that time, a reasonable management strategy would include aggressive medical management of the patient's hypertension, counseling for smoking cessation, and an annual CT scan to evaluate the AAA dimensions

15 Which of the following *is not* typically noted as a complication of AAA endovascular repair?

(A) Leaking of blood into the aneurysmal sac from either the proximal or distal sites of endograft attachment

(B) Accumulation of blood in the aneurysmal sac due to retrograde blood flow from patent lumbar or inferior mesenteric arteries

(C) Increased graft porosity resulting in slow permeation of blood across the endograft into the aneurysmal sac

(D) Renal, mesenteric, or iliac artery ischemia

(E) Spinal cord ischemia (SCI)

16 A 75-year-old man with a history of poorly controlled hypertension, PAD, chronic obstructive pulmonary disease (COPD), and a 60 pack per year history of tobacco abuse presents to his primary care physician's office noting development of dizziness, blurred vision, and gait instability after chopping wood. The patient's wife states that he had difficulty with his speech, and appeared to be disoriented the previous week when he was helping their son move. The patient's neurologic examination is unremarkable, with the exception of diminished radial pulse in the right upper extremity. Which of the following statements regarding this patient is *true*?

(A) A noncontrast head CT would be the most informative diagnostic test and would likely reveal the etiology of the patient's symptoms

(B) The patient should be immediately transferred to the nearest emergency department for urgent neurologic evaluation and thrombolytic therapy

(C) After ordering a sedimentation rate and prescribing a course of oral steroid therapy, the patient should be referred to ophthalmology for an urgent slit lamp examination

(D) After obtaining a baseline electrocardiogram, complete blood count, basic metabolic panel, and coagulation studies ([prothrombin time] PT, [activated partial thromboplastin time] aPTT), the patient should be referred for an arch aortogram as soon as possible

(E) The patient should undergo a transthoracic echocardiogram with agitated saline to rule out patent foramen ovale (PFO).

17 Which of the following does this angiogram show?

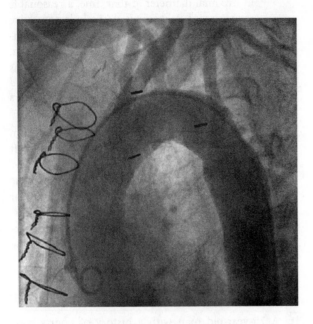

(A) Right-sided aortic arch
(B) Retroesophageal right subclavian
(C) Anomalous origin of the left vertebral
(D) Normal aortic arch

18 A 26-year-old woman presents with low-grade fever over the past 6 to 8 weeks associated with weight loss, malaise, and nocturnal diaphoresis. The patient also notes that her right arm has become painful and "crampy" over the same time course. In addition, the patient states that since the previous week her vision seemed to have become blurred, and she is now concerned that she may be losing her sight altogether. Remarkable findings on examination include a temperature of 38°C, blood pressure 185/100, the presence of a left infraclavicular bruit, and a diminished right radial pulse. The following angiogram is of this patient. Which of the following statements regarding this patient's condition is *false*?

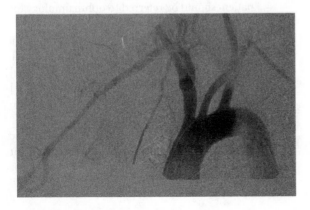

(A) After obtaining a sedimentation rate, VDRL test, rheumatoid factor, antinuclear antibody (ANA), coagulation studies, and baseline blood chemistries, the patient should undergo urgent cerebral and aortic arch angiography
(B) Immediate, aggressive control of the patient's hypertension should be avoided in this situation
(C) Treatment for this condition should consist of high-dose glucocorticoids and cyclophosphamide for an extended period
(D) Primary angioplasty offers a higher rate of cure for this condition
(E) Regardless of the mode of treatment, the patient faces a high relapse rate

19 Which of the following does this angiogram show?

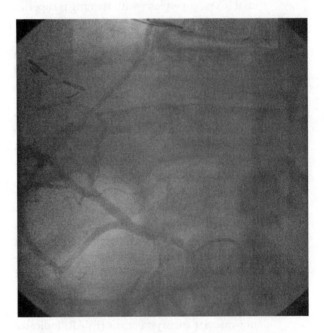

(A) Superior mesenteric artery (SMA)
(B) Inferior mesenteric artery (IMA)
(C) Hepatic and *in situ* right gastroepiploic graft to posterior descending artery (PDA)
(D) Splenic artery
(E) Left gastric and *in situ* right gastroepiploic graft to PDA

20 Observed complications following percutaneous renal artery *stenting* may include which of the following?

(A) Aortic dissection
(B) Renal artery perforation
(C) Renal infarction
(D) Embolization of atheromatous material
(E) Creatinine elevation requiring hemodialysis
(F) All of the above

Answers and Explanations

1 Answer C. Several large registries and one randomized clinical trial have demonstrated that the outcomes following CAS compare favorably with the traditional surgical endarterectomy CEA in select *high-risk* populations. The SAPPHIRE trial (*N Engl J Med.* 2004;351(15):1493–501) randomized 334 patients with symptomatic (>50% stenosis) or asymptomatic (>80% stenosis) carotid disease traditionally considered a high risk for surgical intervention to percutaneous carotid intervention with nitinol stents in conjunction with embolic protection devices (EPD) versus conventional CEA. The results demonstrated the noninferiority of CAS as well as a 39% reduction in the primary endpoint of a composite of death, stroke, and MI within 30 days. Additionally, patients randomized to CAS enjoyed lower rates of target-vessel revascularization, and a shorter hospital stay as well as a significantly greater 1-year event-free survival (88% vs. 79%, $p = 0.048$). On the basis of the balance of evidence, the FDA has approved elective CAS only in the "high-risk" populations with symptoms, listed subsequently. Currently, FDA does not approve asymptomatic patients, though they were included in the SAPPHIRE study. Although trials evaluating lower-risk populations are currently ongoing, only patients meeting one or more of the following criteria are deemed candidates for CAS.

Clinical: Age >80 years, CHF III-IV, known severe left ventricular dysfunction ([ejection fraction] EF <30%), open heart surgery needed within 6 weeks, recent MI (>24 hours and <4 weeks), unstable angina (CCS [Canadian Cardiovascular Society] class III/IV), severe pulmonary disease, contralateral laryngeal nerve palsy.

Anatomic: Previous CEA with recurrent stenosis, high cervical lesions or clear cell acanthoma (CCA) lesions below the clavicle, contralateral carotid occlusion, radiation therapy to the neck, prior radical neck surgery, severe tandem lesions (*Manual of peripheral vascular intervention.* 2005:86–87).

2 Answer E. Data obtained from the high-risk carotid stenting registries indicates that the 30-day incidence of post-CAS stroke approaches 3%. The primary mechanism of procedure-related stroke is thought to be the distal embolization of atheromatous debris dislodged during the procedure. In addition, manipulation of wires, catheters, and guides in the aortic arch and common carotid artery are not protected by EPD, and are frequently responsible for strokes outside the territory of the treated carotid artery.

Distention of the carotid sinus mechanoreceptors by angioplasty and stenting may activate the vasomotor center of the medulla through cranial IX. Subsequent vagal activation results in peripheral vasodilatation with hypotension and bradycardia. This phenomenon is relatively common and occurs in up to 40% of the procedures involving internal carotid lesions. Interestingly, in the restenotic lesions after endarterectomy, this reflex is typically not encountered. Supportive therapy with IV fluids, atropine, pseudoephedrine (60 mg PO b.i.d.) and, infrequently, dopamine are needed to counter hypotension and bradycardia.

The incidence of MI within 30 days of carotid stenting in the high-risk cohort of patients in the SAPPHIRE trial was 1.9%, which was significantly lower than that seen after CEA in that trial (*Manual of peripheral vascular intervention.* 2005:102–106).

In a response to carotid occlusive disease and chronically decreasing cerebral perfusion pressures, the cerebral vessels may undergo a compensatory vasodilatation in an effort to maintain adequate blood flow to the brain. Following intervention to the carotid artery, there is a sudden concomitant increase in blood flow to the dilated vasculature and the net effect can be hyperperfusion to the brain with resultant edema. Presenting symptoms can include a throbbing, retro-orbital headache that lateralizes to the side of the intervention, nausea, vomiting, visual changes, focal motor deficits, and even seizures. Increased flow velocities by transcranial Doppler in symptomatic patients even in the absence of any significant findings on CT imaging are suggestive of hyperperfusion. Aggressive control of blood pressure is necessary to prevent this complication (*J Am Coll Cardiol.* 2004;43:1596–1601).

3 Answer B. The benefits of CEA in select patients with *symptomatic* carotid atherosclerosis (i.e., TIA, nondisabling stroke) have been well-documented by numerous randomized trials. The NASCET (North American Symptomatic Carotid Endarterectomy Trial) (*N Engl J Med.* 1991;325:445–453) was a prospective, multicenter study that randomized 396 patients with a history of hemispheric or retinal TIA or a nondisabling stroke in the 4 months before entry with stenosis of 70% to 99% in the symptomatic carotid artery to either medical therapy or CEA. Although CEA was associated with a significantly higher risk of death or stroke at 30 days (5.8% vs. 3.3%), this was countered by a significantly lower risk of major or fatal ipsilateral stroke (13.1% vs. 2.5%, *p* <0.001) as well as reduced risk of *any* ipsilateral stroke in the CEA group at 2-year follow-up. The overall benefit of CEA persisted even after perioperative stroke and death were included in the end point analysis. The European Carotid Artery Surgery Trial (*Lancet.* 1998;351:1379–1387) randomized 2,518 patients with symptomatic, ipsilateral carotid stenosis, and also found that despite a 7% 30-day rate of stroke or death, patients with severe stenosis (70% to 99%) treated with CEA had a significantly lower risk of ipsilateral stroke (2.8% vs. 16.8%, *p* <0.0001) by 3 years' follow-up. The benefit of CEA persisted even after including all perioperative strokes, death, or any other stroke in the analysis (12.3% vs. 21.9%). It is noteworthy that patients with mild stenosis (0% to 29%) did not realize significant benefit from CEA. Therefore, the patient *is* a good candidate for CEA given his recent TIA, and >80% stenosis of the ipsilateral carotid (A). The preceding data would suggest that he could anticipate a slightly increased risk of perioperative stroke or death, but would then likely be at a significantly reduced risk of ipsilateral or fatal stroke over the next 2 to 3 years (C). Currently, there is no evidence that CEA for *symptomatic* carotid stenosis reduces the risk of contralateral stroke.

4 **Answer E.** The efficacy of performing CEA in asymptomatic patients with significant carotid stenosis has been demonstrated by several randomized, multicenter, and prospective trials. The VA (Veterans Administration) Cooperative Study (*N Engl J Med.* 1993;329:221–227) randomized 444 asymptomatic, male patients shown to have ≥50% stenosis of a carotid artery to either standard medical therapy or CEA plus antiplatelet therapy. This was the first randomized trial to demonstrate a significant reduction in the combined incidence of ipsilateral neurologic events with surgical therapy (8% vs. 20.6%, *p* = 0.001) in the asymptomatic population. Similar findings were reported in the ACAS (Asymptomatic Carotid Atherosclerosis) trial (*JAMA.* 1995;273:1421–1428) where 1,662 asymptomatic patients with >60% carotid stenosis were randomized to CEA plus 325 mg aspirin versus aspirin alone. After nearly 3 years of follow-up, it was estimated that the 5-year aggregate risk of ipsilateral stroke, and any perioperative stroke or death was 5.1% versus 11.0% favoring surgical therapy

(RRR 53%, 95% CI, [22% to 72%]). Contributing further evidence to support surgical therapy in asymptomatic individuals, the ACST (Asymptomatic Carotid Surgery Trial) (*Lancet.* 2004;363:1491–1502) randomized 3,120 asymptomatic patients younger than 75 years with 60% or greater carotid stenosis to either immediate CEA or indefinite referral with similar medical management in both groups. Significant reductions in the net 5-year risk of stroke or perioperative death were reported in the CEA arm (6.4 vs. 11.8, 95% CI, [2.96% to 7.75%]) despite a 30-day, 3.1% risk of perioperative stroke or death. There was also a significant reduction in the rates of *both* ipsilateral, and contralateral stroke in the CEA arm; however, this reduction was not evident until 2 years postprocedurally, and was not significant for patients older than 75 years. Although SAPPHIRE study included asymptomatic patients, FDA has not approved carotid stenting for the treatment of asymptomatic patients.

On the basis of the balance of evidence, the AAN (American Academy of Neurology) has recommended that it is reasonable to pursue CEA in asymptomatic patients with carotid stenosis >60%, *if* surgical risk of stroke or death is <3%, *and* the patient's life expectancy is >5 years. Should the surgical risk approach 3% to 5%, it is appropriate to pursue CEA in patients with *bilateral* carotid stenosis >75%. However, if the risk of surgical revascularization approaches 5% to 10%, CEA should not be offered (*Neurology.* 2005;65:794–801).

5 **Answer D.** Although the rate of periprocedural stroke has been significantly reduced by the use of EPD, this is still a serious complication of CAS. Randomized trials comparing CAS with and without EPDs are not likely because of obvious ethical concerns; however, multiple retrospective studies have suggested efficacy of EPD in the prevention of stroke during CAS (*Stroke.* 2003;34:813–819, *Eur Heart J.* 2004;25:1550–1558).

Although there is a risk of distal embolization of dislodged debris during all the preceding noted portions of the intervention, postdilatation of the stent poses the greatest risk. Although postdilatation of heavily *calcified* lesions can result in the displacement of calcific plaque debris with subsequent embolization, lesions composed of softer plaque materials may respond to overaggressive postdilatation by extrusion of the plaque contents with resultant embolization.

6 **Answer D.** Filter-type devices are usually composed of a polyurethane netting with a fixed pore space (from 80 to 140 micrometers) fitted over a titanium-nickel (nitinol) frame and are currently the most widely used of the EPDs. In practice, the filter is delivered across the carotid lesion in a collapsed form on a 0.014-inch guidewire. Optimum positioning of the filter depends upon deployment in a portion of the vessel that is straight, and free of significant disease. This is frequently found in the prepetrous portion of the cervical ICA, which is usually straight and free of disease. An advantage of the filter-type device is that it allows continuous antegrade blood flow during the intervention. It also allows adequate visualization of the artery during the procedure with dye injection.

Distal occlusion balloon devices are the next most common form of EPD. This device functions through a balloon that is inflated and deflated through a crush-resistant nitinol hypotube situated in a 0.014-inch guidewire. After crossing the stenotic lesion, a marker on the device is placed in the prepetrous portion of the cervical ICA. Subsequent to proper positioning, the balloon is inflated resulting in cessation of all antegrade blood flow. Following the intervention, the column of blood immediately proximal to the balloon is aspirated through a monorail export system thereby removing any debris dislodged during instrumentation.

Yet another system to prevent embolization during procedure includes a proximal occlusion device that creates retrograde flow in the ICA by establishing a continuous pressure gradient between the ICA and the femoral vein. This is accomplished by occluding both the proximal CCA and external carotid artery (ECA) with balloon-mounted catheters resulting in cessation of antegrade flow. Blood is aspirated from the CCA through the catheter tip distal to the balloon, and is returned to the femoral vein through a blood return system resulting in a continuous retrograde flow of blood in the ICA, and removal of all plaque debris from cerebral circulation. However, all of them have a greater number of embolization events as recorded by transcranial Doppler than CEA (*Manual of peripheral vascular intervention*. 2005).

7 **Answer D.** Participation in a formal exercise rehabilitation program results in a significant improvement in the time to claudication pain, and the time to maximal pain as demonstrated by Gardner and Poehlman in their meta-analysis of 33 trials evaluating walking distances in patients with PAD before and after rehabilitation. Program characteristics that were noted to correlate to increased pain-free distances were exercise duration >30 minutes per session, participation in at least three sessions per week, walking as a mode of exercise, and the use of

near-maximal claudication pain as an endpoint, with participation in the program of >6 months. The only independent predictors of increased walking distances were the use of the claudication endpoint, program length, and mode of exercise ($p = 0.001$) (*JAMA*. 1995;274:975–980).

On the basis of the results of numerous studies detailing the elevated crude rates of coronary heart disease (CHD) in patients with PAD, the current NCEP/ATP III (National Cholesterol Education Program/Adult Treatment Panel III) recommendations consider PAD as a CHD *risk equivalent*, and advise that the goal LDL-C be lowered to <100 mg per dL with consideration of drug therapy in addition to lifestyle modifications to achieve this goal (*Circulation*. 2004;110:227–239). The Heart Protection Study (HPS) prospectively randomized 20,536 patients with either CAD, diabetes mellitus (DM), or PAD to either simvastatin 40 mg once daily versus placebo, and reported a reduction in all-cause mortality of 13% ($p = 0.0003$), major vascular events by 24%, coronary death by 18%, and nonfatal or fatal stroke by 25%. Most strikingly, the reduction in the event rates was also observed in the subgroups of patients *without* known coronary disease, including those with diabetes, cerebrovascular disease, and PAD (*Lancet*. 2002;360:1623–1630).

Abnormal ABIs (<0.9), as a noninvasive diagnostic tool for PAD, have been shown to be associated with other traditional cardiovascular risk factors as well as more than a threefold increase in CHD and CVD mortality. In a prospective cohort study of 1,537 patients with systolic hypertension, 25.5% of participants recorded an ABI of <0.9. Abnormal ABI was statistically associated with the presence of other typical CAD risk factors. After 1- to 2-years follow-up, the presence of an abnormal ABI had an increased age–sex adjusted relative risk of mortality because of CHD of 3.8 (95% CI, [2.1 to 6.9]), CVD of 3.7 (95% CI, [1.8 to 7.7]), and total mortality of 4.1 (95% CI, [2 to 8.3]) (*JAMA*. 1993;270:487–489).

Currently, the only FDA-approved medications labeled for the purpose of relief of claudication because of PAD are pentoxifylline and cilostazol. Cilostazol, a type III phosphordiesterase inhibitor with direct action on the platelets and vascular smooth muscle, functions as a potent antiplatelet agent as well as vasodilator. A meta-analysis of eight randomized, placebo-controlled trials encompassing 2,702 patients with moderate to severe claudication demonstrated that cilostazol increased maximal and pain-free walking distances by 50% and 67% respectively (*Am J Cardiol*. 2002;90:1314–1319). Pentoxifylline, known to function by reducing the red blood cell viscosity, was shown to increase the pain-free walking distance by a mean of 29.4 m (95% CI, [13.0 to 45.9 m]), and the absolute claudication distance by a mean of 48.4 m (95% CI, [18.3 to 78.6 m]) in a total of 612 patients with moderate, intermittent claudication symptoms at baseline (*CMAJ.* 1996;155:1053–1059). Another study, however, indicated that cilostazol was more effective than pentoxifylline for increasing pain-free walking distances, but was associated with a greater incidence of side effects such as diarrhea and headache (*Am J Med.* 2000;109:523–530).

8 **Answer D.** The current American Heart Association (AHA) guidelines recommend that percutaneous endovascular interventions be reserved for patients who have developed severe, incapacitating, intermittent claudication that significantly interferes with their lifestyle or work. Additional indications include the development of rest pain, presence of nonhealing ulcerations or wounds, or the development of lower extremity gangrene. Most patients with angiographic evidence of obstructive SFA disease *do not* have significant claudication symptoms and therefore do not warrant peripheral intervention on the basis of the presence of lesions alone (*J Am Coll Cardiol.* 2006;47:1239–1312).

9 **Answer B.** Given that the long-term patency rates following infrapopliteal angioplasty are inferior to that of the larger vessels above the knee, percutaneous transluminal angioplasty (PTA) should be reserved for situations of acute limb ischemia (ALI), nonhealing wounds, or for limb salvage in patients who are not surgical candidates. Medical therapy with antiplatelet agents, such as aspirin, clopidogrel, or cilostazol should be the first line of therapy. In addition to participation in a formal exercise rehabilitation program, risk factor modification including the aggressive management of diabetes, and the cessation of tobacco use are also essential. Although the rate of progression to eventual limb loss or severe ischemia is 2% per year, diabetic patients with claudication symptoms have a greater likelihood of progressing to rest pain, developing gangrene, and eventual limb loss. Smokers also have increased rates of disease progression and have a 20% risk of limb loss if they continue to smoke (*J Am Coll Cardiol.* 2006;47:1239–1312).

Although vessel perforation or thrombosis can occur during any interventional procedure involving a lower extremity vessel, the complication rate of PTA in the infrapopliteal vascular bed is not prohibitively high and, as noted in the preceding text, has clear indications. In a recent study evaluating the efficacy of below-the-knee stent-supported angioplasty to establish inline arterial flow in 82 patients with critical limb ischemia (68%) or lifestyle limiting claudication (32%), the technical success rate was 94% for *de novo* lesions, and there were no major adverse events such as death, MI, or limb loss reported. In addition, there was a significant increase ($p = 0.0001$) in the ABIs of both the groups following intervention, as well as a subjective improvement in wound healing and decreased rest pain (*J Am Coll Cardiol.* 2004;44:2307–2314).

10 **Answer B.** This patient's presentation is consistent with that of ALI and should be treated as a medical emergency. Timely diagnosis and the institution of an appropriate therapy is crucial to prevent limb loss and even death with the 30-day mortality rates approaching 15%, and amputation rates between 15% and 30%. ALI is most frequently because of *in situ* thrombosis in the setting of preexistent atherosclerosis or embolism from a proximal source. All of the treatment modalities listed in the preceding text are utilized for this condition; however, the delivery of thrombolytic therapy for the treatment of ALI should be *catheter-based*, not intravenous. This is because of the data showing increased rates of significant hemorrhage, and less successful target-vessel patency with the use of intravenous thrombolytics as opposed to intra-arterial delivery. Percutaneous mechanical thrombectomy is largely reserved for patients with contraindications to thrombolysis, but is also useful in debulking thrombus mass before thrombolytic therapy or for rescue therapy after failed lysis (*J Vasc Interv Radiol.* 2005;16:585–595). Because of the large number of medical comorbidities that usually accompany patients with ALI, surgical treatment of ALI carries significant risk of mortality with figures approaching 30% in some series (*J Vasc Interv Radiol.* 1996;7:57–63).

11 **Answer E.** The vast majority of RAS is because of either atherosclerotic disease or FMD, and is estimated to be present in up to 5% of hypertensive patients. In addition, RAS may be noted in up to 30% to 40% of patients with documented atherosclerosis of other vascular beds (*N Engl J Med.* 2001;344:431–442). Atherosclerotic renal disease (>90% of RAS) typically involves the ostium or proximal third of the renal artery, progresses with age, and is known to be associated with hypertension and renal insufficiency (*N Engl J Med.* 2001;344:431–442). FMD (<10% of RAS) is most commonly found in women aged 15 to 50 years, and involves the distal two thirds of the vessel with a characteristic "string of beads" appearance on angiography (*N Engl J Med.* 2004;350:1862–1871). In addition to the preceding indications, other indications for renal arteriography include azotemia without clear etiology in a patient with evidence of atherosclerotic disease in other vascular beds, malignant hypertension refractory to the addition of three of more antihypertensive medications, or unexplained renal failure. Although it is generally a safe and well-tolerated procedure, renal arteriography should only be considered for patients in whom the operator has strong clinical suspicion of renovascular disease. Although uncommon, complications of renal arteriography include atheroembolism, renal artery ostial trauma, dissection, and contrast nephrotoxicity. Performing routine angiography of the renal vasculature in a patient without one of the preceding indications is not recommended.

12 **Answer E.** Given the paucity of randomized data comparing percutaneous intervention to medically based therapy for the treatment of RAS, there remains controversy over the exact indications for renal artery intervention. Because of the rather high perioperative mortality rate associated with surgical revascularization (2% to 13% in varying reports), percutaneous revascularization is currently preferred over surgical intervention. In RAS secondary to atherosclerosis, stenting yields superior results to angioplasty alone and is definitely indicated for ostial lesions, restenosis, suboptimal results after angioplasty (>30% residual stenosis, gradient >15 mm Hg), or in cases complicated by dissection (*Lancet.* 1999;353:282–286). In RAS because of FMD, hypertension can typically be managed successfully with medical therapy including angiotensin-converting enzyme (ACE) inhibitors, and percutaneous intervention is not necessary. In situations where intervention is required, *angioplasty alone* provides a cure rate approaching 80%.

Therefore, in the presence of significant RAS (lesion >70% or >15 mm Hg pressure gradient), evidence of CHF, progressive or endstage renal disease and malignant or medically refractory hypertension are the indications to proceed with percutaneous intervention. The mere presence of RAS that is *not* associated with any of the above is not an indication for intervention.

13 **Answer C.** The data on the efficacy of percutaneous revascularization in patients with renovascular hypertension have been conflicting. Van Jaarsveld et al. (*N Engl J Med.* 2000;342:1007–1014) conducted the largest randomized trial where 106 patients with hypertension who had atherosclerotic RAS ≥50%, and a serum creatinine concentration ≤2.3 mg per dL were randomized to receive drug therapy

or percutaneous intervention (balloon angioplasty). The results revealed no significant difference in either systolic or diastolic blood pressure at 3 months; however, the patients in the angioplasty group were taking significantly fewer daily doses of antihypertensive medications as compared with the medical therapy group (2.1 ± 1.3 and 3.2 ± 1.5 respectively; $p \leq 0.001$). At its completion, however, the trial failed to demonstrate any significant difference between the groups with regard to either the amount of antihypertensive medication use or blood pressure control. This could be partly because of the large number of patients (22) who crossed over from the medical therapy group to receive percutaneous intervention because of poorly controlled hypertension despite more than three medications. More recent data from a meta-analysis including 210 patients with >50% unilateral or bilateral atherosclerotic RAS and poorly controlled hypertension found that balloon angioplasty was significantly more effective than medications alone in the reduction of both the systolic (mean difference −7 mm Hg; 95% CI, [−12 to −1]) and diastolic (−3 mm Hg; 95% CI, [−6 to −1]) blood pressure. In addition, at the conclusion of the trial, patients in the angioplasty group were on significantly fewer antihypertensive medications (*Am J Med.* 2003;114:44–50).

Although randomized data is lacking in this population, results from numerous retrospective studies have reported success rates >80% for angioplasty alone in patients (usually women) with renovascular hypertension because of FMD. In a retrospective cohort study following 69 patients with hypertension and FMD undergoing angioplasty, technical success was reported in 95% with a significant decrease in blood pressure at discharge (174 ± 33/100 ± 13 to 138 ± 19/80 ± 15 mm Hg; $p < 0.0001$), and was maintained for >7 years later (140 ± 25/83 ± 12 mm Hg; $p < 0.0001$) (*J Hum Hypertens.* 2005;19:761–767).

Given the suboptimal outcomes often seen with angioplasty of aorto-ostial and proximal renal arterial lesions, the use of angioplasty with stenting has become a common practice in many institutions. In a prospective study of 85 patients with ostial atherosclerotic RAS randomized to either angioplasty plus stenting or angioplasty alone, the primary success rate of angioplasty was 57% as compared with 88% in the stenting group (31%; 95% CI, [12 to 50]) with no significant differences in the complication rate (*Lancet.* 1999;353:282–286). This difference was maintained through the 6-month follow-up with primary patency rate of angioplasty reported at 29% as compared with 75% in the stent group (46%; 95% CI, [24 to 68]). Similar to the clinical experience, restenosis was reported in 48% of the angioplasty group as opposed to only 14% in the stenting group (34%; 95% CI, [11 to 58]); however, after rescue stenting, long-term follow-up of vessel patency was similar in both groups.

It has been shown that among patients with unilateral RAS and renovascular hypertension, the use of ACEIs are particularly effective for blood pressure control, especially in patients with unilateral RAS (*Am J Kidney Dis.* 1999;33:675–681). Although the vasodilatory effect on the glomerular efferent arteriole may result in a transglomerular pressure drop, this is usually compensated for by the contralateral kidney and results in a stable serum creatinine. It should be noted, however, that acute renal failure can result from the use of ACEI in the setting of RAS, and the patients treated in this fashion require a close and serial follow-up.

14 Answer C. The short-term results from the EVAR in patients with AAA (EVAR-1) trial that randomized 1,082 patients aged 60 years and older with aneurysms >5.5 cm in diameter to either surgical or endovascular repair showed a significant reduction in 30-day mortality in the endovascular repair group (1.6% vs. 4.7%, 0.33 [0.15 to 0.74], $p = 0.007$) (*Lancet.* 2004;364:843–848). However, a recent publication of the long-term follow-up data from EVAR-1 revealed that 4 years after randomization, all-cause mortality between the groups was similar with that of the *endovascular* repair group experiencing higher overall rates of complication (17.6/100 person years vs. 3.3/100 person years, 95% CI, [3.5 to 6.8], $p <0.0001$), and needed reintervention (6.9/100 person years vs. 2.4/100 person years, 95% CI, 2.7 [1.8 to 4.1], $p <0.0001$) (*Lancet.* 2005;365:2187–2192). Similar results were reported in the smaller Dutch Endovascular Aneurysm Management (DREAM) trial that randomized 351 patients with an aneurysm >5 cm to endovascular or open surgical repair. As in EVAR-1, there was a significant reduction in 30-day mortality in the endovascular group (1.2% vs. 4.6%; 95% CI, [0.1 to 4.2]), but this difference was no longer significant by 6 months' follow-up (*N Engl J Med.* 2004;351:1607–1618). Although the recently published long-term follow-up results of the DREAM trial revealed a significant reduction in aneurysm-related mortality benefiting the endovascular group (2.1 vs. 5.7; 95% CI, [−0.5 to 7.9]), there was no significant difference in the *cumulative survival* between endovascular and open repair groups (89.7% vs. 89.6%). In contrast to the EVAR-1 trial, however, the rates of severe complication, aneurysm rupture, and reintervention were similar in both groups (*N Engl J Med.* 2005;352:2398–2405).

Clear delineation of aneurysmal anatomy is critical for the proper selection of endovascular repair candidates. The following are anatomic inclusion criteria for endovascular repair: Presence of a patent SMA or celiac trunk, an infrarenal neck diameter <28 mm (to allow for oversizing of the graft by up to 20%, maximal graft size is 32 mm), length of the proximal neck at least 10 to 15 mm to allow for adequate seal of the graft, neck angulation of <45 to 60 degrees to reduce the incidence of endoleak, calcification, or intramural thrombus involving <90 degrees the circumference of the vessel, minimal diameter of the iliac vessels 6 to 7 mm to allow for passage of the delivery system, and distal neck >10 to 15 mm for adequate fixation of the distal portion of the graft (*Manual of peripheral vascular intervention.* 2005:187–188). However, all these are subject to change with the emergence of new devices.

Although there is no randomized data to support the optimum time for aneurysmal repair, general expert opinion suggests that the larger the aneurysm, the greater the risk of rupture. Other independent risk factors for AAA rupture include COPD, hypertension, female gender, smoking, and symptoms including abdominal tenderness or back pain. Additionally, aneurysms that expand >0.6 cm in 1 year are at a high risk of rupture. Therefore, this patient would likely not do well with medical management and should be strongly considered for repair, either surgical or endovascular.

15 Answer E. A dreaded complication, SCI is an infrequent complication of open surgical repair of *thoracic* aortic aneurysm (TAA) repair, although it can be seen following endovascular repair as well. SCI is not a complication of AAA repair. Option A describes a type I endoleak, which can be because of undersizing of the stent, poor proximal or distal fixation, neck dilation, stent fracture or separation, or aneurysms with short, angulated necks. With rare exceptions, the presence of a type I endoleak requires immediate treatment that could include stenting at the location of the leak, further angioplasty of the graft, or open surgical repair. Option B describes a type II endoleak, which is considered a more benign complication with treatment typically reserved for cases where the aneurysmal sac continues to enlarge. Option C describes a type IV endoleak that is most commonly seen in conjunction with thin-walled Dacron grafts, and is also not thought to be at high risk for causing significant clinical complications. Not mentioned in the preceding text is type III endoleak that results from limb separation or fabric wear, and may require the deployment of an additional cuff to adequately treat. As one might expect, embolization of thrombus or plaque debris during EVAR is a feared, but an unfortunately real complication that can result in ischemia of any distal vascular bed. Perforation and/or dissections of the iliac artery are fortunately decreasing in recent years partly because of increased flexibility and easier insertion of the delivery device (*Br J Surg.* 2005;92:937–946).

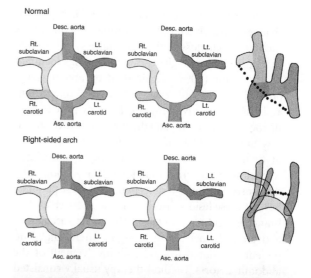

16 Answer D. The group of symptoms described in the preceding text is referred to as the *subclavian steal syndrome*, and can often be confused for TIA, stroke, migraine headache, intracranial mass, or temporal arteritis. The etiology of the symptom complex is vertebrobasilar insufficiency due to the presence of a proximal subclavian stenosis that results in retrograde blood flow in the ipsilateral vertebral artery. In addition to the symptoms mentioned in the preceding text, common presenting symptoms are that of upper extremity claudication, paresthesia, numbness, ataxia, confusion, diplopia, nystagmus, and visual symptoms. A rare, but well-documented phenomenon, is that of coronary steal due to retrograde blood flow in the ipsilateral internal mammary artery thereby causing ischemia in the targeted coronary vascular bed. Indications for revascularization of the subclavian artery include symptomatic steal syndromes, disabling upper extremity weakness, vertebrobasilar insufficiency, preservation of flow to the *in situ* internal mammary grafts, or evidence of embolic phenomenon in the upper extremities thought secondary to the subclavian disease. The presence of subclavian disease in the *absence* of symptoms is *not* an indication for intervention and should be avoided. Although ultrasound and magnetic resonance angiography (MRA) can help diagnose this problem, angiography would be the most efficient and precise strategy to diagnose and treat the subclavian steal syndrome (*Manual of peripheral vascular intervention.* 2005:123–125).

17 Answer A. There are many different variations of the right-sided aortic arch. The most commonly seen right-sided aortic arch has the left carotid as the first branch. The left subclavian is the last branch. The easiest way to understand the right-sided aortic arch is to be familiar with embryology. As shown in the following figures, normally, the segment between the *right subclavian* and the *descending aorta* disappears, but in right-sided arch that is most commonly encountered with in adults, the segment between the *left carotid* and *subclavian* disappears.

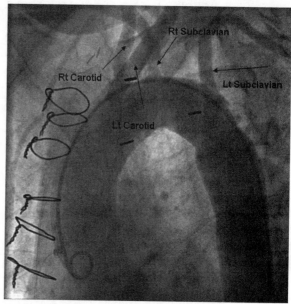

18 Answer D. The clinical presentation described in the preceding text is consistent with Takayasu's arteritis—a chronic, idiopathic disease that is characterized by inflammation of the aorta and its main branches. The disease affects almost exclusively female patients, is more common in Asian persons, and the mean age at presentation is 25 years. The symptoms at clinical presentation are because of the limb or organ ischemia due to the progressive stenosis of involved arteries. In a prospective cohort study of 60 patients with confirmed Takayasu's arteritis after a mean follow-up of 5.3 years (*Ann Intern Med.* 1994;120:919–929) it was reported that the most common presenting symptoms included arm claudication (63%), light-headedness (33%), visual changes (often bilateral), constitutional complaints such as weight loss and fever, and less commonly chest pain and myalgias. Physical findings included carotid bruit (80%), diminished or absent radial pulse (53%), carotodynia (32%), visual aberration, and less commonly aortic insufficiency (due to aortic root inflammation and distention). Hypertension was noted in 33% of the patients at some point of their disease course and was highly associated with either unilateral or bilateral RAS. Angiography demonstrated aortic lesions in 65% of these patients, 32% of these lesions involved the aortic arch and its branches, and 68% involved the aortic vasculature above *and* below the diaphragm. Interestingly, no patient was noted to have sole involvement of the abdominal aorta. Medical therapy usually consisted of oral steroids dosed at 1 mg per kg for up to 3 months with the addition of a cytotoxic agent such as cyclophosphamide or azathioprine, if the steroid dose is unable to be weaned. Surgical treatment was indicated in patients with refractory hypertension due to RAS, extremity ischemia, cerebrovascular ischemia or critical (>70%) stenosis of at least three cerebral vessels, moderate or severe aortic regurgitation, or cardiac ischemia due to angiographically proven coronary artery stenosis. Angioplasty was less commonly performed, and was most often employed in the revascularization of the subclavian and renal vessels. Approximately half of the interventions were successful on the first attempt and only one third on the second with restenosis being a common problem.

19 **Answer C.** Originating from the anterior portion of the aorta inferior to the aortic hiatus of the diaphragm, the celiac artery is a short arterial trunk that courses anteriorly, and divides into three larger branches—the left gastric, the hepatic, and the splenic arteries.

The smallest of the three vessels, the left gastric artery, courses superiorly and branches into numerous subdivisions to provide blood flow to portions of the esophagus and the cardiac portion of the stomach before passing along the less curvature of the stomach to the pylorus where it commonly anastomoses with the right gastric artery.

The hepatic artery courses to the porta hepatis, and branches into the right and left hepatic arteries, thereby supplying blood flow to both lobes of the liver.

Running along the greater curvature of the stomach, the right gastroepiploic artery anastomoses

with the left gastroepiploic branch of the splenic artery and provides blood flow to both surfaces of the stomach. Given its large caliber and close proximity to the inferior aspect of the heart, the right gastroepiploic artery is amenable to grafting to the distal right coronary artery (RCA) and PDA as is seen in the preceding angiogram.

The SMA and IMA are large branches that arise from the aorta inferior to the celiac trunk and are not visualized in this angiogram. (*Anatomy of the Human Body*, 1918).

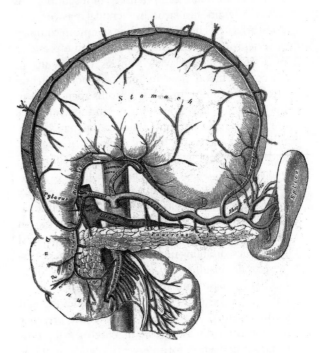

20 **Answer F.** Although the technical success rate for percutaneous renal artery stenting varies according to both operator and institutional experience, all of the preceding events are known complications of this procedure. In one of the largest case series of complications related to renal artery stenting, Ivonovik et al. documented the outcome of 171 patients undergoing 179 consecutive renal artery interventions and reported an overall rate of major complications in >8.4% of cases. Creatinine elevation persisting for >30 days occurred in 5.6% of patients, with 2.2% of patients requiring hemodialysis within that period. Of these cases 4.6% were complicated by pseudoaneurysms of the groin, 2.8% by renal infarction, 2.2% by aortic dissection at the level of the renal artery, and 1.7% by renal artery perforation (*J Vasc Interv Radiol.* 2003;14:217–225).

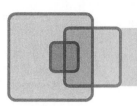

28

Cerebrovascular Interventions

Nezar Falluji and Debabrata Mukherjee

Questions

1 All the following statements pertaining to strokes are true, *except*:

(A) Of all strokes, 88% are ischemic in etiology and 12% are hemorrhagic

(B) When on aspirin, the risk of stroke in an asymptomatic patient with carotid stenosis <60% is 1.6% per year. The risk is approximately 3.2% per year among those with stenosis >60%

(C) Among patients with symptomatic carotid disease (those with prior transient ischemic attack [TIA] or strokes), the risk of recurrence is approximately 30% to 35% at 5 years

(D) Half of the men older than the age of 75 years have carotid atherosclerosis with stenosis over 50% detected in >30% of cases by ultrasound

2 In assessing carotid artery atherosclerosis, all the following statements are true, *except*:

(A) When performed by a trained sonographer, the sensitivity and specificity of Doppler ultrasonography and B-mode imaging approaches 90% accuracy compared with angiography

(B) Peak end-diastolic velocity above 135 cm per second and peak end-systolic velocity above 240 cm per second are suggestive of stenosis >80%

(C) Carotid duplex scans are very useful in assessing near complete occlusive lesions

(D) Contrast-enhanced magnetic resonance angiography is superior to carotid duplex in assessing long internal carotid lesions (>3 cm)

(E) Angiography should be used when the results of the noninvasive tests are inconclusive, yield conflicting results and/or if percutaneous intervention is planned

3 The following are true, *except*:

(A) In the Aspirin in Carotid Endarterectomy (ACE) trial, high dose aspirin (650 to 1000 mg per day) was superior to low dose aspirin (75 to 325 mg per day) in reducing the risk of stroke, myocardial infarction (MI), or death at 30 and 90 days following carotid endarterectomy (CEA)

(B) In the Clopidogrel versus Aspirin in Patients at Risk for Ischemia Events (CAPRIE) trial, clopidogrel (75 mg per day) was not superior to aspirin (325 mg) in reducing the risk of stroke, MI, or vascular death

(C) In the Clopidogrel in Unstable angina to prevent Recurrent Events (CURE) trial, which included 12,562 patients with acute coronary syndrome, the combination of aspirin and clopidogrel (when compared with aspirin alone) resulted in a 20% relative risk reduction of stroke, MI, or vascular death

(D) In the physician health study (a primary prevention study of 22,071 patients), aspirin (325 mg per day) resulted in 10% relative risk reduction of ischemic stroke

4 The following render CEA difficult or not feasible, *except*:

(A) Prior radiation to the neck or previous radical neck surgery

(B) Severe tandem lesion

(C) Aorto-ostial or proximal common carotid artery lesion

(D) Lesion location is distal cervical (C2 level and above)

5 The advantages of the PercuSurge Balloon distal embolization protection device when compared with filter devices include the following, *except*:

(A) Mimics standard guide wires more than other filters
(B) Ability to cross severe lesions
(C) Particles of all sizes can be blocked
(D) Easier to use than most filters

6 A 59-year-old woman with a history of coronary artery disease and prior left CEA presented with a history of two episodes of slurred speech and right-sided weakness. These episodes lasted for <1 hour and the patient recovered completely. The patient's medications include aspirin, lisinopril, and atorvastatin. A carotid angiogram is shown in the following figure. The most appropriate option for management of this patient is as follows:

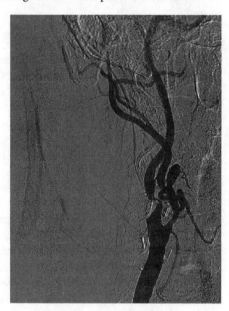

(A) Repeat CEA
(B) Carotid artery stenting (CAS)
(C) Add clopidogrel to the current regimen
(D) Initiate warfarin

7 Predictors of restenosis following carotid artery stenting include the following, *except*:

(A) Age >75
(B) Female sex
(C) Number of stents used
(D) Diabetes

8 The following are considered high-risk factors during CAS, but stenting is still considered feasible, *except* in:

(A) Age >75
(B) Type-3 aortic arch

(C) Pedunculated thrombus
(D) Stenosis involving the ostium of the internal carotid artery (ICA)

9 In patients with vertebrobasilar insufficiency, the following are true, *except*:

(A) The data is limited to case series on the role of percutaneous intervention
(B) Embolic events involving the brain stem can be life threatening
(C) Approximately 25% of patients with vertebrobasilar insufficiency have an associated significant carotid artery disease, the management of which may relieve the symptoms
(D) The risk of recurrent stroke in the acute phase of a vertebrobasilar TIA is low; however, the risk is high for recurrent cerebrovascular diseases (CVA) on longer term follow-up

10 The following factors have been reported as possible predictors of persistent hypotension following carotid stenting, *except*:

(A) History of MI
(B) Distance from the carotid bifurcation <10 mm
(C) History of ipsilateral CEA
(D) Intraprocedural hypotension

11 A 67-year-old man with a history of hypertension, prior radiation to the neck in the context of thyroid cancer, and hyperlipidemia presents with recurrent short-lived episodes of visual loss in his left eye. His electrocardiogram shows normal sinus rhythm with left ventricular hypertrophy. A bilateral carotid duplex study was done, which was suggestive of total occlusion of the right ICA and severe stenosis of the

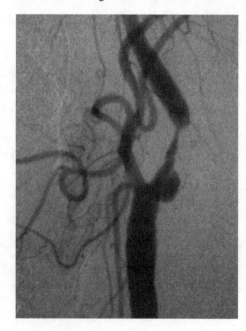

left ICA. A carotid angiogram was done as in the figure on the previous page. What is the best route of action in the management of this patient?

(A) Proceed with CAS

(B) Arrange a vascular surgery consultation for possible CEA

(C) Initiate anticoagulation with heparin followed by Coumadin for 6 weeks with reevaluation and angiography at that time

(D) Initiate anticoagulation and plan reevaluation with angiography in 48 hours

12 A 61-year-old man was referred to the interventional cardiology service for a second opinion regarding the management of a newly diagnosed carotid disease. The patient underwent, before his referral, a carotid duplex study to assess newly recognized bruits over the left carotid artery. This study was soon followed with an angiography by the local cardiology group figure. The patient has been experiencing occasional headache over the past 2 months. His blood pressure (BP) is 140/88 mm Hg in your office. His total cholesterol is 220 and his low-density lipoprotein (LDL) is 150. The patient was advised to consider undergoing CEA. What would be your recommendation to this patient at this point?

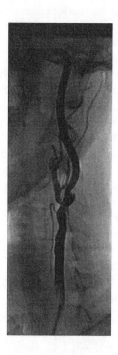

(A) Undergo endarterectomy as he is at a low risk (<4%) for such procedure

(B) Proceed with carotid stenting with the use of a filter wire to protect the distal circulation

(C) Initiate aspirin 162 mg PO q.d., atorvastatin 80 mg PO q.h.s., and ramipril 2.5 mg PO q.d.

(D) Initiate aspirin 162 mg PO q.d., clopidogrel 75 mg PO q.d., atorvastatin 80 mg PO q.h.s., and ramipril 2.5 mg PO q.d.

13 In the Stenting and Angioplasty with Protection in Patients at High Risk for Endarterectomy (SAPPHIRE) trial, carotid stenting was done with the following adjuvant therapy:

(A) Preloading with 300 mg of clopidogrel 24 hours before the procedure and 75 mg thereafter, aspirin 325 mg 24 hours before the procedure, with periprocedural heparin to achieve an activated clotting time (ACT) of 200 to 250 seconds

(B) Clopidogrel 75 mg, 24 hours before the procedure and 2 to 4 weeks thereafter, aspirin 81 to 325 mg per day starting at least 72 hours before the procedure, indefinitely thereafter, and periprocedural heparin to achieve an ACT of 250 to 300 seconds

(C) Loading the patient with clopidogrel 600 mg after placement of the stent, aspirin, weight-based eptifibatide infusion for 12 hours following a loading bolus dose, and periprocedural heparin to achieve an ACT of 275 to 300 seconds

(D) Preloading with 300 mg of clopidogrel 24 hours before the procedure and 75 mg thereafter, aspirin 325 mg, with periprocedural weight-based bivalirudin

14 With regard to the Desmoteplase In Acute ischemic Stroke (DIAS) trial the following statements are true, *except*:

(A) Desmoteplase is a highly fibrin-specific and non-neurotoxic agent

(B) Patients were enrolled if they presented within 3 hours of the onset of their CVA

(C) Patients were enrolled if they presented within 3 to 9 hours of the onset of their CVA

(D) In selecting the patients, a magnetic resonance imaging (MRI) evidence of perfusion/diffusion mismatch was needed to be eligible for enrollment in the trial

15 Following postdilatation of a carotid stent, the patient became acutely hemiparetic and aphasic. The following figure shows the sequence of angiography, stenting, and post dilatation of the stent. What would be the best route of action in this situation?

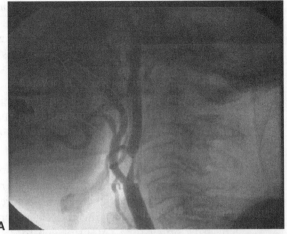

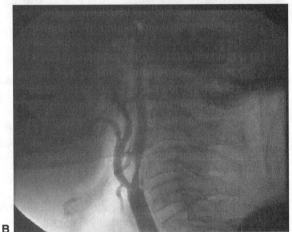

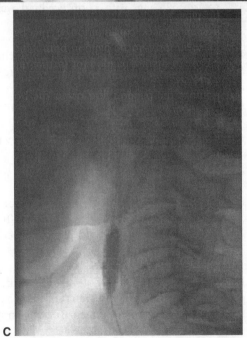

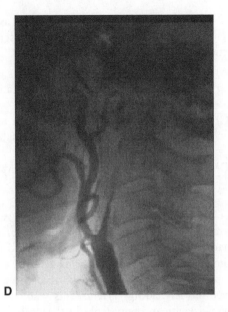

(A) Remove the filter wire and reassess

(B) Inject intra-carotid Urokinase

(C) Use a larger balloon to further dilate the stent

(D) Use an export catheter to aspirate

16 In patients with concomitant coronary artery disease and carotid disease the following are true, *except*:

(A) The risk of perioperative neurologic event following coronary artery bypass graft (CABG) is approximately 9% for individuals with ICA disease with >50% stenosis

(B) Randomized clinical trials have confirmed that carotid stenting followed by CABG (staged) carries the lowest risk for perioperative neurologic events when compared with simultaneous CEA and CABG (combined)

(C) Retrospective reports showed little difference between the staged and the combined approaches for revascularization

(D) Asymptomatic >75% ICA stenosis carries a 14% risk of perioperative stroke in the patient undergoing CABG

17 In assessing carotid artery severity according to the North American Symptomatic CEA Trial (NASCET) all the following statements are true, *except*:

(A) Percent Stenosis = (Presumed Normal Segment Diameter − Diseased Segment Diameter)/ Presumed Normal Segment Diameter × 100

(B) The normal segment is defined as the diameter of the segment just distal to the carotid bulb and not the carotid bulb itself or the poststenotic area distal to the lesion

(C) The normal segment is defined as the estimated diameter of the carotid bulb as it was before the atherosclerotic narrowing

(D) Percent of stenosis by the European Carotid Surgery Trial (ECST) is always more severe than the percent of stenosis given by the NASCET method

18 A 76-year-old diabetic patient with documented three-vessel disease underwent a carotid duplex study that was suggestive of total occlusion of the right ICA and high-grade left carotid artery disease. The surgeons are reluctant to proceed with CABG until the patient's left carotid artery is further assessed and treated. Carotid angiogram confirmed the total occlusion of the right ICA and the noted anatomy on the left carotid artery as in the following figure. What would be the best route of action among the following in this situation?

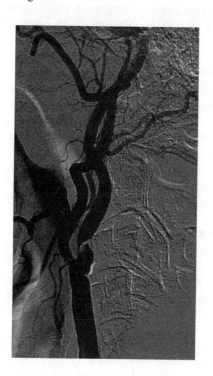

(A) Anticoagulation treatment for 1 month, then reassess the left ICA at that point

(B) Proceed with stenting with the placement of 7 F cook shuttle catheter to be placed in the common carotid artery, then cross the lesion with a 0.014-inch coronary guidewire, with subsequent predilatation, followed by stenting with a self-expanding stent

(C) CEA is the only option for such a lesion as it is unfavorable for carotid stenting

(D) Proceed with stenting with the placement of 7 F cook shuttle catheter to be placed in the common carotid artery, then cross the lesion with a filter based emboli protection device, followed by predilatation and then stenting with a self-expanding stent

19 In performing carotid stenting the following technical principles are recommended, *except*:

(A) A larger catheter should be advanced into the carotid in a step-wise and coaxial manner over a smaller catheter and always over a guide wire

(B) Predilatation is recommended to confirm the ability to adequately dilate the stenosis

(C) Self-expanding stents are preferred for the carotid bifurcation

(D) Self-expanding stents are preferred for ostial common carotid artery

Answers and Explanations

1 Answer D. It is true that half of the men older than age 75 have carotid atherosclerosis, but only 5% have stenosis >50% by ultrasound. The other statements are true (*Circulation.* 2006;113:e85–151).

2 Answer C. Carotid duplex is inferior to contrast-enhanced magnetic resonance angiography in assessing near-complete occlusive disease, calcified lesions, high carotid bifurcation, and long (>3 cm) lesions (*J Vasc Surg.* 2005;41:962–972, *Neuroimaging Clin N Am.* 2005;15:351–365, xi).

3 Answer A. In the ACE trial, the rate of stroke, MI, or death was lower in the low aspirin dose group than the high aspirin group (5% vs. 7% at 30 days and 6.2% vs. 8.4% at 90 days) (*Lancet.* 1999;353:2179–2184).

4 Answer B. CEA is generally technically challenging or not feasible in patients with prior radiation to the neck, prior neck surgery, ipsilateral CEA (the so-called hostile neck), and aorto-ostial or proximal common carotid disease. CEA is associated with higher risk in patients with restenosis following CEA, contralateral ICA occlusion, severe co-morbidities, and contralateral laryngeal nerve palsy. Severe tandem lesions can be effectively treated with endarterectomy.

5 Answer D. All the above are among the advantages of the PercuSurge guard wire balloon protection device, except that its use is rather cumbersome when compared with other filter wire systems (*Ann Thorac Surg.* 1990;49:179–186; discussion 186–187, *J Am Coll Cardiol.* 2002;40:890–895).

6 Answer B. The risk of a stroke is quite high in this patient with recurrent hemispheric TIA and a high-grade ICA disease (10% in the first year and approximately 30% in 5 years). Among the high-risk features for recurrent stroke are hemispheric TIA, recent TIA, increasing frequency of TIA, and high-grade carotid stenosis. The patient's anatomy is suitable for CAS, which may be the best route of action in this scenario. Prior CEA in this patient increases the risk of complications with a second CEA but may also be considered depending on local expertise. The use of clopidogrel or warfarin in addition to aspirin will offer the patients an inferior therapeutic intervention when compared with carotid artery revascularization. Although patients with restenosis following CEA were not included in the North American Symptomatic Carotid Endarterectomy Trial (NASCET) and Asymptomatic Carotid Atherosclerosis Study (ACAS) trials, such a history was a qualifying criterion for inclusion in the SAPPHIRE trial (*N Engl J Med.* 2004;351:1493–1501), which focused on high-risk patients with severe carotid disease and showed that CAS was noninferior to CEA.

7 Answer D. Restenosis (as assessed by ultrasound or repeated angiography) following CAS has been associated with the following variables: Female sex, age >75 and the number of stents used (*Am J Cardiol.* 2003;92:895–897). Of interest is that in CEA, female sex, age <60, hypertension, hyperlipidemia and smoking were associated with restenosis (*Am J Surg.* 1997;174:118–120).

8 Answer D. Presence of thrombus is an absolute contraindication for both CAS and CEA and neither should be attempted till thrombus is resolved.

9 Answer D. On the contrary, the risk of recurrent stroke is extremely high in the acute phase (up to 7 days after the presenting symptoms); however, the risk of death and stroke is relatively low thereafter (*Cochrane Database Syst Rev.* 2005:CD000516).

10 Answer C. Predictors of hypotension during and/or after carotid stenting include a history of MI, proximity to the carotid sinus, and intraprocedural hypotension (*Neurosurgery.* 2005;57:472–477; discussion 472–477, *Am J Surg.* 2005;190:691–695, *Neurosurgery.* 1999;44:1320–1323; discussion 1324).

11 Answer C. Presence of thrombus is an absolute contraindication for both CAS and CEA. Anticoagulation should be initiated and a reassessment with angiography should be postponed for at least 6 weeks.

12 Answer A. Although the efficacy of CAS in the management of low-risk severe asymptomatic carotid atherosclerosis is being evaluated (carotid revascularization endarterectomy versus stenting trial [CREST], Carotid and Vertebral Artery Transluminal Angioplasty Study -2 (CAVATAS-2) and secondary prevention of atherosclerosis through chlamydia pneumoniae eradication [SPACE]), CEA remains at this point the standard of care in the management of patients with severe asymptomatic carotid artery disease who are at an acceptable surgical risk (<4%). The risk of stroke in this patient (with >60% stenosis) is 3.2% per year. In the ACAS, 1,659 patients with asymptomatic carotid stenosis of at least 60% were randomized to CEA versus medical therapy. The perioperative stroke or death reported in this study was 2.3% (*JAMA.* 1995;273:1421–1428).

13 Answer B. Although, in the SAPPHIRE trial the protocol entailed giving the patients 75 mg of clopidogrel and 81 to 325 mg of aspirin 24 hours before the procedure (*N Engl J Med.* 2004;351:1493–1501), preloading with clopidogrel 300 mg and aspirin 325 mg before CAS is recommended (preferably >15 hours before the procedure) on the basis of the evidence derived from coronary artery stenting experience to achieve optimal platelets inhibition. The use of glycoprotein (GP) IIb/IIIa is controversial and is not recommended as routine adjunctive therapy for patients undergoing CAS. The use of bivalirudin in CAS has not been evaluated.

14 Answer B. The DIAS was a placebo-controlled, double-blind, randomized trial of 104 patients with National Institutes of Health Stroke Scale (NIHSS) scores of 4 to 20 and MRI evidence of perfusion/diffusion mismatch. Of these patients, the first 47 (referred to as Part 1) were randomized to fixed doses of desmoteplase (25 mg, 37.5 mg, or 50 mg) or placebo. To enhance recruitment, after the enrollment of nine patients, the baseline NIHSS range was extended from 8 to 20 to 4 to 20 and the onset-to-treatment time window was widened from 3 to 6 to 3 to 9 hours. Because of an excessive rate of symptomatic intracranial hemorrhage (sICH), lower weight-adjusted doses escalating through 62.5 µg per kg, 90 µg per kg, and 125 µg per kg were subsequently investigated in 57 patients (referred to as Part 2). The safety endpoint was the rate of sICH. Efficacy endpoints were the rate of reperfusion on MRI after 4 to 8 hours and clinical outcome as assessed by NIHSS, modified Rankin scale, and Barthel Index at 90 days. Part 1 was terminated prematurely because of high rates of sICH with desmoteplase (26.7%). In Part 2, the sICH rate was 2.2%. No sICH occurred with placebo in either part. Reperfusion rates up to 71.4% ($p = 0.0012$) were observed with desmoteplase (125 µg per kg) compared with 19.2% with placebo. A favorable 90-day clinical outcome was found in 22.2% of placebo-treated patients and between 13.3% (62.5 µg per kg; $p = 0.757$) and 60.0% (125 µg per kg; $p = 0.0090$)

of desmoteplase-treated patients. Early reperfusion correlated favorably with clinical outcome ($p = 0.0028$). Favorable outcome occurred in 52.5% of patients experiencing reperfusion versus 24.6% of patients without reperfusion (*Stroke.* 2005;36:66–73).

15 Answer D. No reflow is a serious complication of carotid stenting. It is attributed to a large thrombus burden that overwhelms the filter wire leading to stagnant forward circulation and essentially no flow distal to target lesion. Aspirating this thrombus column while the filter wire is in place is the recommended strategy in this situation. Retrieving the filter wire will release the thrombotic debris and result in distal embolization. The use of Urokinase can further complicate this precarious situation with intracerebral bleeding. Larger balloon inflation will not resolve this complication and is likely to result in dislodgement of more thrombotic debris distally (*Manual of peripheral vascular intervention.* 2005, *J Cardiovasc Surg Torino.* 2005;46:261–265).

16 Answer B. Evidence for the most appropriate strategy is derived from retrospective analysis. The risk of stroke is reported to be 3% to 4% in the staged approach as opposed to 2.8% to 3.3% in the simultaneous approach. The reversed staged approach (to proceed with CABG followed by CEA) is associated with 14% risk of stroke (*Ann Thorac Surg.* 1999;68: 14–20; discussion 21, *J Am Coll Cardiol.* 2005;45: 1538–1542).

17 Answer C. All the above are accurate statements with the exception of C. In the ECST, normal segment was defined as the estimated diameter of the carotid bulb as it was before the atherosclerotic narrowing as seen in the following figure (*Nebr Med J.* 1992;77:121–123, *J Mal Vasc.* 1993;18:198–201).

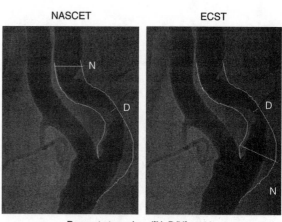

Percent stenosis = ([N–D/N] × 100)

NASCET = 67% stenosis   ECST = 84% stenosis

18 **Answer D.** Several mechanical approaches have been developed in an attempt to prevent distal embolization during carotid stenting. The use of distal balloon occlusive device (PercuSurge Guard-Wire, Medtronic, Santa Rosa, CA) has been studied in a large series of CAS reporting a 30-day stroke and death risk of 2.7% (*Ann Thorac Surg.* 1990;49:179–186; discussion 186–7). The use of Accunet (Guidant, Indianapolis, IN) was assessed in the ARCHER registry of 437 patients with symptomatic stenosis of at least 50% or asymptomatic stenosis of >80% but with high risk features of surgery. The composite risk of stroke, death, or MI at 30 days was reached in 7.8% in the overall cohort but was 1.4% in the 141 patients with restenosis following CEA. The use of embolic protection devices has not entirely eliminated periprocedural strokes. Such devices are not operational during the diagnostic phase of the procedure nor are they operational during the final phase of the procedure. There are also potential complications in the use of such devices, such as hemodynamic intolerance to balloon occlusion (with the PercuSurge), spasm or dissection, filer congestion with filter device, which may result in no reflow. Nevertheless, the use of such devices is widely adopted and recommended during CAS (*Int Angiol.* 2002;21: 344–348, *Indian Heart J.* 2001;53:445–450, *Acta Chir Belg.* 2004;104:65–70, *Ann Thorac Surg.* 1990;49:179–186; discussion 186–7, *Am J Neuroradiol.* 2005;26:854–861).

19 **Answer D.** Balloon expandable stents are for aorto-ostial disease. Self-expanding stents should be used for the carotid bifurcation and other compressible lesions.

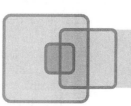

29

Valvuloplasty and Percutaneous Valve Replacement

Thomas Gehrig and Thomas M. Bashore

Questions

1 Each of the following disorders can cause an elevated gradient between the pulmonary capillary wedge pressure (PCW) and the left ventricular diastolic pressure, *except*:

(A) Mitral valve stenosis
(B) Primary pulmonary hypertension
(C) Pulmonary veno-occlusive disease
(D) Cor triatriatum
(E) Pulmonary vein stenosis

2 A 60-year-old woman with prior mitral commissurotomy for rheumatic mitral stenosis (MS) is undergoing percutaneous mitral valvuloplasty. Following an Inoue 28 mm balloon dilation of the mitral valve, the left atrium (LA) mean pressure rises and the accompanying pressure tracing is noted. The next most appropriate course of action is to:

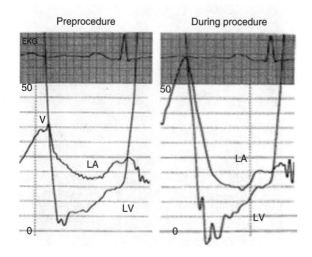

Preprocedure **During procedure**

(A) Remove the balloon and deem the procedure a success
(B) Upsize to a larger balloon for further dilation
(C) Place an intra-aortic balloon pump and obtain urgent surgery consultation if the patient is unstable
(D) Hemodynamically support with phenylephrine
(E) Re-zero the pressure transducer to ensure its accuracy

3 Each of the following characteristics is a component of the Massachusetts General Hospital (MGH) echocardiographic valve score, *except*:

(A) Mitral valve area (MVA)
(B) Leaflet mobility
(C) Valvular thickening
(D) Valvular calcification
(E) Subvalvular thickening and fibrosis

4 The following echocardiogram is obtained on a 40-year-old Hispanic woman with a prior history of rheumatic fever as a child. The echocardiographer noted mild calcium in the leaflet and commented on

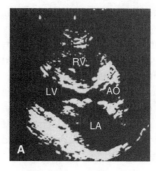
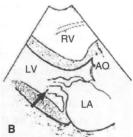

reduced leaflet mobility. The patient is experiencing progressive dyspnea with exertion. She is referred for possible percutaneous mitral valvuloplasty. She has had atrial fibrillation for 2 years. On the basis of the echocardiographic findings, you would suggest:

(A) Proceeding with percutaneous mitral valvuloplasty

(B) Increasing her diuretics and see her back in 4 to 5 weeks

(C) Trying to get her back in normal sinus rhythm by adding amiodarone and attempting direct current cardioversion

(D) Referring her for surgical valve replacement

(E) Referring her for surgical commissurotomy

5 The indications for percutaneous balloon valvuloplasty on a stenotic rheumatic mitral valve include all of the following, *except*:

(A) Progressive dyspnea on exertion

(B) New-onset atrial fibrillation

(C) Progressive increase in pulmonary hypertension

(D) Worsening mitral regurgitation (MR)

(E) Paroxysmal nocturnal dyspnea

6 A 55-year-old man presents to your office with severe right heart failure. He has an extensive history of prior cardiac surgeries, including a coronary artery bypass operation, a mitral valve replacement with a bileaflet mechanical mitral valve and a tricuspid valve replacement with a porcine bioprosthesis. He has no angina but has noted a progressive enlargement of the abdomen and peripheral edema above the knees. His valve surgery was performed 13 years ago, and he has done well until the last 6 to 8 months. An echocardiogram is obtained and his LV and right ventricular (RV) function are preserved, his mechanical mitral valve is functioning normally except for questionable MR and his bioprosthetic tricuspid valve has no regurgitation, but a mean gradient of 12 mm Hg. On the basis of these data, you would suggest:

(A) He needs a cardiac magnetic resonance imaging (MRI) to better assess his RV function, as echocardiography may be misleading in this situation

(B) He needs a cardiac catheterization to assess his pulmonary artery (PA) pressures, his coronary and graft anatomy, and the severity of his tricuspid stenosis. If confirmed, he should undergo percutaneous tricuspid valvuloplasty

(C) He needs a cardiac catheterization to assess his PA pressures, his coronary and graft anatomy, and the severity of this tricuspid stenosis. If confirmed, he should undergo redo tricuspid valve replacement

(D) He needs his diuretics increased, and an exercise sestamibi stress test performed to determine if he has ongoing coronary ischemia

7 Mrs G has had long-standing MS without MR and moderate aortic regurgitation with trivial aortic stenosis. She has had a progressive increase in dyspnea and palpitations and is brought to the cardiac catheterization lab for hemodynamic confirmation of her diagnosis. In the cardiac catheterization laboratory she is noted to have a heart rate of 62, a right atrial mean pressure of 5 mm Hg, a PA pressure of 55/25 with a mean of 35 mm Hg and a PCW pressure of 26 mm Hg. Her left ventricular end diastolic pressure (LVEDP) is 15 mm Hg. A mean mitral gradient of 9 mm Hg and an aortic mean gradient of 10 mm Hg are noted. Her cardiac output is 3 L per minute using Fick oximetry data from PA and femoral artery samples and an assumed oxygen consumption value. A left ventricular angiogram reveals no MR and normal LV systolic function. An aortic root angiogram reveals 2+ aortic regurgitation. The cardiology fellow in the laboratory determines that the MVA is 1.0 cm^2. Which of the following is a correct statement regarding the hemodynamics?

(A) She has both severe aortic stenosis and MS

(B) The MVA of 1.0 cm^2 is probably correct as determined

(C) The MVA is incorrect based on the data and should be approximately 2.1 cm^2 instead of 1.0 cm^2

(D) The associated aortic regurgitation makes it impossible to calculate an MVA by any means and an MVA should not be reported

(E) None of the above statements is correct

8 The accompanying image represents a transesophageal echocardiogram (TEE). There is spontaneous echo contrast noted within the left atrial chamber.

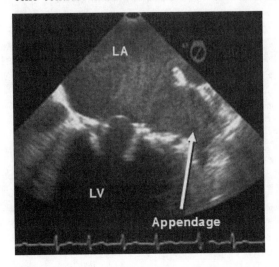

Which of the following is *true* regarding the presence of spontaneous left atrial contrast?

(A) It is most often associated with severe MR

(B) It is an indication of the need for immediate valvuloplasty or valve replacement

(C) It is often associated with a left atrial appendage thrombus

(D) The presence of "smoke" in the LA contraindicates mitral valvuloplasty due to the high risk of embolic stroke

(E) It should be treated with long-term antiplatelet therapy

9 Which of the following is *true* regarding a successful percutaneous mitral valvuloplasty procedure?

(A) It allows for the cessation of antibiotic endocarditis prophylaxis

(B) A successful procedure can be defined as a postprocedural valve area >1.5 cm^2 with no more than 2+ MR

(C) A successful procedure prevents any recurrence of commissural fusion

(D) A successful procedure prevents early occurrence of atrial fibrillation in the future

(E) One can expect a successful result in approximately 50% of cases with an echo valve score <8

10 A 90-year-old former congressman is referred to you for possible aortic valvuloplasty. He has significant chronic obstructive lung disease and has had a prior biventricular pacer with implantable defibrillator placed owing to congestive heart failure and an LV ejection fraction of 28%. The biventricular pacemaker has not improved his symptoms. He had been a heavy alcohol user in the past. Over the last few years he has developed progressive symptoms of dyspnea and chest pressure. A cardiac catheterization in his local community revealed a 20 mm Hg mean aortic gradient with no aortic insufficiency and an aortic valve area of 0.8 cm^2. He has no coronary artery disease. He is referred for a second cardiac catheterization during which time he is given intravenous dobutamine while simultaneously determining his cardiac output and valve gradient. His valve gradient rises to a mean of 30 mm Hg and his aortic valve area increases to 1.2 cm^2. Which of the following statements is *true*?

(A) He should be considered for immediate aortic valve replacement (AVR), though at high risk due to his pulmonary status. A bioprosthetic valve should be used

(B) He should undergo elective AVR with an aortic homograft

(C) He should undergo percutaneous aortic valvuloplasty as a trial to see if he gets better. If he does, then he should go to surgical AVR in the future

(D) He is not a candidate for either surgical or percutaneous valvuloplasty

(E) He should be referred to a center that has access to a percutaneous aortic valve stent

11 A 22-year-old college student is referred because of a murmur. On examination and by echocardiography she has a classic doming pulmonary valve with a peak pulmonary valve gradient by echocardiography of 80 mm Hg. She is minimally symptomatic, but the decision is made to proceed with pulmonary valvuloplasty based on the hemodynamics. The procedure goes smoothly, but she becomes hypotensive immediately after the balloons are removed. The preprocedure and postprocedural right ventriculograms are shown in the following figure. What is the most likely cause for hypotension in this setting?

Preprocedure   Postprocedure

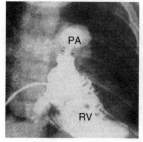 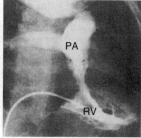

(A) The pulmonary valve has ruptured and there is severe pulmonary regurgitation

(B) A ventricular septal defect has been caused by the procedure

(C) Relief of the pulmonary valve stenosis has resulted in severe subpulmonic dynamic stenosis with low output

(D) There is obvious tamponade due to rupture of the PA

12 Pulmonary hypertension associated with mitral valve stenosis:

(A) Completely resolves following surgical valve correction, but not with percutaneous treatment

(B) Is associated with a soft P2 on physical examination

(C) Is an absolute contraindication to percutaneous valvuloplasty

(D) May lead to a falsely elevated cardiac output by the Fick calculation

(E) Can lead to significant concomitant tricuspid regurgitation (TR)

13 Dr. Y has just performed his second inflation across a congenitally stenotic pulmonary valve using a single balloon technique. The pre- and postprocedural pressure curves are obtained. The next most appropriate action would be to:

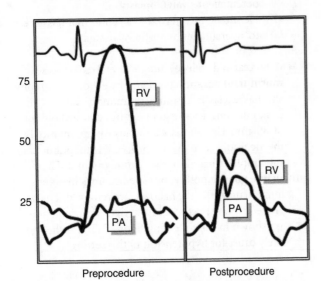

Preprocedure   Postprocedure

(A) Conclude that the procedure is a success
(B) Upsize to a larger balloon to improve the valvular area
(C) Place an intra-aortic balloon pump and call for emergent pulmonary valve replacement
(D) Perform an emergent TEE to assess whether there is severe pulmonary regurgitation
(E) Add low dose dobutamine for support given the drop in the RV pressure

14 A 14-year-old white boy, a member of his high school basketball team, sees you for consultation regarding a murmur. He had been followed up for the murmur by his local pediatric cardiologist but he has recently moved to your town and he thought he would check in. He has been feeling fine, except he notes some increased fatigue lately after an hour or so of pickup basketball with his friends. He denies any chest pressure or presyncope. On examination he has the murmur of aortic stenosis. You obtain an echocardiogram and his LV function is normal. The Doppler gradient across his aortic valve reveals a 4.0 m per second maximal velocity and a calculated valve area of 0.7 cm^2. What should be your next course of action?

(A) He is doing well enough clinically, and he needs no further studies
(B) He should be referred to an invasive pediatric cardiologist for consideration of a percutaneous aortic valvuloplasty procedure

(C) He should undergo a cardiac catheterization to confirm the aortic stenosis and evaluate his coronary arteries
(D) He should be started on β-blockers and followed up with an echocardiogram every 6 months
(E) He should be referred for surgical valve replacement

15 The signs and symptoms of significant MS include all of the following, *except*:

(A) Hemoptysis
(B) Pulmonary hypertension
(C) Platypnea-orthodeoxia
(D) Hepatic congestion
(E) Atrial fibrillation with systemic embolism

16 You are asked to see a 25-year-old woman who is 27 weeks pregnant. She has had little prenatal care. She has no known heart condition but is getting progressively short of breath as the pregnancy continues. She finally saw an internist and obtained an echocardiogram revealing significant MS with trivial MR. When you see her, she is clearly in congestive heart failure but still has normal sinus rhythm. What is the best option?

(A) Aggressive therapy for her heart failure using diuretics, angiotensin-converting enzyme (ACE) inhibitors, β-blockers and digoxin
(B) Put her on complete bed rest until she delivers the baby
(C) Consult cardiac surgery for mitral valve commissurotomy or replacement now
(D) Consider percutaneous balloon valvuloplasty now if the valvular anatomy is suitable
(E) Consider abortion of the pregnancy

17 Percutaneous valve replacement or valve repair procedures are currently under investigation. A variety of procedures are now in phase I trials or soon will be. Select the one procedure from the list below that is *not* being considered:

(A) A percutaneous mitral valve repair approach using a clip device to create a double orifice mitral valve
(B) A percutaneous mitral valve repair approach that reduces the annular size by placing clips along the inner surface of the mitral annulus (from a catheter in the LV guided by one in the coronary sinus), then pulling the mitral annulus toward a central clip to reduce the annular size
(C) A percutaneous semilunar valve mounted in a stent that is derived from the bovine jugular vein

(D) A percutaneous mitral valve repair approach using a catheter in the coronary sinus to reduce the annular size by a cinching method

(E) A percutaneous mitral valve approach to reduce the mitral annular size by placing epicardial buttons on either side of the mitral annulus through a subxiphoid catheter

18 During percutaneous mitral valvuloplasty, the Inoue balloon initially inflates distally, then the balloon is pulled into the mitral annulus and inflation to a maximal balloon diameter is subsequently achieved. The following images reflect a common problem encountered during this procedure. What is the problem that is encountered during this procedure?

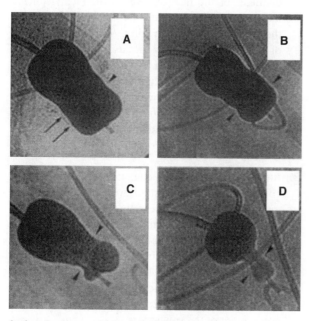

Cathet Cardiovasc Diagn. **1996;37:188–199.**

(A) There is submitral scarring that is preventing the balloon from fully inflating

(B) There is a defect in the distal Inoue balloon that is preventing full inflation

(C) There is an obstruction in the Inoue catheter that is preventing full inflation

(D) The operator is using an improper mixture of radiographic contrast to inflate the balloon

19 Which of the following procedures can routinely be successfully approached by percutaneous balloon valvuloplasty techniques?

(A) Calcific mitral valve stenosis (nonrheumatic)

(B) Parachute mitral valve with stenosis

(C) Subaortic membranous stenosis

(D) Cor triatriatum membrane

(E) None of the above

20 Which of the following statements is *true* regarding percutaneous balloon mitral valvuloplasty?

(A) It is safe to proceed with mitral valvuloplasty in the presence of an atrial thrombus if the patient has been on warfarin for 4 to 6 weeks

(B) The long-term results of surgical commissurotomy for MS are clearly better than those following balloon valvuloplasty

(C) Asymptomatic patients with MS should undergo balloon valvuloplasty if their MVA is <1.5 cm^2 regardless of whether pulmonary hypertension is present or not

(D) The major factors that have been identified as predictive of a successful procedure include a low valvular score and the absence of significant baseline MR

Answers and Explanations

1 Answer B. There are several explanations for an elevated PCW to left ventricle (LV) diastolic gradient. Although rheumatic MS is the leading cause, other rare causes may occur. A mitral web may exist just above the mitral valve and be part of a syndrome with multiple and variable levels of obstruction (*Shone syndrome*) (*Am J Cardiol.* 1963;11: 714–725). This syndrome includes coarctation of the aorta, supravalvular, valvular or subvalvular aortic stenosis, a parachute mitral valve, and/or supramitral valve ring. In *cor triatriatum*, a membrane divides the LA into an accessory venous chamber and an LA chamber contiguous with the mitral valve. *Pulmonary veno-occlusive disease* (*J Am Coll Cardiol.* 2004;43:5S–12S) is an obliterative disease of the pulmonary venous bed or pulmonary veins themselves. In most cases the cause is unknown, but may be related to viral infection or connective tissue diseases such as lupus or Crest syndrome or as a complication of certain blood cancers such as leukemia or lymphoma, or owing to chemotherapy. It presents clinically as pulmonary hypertension, but will show elevated and usually differential gradients throughout the pulmonary vasculature due to the patchy distribution of this illness. *Pulmonary vein stenosis* may also be primary, secondary to fibrosing mediastinitis or iatrogenic related to atrial fibrillation ablations (*Circulation.* 2005;111:546–554), surgical instrumentation (lung transplant) or chest radiation. The presentation may also exhibit differential wedges across the lung bed, as blood flow may only go to the least affected areas. If suspected, it is important to obtain a PCW pressure in all four quadrants of the lung. Wedge angiograms done by initially injecting contrast in the distal PA occluded by a balloon-tipped catheter, and then allowing the contrast to clear in order to visualize each pulmonary vein separately may be helpful in evaluating these disorders. Patients with primary pulmonary hypertension have intrinsic disease of the pulmonary bed and have precapillary smooth muscle hypertrophy. These patients have a normal PCW, an elevated pulmonary vascular resistance and no significant PCW/LV gradient.

2 Answer C. This tracing clearly shows a large V-wave within the atrial tracing consistent with severe MR. Large V-waves may only reflect impaired LA compliance, however, and this would need to be compared with the preprocedural tracing. MR during mitral valvuloplasty is a known complication, occurring in approximately 3% of patients. This is usually because of a rupture of a chord in the heavily scarred subvalvular apparatus or to a tear in the leaflet itself. A progressive increase in the V-wave during the procedure has a sensitivity of 79% and specificity of 89% for worsening MR (*Am J Cardiol.* 1998;82:1388–1393). More than 2+ mitral regurgitation means that the procedure has been unsuccessful. One would not upsize the balloon diameter in the face of severe MR. Phenylephrine increases afterload on the LV and would increase the V-wave in the LA tracing. Although re-zeroing of the transducer may be useful, it would not negate the presence of a V-wave of this magnitude. Depending on the severity and baseline clinical status, the appropriate course would be to place an intra-aortic balloon pump and proceed to urgent surgery if the patient is hemodynamically compromised. Otherwise elective surgery is indicated.

3 Answer A. Four characteristics are taken into account in the scoring system, with each given a 1 to 4 point value based on severity (*Br Heart J.* 1988;60: 299–308). A "0" score implies normal valve morphology. A total valve score of ≤8 implies a mobile valve readily amenable to percutaneous valvuloplasty. Progressively higher total valve scores results in less favorable results, both acutely and in the long term (*J Am Coll Cardiol.* 2002;39:328–334). MVA is not a component of the valve score.

- Leaflet mobility
  - Highly mobile valve with only leaflet tip restriction
  - Midportion and base of leaflets with reduced mobility
  - Valve leaflets move forward in diastole mainly at the base
  - No or minimal forward movement of the leaflets in diastole
- Valvular thickening
  - Leaflets minimally thickened (4 to 5 mm)
  - Midleaflet thickening, pronounced thickening of the margins
  - Thickening extends through the entire leaflet (5 to 6 mm)
  - Pronounced thickening of all leaflet tissue (>8 mm)

- Subvalvular thickening

    - Minimal thickening of chordal structures just below the valve
    - Thickening of the chordae extending up to 1/3 of the chordal length
    - Thickening extending to the distal third of the chordae
    - Extensive thickening and shortening of all chordae extending down to the papillary muscles

- Valvular calcification

    - A single area of increased echo brightness
    - Scattered areas of brightness confined to the leaflet margins
    - Brightness extending to the midportion of the leaflets
    - Extensive brightness throughout most of the leaflet tissue

4 Answer D. On the basis of the echocardiographic scoring system, the still echocardiographic image has significant submitral scarring (see *arrow*) and a thickened mitral valve. This alone would give her an echo score of 7 to 8. Although calcium and mobility cannot be defined from this still frame, the comments of the echocardiographer add further points to the valve scoring system, making it *unlikely* that this is a valve that would respond to percutaneous valvuloplasty methods. Increasing the diuretics may help in the short term, as might the return to normal sinus rhythm if feasible. She is now symptomatic, though, and a surgical intervention is appropriate. The valve morphology for a surgical commissurotomy is precisely the same as for percutaneous valvuloplasty, so that is not an option. The appropriate option is surgical valve replacement at this time.

5 Answer D. The indications for percutaneous balloon valvuloplasty for MS include the presence of moderate to severe MS—defined as an MVA of <1.5 cm^2 and the absence of an LA appendage thrombus and <2+ mitral insufficiency (*J Am Coll Cardiol.* 1998;32:1486–1588).

- Class I indication: Symptomatic (functional class [FC] III or IV) MS with favorable valvular anatomy (Ia)
- Class II indication: Asymptomatic MS with favorable valve morphology and a pulmonary systolic pressure of >50 mm Hg at rest or >60 mm Hg with exercise (IIa)
- Class II indication: Patients with significant symptoms and less favorable valve anatomy who are at high risk for surgery (IIa)
- Class II indication: Patients with new atrial fibrillation (IIb)

6 Answer C. Although a cardiac MRI does provide better information regarding RV mass and function, and RV dysfunction may play a role in his symptoms, a preserved RV by echocardiography is adequate to exclude this and the important finding is the presence of tricuspid stenosis (TS). The normal tricuspid valve area is approximately 10 cm^2 and any gradient over 2 mm Hg is considered abnormal, with severe TS diagnosed when the mean gradient is >5 mm Hg. He clearly has severe TS with right heart failure. Most bioprosthetic valves in the tricuspid position can be expected to remain functional from 10 to 12 years. Degeneration usually results in both TR and stenosis. There is very little experience with percutaneous balloon valvuloplasty for a stenotic tricuspid bioprosthetic valve, but what information is available suggests that there is an extremely high risk of bioprosthetic valvular tearing and that severe TR can be expected. Given his clinical situation, redo tricuspid valve replacement is the best clinical option to resolve his situation. Although constrictive pericarditis may also potentially play an associated role in this situation, the high tricuspid valve gradient points primarily to the tricuspid valve as the main culprit here.

7 Answer B. She has minimal aortic gradient and the aortic stenosis is quite mild. The determination of an estimated valve area depends on knowledge of the amount of forward flow (cardiac output) across the valve in question and the mean gradient across the valve. From the Gorlin equation (*Am Heart J.* 1951;41:1–29):

$$MVA = \frac{cardiac\ output / \left(\frac{diastolic\ filling\ period}{\times\ heart\ rate} \right)}{44.3 \times 0.85 \times (\sqrt{mean\ mitral\ gradient})}$$

Because all these data were not obvious from the information provided, one can estimate the valve area quickly to confirm the fellow's finding by using the Hakki method (*Circulation.* 1981;63:1050–1055). The Hakki method can be applied to other valves and is a simplified calculation. Using this method:

$$Hakki\ MVA = \frac{cardiac\ output}{\sqrt{mean\ gradient}}$$

In this case the cardiac output (3 L/min) is divided by the square root of the mean gradient (3 mm Hg) resulting in a valve area of 1.0 cm^2 and is simpler to remember than the classic Gorlin formula.

Both depend on knowing the true flow across the mitral valve and on determining the mean gradient. The Gorlin formula examines the amount of time in a minute that forward flow is occurring (diastolic filling time × heart rate), uses 44.3 as the gravitational constant, and adds a constant (in this case 0.85 for the mitral valve) that was found to be needed to increase the accuracy of the measurement when the results were compared with autopsy findings.

In this instance, determination of the flow across the mitral valve is not directly impacted by the presence of aortic insufficiency, as the flow across the mitral valve is the same as the Fick determined cardiac output. If there was mitral insufficiency, then the regurgitant flow would need to be added to the Fick forward flow to determine the total flow across the mitral valve during diastole.

8 Answer C. The meaning of spontaneous echo contrast remains obscure. It typically represents slow atrial flow (*Clin Cardiol*. 2000;23:501–506) and although the phenomenon is clearly not circulating thrombi, it is often associated with a left atrial appendage or mural thrombus and a higher risk for embolization (*J Am Coll Cardiol*. 2005;45:1807–1812). At this time there is no specific recommendation for anticoagulation based on this finding unless concomitant thrombus is visualized in the LA or LA appendage or the patient has intermittent or sustained atrial fibrillation. In that situation, warfarin therapy and not antiplatelet therapy is recommended. Patients referred for percutaneous mitral valvuloplasty frequently have spontaneous left atrial contrast and, if there is no evident atrial appendage thrombus, the patient can safely undergo the procedure.

9 Answer B. The risk of endocarditis has *not* been shown to be reduced following mitral valvuloplasty. Successful mitral valvuloplasty should be attained in a high percentage (up to 95%) of cases with the excellent valve morphology that results in a valve score of <8 (*Am Heart J*. 1995;129:1197–1203, *J Am Coll Cardiol*. 2002;39:328–334). Although several definitions of success are possible, a common one defines success as a valve area >1.5 cm^2 with no more than 2+ MR. Others have used >50% increase in the baseline valve area or >50% decrease in the valve gradient. Unfortunately the majority of patients will ultimately have the recurrence of stenosis. In a serial echocardiographic study (*Am Heart J*. 1995;129:1197–1203), as expected, echocardiographic restenosis was more frequent than clinical symptoms of restenosis. By serial echocardiography at 5 years 20% had restenosis if the baseline echo score was <8 but 60% had restenosis if the baseline echo score was >8. Clinical restenosis occurs at a later time, but the anatomic features also predict clinical outcome. In a recent study with a 10-year follow-up, clinical restenosis was present in 23% of those with an echo score of <8, 55% of those

with an echo score of 9 to 11, and 50% of those with an echo score of >12. There are no data to suggest that mitral valve procedures reduce the risk of atrial fibrillation although left atrial size does help predict which patient can maintain sinus (*Am J Cardiol*. 2006;97:1045–1050) and amiodarone has had some success (*J Heart Valve Dis*. 2002;11:802–809) in this population. In addition, it is known that chronic atrial fibrillation portends a poorer long-term result from the procedure compared with those in sinus rhythm (*J Heart Valve Dis*. 2005;14:727–734). Rheumatic carditis has often been postulated as to why the onset of atrial fibrillation does not always correlate with the severity of the MS.

10 Answer D. The surgical risk of AVR in the elderly population has declined considerably and even patients with poor LV systolic function have been shown to benefit from it. His advanced age and lung disease markedly increase the risk of perioperative morbidity and mortality. In this case, the fundamental decision is whether his poor LV function is due to his aortic valve or to his underlying cardiomyopathy. Using nitroprusside or dobutamine to increase the cardiac output is necessary when there is a low gradient but low cardiac output situation. Using dobutamine in this situation increased his gradient slightly, but also significantly increased his aortic valve area. These data suggest that the primary limitation is not the stenotic aortic valve, but rather the underlying cardiomyopathy (*Circulation*. 2002;106:809–813) and he is not a candidate for any valvular procedure including valvuloplasty, a percutaneous stent (even if it were available) or valvular surgery. There are data that suggest that the elderly who best benefit long-term from aortic valvuloplasty are those with a preserved ejection fraction (*Am J Cardiol*. 1991;68:75–80). These are the same patients that do well with surgery. Since aortic valvuloplasty has been shown to provide very limited short or intermediate term survival benefit or symptomatic relief in the elderly (*J Am Coll Cardiol*. 1995;26:1522–1528), its use is very limited and not indicated in the situation described.

11 Answer C. A classic domed pulmonary valve responds excellently to percutaneous balloon valvuloplasty techniques. On an average, the peak gradient can be expected to fall from approximately 90 mm Hg to 29 mm Hg. The procedure has low risk, generally in the range of 1% to 2% and complications include pulmonary edema (presumably from increasing flow to previously underperfused lungs), perforation of a cardiac chamber or vessel, high grade atrioventricular (AV) block, pulmonary valve regurgitation or the "suicide RV" shown in the preceding figure. Sudden relief of the pulmonary valve obstruction can produce transient dynamic RV outflow obstruction as shown in the postprocedural image above. This is usually readily treated with intravenous β-blockers, calcium blockers, and fluids. It is important not to give inotropic agents as these will worsen the dynamic obstruction.

12 Answer E. Pulmonary hypertension in patients with mitral valve stenosis is often higher than one would expect from the passive rise in the pulmonary venous pressure alone (*Am J Cardiol.* 1993;71:874–878). Both reactive vasoconstriction and more fixed morphologic changes may occur. Early in the course of the disease the changes are reversible, with the lowering of the pulmonary venous pressure following mitral valvuloplasty or valve replacement. Later on, the changes become more fixed and are characterized by fibrinoid necrosis, loss of smooth muscle cell nuclei, fibrin deposition, and eventually the plexiform lesion similar to that seen in primary pulmonary hypertension or in Eisenmenger's physiology. The time course of the reduction of pulmonary hypertension is often initially acute with a gradual continued reduction over the ensuing months following the procedure. The elevated pulmonary pressure is associated with a loud or sharp P_2 on physical examination and occasionally pulmonary insufficiency (the Graham–Steele murmur). There is often an associated RV lift and TR. In this setting, the tricuspid valve may develop regurgitation either due to annular dilation and chordal displacement as the RV enlarges or due to rheumatic valvular involvement or a combination. Pulmonary hypertension does not affect the Fick output measures, though associated TR and pulmonary insufficiency can alter cardiac output determined by indicator-dilution methods, such as right heart thermodilution techniques. Although not a contraindication to percutaneous treatment, special care in balloon size and dilation should be made in MS patients with pulmonary hypertension, since they may be less tolerant to any increase in MR that may occur during the procedure.

13 Answer A. This tracing clearly shows a decrease in the gradient, which marks a successful procedure. A successful procedure is generally considered one in which the gradient has been reduced to <20 mm Hg. Pulmonary valvuloplasty has a success rate of over 90% and complications are rare. It is performed by using one or two balloons side-by-side to dilate to annular size of 1.2 to 1.4 times the measured annulus, as there is much elastic recoil in the PA. Recently the Inoue mitral valvuloplasty balloon has

been used with excellent results. The preceding figure represents a successful result and no further action is needed.

14 Answer B. The echo/Doppler reveals a peak aortic velocity gradient of 4 m per second. This corresponds to a peak aortic valve gradient of 64 mm Hg. The calculated valve area of 0.7 cm^2 is also consistent with severe aortic stenosis. On the basis of his activity and goals, he needs an intervention. Although percutaneous balloon aortic valvuloplasty has not proved to be an effective procedure in elderly patients, there are data that suggest it is useful in the adolescent age-group. The successful rate of valvuloplasty in this subset is high (90%) with a procedural mortality of <2% and an average reduction in the aortic gradient of approximately 60% (*Am J Cardiol.* 1996;77:286–293, *Am J Cardiol.* 1990;65:784–789). Progressive regurgitation or restenosis occurs in about half the patients by 8 to 9 years, though, and careful follow-up is warranted. Successful valvuloplasty in this age-group allows deferral of surgical intervention to a later date and is particularly important in young women who wish to have children. He does not need catheterization to confirm the diagnosis or for an evaluation of his coronary artery disease. He should be referred now to a pediatric cardiologist with an interest in percutaneous valvuloplasty techniques based on his early symptoms and the severity of his stenosis. If a percutaneous approach cannot be performed technically, he should consider surgical intervention. This is usually done with a bioprosthetic valve (often an aortic homograft or his own pulmonary autograft as part of the Ross procedure).

15 Answer C. Obstruction at the mitral valve increases LA pressure and subsequently pulmonary venous pressure. Hemoptysis may occur when pulmonary vascular rupture occurs, usually during extreme stress or rapid tachycardia when the pulmonary venous pressure is suddenly increased. Pulmonary hypertension is due to both the high pulmonary venous pressure and a secondary "stenosis" at the pulmonary precapillary level. If the pulmonary pressures are severe enough or if there is associated tricuspid valve involvement, right heart failure from RV dysfunction and TR may develop with subsequent hepatic congestion. Atrial fibrillation is a common finding and is due to both the elevated LA pressure stress on the atrial myocardium and the presence of ongoing rheumatic carditis. Because the LA is markedly enlarged and the flow through the atrium is slowed because of the outflow obstruction created by the MS, the risk of atrial thrombus (primarily in the atrial appendage) is high and systemic embolization is a common occurrence in patients not on anticoagulation. Platypnea-orthodeoxia is a clinical syndrome characterized by dyspnea and deoxygenation accompanying a change to a sitting or standing position from a recumbent one. Two conditions must coexist to cause platypnea-orthodeoxia: An *anatomic* component in the form of an interatrial communication and a *functional* component that produces a deformity in the atrial septum and results in a redirection of shunt flow with the assumption of an upright posture. The anatomic defect can be an atrial septal defect, a patent foramen ovale, or a fenestrated atrial septal aneurysm. The functional component may be cardiac, such as pericardial effusion or constrictive pericarditis; pulmonary, such as emphysema, arteriovenous malformation, pneumonectomy, or amiodarone toxicity; abdominal, such as cirrhosis of the liver or ileus; or vascular, such as aortic aneurysm or elongation. It is not part of the syndromes that occur with MS.

16   Answer D. During pregnancy many hemodynamic events occur, including a 25% increase in the red blood cell mass and a 30% to 50% increase in the blood volume. As a result there is relative anemia. There is a reduction in systemic vascular resistance as well a pulmonary vascular resistance. The cardiac output increases until approximately the 32nd week of pregnancy where it levels out from 30% to 50% higher than at prepregnancy. During the latter stages of pregnancy the stroke volume declines and the cardiac output is maintained by an increase in the heart rate. In MS, the increased blood volume and stroke volume required markedly increases the mitral gradient. In the final trimester, the increasingly rapid heart rate also reduces diastolic time and further increases the mitral gradient. This can lead to progressive symptoms of heart failure. The use of ACE inhibitors is relatively contraindicated in pregnancy, although the risk is less in the last trimester. Complete bed rest has been used in the past, but patients become progressively deconditioned and its use is much less now. Surgical commissurotomy or replacement can be done, but there is substantial fetal loss if the patient is placed on the heart–lung machine for any length of time. Abortion at this stage would not be appropriate because of the advanced age of the fetus. Percutaneous balloon valvuloplasty has been done quite safely during pregnancy and would be the procedure of choice here, as she is already in heart failure and it would be to the fetus' advantage to mature further before delivery.

17   Answer E. All of the first four approaches are being investigated. The preceding figure displays semilunar valves that are being employed for pulmonary and aortic valve replacement. The following figure is representative of several devices being employed for mitral valve repair. A surgical approach that results in septolateral cinching (SLAC) using epicardial buttons connecting a string across the LV at the annulus is being investigated (coapsys). No percutaneous approach is yet available, though SLAC uses a system that pulls the coronary sinus toward the interatrial septum (PS system) has been reported. (*circulation* 2006;113:2329–2334).

There have been multiple attempts at developing a percutaneous semilunar valve, such as might be used in the pulmonary position. The most successful uses the bovine jugular vein valve mounted onto a stent placed in obstructed conduits in children (*Lancet*. 2000;356:1403–1405). Led by their initial positive experience in that setting (*J Am Coll Cardiol*. 2002;39:1664–1669, *Circulation*. 2005;112:1189–1197), the indications have expanded to include valvular pulmonic stenosis.

Using a stented bovine pericardial valve, Cribier et al. from France first reported an initially successful AVR in a desperately ill patient (*Circulation*. 2002;106:3006–3008). Since then both early (*J Am Coll Cardiol*. 2004;43:698–703) and modestly midterm experiences have been published (*J Am Coll Cardiol*. 2006;47:1214–1223). The procedure continues to evolve with both antegrade (through transseptal) (*J Interv Cardiol*. 2003;16:515–521) and retrograde (*Circulation*. 2002;105:775–778) methods being evaluated. Very few patients have been enrolled. The entry criteria for use of the percutaneous AVR approach still focuses on extremely ill, generally nonsurgical patients at high risk for cardiac events.

Percutaneous approaches to MR continue, though there remain little clinical data with only a few patients being reported. One of the more complete trials, the phase I Endovascular Valve Edge-to-edge REpair STudy (EVEREST) I trial enrolled 47 patients (*J Am Coll Cardiol*. 2005;46:2134–2140). It continues into its phase II. Besides the percutaneous clip approach, efforts are continuing to develop coronary sinus cinching devices to reduce the mitral annular size or to attempt annuloplasty using stitches inserted into the mitral annulus from the ventricular side. All of these devices are in very early trials, and the data are too premature as to the advantage, or even the safety and efficacy, of any particular approach. In the transventricular method, a magnetic-tipped catheter is placed into the coronary sinus and used to locate the tip of a second catheter placed through the aortic valve into the LV and shaped to abut against the mitral annulus. Stitches are implanted into the mitral annulus at various locations identified by the two catheters. Each stitch site is then pulled toward each other to reduce the mitral annular size.

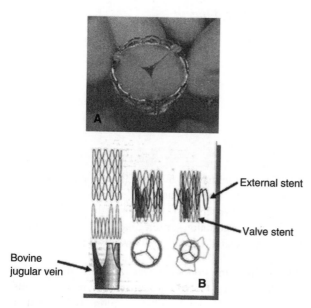

Circulation. 2002;105:775–778.

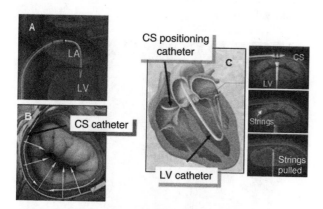

J Am Coll Cardiol. 2005;46:2134–2140.

18 Answer A. In each frame the Inoue balloon is unable to fully inflate owing to rigid submitral apparatus scar and fibrosis. The procedure should be terminated when this is seen to prevent rupture of any of the submitral apparatus and severe MR.

19 Answer E. Calcific MS is the consequence of mitral annular calcium with invasion onto the mitral leaflets. This produces rigidity and creates an obstruction to LV inflow. As the commissures are not fused, the valve is not susceptible to balloon valvuloplasty techniques. A parachute mitral valve includes a single papillary muscle with all the thickened and shortened chordae tendineae inserting onto it. Although attempts have been made to balloon these, they have generally been unsuccessful. A subaortic membrane may be present below the aortic valve with attachments to both the ventricular septum and the anterior leaflet of the mitral valve. It often recurs even after surgical correction, and though attempts have been reportedly successful, it is generally not amenable to percutaneous balloon methods. In cor triatriatum, a membrane separates the pulmonary venous chamber from the LA. Again occasional reports of successful tearing of the opening into the LA have been reported, but this is generally considered a surgical problem.

20 Answer D. Although it may be possible to perform percutaneous mitral valvuloplasty with an atrial appendage thrombus, it not considered wise to do so. One is never sure how well patients have been anticoagulated over time, and the presence of an atrial appendage thrombus is a relative contraindication to the procedure. The long-term results from comparative studies of percutaneous balloon valvuloplasty versus surgical commissurotomy reveal that the valvuloplasty patients have similar or even better improvement in both valve area and symptomatic status, at least up to 7 years. The current guidelines suggest that asymptomatic patients should be considered for percutaneous valvuloplasty with a MVA <1.5 cm^2, but only if there is associated atrial fibrillation or evidence of pulmonary hypertension (peak systolic pressure by echo/Doppler of >50 mm Hg). Consistently the echo valve score for MS morphology has proved to be predictive of outcomes with valve scores <8 corresponding to the greatest immediate and long-term success. In many series, the greater the severity of MR, the worse the immediate and long-term outcome as well.

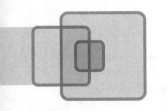

30

Congenital Heart Disease

John Lynn Jefferies, Michael R. Nihill, and Alan W. Nugent

Questions

1 A 3-year-old patient presents to you for evaluation secondary to a referral from his pediatrician for a murmur. You diagnose the patient with a functional murmur. Common characteristics of this murmur include all of the following, *except*:

(A) Often described as musical or "twanging string"
(B) Normal electrocardiogram (EKG) and chest radiograph (CXR)
(C) Also known as a *Still murmur*
(D) Best heard in the upright position
(E) Usual intensity is II-III/VI

2 Which of the following statements is *incorrect* regarding the sinus venosus atrial septal defect (ASD) demonstrated in the angiogram shown?

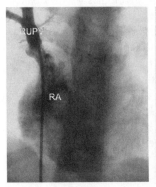 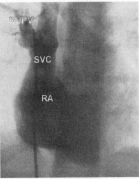

(A) Sinus venosus defects account for <25% of ASDs
(B) Sinus venosus defects are located posterior to the fossa ovalis
(C) Sinus venosus defect is commonly associated with anomalous connection of the left pulmonary veins (PVs)

(D) Approximately, 50% of these patients have a frontal P-wave axis <30 degrees
(E) The Warden procedure may be used to treat the anomalous pulmonary venous drainage associated with the sinus venosus defect

3 The following angiogram was performed on a patient who had fever for 5 days, acute erythema of the palms and soles, bilateral bulbar conjunctival injection without an obvious exudate, a strawberry tongue, and cervical lymphadenopathy. What is the most likely diagnosis?

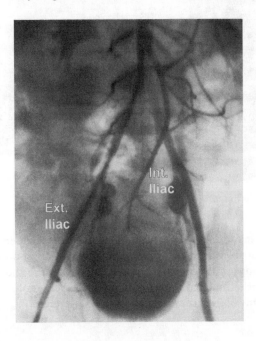

(A) Toxic shock syndrome
(B) Stevens-Johnson syndrome

(C) Takayasu arteritis
(D) Henoch-Schönlein purpura
(E) Kawasaki disease

4 Which of the following statements regarding Kawasaki disease is *false*?

(A) Coronary artery aneurysms or ectasia will develop in approximately 15% to 25% of untreated children with Kawasaki disease
(B) Most children in the United States diagnosed with Kawasaki disease are older than 5 years
(C) Regressed coronary artery aneurysms are not histopathologically normal
(D) In the United States, Kawasaki disease is the leading cause of acquired heart disease in children
(E) In the United States, intravenous immunoglobulin (IVIG) is recommended for all children with Kawasaki disease

5 Congenital rubella is associated with all of the following cardiovascular abnormalities, *except*:

(A) Ebstein anomaly
(B) Patent ductus arteriosus (PDA)
(C) Ventricular septal defect (VSD)
(D) Transposition of the great arteries
(E) Tricuspid atresia

6 A 6-month-old patient presents to your office for evaluation. The mother reports that her child has had poor weight gain, excessive sweating, and poor feeding. You note that the record documents repeated problems with upper respiratory tract infections. On examination, the patient is tachycardic and tachypneic. His pulses are bounding and a thrill is palpable at the left upper sternal border. You obtain a CXR. What is the most likely diagnosis?

(A) Secundum ASD
(B) Patent foramen ovale
(C) PDA
(D) Muscular VSD
(E) Branch pulmonary artery (PA) stenosis

7 The following statements regarding Ebstein anomaly are true, *except*:

(A) There is characteristic displacement of the septal and anterior leaflets into the right ventricle (RV)
(B) There is commonly an ASD or patent foramen ovale present
(C) EKG may reveal right atrial (RA) enlargement
(D) There is an equal frequency between men and women
(E) Of these patients 20% to 30% will also have Wolff-Parkinson-White (WPW) syndrome

8 Which of the following associated cardiac diseases do patients with Duchenne muscular dystrophy commonly have?

(A) Restrictive cardiomyopathy
(B) VSDs
(C) Ebstein anomaly
(D) Dilated cardiomyopathy
(E) Long QT syndrome

9 The following echocardiogram would most likely be associated with which syndrome?

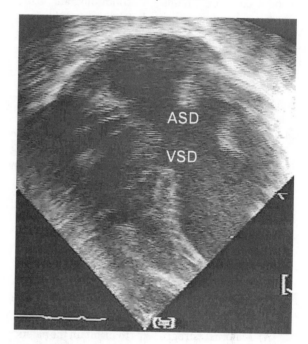

(A) Hurler syndrome
(B) Holt-Oram syndrome
(C) Costello syndrome
(D) Noonan syndrome
(E) Down syndrome

10 Characteristic physical findings of patients with Marfan syndrome include all of the following, *except*:

(A) Malar hypoplasia
(B) Positive thumb and wrist sign
(C) Arm span <105% of their height
(D) Pectus excavatum
(E) Pes planus

11 Blalock-Taussig shunts (BTS) are often used in structural cardiac disease as a palliative procedure to improve pulmonary blood flow. Which of the following anatomic connections describes the BTS anastomotic sites?

(A) Descending thoracic aorta to the main pulmonary artery (MPA)

(B) Subclavian artery to PA

(C) Superior vena cava (SVC) to PA

(D) Ascending aorta to the right pulmonary artery (RPA)

(E) Left ventricular apex to the descending thoracic aorta

12 A 17-year-old patient presents to your office with a history of coarctation of the aorta. He underwent surgical repair as a child and now needs follow-up. He has been asymptomatic otherwise. What would be a common finding on echocardiogram that is most commonly associated with this condition?

(A) Valvar aortic stenosis

(B) VSD

(C) Bicuspid aortic valve

(D) Mitral stenosis

(E) Subvalvular aortic stenosis

13 The patient referred to above asks you what things he should be concerned about in the future regarding his repair. You tell him the most likely complication *is*:

(A) Aortic dissection

(B) Cerebrovascular events

(C) Aortic aneurysm

(D) Recurrent coarctation of the aorta

(E) Diminished left arm growth

14 Regarding PDA, the following statements are true, *except*:

(A) Maternal estrogen helps to maintain the patency of the ductus during pregnancy and following delivery

(B) During fetal life, the ductus arteriosus is exposed to a partial pressure of oxygen of 20 to 25 mm Hg

(C) Changes in pulmonary vascular resistance is the major determinant of left-to-right shunting through a PDA

(D) In a full-term infant, the PDA usually closes in 2 to 3 weeks after delivery

(E) In a patient with a left aortic arch, the PDA connects the MPA with the descending aorta distal to the left subclavian artery

15 Which of the following is the most common coronary anomaly?

(A) Single coronary artery

(B) Origin of the left anterior descending coronary artery from the right sinus of Valsalva

(C) Origin of the left circumflex coronary artery from the right coronary artery

(D) Origin of the left main coronary artery from the right sinus of Valsalva

(E) Origin of the left main coronary artery arising from the PA

16 Spontaneous bacterial endocarditis prophylaxis should be observed in all of the following situations, *except*:

(A) Secundum ASD

(B) Cleft mitral valve

(C) Muscular VSD

(D) Ebstein anomaly

(E) Hypertrophic cardiomyopathy

17 Regarding epidemiology in congenital heart disease, the following statements are true, *except*:

(A) Gender distribution as a whole is equal in patients with congenital heart disease

(B) Approximately between every 5 and 8 of each 1,000 infants are diagnosed with congenital cardiovascular malformations

(C) Maternal exposure to certain environmental agents predisposes the fetus to congenital cardiovascular malformations

(D) Studies of ethnic differences regarding congenital cardiovascular malformations have been largely inconclusive

(E) The most important risk factor for having a child with congenital heart disease is prematurity

18 A person in your office has a screening echocardiogram that reveals dilation of the coronary sinus. The person is otherwise doing well. The most likely cause of this finding is:

(A) Tricuspid stenosis

(B) Tetralogy of Fallot (TOF)

(C) Primum ASD

(D) Persistent left-sided SVC

(E) Maternal alcohol ingestion

19 The following statements regarding balloon atrial septostomy are true, *except*:

(A) Balloon atrial septostomy is indicated for infants with transposition of the great arteries with poor atrial level shunting

(B) Balloon atrial septostomy is indicated for congenital heart lesions that are dependent on traversing the atrial septum for maintenance of circulation such as the hypoplastic left heart syndrome

(C) Balloon atrial septostomy is reliable for children older than 1 month

(D) In infants, the umbilical vein may be used to perform the procedure

(E) Balloon atrial septostomy can be performed safely under echocardiographic guidance

20 A 14-year-old patient presents to your office for chest pain, shortness of breath, and dizziness on exertion. You obtain an echocardiogram that reveals a subaortic stenosis. Your discussion with the patient and his family includes the following statements, *except*:

(A) This lesion is amenable to a percutaneous intervention
(B) This lesion is typically discrete
(C) This lesion can reform following surgical intervention
(D) Surgery is the most effective option for this patient
(E) This lesion can lead to aortic regurgitation that can progress over time

21 Please calculate the pulmonary vascular resistance given the following data: RA: a = 6 mm Hg, v = 5 mm Hg, mean = 4 mm Hg; RV: 20/0, 5 mm Hg; MPA: 20/8, mean = 12 mm Hg; LA: a = 5 mm Hg, v = 7 mm Hg, mean = 6 mm Hg; systemic arterial pressure: 98/56, mean = 75 mm Hg. By thermodilution, the cardiac output was 4 L/min/m². There is no intracardiac shunting.

(A) 0.3 Wood units
(B) 0.6 Wood units
(C) 0.8 Wood units
(D) 1.5 Wood units
(E) 2.4 Wood units

22 The Fontan procedure or total cavopulmonary anastomosis is used as a palliative procedure in patients with single ventricle physiology. All of the following would be clinical evidence of Fontan failure, *except*:

(A) Ascites
(B) High cardiac output heart failure
(C) Atrial arrhythmias
(D) Peripheral edema
(E) Protein losing enteropathy (PLE)

23 A 2-year-old female child with a secundum ASD has the following data by cardiac catheterization: Hemoglobin 11 g HgB, PV O_2 saturation of 98%, PA saturation of 86%, systemic arterial saturation of 98%, and SVC saturation of 74%. The assumed O_2 consumption based on sex, age, and heart rate is 170 mL/minute/m². Please calculate the Qp:Qs.

(A) 0.5:1
(B) 1:1
(C) 1.8:1
(D) 2:1
(E) 2.3:1

24 A 4-year-old male child is referred to you for evaluation. You obtain an echocardiogram that yields the following image. You feel that angiography is indicated. Cardiac catheterization is pursued. The following statements regarding this lesion are true, *except*:

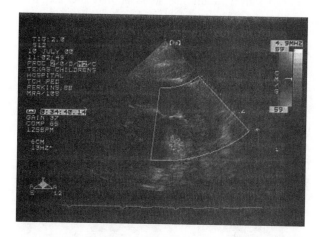

(A) Transcatheter approach to this lesion is typically successful but may require repeat catheterization
(B) This lesion poses no significant risk of endocarditis
(C) Transcatheter closure of this lesion is the management approach of choice
(D) This lesion could lead to pulmonary overcirculation
(E) The transcatheter approach to this lesion may depend on the size of the lesion in different patients

25 A 2-day-old male child is experiencing cyanosis. A transthoracic echocardiogram is performed, which reveals doming of the pulmonic valve and a valvar gradient of 60 mm Hg. The following statements regarding this lesion are true, *except*:

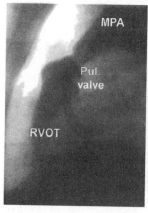
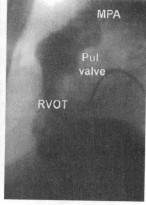

(A) Balloon valvuloplasty should be considered in all asymptomatic patients who have a valvar gradient of >40 mm Hg.

(B) In patients who are cyanotic at rest with severe obstruction, echocardiography accurately estimates the valve gradient

(C) Valvar pulmonic stenosis may be acquired secondary to carcinoid disease

(D) All neonates with critical pulmonary valve stenosis should undergo balloon valvuloplasty

(E) Following balloon valvuloplasty, gradients across the RV outflow may be higher than that before the intervention

26 Angiography is performed on an adolescent patient with shortness of breath. What is the diagnosis?

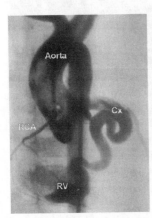 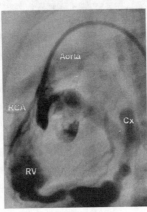

(A) Pulmonary fistula draining into the RV

(B) Pulmonary fistula draining into the left ventricle

(C) Venovenous collateral

(D) Coronary artery fistula draining into the RV

(E) Coronary fistula draining into the coronary sinus

27 This angiogram is performed on a neonate with severe aortic valve stenosis (AS). Regarding this condition the following statements are true, *except*:

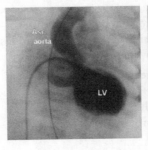 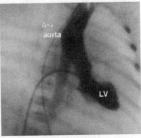

(A) Balloon valvuloplasty should be considered in neonates with critical AS if there is an adequately sized left ventricle

(B) Balloon valvuloplasty in neonates with critical AS is considered curative

(C) Up to 30% of neonates undergoing balloon valvuloplasty for critical AS may develop at least mild aortic regurgitation

(D) Neonates with AS may be asymptomatic after birth

(E) Left bundle branch block or ventricular arrhythmias may develop following balloon valvuloplasty for AS

28 In a postoperative Fontan patient with ongoing cyanosis, the following lesions should be excluded, *except*:

(A) Fontan baffle leak

(B) Venovenous collaterals

(C) Pulmonary arteriovenous malformations

(D) Fontan fenestration

(E) Aortopulmonary collaterals

Answers and Explanations

1 Answer D. The functional murmur, or Still murmur, is the most common innocent systolic murmur. It is known by other names including physiologic murmur and vibratory murmur. It is typically heard in mid systole and is of low frequency in nature. The murmur is best appreciated with the patient in the *supine* position and decreases in intensity with the patient in the upright position. The EKG and CXR are normal.

2 Answer C. Sinus venosus defects account for approximately 5% to 10% of ASDs. They are located posterior to the fossa ovalis and often only have adjacent septal rim tissue anteriorly and inferiorly. Sinus venosus defects are commonly associated with anomalous drainage of the *right-sided* PVs. This connection is often to the right atrium or to the SVC. Approximately half of these patients have an abnormal P-wave axis. The Warden procedure is used to treat anomalous connection of right-sided PVs.

3 Answer E. Kawasaki disease is an acute, self-limited vasculitis that has the clinical characteristics of fever for 5 days, changes in extremities such as erythema of the hands and feet in the acute phase and periungual peeling in the subacute phase, polymorphous exanthem, bilateral bulbar conjunctival injection without exudates, changes in the lips and oral cavity such as lip cracking and strawberry tongue, and cervical lymphadenopathy. Kawasaki disease can result in coronary artery aneurysms and aneurysms in the brachial, axillary, renal, iliac, and femoral arteries. Over several weeks following the acute phase, active inflammatory reactions are replaced by progressive fibrosis with resultant scar formation.

4 Answer B. Most children in the United States diagnosed with Kawasaki disease are younger than 5 years (~75%). Coronary artery aneurysms or ectasia will develop in approximately 15% to 25% of untreated children with Kawasaki disease. Angiographic resolution may occur in up to half of the patients but these segments continue to have functional and histopathologic abnormalities. The aneurysms that persist may have progressive stenosis or occlusion in the future. In the United States, Kawasaki disease has surpassed acute rheumatic fever and is now the leading cause of acquired heart disease

in children. IVIG is recommended for all children diagnosed with Kawasaki disease in the United States within 7 days of illness if possible.

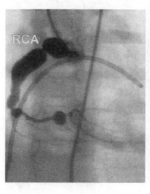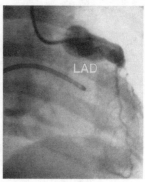

5 Answer A. Congenital rubella is not typically associated with Ebstein anomaly. It is, however, associated with peripheral pulmonary arterial stenosis and PDA and ASDs, VSD, TOF, transposition of the great arteries, tricuspid atresia, and coarctation of the aorta. In addition to cardiovascular abnormalities, congenital rubella is associated with microcephaly, cataracts, and deafness. Rubella has also been documented as a viral cause of myocarditis.

6 Answer C. This patient has findings consistent with a large PDA. These patients will often develop symptoms of left ventricular failure, which include irritability, poor feeding, easy fatigability, and excessive sweating even while in a cold room. Patients with a PDA often have tachypnea and tachycardia and bounding peripheral pulses with a rapid upstroke and widened pulse pressure.

7 Answer A. Ebstein anomaly represents the most common congenital anomaly of the tricuspid valve. In Ebstein, the anterior leaflet arises from the normal position on the tricuspid valve annulus. However, the septal and posterior leaflets are displaced into the RV to varying degrees. This results in a portion of the RV becoming "atrialized." The anterior leaflet may be redundant resulting in a "sail-like" appearance (see following figure). There is an equal distribution between men and women. The EKG typically has prominent P waves consistent with RA enlargement. WPW is seen in 20% to 30% of patients with Ebstein anomaly.

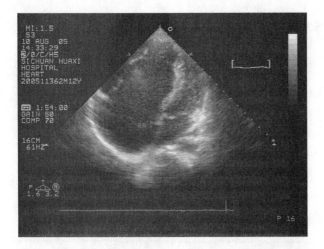

8 **Answer D.** Patients with both Duchenne and Becker muscular dystrophy develop dilated cardiomyopathy. Specifically, at age 21, 100% of Duchenne and 75% of Becker muscular dystrophy patients will have dilated cardiomyopathy. They typically do not develop other forms of cardiomyopathy such as restrictive disease and usually do not have structural heart disease such as VSDs. It is well recognized that patients with muscular dystrophy can develop conduction disease, in particular, heart block. However, there is no recognized association between muscular dystrophy and the long QT syndrome.

9 **Answer E.** The echocardiogram is a four-chamber view depicting a complete atrioventricular (AV) canal defect. This defect is most commonly associated with Down syndrome. As many as 40% of patients with Down syndrome will have some form of congenital heart disease and up to half of these patients will have AV canal defects. Hurler syndrome is a mucopolysaccharidosis that results in chamber and valvar thickening. Holt-Oram syndrome is an autosomal dominant disorder that is often associated with ASDs. Costello syndrome may be associated with pulmonic valve stenosis and mitral valve prolapse. Noonan syndrome is often associated with pulmonic stenosis. It is also associated with hypertrophic cardiomyopathy.

10 **Answer C.** The diagnosis of Marfan syndrome is based on the Nosology of Ghent. These criteria consist of the characteristic cardiac involvement in the disease, which is aortic root dilatation. Patients may also have a history of ectopia lentis. The skeletal abnormalities may include a positive thumb or wrist sign, >20 degrees of scoliosis, pectus carinatum or excavatum, pes planus with demand displacement of the medial malleolus, abnormal upper/lower segment ratio, arm span >105% of height, and typical facies (deep-set eyes, malar hypoplasia, retrognathia). There may also be a history of dural ectasia, which is a ballooning or expansion of the dural sac.

11 **Answer B.** Systemic to pulmonary shunts are placed to provide a source of pulmonary blood flow. See following figure. These may vary in their location and sources of systemic flow (arterial vs. venous). The Glenn anastomosis connects the SVC to the PA resulting in flow only to the right or left PA (classic Glenn) or to both PAs (bidirectional Glenn). The Blalock-Taussig shunt was the first successful palliative procedure for cyanotic congenital heart disease. In the classic Blalock-Taussig procedure, the subclavian artery is connected to the PA directly whereas in the modified Blalock-Taussig, which is the current procedure, a graft is placed from the subclavian artery to the PA. The modified Potts procedure results in a graft from the descending aorta to the left PA. The Waterston shunt (sometimes known as the *Waterston-Cooley shunt*) results in a graft from the ascending aorta to the RPA. Grafts from the apex of the left ventricle to the aorta or apicoaortic conduits have been used to improve systemic flow in the setting of severe left-sided obstructive disease.

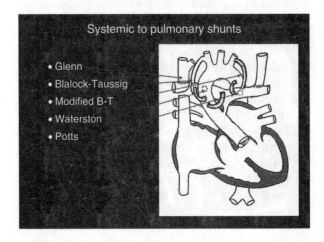

12 **Answer C.** Patients with coarctation of the aorta have a common association with the bicuspid aortic valve. Up to 85% of patients with coarctation of the aorta will have bicuspid aortic valve. They may also have large VSDs, subvalvular aortic stenosis, valvar aortic stenosis, and varying degrees of mitral stenosis. Coarctation represents 6% to 8% of patients with congenital heart disease and is more common in males. A defect in the media of the aorta appears to be the causative mechanism.

13 **Answer D.** All of these conditions may be seen in patients who have undergone surgical repair of coarctation of the aorta. However, residual or recurrent coarctation requiring further intervention may occur in up to 20% of cases. Currently, angioplasty with or without stenting, is advocated at sites of recoarctation as a treatment modality. However, the long-term results of this approach are still not known. In addition, patients are at a higher disposition to develop late postoperative hypertension and at higher risk of developing premature atherosclerotic disease.

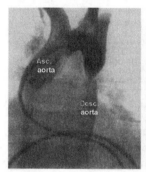 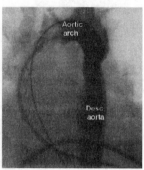

14 **Answer A.** Circulating prostaglandins maintain the patency of the ductus arteriosus. The fetus has relatively high concentrations of prostaglandins secondary to production by the placenta. Following birth, the balance of residual prostaglandins and the constricting effects of oxygen on the ductus decide patency. This balance can be shifted by the infusion of prostaglandin, which is done in congenital lesions that require ductal flow to perfuse either the lungs or the systemic vasculature. In full-term infants, a PDA will usually completely close within 2 to 3 weeks. The PDA is exposed to a partial pressure of oxygen of 20 to 25 mm Hg. The increase in P_{O_2} following birth results in constriction and closure of the duct in term children. The PDA connects the MPA to the descending aorta in a patient with a left arch. With a right aortic arch, the PDA is distal to the right subclavian artery.

15 **Answer C.** Origin of the left circumflex from the right coronary artery is the most common congenital coronary anomaly. Single coronary arteries occur in approximately 5% to 15% of coronary anomalies and are seen in conditions such as truncus arteriosus, transposition of the great arteries, and TOF. Origin of the left main coronary artery from the right sinus of Valsalva carries important clinical significance as the course can lead between the ascending aorta and the MPA. This can result in compression of the artery with resultant sudden cardiac death. Origin of the

left main coronary artery from the PA is also known as *Bland-Garland-White syndrome.*

16 **Answer A.** Secundum ASDs do not require subacute bacterial endocarditis (SBE) prophylaxis. Other types of ASDs, such as primum ASD and sinus venosus defects require prophylaxis. The other lesions all require SBE prophylaxis. The specific therapy is based on the risk of the proposed procedure.

17 **Answer E.** Population-based studies reveal that between 5 and 8 of every 1,000 live births have some form of congenital cardiovascular malformation. However, there are factors that limit this information including the occurrence of lethal defects that result in fetal demise, the relatively broad phenotypic presentation of disease such as in syndromic patients, and the defects that are not detected by clinicians. Gender distribution is essentially equal as a whole but males are at a higher risk of having more serious cardiac lesions such as transposition of the great arteries. There are known agents that can increase risk of malformations such as maternal exposure to drugs such as lithium and diazepam and exposure to hair dyes and certain solvents. The most important risk factor for having a child with a congenital cardiovascular malformation is a positive family history of either a cardiac or noncardiac defect in a parent or sibling.

18 **Answer D.** Dilation of the coronary sinus should prompt the physician to consider the possibility of a persistent left-sided vena cava (LSVC). The physiology of this finding is completely normal and

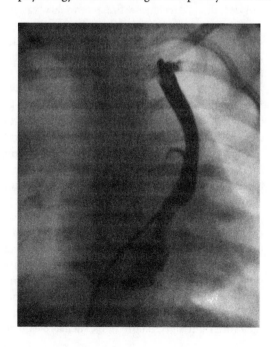

there are no clinical manifestations. Persistent LSVC may also be associated with TOF and other cyanotic cardiac defects but this was not the case in our clinical scenario. Persistent LSVC becomes a consideration if patients are to undergo cardiac surgery or if they were to have a catheterization with a venous approach from the left upper extremity.

19 **Answer C.** Balloon atrial septostomy is one of the few emergency indications for catheterization in infants. The indications for the procedure are as listed in the question. Because septal thickness increases as infants age, the use of a balloon for the technique is only reliable in children <1 month of age. In children older than 1 month, blade atrial septostomy is more reliable. The procedure can be performed through standard venous approaches such as the femoral vein but the umbilical vein is also often utilized. The balloon is pulled back rapidly across the atrial septum from the left atrium to the right atrium in a controlled fashion. This should result in equalization of the atrial pressures. This technique can be performed under fluoroscopic or echocardiographic visualization.

20 **Answer A.** Subaortic stenosis is more common in men and can be difficult to differentiate from valvar aortic stenosis. Echocardiography is the best technique to evaluate this lesion. Surgical intervention is the standard approach as percutaneous techniques have been ineffective. Aortic insufficiency can develop secondary to thickening or impaired mobility of the valve leaflets and can worsen over time. Even with surgical resection, this lesion can recur.

21 **Answer D.** To calculate the pulmonary vascular resistance, the mean left atrial (LA) pressure is subtracted from the mean PA pressure. This value is then divided by the pulmonary flow (Qp). The value is expressed in Wood units.

22 **Answer B.** Single ventricle physiology is marked by the obligation of one functional ventricle (either right or left) to generate sufficient cardiac output to traverse blood through both the systemic and pulmonary vasculature. As there is no generation of force as the blood passes from the systemic venous return into the pulmonary arterial bed through the Fontan circuit or the total cavopulmonary anastomosis, flow into the lungs is passive. Elevation of pressures in the pulmonary vasculature from ventricular failure, AV valve regurgitation, increased pulmonary blood flow or resistance, or arrhythmias can result in congestion in the Fontan circuit and a "failing Fontan." Evidence of Fontan failure can be seen with right-sided failure signs, such as peripheral

edema, ascites, and PLE. PLE is postulated to be secondary to bowel edema and resultant protein loss in the stool. As venous pooling occurs, this can result in low cardiac output states. The stretch of the Fontan circuit or previous surgeries can result in atrial arrhythmias (see following figure).

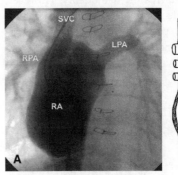 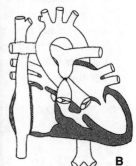

23 **Answer D.** Calculation of pulmonary blood flow or Qp is done by dividing the oxygen consumption by the difference between the pulmonary vein (PV) O_2 content and the pulmonary artery (PA) O_2 content. The systemic blood flow or Qs is calculated by dividing the oxygen consumption by the difference of the systemic arterial O_2 content and the mixed venous O_2 content. The Qp:Qs is calculated by dividing the Qp by the Qs. This value is unitless.

24 **Answer B.** The patient described has a patent ductus arteriosus, as seen by both echocardiography and angiography. These lesions are typically closed in children, as there is a significant risk of spontaneous bacterial endocarditis and pulmonary overcirculation and volume overload. A percutaneous transcatheter approach is the therapy of choice but surgery can still be considered in very small children. Success rates of transcatheter closure are quite good. The size of the lesion can influence the approach. In smaller ducts (<2 mm), coil occlusion would be pursued with the coil being deployed to loop both in the aorta and the PA. The coils are typically deployed in a retrograde manner from the femoral artery. In larger ducts, occlusion would be best performed using an Amplatzer duct occluder from a venous approach.

25 **Answer B.** Severe obstruction secondary to pulmonary valve stenosis may be underestimated by echocardiographic techniques in cyanotic children as there is typically a patent foramen ovale to allow for right-to-left shunting. Therefore, only a fraction of the right-sided cardiac output is traversing the valve. Balloon valvuloplasty should be considered for all patients with a gradient of >40 mm Hg. National health studies have shown that intervention should be pursued for peak systolic gradients of >50 mm Hg. Carcinoid disease can be a cause of acquired pulmonary valve stenosis. However, congenital pulmonary stenosis (PS) would be more common and is a result of commissural fusion. Neonates with critical PS should undergo ballooning. The results are very good and in many patients "curative." Many patients, especially adolescents and adults with PS, have subvalvular or infundibular stenosis. This is unmasked after the valvar obstruction is relieved. This can lead to subpulmonic dynamic obstruction in the face of afterload reduction or the so-called "suicide ventricle" resulting in even higher gradients out of the RV outflow tract than before the intervention.

26 **Answer D.**   This angiogram depicts a coronary artery fistula draining into the RV. These are also known as *cameral fistulas* as they drain into a chamber. Coronary fistulas can drain into the coronary sinus or the PA as well as the right atrium and RV. They may lead to shortness of breath or exercise intolerance. There is also the potential for coronary steal.

27 **Answer B.**   Balloon valvuloplasty in neonates with critical AS is considered a good option for the palliation of this process. Up to 30% of the patients treated will develop at least mild aortic insufficiency within days of the procedure. Femoral artery complications may occur in up to a third of the patients, because many of these patients are small in size. Neonates with critical AS may be asymptomatic after birth as they can receive retrograde perfusion of the ascending aorta and coronaries through the ductus arteriosus. Left bundle branch block and ventricular arrhythmias may occur with the procedure.

28 **Answer E.**   Aortopulmonary collaterals would result in a left-to-right shunt. The other lesions would all result in a right-to-left shunt with resultant cyanosis.

Suggested Readings

Allen HD, Gutgesell HP, Clark EB et al., eds. *Moss and Adams: Heart disease in infants, children, and adolescents*, 6th ed. Philadelphia, PA: Lippincott Williams & Wilkins; 2001.

Baim DS. *Grossman's cardiac catheterization, angiography, and intervention.* Philadelphia, PA: Lippincott Williams & Wilkins; 2005.

Mullins CE. *Cardiac catheterization in congenital heart disease: Pediatric and adult.* Boston, MA: Blackwell Futura; 2006.

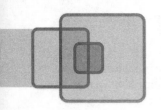

31

Patent Foramen Ovale and Atrial Septal Defect

Howard C. Herrmann

Questions

1 The following figure shows a pictorial diagram of the heart with the patent foramen ovale (PFO) shown by an *arrow*. Which of the following statements correctly identifies other anatomic structures (more than one answer may be correct)?

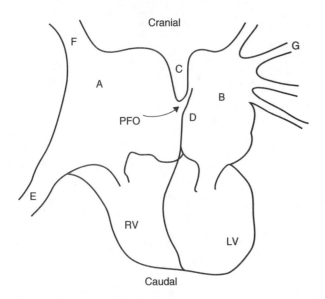

(A) Left atrium
(B) Right atrium
(C) Septum secundum
(D) Septum primum
(E) Inferior vena cava
(F) Right upper pulmonary vein
(G) Left subclavian vein

2 Current indications for closure of a PFO may include all of the following, *except*:

(A) Recurrent paradoxical embolism
(B) Hypoxemia due to right-to-left shunting
(C) Pulmonary hypertension
(D) Decompression illness
(E) Orthodeoxy–platypnea syndrome

3 Which of the following statements describing the United States regulations regarding PFO closure is *true*?

(A) The CardioSEAL closure device is U.S. Food and Drug Administration (FDA)-approved for PFO closure
(B) Several devices have previously had humanitarian device exemption approval for patients with recurrent paradoxical embolism on warfarin anticoagulation, but this approval has recently been revoked
(C) Off-label PFO closure can be performed with any device as long as the physician recommends it and the patient consents
(D) The Institutional Review Board (IRB) approval is needed for any PFO procedure

4 In which of the following patients might percutaneous closure be a reasonable therapeutic option?

(A) A 45-year-old man who has had a presumed embolic stroke with no obvious risk factors for stroke. His magnetic resonance imaging

(MRI) shows a recent as well as a remote infarct in two distinct areas. His transesophageal echocardiogram (TEE) shows a PFO and an atrial septal aneurysm

(B) A 75-year-old man with recurrent transient ischemic attacks (TIAs) despite aspirin therapy. His TTE shows mild mitral stenosis and a PFO

(C) A 42-year-old woman who suffers a stroke and has a PFO. Her workup reveals lupus and a positive anticardiolipin antibody

(D) A 46-year-old man with lung cancer who suffers a stroke and has a deep vein thrombolysis (DVT) in his right leg

5 Which of the following choices is considered to increase the likelihood of recurrent stroke in patients with a paradoxical embolism through a PFO?

(A) Large shunt
(B) Residual shunt after percutaneous closure
(C) Prominent Eustachian valve and right atrium stands
(D) Lipomatous septum secundum
(E) Event occurring on warfarin anticoagulation.

6 The cine image reproduced in the following figure in a patient with PFO illustrates which of the following findings and treatment strategies?

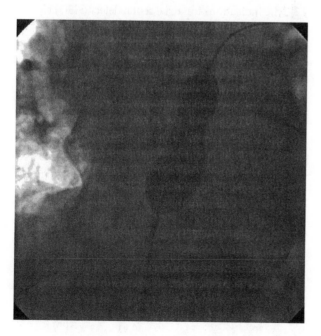

(A) A sizing balloon used to document the absence of a significant left-to-right shunting

(B) A sizing balloon used to stretch or tear a long "tunnel"

(C) A percutaneous occluding device being deployed by balloon inflation

(D) Pulmonary vein isolation to prevent atrial fibrillation (AF) before PFO closure

7 Which of the following is *true* about this echocardiographic image of a markedly positive bubble study for right-to-left shunting through a PFO?

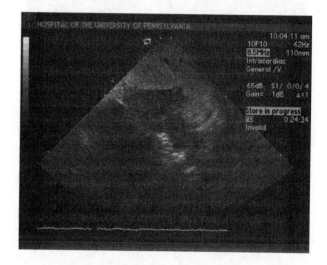

(A) It is an intracardiac echo (ICE) image with the right atrium on top, left atrium below, head to the right, and feet to the left

(B) It is an ICE image with the left atrium on top and right atrium below

(C) It is an ICE image with right atrium on top, left atrium below, head to left, and feet to right

(D) It is a TEE image with left atrium on top

8 Which of the following are possible explanations for the low rates of recurrent stroke and TIA after percutaneous device closure?

(A) The devices prevent thrombi from crossing the PFO

(B) Most trials of device closure have enrolled younger patients than in trials of medical therapy for stroke (selection bias)

(C) Concomitant medical therapy

(D) All of the above

9 Match the following figures with the descriptions given:

(A)

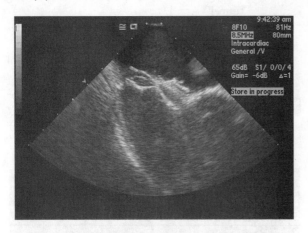

(B)

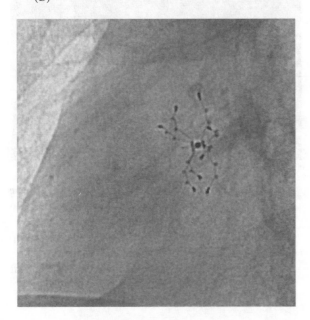

(C)

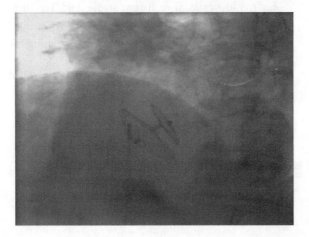

1. Fluoroscopic image of a deployed CardioSeal device

2. Fluoroscopic image of a deployed Amplatzer PFO occluder

3. Intracardiac echo image of a deployed CardioSeal device

10 The most appropriate explanation for a positive bubble contrast echo study in which the bubbles enter the left atrium more than five heart beats after their appearance in the right atrium with an IV injection is:

(A) Coexistent mitral stenosis

(B) Failure of the patient to provide a good Valsalva maneuver

(C) A persistent left superior vena cava

(D) A pulmonary arterial-venous malformation (AVM)

11 Which of the following statements about ASDs is *false*?

(A) Secundum ASDs are the most common type and are usually located in the septum secundum

(B) Sinus venosus ASDs are often associated with one or more anomalous pulmonary veins

(C) Septum primum ASDs may be associated with ventricular septal defects (VSDs)

(D) Most ASDs can now be closed percutaneously

12 The indications for atrial septal defect (ASD) closure may include all of the following, *except*:

(A) Dyspnea

(B) Pulmonary hypertension

(C) Right-sided chamber enlargement

(D) Paradoxical embolism

(E) Qp:Qs >1.8:1, even if asymptomatic

(F) All of the above

13 On the basis of the oximetry measurements (see table), which of the following patients referred for percutaneous ASD closure would cause you to hesitate in proceeding with implantation?

	SVC Saturation (percent)	IVC Saturation (percent)	Pa Saturation (percent)	Aortic Saturation (percent)
A	75	79	85	97
B	72	80	85	100
C	70	71	91	99
D	75	76	81	92

IVC, inferior vena cava; SVC, superior vena cava.

14 The intracardiac echocardiographic image (see following figure) demonstrates which of the following?

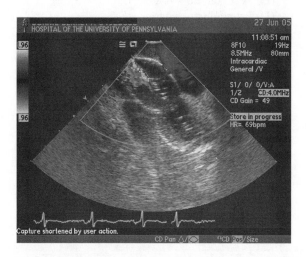

(A) Balloon deployment of an Amplatzer atrial septal occlusion device
(B) Atrial septostomy to increase the ASD size before closure
(C) Percutaneous balloon valvuloplasty for mitral stenosis.
(D) Balloon sizing of an ASD

15 Which of the following statements best describes the ICE image shown in the following figure?

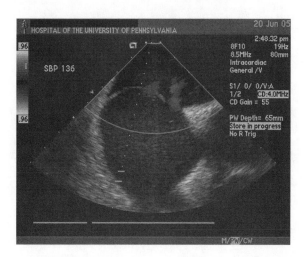

(A) A septum primum defect with both an ASD and a VSD
(B) A fenestrated ASD that will require a surgically placed patch
(C) Two discrete secundum defects closable percutaneously
(D) Echocardiographic reverberations from a bidirectional ASD

16 Which of the following complications (<30 days) and their incidence is *incorrect* for Amplatzer ASD closure procedures?

(A) Unsuccessful procedure, 2% to 3%
(B) Stroke, <1%
(C) Device embolization, <1%
(D) Cardiac arrhythmia, approximately 5%
(E) Perforation/Tamponade, <1%
(F) Allergic reactions to nickel, approximately 5%

17 Which of the following statements is *true* in short-term and medium-term follow-up after percutaneous ASD closure?

(A) Most patients will eventually require surgery to permanently close their defects
(B) Pulmonary hypertension will return to normal over 1 to 3 months
(C) Most patients will not experience further enlargement or deterioration in right ventricular (RV) function
(D) Endocarditis prophylaxis and anticoagulation is required life-long

18 Match the complications of ASD closure with their most likely mechanism:

(A) Inferior ST-segment elevation during the procedure
(B) Pericardial tamponade 18-hour postprocedure
(C) AF 30-day postprocedure
(D) Recurrent, nonsustained venous thrombus (VT) 4-hour postprocedure

1. A pulse transit time (PTT) >150 seconds
2. Common, transient response to healing
3. Compression of the left circumflex coronary artery
4. Irritation of the left upper pulmonary vein
5. Air embolism
6. Device perforation
7. Thrombotic embolism to left anterior descending (LAD)
8. Device embolization

19 Which of the following tests can be used to detect a right-to-left shunt?

(A) Transthoracic echo with peripheral intravenous contrast (e.g., agitated saline microbubbles) injection
(B) Transesophageal echo with contrast injection
(C) Transcranial Doppler (power mode) ultrasonography with contrast injection
(D) Green dye indicator dilution curves

(E) Intracardiac echocardiography with femoral venous contrast injection

(F) All of the above

20 Which of the following structural heart defects have now been successfully closed with percutaneous devices (more than one answer is possible)?

(A) Secundum ASD
(B) Muscular VSD
(C) Postinfarction VSD
(D) Patent ductus arteriosus
(E) Primum ASD
(F) Sinus venosus ASD

Answers and Explanations

1 Answer C, D, and E. The foramen ovale is an interarterial communication defect present in up to 20% of normal adults. It is a small channel between the septum secundum and septum primum that may allow passage of blood or thrombotic emboli from the right part to the left part of the heart.

2 Answer C. Most patients who undergo percutaneous (or surgical) PFO closure do so to prevent recurrent paradoxical embolism of a VT. However, a less common indication is hypoxemia due to positional right-to-left shunting (orthodeoxy-platypnea) (*J Interv Cardiol.* 2005;18:227–232). Right-to-left shunting of dissolved gas after deep scuba diving can result in decompression illness and may be an indication for closure in some technical divers. Pulmonary hypertension alone is not an indication to close a PFO unless it results in hypoxemia due to right-to-left shunting. It may result secondarily because of left-to-right shunting through an ASD, but left-to-right shunting through a PFO is never severe enough to cause pulmonary hypertension.

3 Answer B. No device is fully FDA-approved for PFO closure. The HDE exemption allows closure with either the CardioSEAL or Amplatzer PFO devices for patients with recurrent paradoxical embolism following failure of warfarin anticoagulation under IRB supervision. The CardioSEAL VSDs and Amplatzer ASD occluders can be utilized by a physician in an off-label fashion to close a PFO, and IRB approval in addition to standard procedural consent is not required for this situation.

4 Answer A. This patient has evidence for recurrent paradoxical embolism with a high-risk anatomy. However, it must be recognized that no randomized trial has been completed to demonstrate that percutaneous closure is superior to medical therapy with either antiplatelet or anticoagulant therapy. The other patients have other potential causes for their strokes and also have indications for chronic anticoagulation.

5 Answer D. All of the other characteristics have been associated with recurrent paradoxical embolism.

6 Answer B. The segment of overlap between septum primum and secundum may be discrete, or have substantial overlap. In the latter case, the overlap segment or "tunnel" may be quite stiff thereby preventing optimal deployment of a device. In this case, stretching or tearing of the tunnel with a balloon can facilitate device placement.

7 Answer A. This is a standard ICE image projection with the transducer in the right atrium (top of image) looking across the septum to the left atrium. It is oriented with the feet to the left and the head of the patient to the right. The entire right atrium is opacified with contrast, which is flowing briskly through the PFO into the upper portions of the left atrium.

8 Answer D.

9 Answer. The figure in A is an ICE image of a deployed CardioSEAL device. The figure in B is the fluoroscopic image of the same device. The figure in C is a fluoroscopic image of an Amplatzer PFO occluder.

10 Answer D. Although a Valsalva maneuver (or sniffing) can increase the detection of a PFO by increasing right atrium (relative to left atrium) pressure, most shunts will be visible because of normal respiratory variation within five cardiac cycles. Patients with a pulmonary AVM may have an extracardiac shunt that is only visible once contrast has traversed the pulmonary circulation. These can also be a cause of paradoxical embolism and can be diagnosed by chest computed tomography (CT) and MRI.

11 Answer A.

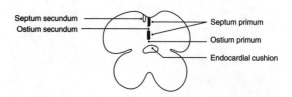

Secundum ASDs are the most common form of ASD (70%) and most can now be closed percutaneously (hence, D is true). Secundum ASDs are (paradoxically) located in the primum portion of the atrial septum (see preceding figure). The ostium primum defects are associated with abnormalities of the endocardial cushion, and may involve the upper portion of the ventricular septum.

12 **Answer F.** All of these are reasonable indications for ASD closure in the presence of a significant left-to-right shunt. Traditionally, a Qp:Qs ratio >2 has been considered a cutoff for surgical closure in asymptomatic patients. However, it has been shown that percutaneous closure can increase peak oxygen consumption during exercise even in some apparently asymptomatic patients with Qp:Qs <2 (*J Am Coll Cardiol.* 2004;43:1886–1891).

13 **Answer D.** Patients A, B, and C all have significant left-to-right shunts ranging from 1.7 to 3.6 (calculated using a mixed venous saturation $= ([3 \times SVC + IVC])/4$ and the shunt formula of $Qp:Qs = (Ao\,sat - MV02)/(Ao\,sat–Pa\,sat)$. Patient D has a systemic desaturation that can reflect associated lung disease or right-to-left shunting. In the latter case, the bidirectional shunt formula must be utilized. Eisenmenger syndrome (right heart failure leading to reversal of flow across the ASD) must be assessed to ensure that the closure does not result in progressive right heart failure.

14 **Answer D.** This ICE image shows a balloon inflated in a secundum ASD, which is an important part of percutaneous ASD closure. The balloon forces the defect into a circular configuration, and is expanded until the color flow Doppler evidence of left-to-right shunting ceases. An Amplatzer atrial septal occluder is then chosen so that its central diameter is 1 to 2 mm greater than the waist measurement on the balloon.

15 **Answer C.** Secundum ASDs may have multiple defects or fenestrations. In some cases, defects can be closed percutaneously by placing an ASD device in the largest fenestration or using multiple devices. In the illustrated case, these two discrete defects were closed using two ASD devices placed in an overlapping or "sandwich" approach (see figure below).

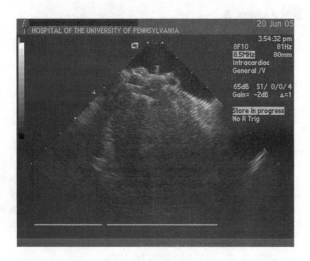

16 **Answer F.** Procedural success in the pivotal study was >97%, but does depend on how patients are selected preprocedure (should have at least 5 mm of tissue rim on all sides and diameter <38 mm). Major complications are rare, with minor atrial arrhythmias occurring in up to 5% of patients within the first month. Allergic reactions are usually related to concomitant medications (especially clopidogrel) and true allergies to the nickel contained in the device that is made of a nickel-titanium alloy (titanium) is extremely rare (<1/1,000). (*AGA physician manual http://www.Fda.gov/ohrms/dockets/ac/01/briefing/ 3790b1_02_sponsor.doc*).

17 **Answer C.** In general, percutaneous closure of the ASD is definitive therapy that eliminates the left-to-right shunt causing RV enlargement, pulmonary hypertension, and the stimulus to RV hypertrophy. However, some patients with pulmonary hypertension would have developed permanent changes that prevent the pressure from returning to normal (fixed pulmonary hypertension). Antiplatelet medications are usually administered for 6 months following device closure after which endothelialization reduces the risk of thrombus formation and infection. Anticoagulation is rarely necessary unless there is a separate indication such as chronic AF.

18 **Answer.** A-5, B-6, C-2, D-8.

19 **Answer F.** A, B, and C are the usual preprocedure methods utilized. ICE is often used during the procedure to confirm the shunt before closure. Indocyanine green dye dilution curves can also be used to assess cardiac output and to detect shunts. If dye is injected into the femoral vein, early appearance in a femoral artery sample due to bypass of the pulmonary circulation is evidence of a right-to-left shunt (see following figure) (*Diagnostic and Therapeutic Catheterization.* 1994; 388–390).

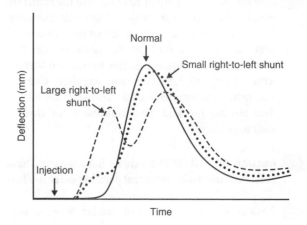

Because these calculations are somewhat cumbersome, this method has been replaced by imaging modalities with contrast injections. Currently, power mode transcranial Doppler and TEE are considered more sensitive than TTE, though the patient position, injection site, and the use of maneuvers (e.g., Valsalva and Mueller) affect the sensitivity and specificity of shunt detection (*J Neuroimaging*. 2004;14:342–349, *J Neuroimaging*. 2003;13:356–358).

20 **Answer E and F.** Primum ASD defects are located in the lower portion of the septum at the endocardial cushion and are often associated with abnormalities of the atrioventricular valves and/or ventricular septum making placement of a closure device dangerous as it could interfere with valvular function. Sinus venous defects are in the upper portion of the septum and are often associated with an anomalous pulmonary vein in the right atrium. The lack of a rim of tissue superiorly and the frequent need to baffle the anomalous pulmonary venous flow to the left atrium makes these defects not suitable for currently available closure devices.

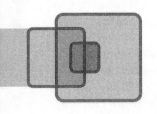

32

Percutaneous Balloon Pericardiotomy for Patients with Pericardial Effusion and Tamponade

Andrew O. Maree, Hani Jneid, and Igor F. Palacios

Questions

1 A 61-year old woman with recent tricuspid valve repair presents with increasing dyspnea, orthopnea, and presyncope. The patient was hypotensive, with distended jugular veins, and distant heart sounds on physical examination. On the basis of the hemodynamic tracing from the right ventricle (RV) shown in the following figure, which of the following statements is *incorrect*?

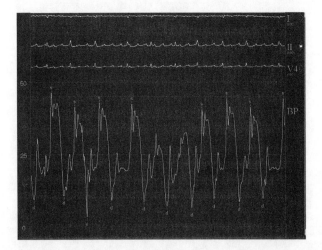

(A) Pulsus paradoxus is likely to be present
(B) Presence of right ventricular collapse lasting more than one third of diastole is a more

sensitive echo finding in this condition than right atrial collapse
(C) Blunt or absent Y descent on the right atrial pressure tracing is typically described in this condition
(D) Ventricular interdependence may be accentuated

2 Cardiac tamponade in the absence of pulsus paradoxus is described with all of the following, *except*:

(A) Aortic incompetence
(B) Severe rheumatoid spondylitis
(C) Constrictive pericarditis
(D) Large atrial septal defect

3 Regarding the intervention depicted in the figures, which of the following statements is *incorrect*?

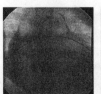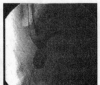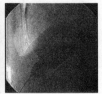

(A) Left pleural effusion occurs in 1% to 2% of cases

(B) A pericardiocutaneous fistula is a potential complication

(C) It is recommended that the balloon be inflated until the waist disappears

(D) Biplane fluoroscopy is recommended

4 All of the following are relative contraindications to percutaneous balloon pericardiotomy, *except*:

(A) Marginal respiratory reserve

(B) Presence of a large pleural effusion

(C) Thrombocytopenia

(D) Malignant pericardial effusion

5 Which of the following catheterization finding most reliably *supports* a diagnosis of pericardial constriction over restrictive cardiomyopathy?

(A) Pulmonary artery systolic pressure <50 mm Hg

(B) A prominent Y descent

(C) Equalization of right and left heart late diastolic pressures

(D) Ventricular interdependence

6 Regarding pericardiocentesis, which of the following statements is *most accurate*?

(A) It is advisable to drain <500 mL at a time to avoid acute right ventricular dilatation

(B) Recurrence rate with drainage of large idiopathic pericardial effusions is no better than with conservative management

(C) Major complications occur during 1.3% to 1.6% of pericardiocenteses

(D) Effusions measured by echo tend to be larger than those measured by computed tomography (CT) or magnetic resonance imaging (MRI)

7 In the setting of aortic dissection, which of the following statements is *incorrect*?

(A) Pericardial effusion coincides with 17% to 45% of cases

(B) Pericardial tamponade occurs most frequently with a De-Bakey type I dissection

(C) Pericardiocentesis may cause extension of the dissection

(D) Surgery should be performed as soon as possible

8 In patients with large malignancy-related pericardial effusion treated with percutaneous balloon pericardiotomy, which of the following is *incorrect*?

(A) Fever occurs in approximately one third of patients post procedure

(B) Recurrence rate at 4 months is approximately 50%

(C) Results with immediate and deferred procedures are similar

(D) Lung and breast cancer associated effusions are most common

9 A 64-year-old man with a history of alcohol dependency presented to the emergency room with increasing dyspnea, chronic cough, hemoptysis, and persistent fever. Echocardiography confirms the presence of a large pericardial effusion. Simultaneous right atrial pressure and pericardial opening pressure are shown in the following figure. Regarding this hemodynamic tracing, which of the following statements is *incorrect*?

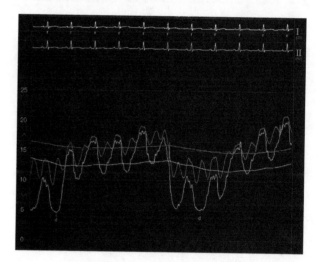

(A) The X descent during ventricular systole is the dominant waveform

(B) The right atrial and pericardial pressures fall during inspiration

(C) With increased pericardial fluid accumulation, the X descent will become less prominent and the Y decent more pronounced

(D) RV mid-diastolic pressure may be elevated and equal to the right atrial and pericardial pressure

10 The patient discussed in Question 9 had a cardiac CT (short axis shown in the following figure) on admission. He had a reasonable symptomatic response to pericardiocentesis and his pericardial pressure returned to zero post-tap; however, his right atrial pressure remained elevated. On the basis of his findings on cardiac CT scan and his hemodynamic parameters, a presumptive diagnosis of effusive-constrictive pericarditis was made. Which of the following findings does *not* support this diagnosis?

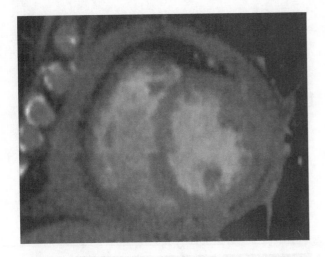

(A) Equalization of the right and left ventricular end diastolic pressures

(B) A prominent dip and plateau waveform in the right ventricular tracing

(C) Concordance between the left and right ventricular systolic pressures

(D) Right ventricular end systolic pressure <50 mm Hg

11 *Mycobacterium tuberculosis* was found in the same patient's (discussed in Questions 9 and 10) pericardial fluid. Which of the following statements regarding tuberculous pericarditis is *incorrect*?

(A) Pericardial constriction occurs in 10% to 15% of cases

(B) The mortality rate approaches 85% in untreated cases

(C) A rapid diagnosis can be made from a small volume fluid sample by polymerase chain reaction (PCR)

(D) The tuberculin skin test is falsely negative in 25% to 30% of cases

12 A patient with a history of tuberculous pericarditis presents with progressively increasing dyspnea and undergoes the noninvasive study depicted in the following figure. Regarding this investigative study, which of the following statements is *correct*?

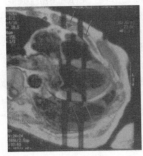 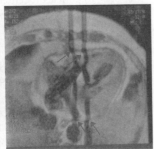

(A) The image on the left represents evidence of pericardial constriction and tethered movement of the heart

(B) The images represent CT scan tagging, which can be used to diagnose pericardial constriction

(C) Pericardial thickening is absent in approximately 18% of cases of constrictive pericarditis

(D) Pericardiectomy for constrictive pericarditis has a mortality rate of 1% to 2%

13 Which of the following statements regarding endomyocardial biopsy or temporary pacemaker lead placement is *false*?

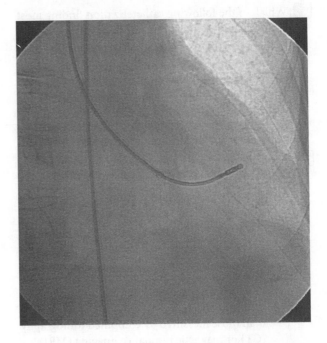

(A) The rate of perforation during right ventricular biopsy is 0.3% to 5%

(B) Tamponade and circulatory collapse follow right ventricular perforation 75% of the time

(C) Pericardial haemorrhage complicates 0.1% to 3.3% of left ventricular biopsies

(D) Presence of right rather than left bundle branch block configuration suggests pacemaker lead penetration of the RV

14 During insertion of an implantable cardioverter defibrillator the patient becomes acutely hypotensive and an echo confirms the presence of an effusion. Which finding in the hemodynamic tracing in the following figure does *not* support a diagnosis of pericardial tamponade?

(A) Presence of an elevated right atrial pressure

(B) Blunting of the Y descent in expiration

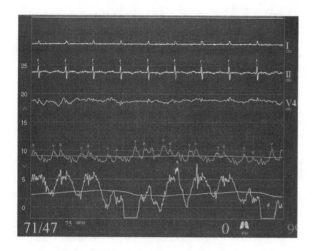

(C) Absence of respiratory variation in the right atrial tracing

(D) Pericardial pressure approaching right atrial diastolic pressure in expiration

15 Which of the following statements regarding the pericardium is *incorrect*?

(A) The pericardial space contains 15 to 35 mL serous fluid

(B) Pericardial inflammation may produce vagal mediated responses

(C) The parietal pericardium is attached to both the diaphragm and the sternum

(D) Aspirin is more effective at reducing symptoms and recurrence of acute pericarditis than colchicine

16 With regard to an association between the procedure depicted in the following figure and pericardial tamponade, which of the following is *true*?

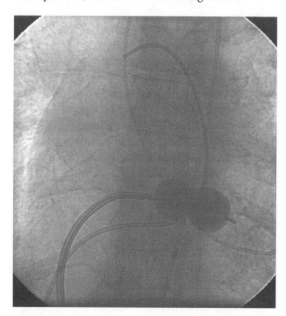

(A) Performing the procedure in a biplane catheterization laboratory does not reduce the association with tamponade

(B) Presence of a small left atrium is associated with a greater incidence of tamponade

(C) Onset of symptoms of tamponade rarely occur more than an hour after the procedure

(D) Tamponade occurs without associated chest pain in most cases

17 Which of the following parameters significantly determines pericardial pressure in the setting of a pericardial effusion?

(A) Volume of the effusion

(B) Rate of accumulation of the effusion

(C) Pericardial elasticity

(D) All of the above

18 Among patients with an active malignancy or a history of cancer and a significant pericardial effusion, which of the following statements is *correct*?

(A) Pericardial disease is the most common indication for cardiology consultation among patients with cancer who are hospitalized

(B) Presence of abnormal fluid cytology is not associated with a significant reduction in survival

(C) Patients with malignancy-related pericardial effusions are twice as likely to require repeat pericardial intervention as those with nonmalignancy-related effusions

(D) Pericardial fluid cytology is abnormal in approximately 75% of cases

19 Regarding percutaneous approach to pericardiocentesis, which of the following statements is *false*?

(A) A right xiphocostal approach is associated with right atrium and inferior vena cava injury

(B) Puncture of the left pleura and lingual is more frequent with an apical approach

(C) Puncture of the left anterior descending coronary artery and left internal mammary artery is more common with the parasternal approach

(D) Left chest wall approach should not be used when performed with echo-guided procedures

20 Regarding percutaneous balloon pericardiotomy, which of the following is *incorrect*?

(A) Thoracocentesis is required following balloon pericardiotomy in 30% to 40% of cases

(B) Drainage of >100 mL fluid per 24 hours, 3 days after standard catheter drainage indicates the need for more definitive intervention

(C) Surgical window may be preferred if a loculated fibrinous effusion is present

(D) Reaccumulation of pericardial fluid with recurrent tamponade is considered a strong indication for performing percutaneous balloon pericardiotomy

Answers and Explanations

1 **Answer B.** The hemodynamic trace depicts an elevated RV pressure with exaggerated respiratory variation consistent with pericardial tamponade. Echocardiographic evidence of right ventricular collapse lasting more than one third of diastole is a more specific but less sensitive sign of cardiac tamponade than right atrial collapse (*Circulation.* 1984;70: 966–971). Pulsus paradoxus, which is an exaggeration of the normal respiratory variation in blood pressure and is defined as a >10 mm Hg drop in the systolic arterial pressure during inspiration, is likely to be present. Blunting or loss of the right atrial pressure Y descent with a well-preserved X descent and enhanced ventricular interdependence are well-described findings in pericardial tamponade.

2 **Answer C.** Constrictive pericarditis is a well-described cause of pulsus paradoxus. Pericardial tamponade in the presence of the other three conditions may occur in the absence of pulsus paradoxus. In the presence of aortic incompetence, which may accompany aortic dissection, the left ventricle fills from the aorta during inspiration. The increase in systemic venous return during inspiration is balanced by a decrease in left-to-right shunting by a large atrial septal defect, which results in minimal change in the right ventricular volume and thereby a minimal displacement of the interventricular septum. Severe thoracic skeletal disease prevents wide changes in intrathoracic pressure (*J Postgrad Med.* 2002;48:46–49).

3 **Answer A.** Left pleural effusion occurring within 24 to 48 hours of percutaneous balloon pericardiotomy is a common occurrence, which occurs in up to 50% of patients. Thoracentesis or chest tube placement is required in up to 16% of cases (*J Am Coll Cardiol.* 1993;21:1–5). When carrying out the procedure, care must be taken to advance the balloon so that it straddles the parietal pericardium, however, its proximal end needs to be clear of the skin and subcutaneous tissue to avoid pericardiocutaneous fistula formation. Biplane fluoroscopy is recommended to confirm the position of the balloon in two planes before inflation. Two to three balloon inflations are generally performed ideally resulting in complete obliteration of the waist caused by the parietal pericardium (*Textbook of interventional cardiology.* 1999;869–877).

4 **Answer D.** If a large pleural effusion precedes percutaneous balloon pericardiotomy then the chances of requiring thoracocentesis are high and procedure benefit must outweigh this risk. It is ill advised to perform the procedure in patients with marginal pulmonary reserve such as in those post pneumonectomy owing to the risk of further compromise by a pleural effusion. Platelet or coagulation abnormalities are relative contraindications for the procedure because excessive bleeding from trauma to pericardial vessels may require surgical intervention (*J Am Coll Cardiol.* 1993;21:1–5). The procedure is of particular benefit in patients with recurrent malignant pericardial effusions (*Cathet Cardiovasc Diagn.* 1991;22:244–249). In the presence of a pyopericardium due to bacterial or fungal infection percutaneous balloon pericardiotomy should not be performed.

5 **Answer D.** Dynamic respiratory variation consistent with ventricular interdependence is the best hemodynamic parameter for distinguishing pericardial constriction from a restrictive cardiomyopathy. During inspiration the right ventricular systolic pressure increases and the left ventricular systolic pressure decreases and the inverse occurs during expiration. This finding is >90% sensitive and specific in distinguishing the two conditions (*Circulation.* 1996;93:2007–2013). A prominent Y descent in the right atrial pressure tracing is described with constriction along with equalization of right and left heart diastolic pressures; however, these are less reliable distinguishing parameters. In the presence of a restrictive cardiomyopathy, the left ventricular end diastolic pressure generally exceeds that of the RV. Pulmonary hypertension with a pulmonary artery systolic pressure <50 mm Hg is more typical of a restrictive process (*Circulation.* 2006;113:1622–1632).

6 **Answer C.** Major complications are reported in 1.3% to 1.6% of cases of pericardiocentesis (*Eur Heart J.* 2004;25:587–610). Drainage of more than 1L of pericardial fluid at a time may be associated with right ventricular dilatation (*Am Heart J.* 1984;107:1266–1270). Pericardial catheter drainage on large idiopathic effusions is associated with lower recurrence rate than with conservative treatment (*Am J Cardiol.* 2002;89:704–710). Effusions measured by

CT or MRI tend to be larger than when studied by echocardiography.

7 Answer B. Tamponade is more common with De-Bakey type II (18% to 45%) than type I (17% to 33%) or type III (6%) aortic dissections (*N Engl J Med.* 1992;327:500–501). Pericardial effusions are confirmed in 17% to 45% of patients presenting with aortic dissection and in 48% at autopsy (*Heart.* 2001;86:227–234). Pericardiocentesis is contraindicated in these patients due to the risk of further haemorrhage and extension of the dissection (*Eur Heart J.* 2001;22:1642–1681).

8 Answer B. Percutaneous balloon pericardiotomy in patients with large malignancy-related pericardial effusions is highly successful with approximately 88% freedom from recurrence at 4 months. Malignancy-related effusions are most commonly associated with lung and breast cancer. Results with immediate or deferred intervention are comparable and the procedure is associated with fever in approximately one third of patients (*Chest.* 2002;122:893–899).

9 Answer C. The patient has elevated right atrial and pericardial pressures. The pericardial pressure approaches right atrial pressure in expiration and thereby represents early pericardial tamponade. The X descent, which occurs after the a wave and before and after the C wave represents systolic decline in atrial pressure. It is well preserved during cardiac tamponade unlike the Y descent. The Y descent follows the V wave (venous filling of atrium in late systole) and represents diastolic decline in atrial pressure. The Y descent is initially blunted and then obliterated as pericardial pressure rises with increasing pericardial fluid accumulation. Both pericardial and right atrial pressures fall during inspiration and increase during expiration. Right ventricular mid-diastolic pressures are elevated and may equal the right atrial and pericardial pressures. Ultimately diastolic equalization of pressures occurs and interventricular dependence becomes more apparent.

10 Answer C. Effusive-constrictive pericarditis exists when constrictive pericardial hemodynamic findings result after a pericardial effusion is treated. Pericardial constriction results in increased ventricular interdependence and discordance between the right and left ventricular pressures. This is the best hemodynamic parameter for distinguishing constriction from a restrictive cardiomyopathy. The right and left ventricular end diastolic pressures usually differ by <5 mm Hg and a classic dip and plateau pattern is seen in diastole. Right ventricular end systolic pressure is usually <50 mm Hg unlike in restrictive cardiomyopathy where it can often be higher (*Curr Treat Options Cardiovasc Med.* 1999;1:63–71).

11 Answer A. Pericardial constriction occurs in 30% to 50% of patients with tuberculous pericarditis. Mortality rate can be as high as 85% if untreated and the disease follows a relapsing and remitting course. Use of PCR to identify *M. tuberculosis* deoxyribonucleic acid (DNA) is rapid and highly sensitive and can be performed on very limited samples. The tuberculin skin test is falsely negative in 25% to 33% of patients (*J Am Coll Cardiol.* 1988;11: 724–728).

12 Answer C. Pericardial thickening (>2 mm) was found to be absent in 18% of operatively proven cases of constrictive pericarditis (*Circulation.* 2003;108: 1852–1857). The mortality rate for pericardiectomy to treat constrictive pericarditis is approximately 6% to 12% (*Circulation.* 1999;100:1380–1386). The images represent MRI tagging and show a normal heart on the left and an example of pericardial constriction on the right. The arrows accompanying the image on the left indicate normal pericardial sliding and those on the right indicated tethered pericardium in the presence of constriction. The ventricles on the right are classically tubular in appearance supporting the diagnosis.

13 Answer B. Tamponade and circulatory collapse follow right ventricular perforation in <50% of cases. Endomyocardial biopsy is complicated by right ventricular perforation in 0.3% to 5% of cases and left ventricular perforation in 0.1% to 3.3% of cases. Perforation of the RV by a pacemaker lead results in a right rather than left bundle branch block pattern (*Eur Heart J.* 2004;25:587–610).

14 Answer C. Exaggerated respiratory variation in the right heart pressure trace is expected in the setting of pericardial tamponade. Elevated right atrial pressure, blunted Y descent and gradual narrowing in the difference between the pericardial and right atrial pressures are all consistent with early evidence of pericardial tamponade.

15 Answer D. Pericardial pain is typically referred to the scapular ridge through the phrenic nerve and is relieved by sitting forward. Use of colchicine is supported by the results of the recent Colchicine for Acute Pericarditis (COPE) Trial, in which colchicine gave greater symptom relief and was associated with less recurrence than aspirin (*Circulation.* 2005;112:2012–2016).

16 **Answer B.** The image depicts mitral valvuloplasty, which requires puncture of the interatrial septum. Presence of a small left atrium and performance of the procedure without biplane imaging are associated with increased incidence of pericardial tamponade. Puncture of the left atrial free wall is associated with immediate chest pain; however, symptoms of tamponade may be delayed for 4 to 6 hours.

17 **Answer D.** Pericardial pressure increases in proportion to the effusion volume. Rapidly accumulating effusions can cause tamponade at a relatively low volume, whereas a slowly accumulating large volume chronic effusion is often well tolerated (*N Engl J Med*. 2004;351:2195–2202). The parietal pericardium is fibroelastic; however, it can become fibrotic and less distensible with chronic inflammatory processes. Pericardial pressure increases more acutely if the pericardium is inelastic.

18 **Answer A.** Pericardial disease, either related or unrelated to malignancy or radiotherapy, is the most common indication for cardiology consultation among patients with cancer who are hospitalized. Pericardial fluid cytology is abnormal in approximately 50% of cases and presence of abnormal cytology is a significant predictor of decreased survival.

These patients are five times more likely to require repeat intervention when compared with those with nonmalignancy-related effusions (*J Clin Oncol*. 2005;23:5211–5216).

19 **Answer D.** Multiple approaches to pericardiocentesis can be taken and include subxiphisternal, right xiphocostal, apical, and parasternal approaches. The left chest wall approach is often favored with echo-guided pericardiocentesis. Trauma to the right atrium and inferior vena cava is more with right xiphocostal approach, trauma to the left pleura and lingual with the apical approach, and puncture of the left anterior descending coronary artery and left internal mammary artery with the parasternal approach.

20 **Answer A.** Thoracocentesis is required following approximately 10% to 15% of cases of percutaneous balloon pericardiotomy. Continuous drainage of >100 mL in 24 hours, 3 days post procedure or reaccumulation of an effusion with tamponade both indicate the need for a more definitive percutaneous or surgical procedure. A primary surgical approach may be preferred if a loculated fibrinous effusion is present (*Cathet Cardiovasc Diagn*. 1991;22: 244–249).

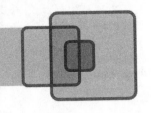

33

Percutaneous Alcohol Septal Ablation for Hypertrophic Cardiomyopathy

Amy L. Seidel and E. Murat Tuzcu

Questions

1 A 43-year-old man with hypertrophic cardiomyopathy (HCM) and a resting left ventricular outflow tract (LVOT) gradient of 60 mm Hg is referred to you for alcohol septal ablation. He has dyspnea when walking rapidly up a flight of stairs or more than two blocks on level ground. His blood pressure is 140/80 mm Hg and his heart rate is 85 bpm. His examination is consistent with dynamic LVOT obstruction; however, there are no signs of heart failure. He is taking 12.5 mg of Toprol XL daily. You should:

(A) Arrange for left heart catheterization, to be followed by alcohol ablation if severe coronary artery disease is not present

(B) Increase his Toprol XL to 25 mg daily and have him follow-up with his cardiologist for up-titration of β-blockers as tolerated and then reevaluate the symptom

(C) Refer him for surgical consultation because he is too young for alcohol ablation

(D) Tell him that he should not be considered for alcohol ablation unless he develops New York Heart Association (NYHA) Class IV symptoms

2 A 57-year-old patient with HCM presents to your office because she is short of breath upon minimal exertion. Echocardiography demonstrates mild systolic anterior motion (SAM) of the mitral valve leaflet tips, mild mitral regurgitation (MR), and a resting LVOT gradient of 10 mm Hg. What should you do next?

(A) Perform alcohol septal ablation

(B) Refer her for myectomy

(C) Ask the sonographer to administer inhaled amyl nitrate and/or arrange for a stress echocardiogram to determine if the LVOT gradient increases with exercise

(D) Tell her that her symptoms are unlikely to be related to LVOT obstruction

3 A 70-year-old patient with HCM with resting and provocable LVOT gradients of 30 and 160 mm Hg, respectively, comes to you for alcohol septal ablation. She has NYHA functional Class IV symptoms in spite of maximal medical therapy. Her echocardiogram demonstrates normal left ventricular function, severe asymmetric left ventricular hypertrophy with an upper septal diameter of 2.0 cm, and SAM of the anterior mitral valve leaflet. The anterior mitral valve leaflet is excessively long and there is posterior mitral valve leaflet override as a result. There is moderate to severe MR at rest. Left heart catheterization shows mild, nonobstructive coronary artery disease. You should:

(A) Refer her for myectomy and repair of the mitral valve

(B) Proceed with alcohol septal ablation because you feel that her septal and valvular anatomy is ideal for this form of therapy

(C) Proceed with alcohol septal ablation because she does not have significant obstructive coronary artery disease that requires coronary artery bypass graft (CABG) surgery

4 Mortality following myectomy is much higher than that following alcohol septal ablation.

(A) True
(B) False

5 A 75-year-old man with HCM and severe LVOT obstruction comes to you because he wants alcohol septal ablation. He heard that it was a noninvasive procedure that will provide him with complete and immediate relief of his symptoms. He is NYHA functional Class III on maximum tolerated doses of verapamil and disopyramide, has SAM of the anterior mitral valve leaflet that is responsible for his LVOT obstruction, and has no unfavorable anatomic features to suggest that he would be better served by myectomy. You should:

(A) Schedule him for alcohol septal ablation because you feel confident that it will result in an immediate reduction in his LVOT gradient and, therefore, immediate resolution of his current symptoms
(B) Explain to him that while alcohol septal ablation is less invasive than myectomy, the reduction in LVOT gradient is not as complete immediately after alcohol ablation as that following myectomy. As a result, he may not initially experience a dramatic decrease in his symptoms
(C) Tell him that LVOT gradients are reduced significantly following alcohol septal ablation; however, the gradients gradually increase to preprocedure levels within a year's time

6 The most common conduction abnormality following percutaneous transluminal septal myocardial ablation (PTSMA) is:

(A) Complete heart block
(B) Left bundle branch block
(C) Right bundle branch block
(D) Alternating right and left bundle branch block

7 Which patients should have a temporary transvenous pacemaker placed before performing alcohol septal ablation?

(A) Patients without preexisting conduction abnormalities on electrocardiogram (EKG)

(B) Patients in whom you feel you may need to ablate more than one septal perforator
(C) Patients with a preexisting left bundle branch block on EKG
(D) All of the above

8 What imaging modality has become standard practice to help with the identification of the most appropriate septal branch targets for alcohol septal ablation?

(A) Intracardiac echocardiography (ICE)
(B) Cardiac computed tomography (CT)
(C) Myocardial contrast echocardiography (MCE)
(D) Cardiac magnetic resonance imaging (MRI)

9 What step is necessary before instillation of alcohol into the targeted septal branch?

(A) No steps are necessary once the targeted branch is identified
(B) Contrast must be injected into the central lumen of the balloon
(C) A second flexible guidewire must be placed into the distal left anterior descending (LAD) artery, and a balloon inflated over that wire, just distal to the origin of the targeted septal artery. This will prevent extravasation of alcohol into the middle and distal portions of the LAD beyond the targeted branch
(D) None of the above

10 Approximately 10 mL of ethanol is necessary for successful ablation of a single septal perforator.

(A) True
(B) False

11 Once the procedure is complete the operator must do all of the following, *except*:

(A) Place the patient in the intensive care unit for at least 24 to 48 hours
(B) Remove the temporary pacemaker wire if complete heart block did not occur during the course of the procedure
(C) Cycle cardiac biomarkers until they have peaked
(D) Obtain a transthoracic echocardiogram before discharge for postprocedure gradient measurements

12 What features of this hemodynamic tracing distinguish it as HCM with LVOT obstruction rather than aortic stenosis?

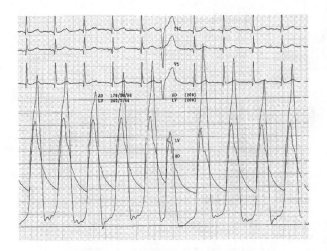

(A) There is a decrease in aortic pulse pressure following a premature ventricular contraction (PVC)

(B) There is an increase in the gradient between the left ventricle and aorta following PVC

(C) There is a significant reduction in the gradient between the aorta and left ventricle in the beat of the PVC

(D) A and B

13 A 30-year-old woman with HCM and a resting LVOT gradient of 70 mm Hg comes to you for alcohol septal ablation. She is otherwise healthy and has NYHA Class III symptoms in spite of maximal medical therapy. There are no anatomic reasons to suggest that she would be better served by a myectomy. You should:

(A) Schedule her for alcohol septal ablation and explain that the risk of her developing a lethal ventricular arrhythmia is equivalent to that following myectomy

(B) Schedule her for a myectomy because there is a much higher risk of developing lethal ventricular arrhythmias following alcohol septal ablation

(C) Discuss with her that we do not yet know the true risk of lethal ventricular arrhythmias following alcohol septal ablation. Long-term data about the myectomy is more robust. She is young and at a surgical center that has extensive experience and excellent outcomes following myectomy, therefore you would recommend at this point in time that she has a myectomy

(D) Schedule her for alcohol septal ablation because the risk of lethal ventricular arrhythmias

following myectomy is much higher in young patients

14 Which of the following Guidant guidewires would be the least acceptable for use during alcohol septal ablation?

(A) HI-Torque Balance Middle Weight Wire

(B) HI-Torque Whisper Wire

(C) HI-Torque Cross-IT 200XT Wire

(D) HI-Torque Balance Heavy Weight

15 The following angiograms were taken to document the key steps used during alcohol septal ablation in a 60-year-old patient with HCM and severe LVOT obstruction. A 0.014-inch flexible guidewire followed by an over-the-wire balloon (2 × 10 mm) was introduced into the first major septal perforator before documenting the following angiograms. Before alcohol injection, the operator used MCE to confirm septal perfusion at the appropriate locations. The patient developed severe chest pain and an anterior ST elevation in multiple anterior leads following alcohol injection. On the basis of the preceding information and the following angiograms, what was the most likely cause?

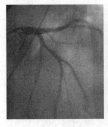 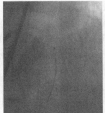 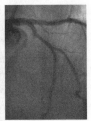

(A) Plaque in the proximal LAD was disrupted by the guidewire during initial wiring of the septal perforator

(B) The guidewire caused dissection of the proximal LAD

(C) There was spillover of alcohol into the LAD beyond the septal perforator

(D) The septal perforator supplied portions of the anterior wall of the left ventricle

16 Looking at the following angiograms, which patient will likely have the best result in terms of LVOT gradient reduction following alcohol septal ablation?

(A)

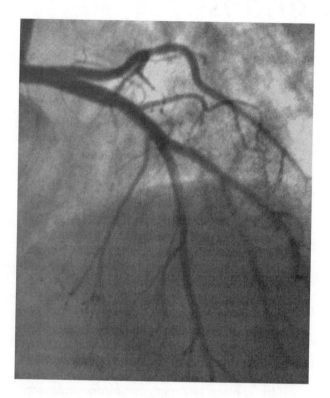

(B)

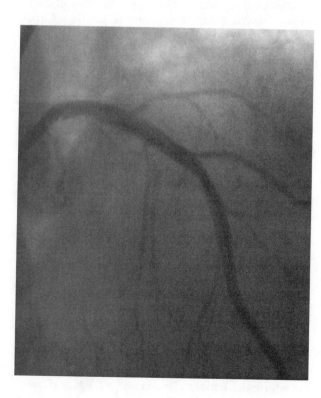

(C)

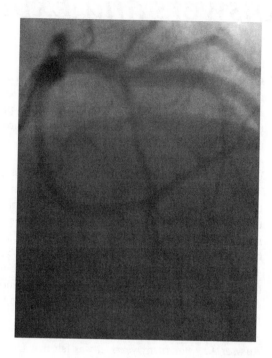

(D) Unable to determine

17 Alcohol septal ablation has surpassed myectomy as the gold standard mechanical intervention for treatment of HCM with LVOT gradient obstruction.

(A) True
(B) False

18 Specific hemodynamic criteria exist to determine when the procedure is complete.

(A) True
(B) False

19 If a patient experiences chest pain and transient ST elevation in V1 and V2 during alcohol infusion, you should:

(A) Immediately stop the infusion of alcohol
(B) Immediately deflate the balloon
(C) Administer an intravenous analgesic agent like fentanyl
(D) Administer sublingual nitroglycerin

20 How should alcohol be administered into the central lumen of the balloon?

(A) As a rapid bolus injection
(B) At a rate of 1 mL per 60 to 120 seconds
(C) At a rate of 1 mL per 30 seconds

Answers and Explanations

1 **Answer B.** PTSMA for the relief of LVOT obstruction in HCM should not be considered until a patient develops severe drug refractory symptoms. This patient is currently NYHA functional Class II without optimal medical therapy, which makes him an inappropriate candidate for mechanical intervention. Up-titration of Toprol XL would be the next step. This is important because drug refractory symptoms, a criteria for mechanical intervention, implies that the patient is on maximum tolerated doses of negative inotropic agents used to reduce the degree of LVOT obstruction (*Circulation.* 2004;109:452–456, *JAMA.* 2002;287:1308–1320, *J Am Coll Cardiol.* 2003;42:1687–1713). These medications include β-blockers, non-dihydropyridine calcium channel blockers, and the antiarrhythmic disopyramide.

2 **Answer C.** For many years, it was felt that LVOT obstruction occurred in 25% of the HCM population. However, recent literature and expert opinion suggest that it is much more common and occurs in up to 70% of patients with HCM when both resting and provocable gradients are considered (*J Am Coll Cardiol.* 2005;45:161). It is always important to assess for provocable LVOT gradient obstruction. This can be done with provocative maneuvers designed to decrease preload, decrease afterload, or increase cardiac contractility. Amyl nitrate, which decreases afterload, is routinely used with echocardiography to assess for a provocable LVOT gradient in patients with HCM. Stress echocardiography is also helpful because changes in the degree of LVOT obstruction and MR at peak stress can be correlated with a patient's symptoms. Alcohol septal ablation should only be considered when there is a resting or provocable LVOT gradient of 50 mm Hg or more (*JAMA.* 2002;287:1308–1320).

3 **Answer A.** In spite of maximal medical therapy, 15% of patients with HCM with LVOT obstruction will develop debilitating heart failure and should be considered for mechanical intervention designed to relieve outflow tract obstruction (*Am J Cardiol.* 1992;70:657–660). Several factors must be considered to determine the most appropriate form of mechanical intervention. For PTSMA to be effective, the mechanism of LVOT obstruction must be SAM of the anterior mitral valve leaflet with leaflet to ventricular septal contact (*J Am Coll Cardiol.*

2003;42:1687–1713). In addition, there should be no structural abnormalities of the mitral valve and/or its apparatus, severe coronary artery disease amenable to CABG, or atypical patterns or excessive degrees of septal hypertrophy (*J Am Coll Cardiol.* 2003;41:145, *Circulation.* 2004;109:452–456, *J Am Coll Cardiol.* 2003;42:1687–1713). While this patient does have LVOT obstruction secondary to SAM of the anterior mitral valve leaflet, the leaflet is excessively long and allows for posterior mitral valve leaflet override. This contributes to the degree of MR and cannot be corrected by alcohol septal ablation. Therefore, this patient would be better served with myectomy and valvular repair or replacement.

4 **Answer B.** False. While mortality associated with both myectomy and alcohol septal ablation is center dependent, both are similar. The mortality associated with myectomy is 0% to 3%, while that associated with alcohol septal ablation is 1% to 4% with incidences of 0% to 2% at more experienced centers (*Circulation.* 1999;100:1380–1386, *J Am Coll Cardiol.* 2003;42:1687–1713, *J Am Coll Cardiol.* 2005; 46:470–476, *Circulation.* 1994;90:1781–1785, *Circulation.* 2005;111:2033–2041).

5 **Answer B.** Since the start of alcohol septal ablation in 1995, several observational studies have shown that both resting and provocable gradients following the procedure are reduced by >50%, with a majority being reduced by 90% or more (*Heart.* 2000; 83:326–331, *Circulation.* 1999;98:2415–2421, *Eur Heart J.* 1999;20:1342–1354, *Circulation.* 1997;95: 2075–2081, *J Am Coll Cardiol.* 2000;36:852–855, *Circulation.* 1998;98:1750–1755, *Circulation.* 2001; 103:1492–1496, *J Thorac Cardiovasc Surg.* 1999;47: 94–100, *Lancet.* 1995;346:211–214). However, the decrease in LVOT gradient following myectomy is more complete and immediate than that following alcohol septal ablation (*J Am Coll Cardiol.* 2001;38: 1994–2000). Two studies have compared outcomes in patients following alcohol septal ablation and surgical myectomy. The first of these compared 1-year outcomes of 41 consecutive patients who underwent alcohol septal ablation at Baylor College of Medicine to 41 years of age and gradient-matched patients who underwent septal myectomy at the Mayo Clinic. The decrease in LVOT gradient at 1 year was not significantly different between the two procedures

(*J Am Coll Cardiol*. 2001;38:1701–1706). A second study compared immediate and 3-month outcomes of 25 patients with alcohol septal ablation with those of 26 patients with myectomy at the Cleveland Clinic Foundation. This study demonstrated that while there were significant reductions in the LVOT gradient following alcohol septal ablation immediately and at 3 months, those following myectomy were significantly lower at these time points (*J Am Coll Cardiol*. 2001;38:1994–2000). In addition, a significant degree of provocable LVOT obstruction remained in the patients who underwent alcohol septal ablation 3 months following the procedure. Therefore, while LVOT gradient reductions following alcohol septal ablation are significantly lower immediately following the procedure, they are not as pronounced as those seen following myectomy. While there is a gradual decrease in the remaining LVOT gradient over time, a significant degree of provocable obstruction may remain. It is, therefore, important to consider the patient's expectations along with the need for rapid hemodynamic improvement.

6 Answer C. The most common conduction abnormality following alcohol septal ablation is right bundle branch block. Its high incidence of approximately 60% can be explained by the location of the right bundle branch in relation to the myocardial infarction created by alcohol septal ablation (*Am J Cardiol*. 2004;93:171–175, *J Am Coll Cardiol*. 2004;44:2329–2332). Unlike the left bundle, when the right bundle enters the muscular portion of the interventricular septum, it remains as a discrete cord-like structure located deep within its midportion and does not begin to branch until it reaches the level of the papillary muscles. This is unlike the left bundle branch, which enters the muscular portion of the interventricular septum as multiple branches in a sheet-like array that are located much closer to the septum's endocardial surface throughout its anterior, mid, and inferior portions (*J Am Coll Cardiol*. 2004;44:2329–2332). During alcohol septal ablation, a transmural infarction is created in the midportion of the septum that often contains the right bundle branch and spares the more subendocardially located left bundle branch. It is important to keep in mind, however, that individual septal perfusion patterns do vary and a variety of conduction abnormalities can occur.

7 Answer D. A temporary pacemaker wire must be placed in the right ventricular apex before alcohol septal ablation in all patients, regardless of whether there is preexisting conduction disease and/or the operator feels that it may be necessary to ablate

additional septal perforators. This is because complete heart block can occur transiently in up to 50% of patients undergoing the procedure (*J Am Coll Cardiol*. 2003;42:296–300). Stable and reliable pacing thresholds are of utmost importance and some operators will utilize screw-in leads for this purpose. While all patients can develop this complication, there are risk factors for its development. Preexisting conduction disease, particularly, preexisting left bundle branch block, appears to place patients at greatest risk (*J Am Coll Cardiol*. 2003;42:296–300, *Am J Cardiol*. 2004;93:171–175). In addition, female gender, rapid injection of ethanol, and ablation of more than one septal perforator have been associated with higher incidences of complete heart block (*J Am Coll Cardiol*. 2003;42:296–300).

8 Answer C. Before the use of MCE, operators determined the most appropriate septal branches by assessing the impact that temporary balloon occlusion had on the LVOT gradient. If balloon occlusion caused an acute and significant reduction in the LVOT gradient, typically ≥50%, the branch was selected if unwanted areas of myocardium were not at risk (*Eur Heart J*. 1999;20:1342–1354). In addition to this technique, MCE has become the standard to aid in selecting the most appropriate target branches. After the septal branch has been wired and a balloon placed over the wire in its most proximal portion, the guidewire is removed and the balloon inflated. One to 2 mL of an echocardiographic contrast agent is then injected into the balloon's central lumen and transthoracic echo images are obtained (*Circulation*. 1999;98:2415–2421, *J Am Coll Cardiol*. 1998;32:225–229, *Textbook of interventional cardiology*. 2003:987–995). The contrast defines the myocardial territory supplied by the branch and delineates the area of planned infarction. The branch is chosen if the area of SAM–septal contact is opacified at the area of maximal flow acceleration and remote regions of the left and right ventricle are not involved (*Circulation*. 1999;98:2415–2421, *Textbook of interventional cardiology*. 2003:987–995). When compared with routine probatory balloon occlusion, ablations utilizing MCE result in smaller infarcts, greater LVOT gradient reductions, faster atrioventricular nodal recovery times, more significant reductions in NYHA functional class, and reduced incidences of recurrent LVOT obstruction. (*Textbook of interventional cardiology*. 2003:987–995).

9 Answer B. If spillover of alcohol occurs during infusion, a myocardial infarction secondary to abrupt closure of the LAD distal to the targeted branch can occur (*Circulation*. 1997;95:2075–2081, *J Am Coll Cardiol*. 2001;38:1707–1710). This highlights the need to confirm precise balloon positioning in the proximal portion of the branch and exclude reflux of dye into the LAD through contrast injection while the balloon is inflated, before alcohol infusion.

10 Answer B.   False. Ten milliliters of ethanol is excessive for alcohol ablation. There is a higher incidence of complete heart block and permanent pacemaker implantation when large volumes are used and typically, 1 to 2 mL is adequate per artery (*J Am Coll Cardiol*. 2003;42:296–300, *J Am Coll Cardiol*. 2003; 42:1687–1713, *Textbook of interventional cardiology*. 2003:987–995).

11 Answer B.   Following completion of the procedure, the temporary pacemaker wire must remain in place due to the high incidence of complete heart block that can occur transiently, during or following the procedure. If complete heart block is going to occur, it typically does so within the first 72 hours of the procedure (*J Am Coll Cardiol*. 2003;42:296–300, *Circulation*. 1999;98:2415–2421, *J Am Coll Cardiol*. 2000;36:852–855, *Circulation*. 1998;98:1750–1755). If the patient remains free of any concerning arteriovenous (AV) conduction abnormalities for up to 72 hours, the temporary wire can be removed. Monitoring should occur in an intensive care unit for the first 48 hours, and telemetry continued for the duration of the patient's stay. Cardiac biomarkers should be cycled and follow a pattern similar to that seen following an acute myocardial infarction. It is important to obtain a transthoracic EKG to assess baseline postprocedure gradients before the patient's discharge.

12 Answer D.   This hemodynamic tracing demonstrates many of the features characteristic of the dynamic LVOT obstruction that occurs with HCM. What distinguishes it from aortic stenosis, which is a fixed obstruction to left ventricular outflow is the decrease in the aortic pulse pressure and increase in LVOT gradient in the beat following a PVC. The former is referred to as the *Brockenbrough-Braunwald-Morrow sign*. When a PVC occurs, there is an increase in cardiac contractility and typically, although not present in this tracing, a compensatory pause that allows for an increase in left ventricular end-diastolic volume. In a patient without a dynamic LVOT obstruction or in a patient with a fixed obstruction at the level of the aortic valve, the increase in contractility and increased end-diastolic volume will lead to an increase in the aortic pulse pressure. In HCM with LVOT obstruction, the increase in cardiac

contractility following PVC increases the degree of LVOT obstruction and the aortic pulse pressure decreases. This will occur even in situations where a compensatory pause allows for increased LV filling. The other feature in this tracing that will distinguish it from a patient with a fixed outflow obstruction as in aortic stenosis is the tremendous increase in the left ventricular to aortic gradient following a PVC. This too is a result of a worsening of the outflow tract obstruction with an increase in cardiac contractility.

13 Answer C.   The risk of sudden death following alcohol septal ablation is currently unknown. There is concern that scar tissue as a result of the infarction may serve as a substrate for the development of lethal ventricular arrhythmias, which would be an undesirable complication in a group of patients already prone to their occurrence (*Circulation*. 2004; 109:452–456, *JAMA*. 2002;287:1308–1320, *J Am Coll Cardiol*. 2003;42:1687–1713). The results of programmed electrical stimulation in a group of patients before and after alcohol septal ablation are mixed and there have been two case reports of patients developing monomorphic ventricular tachycardia 1 to 2 weeks following alcohol septal ablation (*N Engl J Med*. 2004;351:1914–1915, *Eur Heart J*. 1999;20:1342–1354, *Am J Med Sci*. 2004;328:185–188). Therefore, while there is currently not enough information available to suggest that alcohol septal ablation increases the risk of sudden death, a longer duration of follow-up is needed to assess the true potential of this complication. There has not been an increased risk of lethal ventricular arrhythmias in patients who have undergone myectomy, a procedure for which there is more than four decades of follow-up. Therefore, because she is young, otherwise healthy, and has access to an experienced surgical myectomy center, it would be prudent to refer her for myectomy.

14 Answer C.   Appropriate guidewire selection for alcohol septal ablation is of great importance for procedural success. Engaging and navigating through the septal branches can be challenging because they often take off at a 90-degree or greater angle from the LAD. In addition, the vessels can be small and tortuous. Ideally, one would like to use the safest guide wire with gradual tapering of its core that will provide flexibility and allow for the balloon to be inserted into and easily manipulated within the target vessel (*Textbook of interventional cardiology*. 2003:987–995). The HI-Torque Cross-IT 200XT Wire is a poor choice for alcohol septal ablation because it has the least degree of flexibility of any of the wires listed. Not only will this increase the risk of vessel dissection and perforation, engaging the vessel will also be quite challenging.

15 Answer C.   Although it was not frequently reported myocardial infarction, most commonly involving the LAD territory, can occur at sites beyond the intended septal region (*J Am Coll Cardiol*. 2001;38:1707–1710). The operator in this scenario failed to ensure proper balloon positioning within the proximal portion of the septal artery and did not ensure that there was no spillover of contrast into the LAD before injecting alcohol. A short balloon was used, and this is important because these are easier to position solely within septal branches, which will decrease the risk of LAD dissection upon balloon inflation. Positioning of the balloon can then be confirmed by inflating the balloon within the septal branch and injecting contrast into the left main trunk (LMT). It is also important to confirm that the diameter of the balloon is adequate to completely occlude the proximal portion of the septal branch during alcohol injection. This is done by injecting contrast into the central lumen of the balloon while it is inflated. This step, which was not performed during this procedure, will exclude the reflux of contrast into the LAD.

16 Answer D.   Not only is it impossible to determine the degree of LVOT gradient reduction one can achieve with alcohol septal ablation by looking at an angiogram alone, but it is also impossible to determine which vessel(s) is(are) appropriate for ablation. Individual septal perfusion patterns vary widely, as do the anatomic features related to LVOT obstruction. This is why it is important to assess the physiologic impact that temporary balloon occlusion has on the LVOT gradient, in addition to employing MCE, which will confirm that the septal artery(ies) supplies(supply) the region where the mitral valve leaflets contact the septum and maximal flow acceleration occurs.

17 Answer B.   The current gold standard mechanical intervention remains surgical myectomy. It involves excision of approximately 5 g of muscle from the basal anterior portion of the interventricular septum to just beyond the distal margins of the mitral valve leaflets. (*Circulation*. 2004;109: 452–456, *JAMA*. 2002;287:1308–1320, *J Am Coll Cardiol*. 2003;42:1687–1713). Removal of the hypertrophied tissue decreases the degree of outflow tract obstruction and frequently improves the severity of MR secondary to SAM. Mortality is 0% to 3% and patients experience long-lasting symptomatic improvement that often includes an enhanced exercise capacity (*Am J Cardiol*. 1992;70: 657–660, *JAMA*. 2002;287:1308–1320, *J Am Coll Cardiol*. 2003;42:1687–1713, *J Am Coll Cardiol*. 2005;46: 470–476, *Circulation*. 1994;90:1781–1785, *Circulation*. 2005;111:2033–2041). Alcohol septal ablation was developed as a less invasive alternative to this procedure because elderly patients and those with multiple comorbidities are not always optimal candidates for surgery. In addition, the excellent results following myectomy come from a small number of North American and European medical centers, which highlights the fact that there is limited accessibility to this modality of treatment. Therefore, while alcohol septal ablation appears to be a safe and effective technique, until long-term follow-up and randomized controlled studies are available, it is most useful in patients with high surgical risk or those without access to a high volume surgical center with documented excellent outcome measures, including a surgical mortality of ≤2%.

18 Answer B.   No specific criteria are used to determine when to end the procedure, and practice patterns differ. Some interventionalists continue to ablate additional branches until the LVOT gradient is at a particular value, typically <50% of its baseline or <20 mm Hg (*Circulation*. 2004;109:452–456, *J Am Coll Cardiol*. 2000;36:852–855). Others stop the procedure after some reduction in the gradient as long as they are satisfied that the anatomic location of the alcohol bathed territory, as demonstrated by MCE, involves the area of SAM–septal contact and maximal flow acceleration.

19 Answer C.   It is not uncommon for patients to experience chest pain during and several hours following alcohol infusion. This typically responds to intravenous analgesic agents, not sublingual nitroglycerin. Alcohol infusion should only be stopped if there is evidence of acute infarction in territories other than the septum. The balloon should not be deflated in response to chest pain because alcohol in the septal perforator can spill into the LAD and can cause abrupt occlusion of this vessel.

20 Answer B.   Alcohol is not given as a rapid bolus injection as this leads to higher incidences of complete heart block (*J Am Coll Cardiol*. 2003;42:296–300). Rather, alcohol is infused into the central lumen of the balloon at a rate of 1 mL per 60 to 120 seconds and the balloon should remain inflated for 5 to 10 minutes (*Textbook of interventional cardiology*. 2003: 987–995).

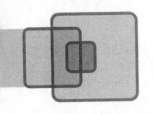

34

Chronic Stable Angina: American College of Cardiology/ American Heart Association Guidelines

Paul Sorajja and Bernard Gersh

Questions

1 A 40-year-old female airline pilot is seeing you for recent-onset chest pain. Her symptoms arise in her left inframammary region. They are reproducible with physical exertion, but can be prolonged despite rest. She inquires whether she should have a coronary angiogram. Which of the following is the correct answer?

(A) You reassure her that her symptoms are not typical for angina pectoris

(B) A normal stress test would obviate the need for a coronary angiogram

(C) You proceed directly to invasive coronary angiography

(D) You have her undergo a chest computerized tomography (CT) coronary angiogram

2 A 74-year-old man with stable angina and diabetes is found to have the findings shown on coronary angiography (see following figures). Select the best answer with regard to this patient:

(A) Coronary artery bypass grafting (CABG) is preferred over percutaneous coronary intervention (PCI)

(B) An initial revascularization strategy of CABG or balloon angioplasty results in similar survival

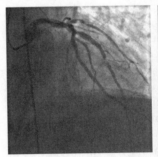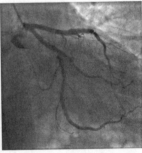

(C) The use of sirolimus-eluting stents has resulted in similar long-term survival compared with bypass grafting

(D) None of the above

3 A 55-year-old woman is referred to your office with mild dyspnea. Six weeks ago, she had suffered a myocardial infarction and did not undergo reperfusion therapy. Her referring physician had obtained a nuclear viability study and those images are shown in the following figure. The study is interpreted as showing a large area of nonviable myocardium involving the anterior, apical, septal, and inferior regions. There was also severe left ventricular and moderate right ventricular enlargement. No myocardial ischemia is found. Her ejection fraction is calculated to be 22%. Select the best management for this patient:

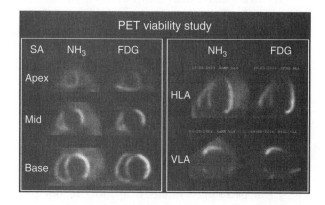

(A) Coronary angiography, followed by PCI of high-grade stenoses

(B) Coronary angiography, followed by bypass grafting of high-grade stenoses

(C) Medical therapy only

(D) None of the above

4 A 69-year-old man is referred to you for coronary angiography. He exercises frequently, and his symptoms of angina occur near the completion of his regular 3-mile run. Before seeing you, the referring physician has the patient undergo a treadmill study, where he exercises for 7 minutes on the Bruce protocol with no electrocardiogram (EKG) evidence of ischemia or precipitation of angina. The patient takes no medications. His angiogram is shown in the following figure. Select the best management for this patient:

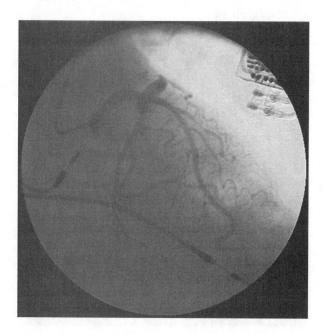

(A) Initiation of a statin drug

(B) Referral to a cardiac surgeon

(C) PCI

(D) Stress echocardiography

5 A 60-year-old man with angina is referred to you. His symptoms have been stable, but in the past month they have begun to interfere with his job as a construction worker. Apart from nicotine dependence, he has no other health problems. A recent echocardiogram showed his ejection fraction to be 50%. His coronary angiogram is shown below. Select the *false* statement:

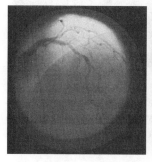
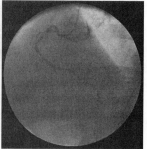

(A) Randomized trials have shown equivalent long-term survival with PCI versus CABG as the initial strategy for these patients

(B) Data from trials of PCI versus CABG do not apply to this case because those studies frequently enrolled much older, more severely symptomatic patients with abnormal ventricular function

(C) Balloon angioplasty alone results in more repeat procedures, whose cumulative costs are equivalent to those of an initial strategy of bypass grafting

(D) PCI is indicated

6 A 78-year-old man is referred after a treadmill study. During exercise, his EKG became positive for ischemia in conjunction with the onset of angina soon after he had reached Stage 2 of the Bruce protocol. His comorbidities include hyperlipidemia and chronic obstructive pulmonary disease, which has been stable with steroid inhalers. His coronary angiogram is shown in the following figure. Which of the following is *correct*?

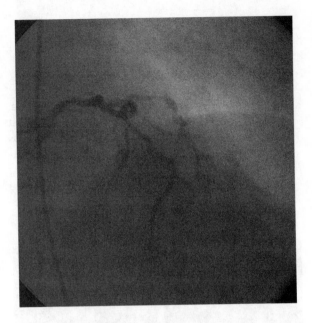

(A) PCI can be undertaken because the lesion does not involve the distal left main or bifurcation of the left anterior descending (LAD) and circumflex arteries

(B) PCI can be performed if the minimal lumen area measured by intravascular ultrasound is $<7.5 \text{ mm}^2$

(C) PCI should not be performed

(D) PCI is indicated if a fractional flow reserve measurement of the lesion is <0.75 or additional noninvasive stress imaging shows myocardial ischemia

7 Among randomized trials of PCI versus CABG for patients with multivessel disease, what is the frequency of repeat revascularization in those undergoing surgery during long-term follow-up?

(A) 15%

(B) 10%

(C) 5% to 6%

(D) 1% to 2%

8 Which of the following is a *true* statement with regard to periprocedural rise in cardiac biomarkers among patients undergoing elective PCI?

(A) A positive linear relation exists between the risk of cardiac mortality and peak creatinine kinase (or CK-MB) for intermediate (1.5 to 3.0 times normal) and higher (>3 times normal) levels of rise

(B) A positive linear relation exists between the risk of cardiac mortality and elevation of troponin isoforms (I or T) at intermediate levels of rise (<5 times normal)

(C) Elevation of troponin isoforms is common and not of prognostic value

(D) In comparisons of CABG with PCI, studies have utilized the same levels of cardiac biomarker rise in defining the rates of periprocedural myocardial infarction for both procedures

9 In reference to the randomized trials of stenting versus bypass surgery for multivessel disease, select the *true* statement:

(A) Comparable 1- to 3-year survival has been observed, including among patients with severe ischemia and high-risk features for adverse outcomes with surgery

(B) Bypass surgery results in superior freedom from death or myocardial infarction

(C) In comparison with previous balloon angioplasty trials, there has been approximately an 80% reduction in the need for repeat revascularization

(D) Because of the need for repeat procedures, patients undergoing PCI have demonstrated a small, but statistically significant, worse survival

10 A 57-year-old man is referred for angina. His symptoms began 2 months ago when he began shoveling heavy snow. He is able to clear his driveway without stopping, but he is worried that he could "drop dead." On a treadmill exercise study with the Bruce protocol, he exercised for 12 minutes and developed 1-mm horizontal ST-segment depression without chest pain. His only medication is atenolol, which he takes for hypertension. His angiogram is shown in the following figure. Select the best management:

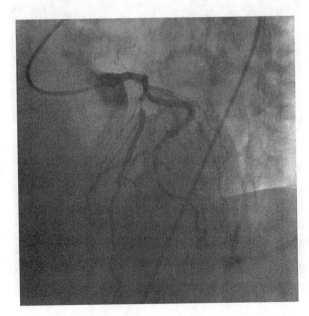

(A) You tell him his symptoms are mild and that additional medical therapy and lifestyle modification afford the same prognosis as revascularization

(B) You recommend bypass surgery, as placement of an internal mammary graft will reduce his risk of sudden death

(C) You tell him that the burden of his antianginal medications will be the same if he undergoes bypass surgery or medical therapy alone

(D) None of the above are correct statements

11 A 64-year-old woman undergoes angiography for recent onset of mild angina. A tubular 70% stenosis in her mid LAD is found, and she undergoes successful percutaneous treatment with a 4.0 × 12 mm bare-metal stent. What is the probability that repeat target lesion revascularization will be needed in the next 4 years?

(A) ≤5%

(B) 8% to 20%

(C) >20%

(D) None of the above

12 A 45-year-old male executive undergoes a treadmill study with nuclear perfusion imaging as part of an annual examination. Recently he began exercising for maintaining his health, and has no cardiovascular symptoms. He exercises for 4 minutes and develops 1.5-mm horizontal ST-segment depression that returns to normal after 5 minutes of recovery. He has no chest pain during the study. His nuclear imaging demonstrates impaired coronary flow reserve in the anterior and anterolateral walls of his left ventricle with mild dilatation on the poststress images. Select the best management:

(A) Because he is asymptomatic, you recommend continued medical therapy with an emphasis on primary preventive measures

(B) You order a cardiac MR perfusion study to confirm the myocardial ischemia detected on the nuclear scan

(C) You schedule a coronary angiogram and revascularization

(D) None of the above

13 A 64-year-old diabetic woman returns for follow-up after elective PCI for stable angina. She has been free of angina following the successful intervention. Currently indicated pharmacotherapy to prevent death or myocardial infarction in this patient includes all of the following, *except*:

(A) Aspirin

(B) β-Receptor antagonists

(C) ACE inhibitors

(D) Calcium channel blockers

(E) Lipid-lowering therapy

14 A 56-year-old woman returns to see you 6 months after having elective PCI of a proximal left circumflex lesion. She had entered a cardiovascular health program near her home after the procedure, and reports no symptoms. Before the intervention, you had told her about the possibility of restenosis during follow-up. She wants to have a stress test to evaluate the status of the intervention. Select the best next step:

(A) Exercise EKG

(B) Exercise EKG with nuclear perfusion imaging or stress echocardiography

(C) Coronary angiography

(D) None of the above

15 Each of the following statements is true, *except*:

(A) 6% to 11% of saphenous vein grafts become occluded within 1 year of surgery

(B) Perioperative and long-term treatment with platelet inhibitors significantly improves the patency rate of saphenous vein grafts

(C) Use of the internal thoracic artery in place of a saphenous vein has slightly, but significantly, improved long-term graft patency

(D) Aggressive lipid-lowering therapy significantly decreases vein graft atherosclerosis

16 A 66-year-old man recently underwent successful balloon angioplasty of a mid-LAD lesion after having had a 2-month history of severe angina. His past medical history consisted of hyperlipidemia, but there was no history of diabetes or heart failure. Currently, he is asymptomatic with an excellent functional capacity. His EKG is shown in the following figure. Select the best management:

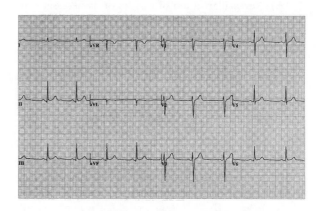

(A) Echocardiogram or radionuclide angiogram to examine left ventricular function for prognosis

(B) Cardiac magnetic resonance imaging (MRI) with gadolinium hyperenhancement to examine left ventricular function and myocardial scarring

(C) Left ventriculography

(D) None of the above

17 A 72-year-old asymptomatic man comes to you for a second opinion regarding his coronary artery disease (CAD). As part of a routine evaluation, he underwent a treadmill study, where he exercised on the Bruce protocol for a total of 11 minutes. His EKG became positive for ischemia at 9 minutes of exercise with 1 mm, horizontal ST-segment depression. There was no accompanying chest pain. He underwent angiography as shown in the following figure. He was advised to undergo PCI of this lesion, but was reluctant because he felt that the interventionalist was being "pushy." You tell him:

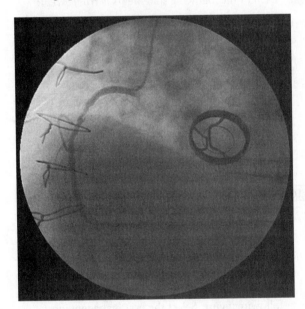

(A) Revascularization of this lesion is necessary to reduce his risk of nonfatal infarction

(B) Surgery is preferred for revascularization because of the complexity of the lesion

(C) PCI with drug-eluting stenting will not improve his prognosis

(D) Surgery is preferred because treatment with angioplasty and/or stenting would not improve his prognosis

18 Each of the following findings on noninvasive testing is consistent with a high rate of annual cardiovascular events (>3% per year), *except*:

(A) Left ventricular ejection fraction (LVEF) <35%

(B) Large fixed defect with increased pulmonary uptake on stress thallium imaging

(C) New apical and inferior hypokinesis occurring at a heart rate of 130 bpm during dobutamine echocardiography

(D) A Duke treadmill score of −11

19 A 78-year-old man with a history of stable angina suffers an out-of-hospital cardiac arrest due to ventricular fibrillation. He was resuscitated immediately and has suffered no neurologic sequelae. His medical history consists of hypertension, hyperlipidemia, and nicotine dependence. He undergoes coronary angiography. Select the correct statements:

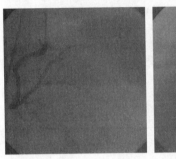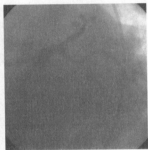

(A) PCI is preferred over surgery

(B) Surgical revascularization is preferred over PCI

(C) Surgical revascularization and PCI are equally preferred

(D) Defibrillator implantation with or without revascularization is recommended

20 A 43-year-old man is referred for coronary angiography. He recently underwent an exercise echocardiogram. During exercise, he had developed mild pain in his right lower chest after 8 minutes of exercise on the Bruce protocol. Both the exercise EKG and stress echocardiographic images showed no evidence of ischemia. The exercise test is interpreted as equivocal, and he undergoes angiography. This demonstrates a 40% to 50% left main lesion. Using intravascular ultrasound, the minimal lumen area is determined to 8.9 mm^2. Select the best management:

(A) CABG

(B) Balloon angioplasty only

(C) PCI with drug-eluting stenting

(D) Reassurance and no revascularization

21 All of the following statements are true concerning the randomized trials of CABG versus medical therapy, *except*:

(A) Most patients had moderate or severe symptoms

(B) The survival advantage of the patients initially treated with surgery became less by 10 postoperative years

(C) There was a 40% crossover rate to surgery by the medical therapy patients during follow-up

(D) Patient subgroups at high risk of death without surgery were those with left main disease, three-vessel disease and abnormal left ventricular function, two- or three-vessel disease with significant proximal LAD disease, a markedly positive exercise test, or an abnormal baseline EKG

22 A 58-year-old healthy man comes to you for a second opinion. He recently underwent a CT scan of his chest, which suggested significant coronary atherosclerosis and prompted angiography. This demonstrates a 50% to 60% lesion in the left main with good distal targets. Intravascular ultrasound of the left main lesion demonstrates the minimal lumen area to be 5.0 mm^2. The patient states that he exercises regularly and reports no cardiovascular symptoms. He has a remote history of smoking but no other comorbidities. Select the best management:

(A) CABG

(B) PCI using a 3.5-mm diameter drug-eluting stent with planned postdilatation

(C) PCI with a 4.5-mm diameter bare-metal stent

(D) No revascularization

23 A 62-year-old woman is referred for a 3-month history of worsening angina. Two years ago, she had undergone PCI of a diagonal lesion with placement of a 3.0 × 13 mm sirolimus-eluting stent. Presently, walking a distance of 15 feet from her front door to the mailbox reliably precipitates her symptoms, but there are no unstable features. She has been faithfully taking her previously prescribed medications, including metoprolol (75 mg twice daily), isosorbide dinitrate (40 mg twice daily), aspirin (81 mg daily), atorvastatin (20 mg daily), and clopidogrel (75 mg daily). Select the next best step in her management:

(A) Treadmill study

(B) Stress radionuclide imaging

(C) Coronary angiography

(D) Either B or C

24 A 77-year-old man with a 4-year history of stable angina is admitted to your hospital with dyspnea. On examination, crackles are auscultated in the lower halves of both lung fields. The first heart sound is slightly diminished, and a third heart sound is heard. His chest x-ray shows a cardiothoracic ratio of 0.6 with mild bilateral pulmonary infiltrates. Which of the following would be appropriate?

(A) Intravenous diuresis

(B) Initiation of an ACE inhibitor

(C) Coronary angiography

(D) All of the above

25 A 78-year-old man with a history of CABG 9 years ago comes to you for recent-onset angina. His symptoms have steadily progressed over the past 6 months. His angiogram is shown in the following figure. The comorbidities of the patient include chronic obstructive pulmonary disease, obesity, and renal insufficiency. Which of the following is *true* regarding revascularization of this lesion?

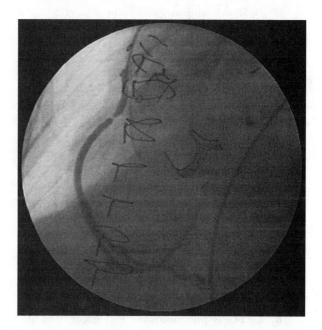

(A) Reoperation with bypass grafting is strongly indicated and preferred over PCI

(B) Because of the comorbidity of the patient, PCI is preferred over CABG

(C) No randomized trials have compared PCI with reoperation with bypass grafting

(D) None of the above

26 A 72-year-old woman with diabetes is referred to you for angina, which began 2 months ago. Her cardiopulmonary examination is consistent with mild mitral regurgitation. An echocardiogram shows her LVEF to be 55%. During exercise echocardiography, her midanterior, apical, and inferoapical walls become hypokinetic following 6 minutes of exercise on the Bruce protocol. She undergoes coronary angiography, which is shown in the following figure. Select the next best step:

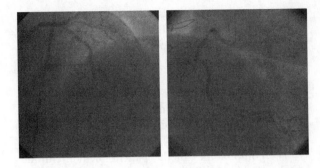

(A) PCI with drug-eluting stents
(B) CABG
(C) Balloon angioplasty with bail-out stenting
(D) Intense medical therapy and reevaluation in 6 months

27 A 58-year-old man with a known history of CAD has recurrent angina. He has undergone three prior percutaneous procedures on his middle LAD, including previous balloon angioplasty on two occasions, and placement of a drug-eluting stent. During exercise radionuclide imaging, his EKG shows 1.5 mm horizontal ST-segment depression at 3 minutes of exercise with development of chest pain. The radionuclide images show a moderately large area of ischemia in the anterior and anterolateral walls. Repeat angiography shows a 95% lesion of restenosis at the edge of the previously stented segment. Which of the following is *true*?

(A) PCI is contraindicated because of the multiple prior episodes of restenosis in his LAD
(B) CABG is preferred over PCI because of the multiple prior episodes of restenosis in his LAD
(C) Either CABG or PCI may be performed
(D) None of the above

28 A 72-year-old man with a history of prior myocardial infarction 8 years ago undergoes coronary angiography. He has had symptoms of stable angina for the past 2 years that occur with moderate exertion, such as climbing several flights of stairs. There are no unstable features of his chest pain. Coronary angiography demonstrates a 20-mm long, calcific total occlusion of the middle right coronary artery with bridging collaterals and Rentrop grade 2 collateralization of the distal vessel from the distal LAD. Select the best management:

(A) Rotational atherectomy followed by drug-eluting stenting
(B) Predilatation with drug-eluting stenting
(C) Local infusion of fibrinolytic agents
(D) None of the above

29 Select the *correct* Canadian Cardiovascular Society (CCS) classification as per the symptoms of each patient:

(A) Class I: Angina occurs while walking uphill or climbing stairs rapidly
(B) Class II: Angina occurs on walking or climbing stairs after meals
(C) Class III: Angina occurs on walking more than two blocks on the level or climbing more than one flight of stairs
(D) Class IV: Angina occurs on walking one to two blocks on the level or with climbing one flight of stairs under normal conditions and at normal pace

30 A 78-year-old woman undergoes coronary angiography for new, stable symptoms of angina. She has a history of hypertension, but has no other comorbidities. Her angiogram (shown in the following figure) demonstrates a lesion that is treated percutaneously with a 2.75 × 18 mm sirolimus-eluting stent. The following statements are true regarding this patient, *except*:

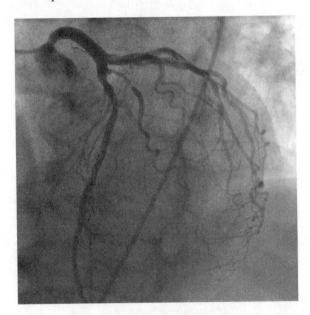

(A) PCI of the lesion likely will afford superior symptom relief than that achieved with medical therapy alone
(B) The rate of target vessel failure for PCI of this lesion ranges from 14% to 18%
(C) Stenting of the lesion likely will result in greater exercise performance on objective testing than with medical therapy alone
(D) Medical therapy alone would have resulted in the same rates of death and nonfatal infarction as that achieved by PCI

Answers and Explanations

1   Answer C.   Because the symptoms of the patient do not meet the criteria for typical angina pectoris, noninvasive assessment is appropriate for many patients with symptoms of chest pain. However, in the case of this patient, the nature of her occupation warrants definitive assessment of coronary arteries (ACC/AHA Class IIa recommendation).

2   Answer A.   The randomized Bypass versus Angioplasty Revascularization Investigation (BARI) study demonstrated equivalent long-term survival for PCI and bypass grafting among patients with multivessel disease. However, superior survival was observed in diabetic patients who had received an internal mammary graft to their left anterior descending (LAD) artery. This finding, which has been corroborated in the Emory Angioplasty versus Surgery Trial (EAST), supports the ACC/AHA guideline recommendation that CABG is preferred over PCI for diabetics with multivessel disease (Class I recommendation). The efficacy of drug-eluting stents versus bypass grafting in diabetic patients is the subject of ongoing study (the FREEDOM trial).

3   Answer C.   The nuclear study demonstrates a large area of nonviable myocardium and no areas of ischemia. Currently, revascularization with either PCI or bypass grafting is not recommended in the absence of demonstrable ischemia on noninvasive testing, irrespective of the findings on angiography. The topic of revascularization late after infarction is the subject of ongoing investigation (the OAT study).

4   Answer A.   Revascularization is not indicated for patients with one- or two-vessel disease without proximal LAD involvement who have not received an adequate trial of medical therapy and have no demonstrable evidence of ischemia (ACC/AHA Class III recommendation).

5   Answer B.   Patients with multivessel disease with anatomy suitable for either PCI or CABG can undergo either procedure with equivalent long-term survival (with the exception of diabetic patients). Characteristically, patients enrolled in such randomized trials were relatively young (60 years old), and most frequently had two-vessel disease, preserved ventricular function, and stable symptoms, although some studies enrolled patients with unstable angina.

A cost-effective analysis of the BARI trial demonstrated equivalent costs for angioplasty versus CABG after 12 years, principally because of the need for repeat procedures in the angioplasty group.

6   Answer C.   Although the left main lesion is approachable by PCI because of its distance from the bifurcation of the LAD and circumflex, current guidelines recommend bypass grafting over PCI in patients who are suitable for surgery. PCI with drug-eluting stenting versus bypass grafting for patients with left main disease is the subject of ongoing trials (e.g., SYNTAX).

7   Answer C.   PCI is the most frequent mode of repeat revascularization among patients undergoing CABG with rates of 5% to 6% over follow-up periods of 2 to 3 years.

8   Answer A.   A linear relation between adverse outcomes and all levels of creatinine kinase rise has been demonstrated, though not for mild elevations of troponin isoforms. However, marked troponin elevations (>5 times normal) are associated with increased mortality. In comparison studies, definitions of periprocedural infarction typically use higher levels of biomarker rise (five to ten times normal) for CABG procedures compared with PCI.

9   Answer A.   Comparable survival and freedom from infarction have been observed in most of the major trials of stenting versus CABG (ARTS, ERACI II, SoS, MASS II), including high-risk patients (AWESOME). In SoS, there was a higher mortality in the PCI arm, mainly because of a particularly low surgical mortality and high rate of noncardiac death in patients with stents. Stenting has reduced the need for repeat revascularization by 50% in comparison with rates observed in percutaneous transluminal coronary angioplasty (PTCA) trials.

10   Answer A.   The MASS study demonstrated comparable survival for patients with LAD disease, irrespective of whether they received medical therapy, PCI, or CABG. However, revascularization was associated with superior relief of angina and reduced need for antianginal medications. On the treadmill study, the Duke score of the patient was +7, which has been associated with a low annual risk of cardiovascular events (<1% per year).

11 Answer B. Few studies have examined the rates of repeat PCI after bare-metal stenting in ≥4.0 mm vessels. In TAXUS V, which compared the paclitaxel-eluting stent with bare-metal stenting in complex CAD, 17% of patients were treated with a 4.0-mm stent. The 9-month target lesion revascularization rates were 5% for the bare-metal arm, and 0% in the paclitaxel-eluting stent arm.

12 Answer C. Although the patient is asymptomatic, there are high-risk features on his nuclear stress study that suggest significant left main or multivessel disease. Few studies have included or focused on asymptomatic patients (e.g., CASS registry, ACIP). The ACC/AHA guidelines recommend coronary angiography for risk stratification with high-risk criteria on noninvasive testing irrespective of anginal severity. As in symptomatic patients, revascularization is indicated for asymptomatic patients when a large ischemic burden is present.

13 Answer D. Whereas the benefit of aspirin and β-receptor antagonists in patients with CAD is greater in those with prior infarction, patients with stable angina also likely derive benefit, and the ACC/AHA guidelines recommend their routine use in patients with CAD irrespective of symptoms. Therapy with ACE inhibitors reduces diabetic complications and cardiovascular events, particularly if hypertension or heart failure is present. Although calcium channel blockers are highly effective for the relief of angina, their use in patients with CAD has led to higher rates of adverse cardiovascular events in comparison with other therapies, such as ACE inhibitors (e.g., ABCD, FACET studies).

14 Answer D. Although restenosis may be clinically silent, the prognostic benefit of controlling silent ischemia remains unproven. Therefore, stress testing after revascularization may only be considered in patients with a significant change in their angina pattern (ACC/AHA Class IIb recommendation). If stress testing is undertaken, adjunctive imaging is recommended to improve the sensitivity of the test and to help localize the site of ischemia.

15 Answer C. Use of the internal thoracic artery has greatly improved graft patency with 90% of grafts still functioning >10 years after surgery. Over the same time, saphenous vein grafts have an occlusion rate of 40%, with significant atherosclerosis being present in 50% of those that are still patent.

16 Answer D. In patients with a normal EKG, no prior myocardial infarction, and no heart failure, routine assessment of left ventricular function is not recommended (ACC/AHA Class III recommendation). It is of note that several large studies of patients with CAD have shown that >90% of patients with a normal EKG have normal left ventricular function.

17 Answer C. On the basis of his performance on the treadmill, the prognosis of the patient is excellent (Duke score = 6; annual cardiac mortality <1%) and cannot be improved with revascularization by any means. Revascularization has not been shown to decrease rates of nonfatal infarction.

18 Answer C. The table below lists noninvasive criteria for prognosis in patients with CAD.

Noninvasive Risk Stratification

High Risk (greater than 3% annual mortality rate)

1. Severe resting left ventricular dysfunction (LVEF <35%)
2. High-risk treadmill score (score ≤ − 11)
3. Severe exercise left ventricular dysfunction (exercise LVEF <35%)
4. Stress-induced large perfusion defect (particularly if anterior)
5. Stress-induced multiple perfusion defects of moderate size
6. Large, fixed perfusion defect with left ventricular dilation or increased lung uptake (thallium-201)
7. Stress-induced moderate perfusion defect with left ventricular dilation or increased lung uptake (thallium-201)
8. Echocardiographic wall motion abnormality (involving greater than two segments) developing at low dose of dobutamine (≤10 mg/kg/min) or at a low heart rate (<120 bpm)
9. Stress echocardiographic evidence of extensive ischemia

Intermediate Risk (1%–3% annual mortality rate)

1. Mild/moderate resting left ventricular dysfunction (LVEF = 35%–49%)
2. Intermediate-risk treadmill score (−11 < score < 5)
3. Stress-induced moderate perfusion defect without LV dilation or increased lung intake (thallium-201)
4. Limited stress echocardiographic ischemia with a wall motion abnormality involving less than or equal to two segments only at higher doses of dobutamine

Low Risk (less than 1% annual mortality rate)

1. Low-risk treadmill score (score ≥5)
2. Normal or small myocardial perfusion defect at rest or with stress[a]
3. Normal stress echocardiographic wall motion or no change of limited resting wall motion abnormalities during stress[a]

[a]Although the published data are limited, patients with these findings will probably not be at low risk in the presence of either a high-risk treadmill score or severe resting left ventricular dysfunction (LVEF <35%).

LVEF, left ventricular ejection fraction; LV, left ventricular.

19 **Answer B and D.** For patients with CAD who survive sudden cardiac death, surgical revascularization is recommended over PCI if there is not proximal LAD involvement (ACC/AHA Class I recommendation).

20 **Answer D.** Although there are no strict criteria for defining a significant left main lesion, most studies have supported a minimal lumen area of <7.5 to 8.0 mm². In this patient, revascularization with either CABG or PCI is contraindicated in the absence of demonstrable ischemia on noninvasive testing (ACC/AHA III recommendation).

21 **Answer A.** Most patients enrolled in these trials had mild or moderate symptoms.

22 **Answer A.** Even in the absence of symptoms, CABG is recommended for patients with significant left main disease (ACC/AHA Class I recommendation). PCI is contraindicated in patients who are otherwise healthy candidates for CABG (ACC/AHA Class III recommendation).

23 **Answer D.** Stress testing with adjunctive imaging is recommended over treadmill study alone in patients with prior revascularization who have had a change in clinical status (ACC/AHA Class I recommendation). Coronary angiography may also be performed as the initial step in patients with CCS Class III angina despite maximal medical therapy (ACC/AHA Class I recommendation).

24 **Answer D.** Coronary angiography, in addition to medical therapy, is indicated for patients with angina and symptoms of congestive heart failure (ACC/AHA Class I recommendation).

25 **Answer C.** Despite the large number of patients with previous CABG, no randomized trial has compared PCI versus CABG in this patient subset. In one observational study comparing CABG and medical therapy, patients with late vein graft stenoses (>5 postoperative years) did better with CABG, particularly if the vein graft supplied the LAD. Decisions about revascularization in such patients should be made by experienced cardiac surgeons and interventional cardiologists.

26 **Answer B.** Both the BARI trial and the EAST study demonstrated that diabetic patients have superior survival with CABG versus PCI, particularly when a left internal mammary artery (LIMA) graft is placed on the LAD. Therefore, as per the ACC/AHA guidelines, CABG is preferred over PCI in diabetic patients (Class I recommendation). Nonetheless, registry data have shown that, when procedural choice is left to the discretion of physicians, comparable survival for CABG and PCI results.

27 **Answer C.** In patients with prior PCI, either CABG or PCI may be performed if a restenosis is associated with a moderate-to-large area of viable myocardium or high-risk criteria on noninvasive testing is present (ACC/AHA Class I recommendation).

28 **Answer D.** PCI is not recommended for lesions with mild symptoms and a low likelihood of success (ACC/AHA Class III recommendation).

29 **Answer B.** Grading of angina pectoris according to CCS classification is shown in the table below.

Class	Description of stage
I	"Ordinary physical activity does not cause angina," such as walking or climbing stairs. Angina occurs with strenuous, rapid, or prolonged exertion at work or recreation.
II	"Slight limitation of ordinary activity." Angina occurs on walking or climbing stairs rapidly; walking uphill; walking or climbing stairs after meals; walking in cold, in wind, or under emotional stress; or only during the few hours after awaking. Angina occurs on walking more than two blocks on the level and climbing more than one flight of ordinary stairs at a normal pace and under normal conditions.
III	"Marked limitations of ordinary physical activity." Angina occurs on walking one to two blocks on the level and climbing one flight of stairs under normal conditions and at a normal pace.
IV	"Inability to carry on any physical activity without discomfort—anginal symptoms may be present at rest."

30 **Answer B.** Randomized trials of PCI versus medical therapy have consistently shown superior symptom relief, less antianginal medications, and greater functional capacity on objective exercise testing with PCI. No difference in survival or nonfatal infarction has been observed for either PCI or medical therapy in these studies. The rate of target vessel failure for comparable lesions treated with the sirolimus-eluting stent in the SIRIUS trial was 5.2% in nondiabetics.

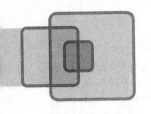

35

Practice Guidelines in Non–ST-Elevation Acute Coronary Syndromes

Juhana Karha and Eric J. Topol

Questions

1. A 65-year-old man with a history of hyperlipidemia presents to the emergency room with 2 hours of chest heaviness. His electrocardiogram (EKG) reveals sinus rhythm with anterolateral ST-segment depressions. His physical examination and initial blood work are unremarkable. He is diagnosed with non–ST-elevation acute coronary syndrome (ACS) and preparations are being made to perform coronary angiography in the next hour. His only medication is atorvastatin 20 mg daily. What antiplatelet agents should be administered to him?

   (A) Aspirin and abciximab
   (B) Aspirin, clopidogrel 600 mg, and plans for abciximab if a decision is made to proceed to percutaneous coronary intervention (PCI)
   (C) Aspirin and eptifibatide
   (D) Aspirin and plans for abciximab if a decision is made to proceed to PCI
   (E) Aspirin, clopidogrel 600 mg, and eptifibatide

2. A 54-year-old woman with a history of type 2 diabetes on metformin is being transferred to undergo urgent coronary angiography and possible PCI after being diagnosed with non–ST-elevation myocardial infarction (NSTEMI) at an outside facility. She arrives in the catheterization laboratory without ongoing chest pain and no signs of heart failure. The onset of chest pain was 8 hours ago, and the cardiac biomarkers from the outside facility are positive. Serum creatinine is normal. She received aspirin 325 mg and enoxaparin 1 mg per kg SQ at the outside hospital 8 hours ago. Coronary angiography reveals mid-LAD culprit lesion with a severe thrombotic stenosis. What is the optimal anticoagulation strategy during the upcoming PCI?

   (A) No further heparin
   (B) Enoxaparin 0.3 mg per kg IV
   (C) Unfractionated intravenous heparin

3. A 41-year-old man with a past medical history of asthma presents to the emergency department with an acute onset of severe retrosternal discomfort approximately 10 hours ago. His echocardiogram reveals sinus tachycardia and nonspecific T-wave changes. Which of the following are appropriate cardiac biomarkers to assist in risk stratification?

   (A) Creatine kinase (CK), creatine kinase–myocardial band (CK-MB), and a cardiac-specific troponin
   (B) Myoglobin only
   (C) C-reactive protein and myoglobin
   (D) Myeloperoxidase and aspartate aminotransferase (AST)
   (E) CK without CK-MB and a cardiac-specific troponin

4. A 71-year-old man with a history of coronary artery disease and prior coronary artery bypass graft (CABG) surgery presents to the emergency department with chest discomfort and dyspnea. The

symptoms started approximately 5 hours before his arrival. On physical examination, blood pressure (BP) is 95/55 mm Hg and heart rate (HR) is 110 bpm. Pulsoximetry reveals 88% on room air. The patient is diaphoretic. He has elevated jugular venous pulsations and bilateral wet crackles midway up the lung fields. His cough is productive of pink sputum. His EKG reveals sinus tachycardia with anterolateral T-wave inversions. His outpatient medications are aspirin and simvastatin. He is diagnosed with unstable angina. In this patient's presentation, which of the following portends the *highest* short-term risk of death or myocardial infarction (MI)?

(A) Age >70 years
(B) History of a prior CABG surgery
(C) Pulmonary edema most likely because of ischemia
(D) History of prior aspirin use
(E) T-wave inversions on the EKG

5 Which of the following anti-ischemic medications does *not* have an American College of Cardiology/American Heart Association (ACC/AHA) Class I indication for patients with non–ST-elevation ACS?

(A) Nitroglycerin
(B) Morphine sulfate
(C) ACE inhibitor
(D) β-adrenergic antagonist.
(E) Dihydropyridine calcium channel blocker

6 Which of the following antiplatelet or anticoagulant medications does *not* have an ACC/AHA Class I indication for patients with non–ST-elevation ACS?

(A) Low molecular weight heparin (LMWH) subcutaneously
(B) Unfractionated heparin intravenously
(C) Fondaparinux
(D) Aspirin
(E) Clopidogrel for patients who have a documented allergy to aspirin

7 A 68-year-old man with no previous history of bleeding sustains an NSTEMI and undergoes coronary angiography that reveals a recanalized right coronary artery (RCA) culprit lesion with only mild residual stenosis. No PCI is performed. His echocardiogram reveals normal ventricular function. His BP is 106/68 mm Hg. A lipid profile reveals total cholesterol of 214 mg per dL, high-density lipoprotein (HDL) of 50 mg per dL, low-density lipoprotein (LDL) of 140 mg per dL, triglycerides of 120 mg per dL. He is discharged home on aspirin and atorvastatin. Should he also be prescribed clopidogrel?

(A) No
(B) Yes, for 1 month
(C) Yes, for 9 months
(D) Yes, for 2 years
(E) Yes, indefinitely

8 A 72-year-old woman with a previous history of CABG surgery and severe dementia is admitted to the hospital with unstable angina. Her EKG reveals sinus rhythm and dynamic ST depressions. Her HR is 64 bpm and BP is 110/55 mm Hg. Her troponin T level is 0.05 ng per mL. She and her family adamantly refuse cardiac catheterization. She is started on aspirin, enoxaparin, simvastatin, IV nitroglycerin, and IV metoprolol. She denies any chest discomfort at present. To improve her medical regimen:

(A) Add abciximab
(B) Add eptifibatide
(C) Add tirofiban
(D) Add clopidogrel
(E) Substitute enoxaparin with unfractionated heparin

9 A 59-year-old woman presents to the emergency department with 12 hours of severe unremitting chest heaviness with onset at rest. Her past medical history is remarkable for hypertension, type 2 diabetes mellitus, obesity, hyperlipidemia, obstructive sleep apnea, and renal insufficiency. Her EKG reveals sinus rhythm and a normal tracing. Her CK is 500, CK-MB is 43.4, TnT is 1.88. Her creatinine is 1.6 mg per dL. After receiving aspirin, heparin, and nitroglycerin in the emergency department, her discomfort is relieved. The most appropriate next step in management is:

(A) Continued monitoring of her renal function with plans for coronary angiography if renal function improves
(B) Early invasive strategy with plans for urgent left heart catheterization
(C) Early conservative strategy given the absence of chest discomfort and a normal EKG
(D) Echocardiogram to evaluate the left ventricular function
(E) Resting nuclear sestamibi scan to evaluate for a perfusion abnormality at rest

10 A 74-year-old man is admitted to the hospital with NSTEMI. His prior medical history is significant for a remote coronary artery balloon angioplasty (with no stenting). He also has hyperlipidemia and gout. His echocardiogram reveals sinus rhythm with nonspecific T-wave changes. His cardiac biomarkers are positive. The coronary angiogram reveals a right-dominant system with severe stenoses in the proximal left anterior descending (LAD) and in the mid-RCA. The proximal LAD lesion does not involve the ostium of the LAD and is not near any diagonal or septal branches. It appears to be a discrete lesion obstructing approximately 75% of the lumen diameter. It does not appear thrombotic and it seems to be only mildly calcified. The mid-RCA stenosis appears hazy, but has TIMI grade 3 flow. It is near a small marginal branch. Ventriculography reveals inferior hypokinesis with an estimated left ventricular ejection fraction (LVEF) of 40%. An EKG performed in the emergency department also estimated LVEF at 40%. What is the most appropriate revascularization strategy for this patient?

(A) PCI to LAD and RCA
(B) Balloon angioplasty to RCA followed by CABG to LAD and right posterior descending artery (RPDA)
(C) CABG to LAD and RPDA
(D) PCI to RCA with a bare-metal stent implantation followed by 1 month of clopidogrel therapy and CABG to LAD
(E) No revascularization therapy unless further ischemia is detected

11 A 60-year-old woman presents to the emergency department with chest discomfort and is diagnosed with unstable angina. She undergoes coronary angiography that reveals a right-dominant system with a hazy ulcerated lesion in the RPDA. In the area of the lesion, the most severe percent diameter stenosis is 40% and the blood flow is TIMI grade 3 flow. The left coronary artery has mild diffuse disease and does not supply any collaterals to the RPDA. What is the optimal strategy?

(A) PCI with stenting to the RPDA given the hazy culprit appearance
(B) Medical therapy of carotid artery disease (CAD) given that no stenosis is at least 50%
(C) Catheter-based thrombectomy procedure without balloon or stent implantation
(D) Intravascular ultrasound (IVUS) examination of the lesion
(E) Determination of fractional flow reserve (FFR) of the lesion

12 A 42-year-old woman with familial hypercholesterolemia and a previous history of anterior MI (at age 25) and lateral MI (at age 37) presents to your office for follow-up. She has been doing well and denies chest pain or shortness of breath. She states that she wishes to get pregnant. She is currently on clopidogrel due to her severe aspirin allergy, lipitor 80 mg,

zetia 10 mg, metoprolol 50 mg b.i.d., and ramipril 5 mg a day. Which of the following medications should she be on during pregnancy?

(A) Desensitize her aspirin allergy because aspirin is the only safe drug during pregnancy
(B) Clopidogrel and metoprolol
(C) Clopidogrel, metoprolol, and zetia
(D) Clopidogrel, metoprolol, and lipitor
(E) Clopidogrel, ramipril, and zetia

13 A 69-year-old man with a prior CABG surgery 8 years ago (LIMA-LAD, SVG-OM2, SVG-RPDA) presents with unstable angina and a troponin T of 0.07 ng per mL. His EKG reveals 2 mm ST-segment depressions in leads I and aVL during chest discomfort. Coronary and graft angiography reveals severe left main trunk disease, occluded mid-LAD, severe proximal circumflex stenosis, and occluded dominant RCA. The grafts to LAD and RCA are patent. The vein graft to obtuse marginal branch has a severe ulcerated stenosis in its midportion with TIMI grade 2 flow. There appears to be an adequate landing zone for a distal emboli protection device. What is the optimum treatment strategy for this patient?

(A) PCI to SVG with distal emboli protection
(B) PCI to SVG with adjunctive glycoprotein (GP) IIb/IIIa
(C) PCI to left main trunk and proximal circumflex
(D) Redo-CABG to OM2
(E) Medical therapy given that LAD and RCA grafts are patent

14 A 55-year-old man with hyperlipidemia and obesity undergoes PCI with sirolimus-eluting stenting to LAD to treat his NSTEMI. The PCI is successful. His BP is not elevated. Post-PCI echocardiogram reveals normal ventricular function and mild mitral regurgitation. His discharge medications should include:

(A) Aspirin 325 mg daily, clopidogrel 75 mg daily, a statin, and a β-adrenergic blocker
(B) Aspirin 81 mg daily, clopidogrel 75 mg daily, a statin, and an ACE inhibitor
(C) Aspirin 325 mg daily, clopidogrel 75 mg daily, and a statin
(D) Aspirin 81 mg daily, clopidogrel 75 mg daily, a statin, and a β-adrenergic blocker
(E) Aspirin 325 mg daily, clopidogrel 75 mg daily, a statin, a β-adrenergic blocker, and an ACE inhibitor

15 A 52-year-old woman is transferred after presenting to an outside hospital with chest discomfort and being diagnosed with an NSTEMI. She then undergoes

PCI with implantation of three sirolimus-eluting stents to the RCA. She is not at an increased risk of bleeding. Her EKG demonstrates sinus rhythm. In addition to low-dose aspirin, how should she be prescribed clopidogrel?

(A) 75 mg daily indefinitely
(B) 75 mg daily for 1 month
(C) 75 mg daily for 9 to 12 months
(D) 150 mg daily for 2 years
(E) 150 mg daily for 9 to 12 months

16 A 60-year-old man with prior drug-eluting stent placement to mid-LAD has been having crescendo angina over the last 2 months. He is not a diabetic patient. He comes to the emergency department after a particularly severe episode of exertional angina. The discomfort was relieved by two sublingual nitroglycerin tablets (as opposed to the usual one tablet). His outpatient medications consist of aspirin, clopidogrel, atorvastatin, and a long-acting niacin. His EKG is sinus rhythm with normal tracing and his blood work including CK-MB and TnT is normal. The emergency department physician diagnoses him with unstable angina and he undergoes coronary angiography. The mid-LAD stent is patent with no evidence of in-stent restenosis. A large OM2 branch has a severe stenosis. It is a type A lesion. What is the optimal adjunctive medical therapy during the upcoming PCI with stenting?

(A) Bivalirudin only
(B) Heparin only
(C) Heparin and abciximab
(D) Heparin and eptifibatide
(E) Heparin and tirofiban

17 A 62-year-old diabetic woman undergoes PCI to LAD and D1 with paclitaxel-eluting stenting. She has moderate LV dysfunction with LVEF 35%. Her HbA_{1c} is 7.3%. Her BP is 135/87 mm Hg. Her lipid profile shows total cholesterol of 153 mg/dL, HDL of 38 mg/dL, LDL of 90 mg/dL, and triglycerides of 125 mg/dL. Her inpatient medications include aspirin, clopidogrel, atorvastatin 40 mg, metoprolol, and a multivitamin. Which of the following is *not* recommended adjustment in her discharge medications?

(A) Add short-acting nifedipine to lower her BP
(B) Add a fibrate or niacin to increase HDL
(C) Increase atorvastatin dose to lower LDL
(D) Add an ACE inhibitor to lower her BP and to afford benefits given her diabetes and depressed LVEF
(E) Add metformin to lower HbA_{1c}

18 A 43-year-old woman presents with episodic rest angina. Her past medical history is unremarkable. Her EKG shows normal sinus rhythm. An EKG obtained during an episode of chest discomfort in the emergency room reveals dynamic ST-segment elevation in leads V_3 through V_4. The discomfort resolves spontaneously. She declines urine toxicology screen. The cardiac markers are within normal limits and an echocardiogram is normal except for mild posterior mitral valve leaflet prolapse (MVP) without evidence of mitral regurgitation. Coronary angiography demonstrates mild coronary disease with no flow-limiting lesions. The most appropriate next step is:

(A) No further therapy for heart disease
(B) Exercise stress test to evaluate for ischemia
(C) Provocative testing during left heart catheterization with IC methylergonovine, followed by therapy with nitrates and calcium antagonists if the challenge is positive
(D) Provocative testing during left heart catheterization with IV methylergonovine, followed by therapy with nitrates and calcium antagonists if the challenge is positive
(E) Patient education regarding MVP associated chest pain and instructions for antibiotic prophylaxis with dental procedures

19 A 45-year-old man with previous stenting of proximal RCA with a sirolimus-eluting stent presents to the emergency department with new onset chest discomfort at rest. The discomfort is atypical. He has severe degenerative lumbar disc disease and is scheduled to undergo L4/L5 discectomy in 2 weeks. Coronary angiography demonstrates patent RCA stent and mild left coronary artery (LCA) disease. His cardiac medications are aspirin and clopidogrel. His ventricular function is normal. After discussion with the patient and the orthopaedic surgeon, it is clear that the surgery needs to occur in the near future to relieve his debilitating symptoms. In addition to perioperative β-blockade and minimizing the discontinuation period of aspirin and clopidogrel, what should be the perioperative recommendations?

(A) None
(B) Pharmacologic stress test with either an echo or nuclear imaging
(C) In-hospital GPIIb/IIIa therapy during the period of aspirin and clopidogrel discontinuation
(D) Intraoperative monitoring with Swan-Ganz catheter
(E) Continuous ST-segment monitoring following the operation

20 A 36-year-old man presents to the emergency department with 1 hour of acute-onset chest discomfort at rest. The pain started approximately 10 hours after he snorted cocaine. The past medical history is unremarkable except for polysubstance abuse. His EKG demonstrates sinus tachycardia with upsloping 2 mm ST-segment depression inferolaterally. Cardiac biomarkers are negative. Physical examination is remarkable for BP of 175/95 mm Hg (equal in both arms) and clear lungs. Chest x-ray is normal. The most appropriate management is:

(A) IV metoprolol
(B) IV morphine
(C) IV esmolol
(D) IV labetalol
(E) IV nitrates and calcium antagonists, followed by coronary angiography if discomfort persists

21 A 38-year-old woman who is 28 weeks pregnant presents to the emergency room complaining of chest pain for the last 10 hours. She is noted to have T-wave inversions in leads II, III, and aVF. Her BP is 100/60 with HR of 100. Her initial troponin is 10. She has no other medical problems in the past. She is still having chest pain. The emergency department doctors would like your advice. Which would be the most appropriate advice?

(A) Proceed to the catheterization laboratory for emergent angiogram and possible PCI with heparin only because GPIIb/IIIa inhibitors are contraindicated in pregnant women
(B) Medical management with GPIIb/IIIa inhibitor, unfractionated heparin, clopidogrel, aspirin, and statin therapy
(C) Medical management with GPIIb/IIIa inhibitor, LMWH, clopidogrel, aspirin, and statin therapy
(D) Proceed to catheterization laboratory for emergent angiogram with possible PCI with heparin and GPIIb/IIIa inhibitor

22 The patient referred in Question 21 does well and is discharged. She was diagnosed as having coronary artery dissection. What are the known risk factors for developing coronary artery dissection?

(A) Advance maternal age
(B) Third trimester of pregnancy
(C) Multigravida
(D) All of the above
(E) No known risk factors

23 A 48-year-old woman with recent resection of colorectal cancer (and an upcoming reversal of ileostomy) is hospitalized with a diagnosis of unstable angina. Her left heart catheterization reveals a 90% stenosis in a large diagonal branch (the reference vessel diameter is estimated at 3.0 mm). The remainder of her coronary arteries have mild disease. Which would be the most appropriate treatment plan for this lesion?

(A) PCI with sirolimus-eluting stent
(B) PCI with paclitaxel-eluting stent
(C) PCI with balloon angioplasty with no stenting
(D) PCI with bare-metal stenting
(E) Single-vessel CABG surgery

24 A 78-year-old man with a previous history of inferior MI presents to an outside freestanding emergency department with chest pain for 4 hours. His EKG reveals inferior Q waves and 3-mm ST-segment depressions in leads V_3 through V_6. He is treated with 5 units of reteplase, tirofiban, enoxaparin, aspirin, and clopidogrel. His chest discomfort resolves and there is complete resolution of his ST-segment depressions. He is transferred to the intensive care unit (ICU) and has no discomfort. His echocardiogram reveals inferior wall hypokinesis. Clinically, there is no evidence of heart failure. What is the most appropriate management step?

(A) Immediate coronary angiography
(B) Discontinuation of tirofiban, followed by coronary angiography the next day once the fibrinolytic effect has dissipated
(C) Continued tirofiban, enoxaparin, aspirin, and clopidogrel, followed by stress testing in 4 to 6 days
(D) Discontinuation of clopidogrel given the high likelihood of urgent CABG
(E) Stress testing to evaluate for inferior wall ischemia

25 A 59-year-old woman is admitted to the hospital with NSTEMI. Her EKG demonstrates inferior ST-segment depression. Her coronary angiogram reveals hazy appearing 80% mid-RCA obstruction with TIMI grade 2 flow. The mid-LAD has a severe 70% stenosis and the small circumflex artery lateral branch has two serial 70% lesions supplying a moderate territory. The patient is hemodynamically stable with left ventricular end diastolic pressure (LVEDP) of 16 mm Hg. Ventriculography demonstrates inferior hypokinesis, but preserved wall motion in the anterior wall. What is the optimal revascularization strategy?

(A) PCI with drug-eluting stenting to mid-RCA and mid-LAD, and later evaluation of the severity of the OM2 stenosis

(B) PCI with bare-metal stenting to mid-RCA with plan for CABG in 6 weeks (4 weeks of clopidogrel) to LAD and OM2

(C) Balloon angioplasty without stenting to mid-RCA with plan for CABG to LAD, RCA, and OM2

(D) PCI with drug-eluting stenting to mid-RCA, mid-LAD, and OM2

(E) PCI with drug-eluting stenting to mid-RCA, staged PCI with drug-eluting stenting to mid LAD, and an evaluation of the severity of the OM2 stenosis

26 A 84-year-old man is admitted at midnight with NSTEMI. He is pain-free and hemodynamically stable. A plan is formulated to perform coronary angiography in the morning. He has long-standing diabetic nephropathy, and his creatinine is 1.9 mg per dL. In addition to minimizing the amount of contrast dye used during the procedure, which of the following is the optimal way to minimize the extent of contrast dye-induced renal injury?

(A) Hydration with normal saline and mucomyst 600 mg

(B) Bicarbonate infusion

(C) The use of iodixanol dye along with biplane imaging system

(D) Mucomyst and bicarbonate infusion

(E) Hydration with normal saline and the use of iodixanol dye

27 A 52-year-old man with a history of obesity, hyperlipidemia, hypertension, and chronic renal insufficiency presented with new-onset exertional chest heaviness. He was admitted to the hospital with unstable angina. His EKG revealed sinus rhythm and a normal tracing. CK, CK-MB, and troponin T were within normal limits. At rest, he was asymptomatic and physical examination was notable for HR of 76 bpm, BP of 128/88 mm Hg, clear lungs, normal cardiac examination, and no peripheral edema. He was not on medication before the hospitalization. His creatinine was elevated at 2.4 mg per dL. Which is the optimal plan for risk stratification?

(A) Symptom-limited exercise stress test (without an echo or nuclear imaging) 2 to 3 days after admission

(B) Symptom-limited exercise stress test (without an echo or nuclear imaging) 7 to 10 days after admission

(C) Symptom-limited exercise stress test (with an echo or nuclear imaging) 4 to 6 days after admission

(D) Submaximal exercise stress test 2 to 3 days after admission

(E) Pharmacologic stress test 4 to 6 days after admission

28 A 50-year-old man with a history of hyperlipidemia and prior coronary angiogram with moderate coronary disease presents to the emergency department with chest discomfort of 15 hours' duration. His EKG shows normal sinus rhythm with no ischemic changes. The cardiac biomarkers are positive. He is admitted to the hospital with a diagnosis of NSTEMI and undergoes PCI with drug-eluting stenting to proximal circumflex artery. His outpatient medications had been aspirin, atorvastatin, and enalapril. His admission lipid profile fasting showed total cholesterol of 187 mg per dL, HDL of 38 mg per dL, LDL of 99 mg per dL, triglycerides of 250 mg per dL. Which of the following statements is *true*?

(A) His LDL is at goal

(B) The LDL value calculation may be incorrect because of the high triglyceride level

(C) His HDL is too low

(D) His total cholesterol of <200 mg per dL is more important than the rest of the panel

(E) His triglycerides are within acceptable range

29 A 76-year-old woman is admitted with NSTEMI and undergoes left heart catheterization. The diagnostic angiogram is followed by PCI with stenting to mid-LAD. Ventriculography demonstrates normal LV function. Before discharge, the physician caring for the patient orders an echocardiogram. Which of the following statements is *true*?

(A) Given that ventriculogram was normal, there is no need for an echocardiogram

(B) An echocardiogram is only warranted if there is an audible murmur

(C) In non–ST-elevation ACS, an echocardiogram is only indicated if the biomarkers are positive

(D) All patients with ACS should undergo an echocardiogram before discharge

(E) An echocardiogram EKG is necessary to rule out pericardial effusion given the recent angioplasty

30 A 51-year-old man is admitted with unstable angina. His past medical history is significant for remote tobacco use and a positive family history of sudden cardiac death. He prefers not to undergo heart catheterization despite the recommendation of the treating physician. A nuclear stress test reveals no scar and an area of inferior wall ischemia versus artifact. His BP is within normal limits and his lipid profile shows total cholesterol of 163 mg/dL, HDL of 55 mg/dL, LDL of 80 mg/dL, triglycerides of 140 mg/dL. His fasting glucose is within normal limits and his ventricular function by echocardiogram is normal. Is the measurement of high-sensitivity C-reactive protein (hsCRP) of additional benefit in assessing his risk of adverse cardiac outcomes?

(A) Yes, no other information captures the inflammatory component of coronary artery disease

(B) Yes, because he is at an intermediate risk on the basis of the rest of his health information, hsCRP adds incremental prognostic value

(C) Yes, but the high cost of the assay outweighs the beneficial information that it yields

(D) No, given his low overall risk, hsCRP is not helpful

(E) No, his fasting lipid profile is so good that hsCRP would not add value

Answers and Explanations

1 Answer B. All patients with an ACS should be treated with nonenteric-coated aspirin 162 to 325 mg. The only exceptions are patients who are known to be intolerant of aspirin. In patients for whom PCI is planned, an oral loading dose of clopidogrel 300 to 600 mg is recommended (the Intracoronary Stenting and Antithrombotic Regimen: Rapid Early Action for Coronary Treatment 2 [ISAR REACT 2] trial used a loading dose of 600 mg). Although higher loading doses such as 900 mg may provide greater platelet inhibition, the additive efficacy of this has not been rigorously established. The clopidogrel-loading dose may be administered either following the diagnostic angiography but before the PCI, or in cases where the estimated likelihood of the need for urgent open heart surgery is low; the loading dose may be administered before the diagnostic angiography. This patient represents low probability of need for urgent surgery. Platelet GPIIb/IIIa receptor antagonists afford further benefit in patients with an ACS undergoing PCI. The data in support of their use is strongest for abciximab. After a firm plan is made to perform PCI, abciximab should be administered. Ongoing trials will compare the strategies of starting abciximab in the emergency room versus in the catheterization laboratory. Of note, abciximab is contraindicated in patients in whom medical management only (and no PCI) is planned.

2 Answer C. Unfractionated intravenous heparin remains the recommended anticoagulation regimen during PCI at this point. The SYNERGY (Superior Yield of the New strategy of Enoxaparin, Revascularization, and Glycoprotein inhibitors) trial compared enoxaparin with unfractionated heparin among non–ST-elevation ACS patients undergoing PCI. There was no significant difference in the ischemic efficacy end points, but more bleeding was noted in the enoxaparin group. Although a *post hoc* analysis suggested that this may be explained by the higher rate of bleeding among patients who were switched from enoxaparin to heparin during the PCI, this finding requires prospective validation before it can be applied in practice. Another interesting development in the field is the ACU-ITY (Acute Catheterization and Urgent Intervention Triage strategY) trial, which demonstrated upon initial review that bivalirudin may be equally efficacious,

but safer than a strategy on the basis of heparin in patients undergoing PCI for non–ST-elevation ACS.

3 Answer A. CK and CK-MB are the principal serum cardiac biomarkers used in evaluation of ACS. Cardiac troponin I and T are cardiac-specific and more sensitive for myocardial necrosis compared with CK-MB. On the other hand, CK-MB provides better information about infarct extension and myocardial damage following PCI. Elevated levels of CK, CK-MB, and cardiac-specific troponins are all associated with worse prognosis. Myoglobin is released from injured myocytes earlier than CK and troponin. It may be detectable as early as 2 hours after the onset of myonecrosis. However, myoglobin is not cardiac-specific as it is also found in skeletal muscle, and therefore, it should not be used as a sole biomarker for evaluation of ACS. Both C-reactive protein and myeloperoxidase have incremental prognostic information in patients with stable and unstable coronary artery disease. AST is elevated with large amounts of myocardial damage, but is not as sensitive as CK and troponin in detecting myonecrosis.

4 Answer C. Pulmonary edema in the setting of ACS portends a high short-term risk of death or MI. The other available choices are associated with intermediate risk. Low-risk features would be, for instance, normal levels of cardiac biomarkers and normal (or unchanged) EKG during chest discomfort.

5 Answer E. Long-acting dihydropyridine calcium channel blockers have a Class IIa indication and the immediate release ones have a Class IIb indication according to the ACC/AHA guidelines.

6 Answer C. The current ACC/AHA guidelines do not list administration of fondaparinux among the Class I indicated interventions.

7 Answer C. The CURE and CREDO studies have demonstrated the benefit of dual antiplatelet therapy with aspirin and clopidogrel for patients with ACS. In these trials the benefit was seen with 9 to 12 months of clopidogrel use. The ACC/AHA guidelines make no distinction between medically managed patients versus those who underwent revascularization in terms of the length of clopidogrel treatment. It is of note that the recently conducted Clopidogrel for High Atherothrombotic Risk and Ischemic Stabilization, Management and Avoidance (CHARISMA) trial found no benefit in adding clopidogrel to aspirin among patients with stable cardiovascular disease. The placement of a drug-eluting coronary stent requires long-term clopidogrel therapy without interruption, but it is not applicable in this clinical scenario.

8 **Answer D.** Abciximab should not be administered to patients in whom PCI is not planned (the Global Use of Strategies To Open occluded coronary arteries, number IV (GUSTO IV) trial demonstrated harm with this strategy). The administration of tirofiban or eptifibatide is not likely to provide a benefit among patients with ACS who are medically treated, with no signs of ongoing ischemia. Addition of clopidogrel is associated with lower incidence of adverse ischemic events compared with aspirin only in the CURE trial. In this case, clopidogrel should be started and continued for 9 to 12 months. Enoxaparin is superior to unfractionated heparin among patients with ACS who are medically treated.

9 **Answer B.** Early invasive strategy is associated with a lower incidence of major adverse cardiac events compared with conservative strategy among patients with NSTEMI. This was noted, for example, in the TACTICS TIMI 18 trial. Other features that would favor invasive strategy are ongoing ischemic symptoms, ischemic EKG changes, evidence of hemodynamic instability or heart failure, and electrical instability. Attention to renal function and eventual assessment of ventricular function are both reasonable, but secondary in importance to coronary angiography in this case.

10 **Answer C.** On the basis of the available comparative data, CABG surgery is the recommended revascularization strategy for patients with NSTEMI with two-vessel disease involving the proximal LAD and abnormal (<50%) LVEF. Admittedly, the recent advances in PCI with adjunctive pharmacotherapy and drug-eluting stent design have not been evaluated against surgery. Because the flow through the apparent culprit RCA lesion is TIMI grade 3 flow, it is not necessary to perform balloon angioplasty or bare metal stenting before CABG.

11 **Answer B.** Revascularization of lesions with <50% stenosis is not recommended. No data support the use of a thrombectomy device in this case. An IVUS might be reasonable in cases where there is a question

about the severity of the stenosis. An FFR may be useful to evaluate intermediate stenoses (50% to 70% diameter stenosis).

12 **Answer B.** The U.S. Food and Drug Administration (FDA) has established five categories (A, B, C, D, and X) to indicate a drug's potential for causing teratogenicity:

- A—Controlled studies in women fail to demonstrate a risk to the fetus in the first trimester (and there is no evidence of a risk in later trimesters) and the possibility of fetal harm appears remote.
- B—Either animal-reproduction studies have not demonstrated a fetal risk, but there are no controlled studies in pregnant women or animal-reproduction studies that have shown adverse effect (other than a decrease in fertility) that was not confirmed in controlled studies in women in the first trimester (and there is no evidence of a risk in later trimesters).
- C—Either studies in animals have revealed adverse effects on the fetus (teratogenic or embryocidal or other) and there are no controlled studies in women or studies in women and animals are not available. Drugs should be given only if the potential benefit justifies the potential risk to the fetus.
- D—There is positive evidence of human fetal risk, but the benefits from use in pregnant women may be acceptable despite the risk (e.g., if the drug is needed in a life-threatening situation or for a serious disease for which safer drugs cannot be used or are ineffective).
- X—Studies in animals or human beings have demonstrated fetal abnormalities or there is evidence of fetal risk on the basis of human experience or both, and the risk of the use of the drug in pregnant women clearly outweighs any possible benefit. The drug is contraindicated in women who are or may become pregnant.

Lipitor and zetia are Category X drugs, whereas ramipril is a Category D drug during the second and third trimester. Clopidogrel is Category B and Metoprolol is Category C.

13 **Answer A.** Although no specific data guide us to recommend revascularization of the SVG versus medical therapy only, it is reasonable to expect the PCI to provide superior preservation of myocardial function given that the graft appears to be on the brink of closing. Reoperation for a single circumflex territory target would have unfavorable risk-to-benefit ratio and PCI to native coronaries, while perhaps an option later, would be more difficult than PCI to SVG. Adjunctive IIb/IIIa inhibitors do not offer any benefit in vein graft angioplasty in a stable situation, but may offer modest benefit in a patient with ACS, like this one. The use of a distal emboli protection device has been shown to reduce ischemic complications during vein graft angioplasty. Given the large amount of thrombotic debris, its use is particularly advisable in this case.

14   Answer D. Aspirin and clopidogrel are essential medications following PCI with drug-eluting stenting. For long-term use, aspirin at 81 to 162 mg daily doses is equally efficacious and associated with fewer bleeding complications versus 325 mg daily. More information is required regarding the optimal clopidogrel dose. It is also possible that in the future testing for aspirin and clopidogrel resistance may yield personalized dosing recommendations for patients. Given this patient's hyperlipidemia, it is critically important to discharge him on a statin drug with a goal LDL level <70 mg per dL. All patients should be treated with a β-adrenergic blocker following MI, unless contraindications exist. ACE inhibitors are appropriate discharge medications for patients with ventricular systolic dysfunction, hypertension, or diabetes mellitus. The patient in this vignette does not require an ACE inhibitor.

15   Answer A. The feature that guides the decision regarding the length of clopidogrel therapy in this case is the implantation of a sirolimus-eluting stent. As the endothelialization of the stent is retarded to variable degrees with drug-eluting stents, it is most prudent to continue clopidogrel indefinitely. It is not known when, if ever, it is safe to discontinue clopidogrel, but case reports have documented stent thromboses even years after the procedure. Clearly, more investigation is needed to answer this controversial question. No data exist about the appropriate maintenance dose and most physicians use the standard dose of 75 mg daily.

16   Answer A. The ACUITY trial demonstrated that among patients with non–ST-elevation ACS undergoing PCI, bivalirudin is similar to a strategy of heparin plus GPIIb/IIIa inhibitor in terms of ischemic endpoints, but safer with respect to bleeding. The performance of bivalirudin was especially good in the setting of clopidogrel pretreatment. The ISAR REACT 2 trial evaluated a similar patient population receiving aspirin, clopidogrel loading, and heparin, and demonstrated that among troponin-positive patients addition of a GPIIb/IIIa inhibitor

was beneficial. Therefore, in this patient with unstable angina and a culprit lesion, which does not appear thrombotic, the optimal adjunctive pharmacotherapy is bivalirudin.

17   Answer A. Short-acting nifedipine has been associated with adverse outcomes among patients with coronary disease. Lipid management is clearly very important for this patient and the efforts to raise HDL and further lower LDL are reasonable. Her goal HbA$_{1c}$ is <7%, and addition of metformin has a good chance of achieving that goal. ACE inhibitors are particularly beneficial for diabetic patients, especially if BP continues to be elevated or if the ventricular systolic function is depressed.

18   Answer D. Provocative testing with IV methylergonovine is safe and will likely yield a diagnosis of Prinzmetal angina. Methylergonovine should never be administered through the intracoronary route as it may precipitate irreversible spasm and electric instability. Once diagnosed, coronary vasospasm is readily treatable with nitrates and calcium channel blockers. Given the coronary anatomy, a stress test would be unremarkable. No antibiotic prophylaxis is required given the absence of mitral regurgitation with MVP.

19   Answer A. The patient's discomfort does not represent myocardial ischemia due to epicardial coronary stenosis. The upcoming cessation of antiplatelet therapy along with the prothrombotic storm that accompanies the surgery presents a real risk for stent thrombosis. Stress testing will not be helpful as there are no flow-limiting coronary stenoses. It is also not clear whether more careful monitoring or treatment with GPIIb/IIIa inhibitors might reduce the risk.

20   Answer E. Cocaine use is associated with multiple cardiac illnesses including coronary vasospasm, accelerated atherosclerosis, increased incidence of MI, and elevated BP (along with an increased incidence of aortic dissection). In this case, the most important management step is cautious lowering of BP. The concern in using β-adrenergic blockers is the unopposed α action that may result. From this perspective, labetalol may be preferable (with its concomitant α-blocking action). However, in this case where the concern is more for myocardial ischemia, especially vasospasm, and less for dissection, nitrates and calcium channel blockers are more likely to be effective. Importantly, if the discomfort persists after optimization of hemodynamics, coronary angiography is advisable.

21 Answer D. This patient needs to be taken to the catheterization laboratory. She has an elevated troponin and is having ongoing ischemia. The likelihood of fetal damage from radiation exposure is lower after the first trimester. Fortunately, anticoagulation drugs used during PCI are either Category B or C. For instance, bivalirudin, tirofiban, eptifibatide, and enoxaparin are all Category B drugs whereas abciximab and heparin are Category C drugs.

22 Answer D. On the basis of current literature, coronary artery dissection has been associated with advance maternal age, in multigravida women, near term or within 3 months postpartum.

23 Answer D. Given the upcoming interruption in clopidogrel therapy with the surgery (along with the prothrombotic state), drug-eluting stenting is not recommended for this large diameter diagonal branch. The optimal strategy is bare-metal stenting followed by 1 month of clopidogrel, followed by the surgery. The risk of acute closure and restenosis will be significantly less than with balloon angioplasty only (with no stent deployment). There is no indication for a single-vessel surgery.

24 Answer B. Apparently the medical therapy successfully treated the ACS. It is worth noting that in this case, the fibrinolytic agent was administered without appropriate indication (ST elevation or equivalent). Given that this elderly patient received three antiplatelet medications, heparin, and a fibrinolytic agent, the risk of bleeding complications is high. Therefore, the GPIIb/IIIa inhibitor should be discontinued and coronary angiography delayed until the fibrinolytic has worn off. Although no definitive data guide the routine angiography following successful fibrinolysis, it may reduce ischemia. In this case, the EKG abnormality was quite impressive shifting the balance in favor of angiography (vs. stress testing). The likelihood of urgent CABG is actually low and therefore, clopidogrel should be continued.

25 Answer E. The mid-RCA culprit lesion requires immediate therapy. This is best achieved by PCI with drug-eluting stenting. Given that the patient is hemodynamically stable, the prudent strategy is to stage PCI to mid-LAD and the assessment of the functional importance of the circumflex lesions is to be performed later. Had the LAD lesion been in the proximal portion of the vessel, one could have considered palliation of the culprit lesion percutaneously, followed by CABG.

26 Answer E. The two most important measures in limiting the injury to kidney are preprocedural hydration with saline and the use of iodixanol (or similar) dye. *N*-acetylcysteine (mucomyst) and bicarbonate infusion may also provide incremental protection, but this is less well established. Biplane imaging often allows for fewer injections thereby affording further nephroprotection.

27 Answer A. In a patient who is able to exercise, the stress test that provides the most prognostic information is a symptom-limited exercise test. No additional echo or nuclear imaging is required given that the baseline EKG is normal. Although an echo or nuclear imaging might provide useful additional information, it would not be cost-effective in this case. It is safe to perform the stress test 2 to 3 days after admission, provided that there has been no recurrent ischemia during the hospital stay.

28 Answer C. The components of total cholesterol are the most important information in a lipid panel. The LDL goal among patients who have coronary artery disease is <70 mg per dL. The HDL should be >40 mg per dL for men and >50 mg per dL for women, and hypertriglyceridemia should be treated if the level is >200 mg per dL. The calculated LDL value may be inaccurate if the triglyceride level exceeds 400 mg per dL.

29 Answer D. The most important ultimate goal in managing ACS is to prevent the development of ventricular dysfunction. Although ventriculography is decent in assessing LV function, the best test for this is an echocardiogram. All the myocardial segments can be evaluated over many heartbeats. In addition, an echocardiogram is excellent in evaluating valvular dysfunction (for instance, mitral insufficiency which may result from MI). Therefore, all patients with ACS should have a transthoracic echocardiogram.

30 Answer A. This patient is at low risk of future adverse cardiac events on the basis of his ventricular function and lipid profile. However, the positive family history and the uncertainty about the stress test result make risk assessment more difficult. It is possible that he has mild coronary disease with significant plaque burden, but no flow-limiting lesions. In that case, his risk is governed by his propensity for plaque rupture and resultant ACS. The process of plaque instability may be related to endothelial inflammation. In addition, it is possible that hsCRP level, unlike the other tests mentioned, would capture these important data.

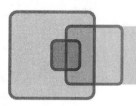

36

Percutaneous Coronary Intervention: American College of Cardiology/American Heart Association Guidelines 2005

Leslie Cho

Questions

1. A 67-year-old woman with a history of hypertension (HTN) and hyperlipidemia who underwent left anterior descending (LAD) stenting 2 years ago for angina presents to your office for a second opinion. She has been on atenolol, Norvasc, Lipitor, aspirin (ASA), and Imdur with minimal angina. She underwent her annual stress test where she exercised for 10 minutes on modified Bruce protocol and achieved 10 METS. Her ejection fraction (EF) at rest was 60%. There was no evidence of ischemia at stress. She underwent cardiac computed tomography (CT) at her own request and was found to have significant stenosis in her circumflex (CX) artery. She then underwent catheterization, which showed 30% mid-LAD stenosis, large dominant right coronary artery (RCA) with 40% distal RCA stenosis and 80% proximal stenosis in moderate size CX artery. On examination, her blood pressure (BP) is 104/68 with heart rate (HR) of 58 without any evidence of heart failure. She wants your opinion regarding revascularization. You would advise:

    (A) Continue current medication regimen but not revascularization
    (B) Fractional flow reserve (FFR) of CX artery and if <0.75 proceed to percutaneous coronary intervention (PCI)

    (C) PCI of CX artery
    (D) Add Plavix therapy but no revascularization

2. The patient in Question 1 is not satisfied with your answer and goes to another cardiologist in town. She undergoes FFR of CX artery which was 0.86 and intravascular ultrasound (IVUS) of the lesion showed 70% stenosis. She is still asymptomatic. She then returns to your office and wants your opinion regarding revascularization.

    (A) There is data to support IVUS over FFR, therefore, should proceed with PCI to CX
    (B) Clinical outcome of a significant lesion based on IVUS is poor, therefore, the FFR result should be ignored and PCI to CX should be planned
    (C) Clinical outcome of deferring coronary intervention for stenosis with normal physiology shows low clinical event rates, so there is no need for PCI

3. A 76-year-old man with HTN, diabetes mellitus (DM), coronary artery disease (CAD), hyperlipidemia, and history of congestive heart failure (CHF) presents to the emergency room (ER) with increasing shortness of breath (SOB) and chest pain. His past medical history is notable for coronary artery bypass

graft (CABG) performed 5 years ago. He has been doing well until recently when a few weeks ago he experienced mild chest pain while mowing his lawn. Since then he has noticed increasing chest pain with exertion. On the day of admission, he had chest pain at rest with increasing SOB and called 911. In the ER, his electrocardiogram (EKG) showed ST elevation in leads II, III, and a VF. His BP was 126/90 with a HR of 100, and examination showed regular rhythm and rate, S1, S2 with S3 and elevated jugular venous pressure (JVP). He is taken to the catheterization laboratory. His catheterization reveals normal left main trunk (LMT), 100% mid-LAD, 60% proximal CX stenosis, 100% RCA, patent left internal mammary artery (LIMA) to LAD with minimal distal LAD stenosis, 95% stenosis in saphenous vein graft (SVG) to posterior descending artery (PDA) with thrombolysis in myocardial infarction (TIMI) I flow and 90% SVG to D1 lesion. His EF is 55% with 2 to 3+ MR. SVG to PDA is thought to be the culprit lesion and successful PCI is performed using an emboli filter device and stent. His general cardiologist would like you to fix his SVG to D1 lesion as well. Do you agree?

(A) Yes, in light of his heart failure symptoms, it is best to open all significant lesions based on the SHOCK trial

(B) No, elective PCI should not be performed in a noninfarct-related artery at the time of primary PCI of the infarct-related artery in patients without hemodynamic compromise

(C) Yes, elective PCI should be performed in a noninfarct-related artery at the time of primary PCI of the infarct-related artery in patients without hemodynamic compromise

(D) No, the patient is older than 75 years, and in the SHOCK trial, multivessel revascularization was only beneficial to patients younger than 75 years

4 A 46-year-old man with history of hyperlipidemia is an active smoker and presents with chest pain for 3 months. He undergoes a stress thallium where he exercised to 11 METS and at stress showed large anterior wall ischemia. His EF is 70%. The patient undergoes cardiac catheterization, which shows 75% mid-LAD, noncalcified, nontortuous stenosis. The lesion appears to be at low risk. He is scheduled for PCI at the same hospital. While you are explaining the risks and benefits of PCI, he becomes concerned about the risk of possible urgent CABG. What is the exact percentage of this risk?

(A) 1% to 2%

(B) 3% to 5%

(C) 5% to 7%

(D) 0.1% to 1.0%

5 The patient referred in Question 4 undergoes successful PCI to LAD with a sirolimus stent and is now ready for discharge. The nurse practitioner wants to talk to you about his discharge medication. The patient and his wife are extremely worried about bleeding complications after reading about clopidogrel on the web. They want to take the minimal length of antiplatelet therapy. On the basis of current recommendation, what should his oral antiplatelet regimen be?

(A) ASA 325 mg a day for 1 month, then ASA 81 mg a day for life, and clopidogrel 75 mg a day for at least 3 months

(B) ASA 81 mg a day for life and clopidogrel 75 mg a day for 3 months

(C) ASA 325 mg a day for 1 month, then ASA 81 mg a day for life, and clopidogrel 75 mg a day for at least 9 months

(D) ASA 81 mg a day for life and clopidogrel 75 mg a day for 9 months

6 A 54-year-old woman presents to the ER with chest pain and is found to have nonspecific scapulothoracic (ST) changes in leads II, III, and aVF, and a troponin I level of 2.3 ng per mL. Her medical history is notable for morbid obesity, DM, HTN, and active smoking. She is given ASA 325 mg and 5,000 units of IV heparin in the ER. She is taken immediately to the catheterization laboratory. Her diagnostic catheterization reveals 99% mid-RCA stenosis with 60% proximal CX lesion and 60% mid-LAD lesion. You proceed with PCI of RCA. The best antiplatelet and antithrombotic regimen for this patient based on the current body of evidence would be:

(A) Clopidogrel load of 600 mg and bivalirudin

(B) Heparin and glycoprotein (GP) IIb/IIIa inhibitor

(C) Heparin, clopidogrel 600-mg load, and GP IIb/IIIa inhibitor

(D) Low molecular weight heparin (LMWH), clopidogrel 600 mg load, and GP IIb/IIIa inhibitor

7 This same woman does well after her successful PCI to RCA and is found to have a platelet count of 50,000 the next day. She does not have any evidence of ischemia and appears to be well. An intern on your service requests a serotonin release assay test as well as solid phase immunoassay for heparin-induced antibodies. The results of the serotonin assay test comes back positive, whereas those of the solid phase immunoassay returns negative. The patient continues to do well and is discharged and returns to your office in 2 weeks. At that time, her platelet count is 100,000 and she is asymptomatic but continues to smoke and is not interested in losing weight. Her medication regimen includes ASA, clopidogrel, atorvastatin, atenolol, and lisinopril. Eight months later, on the same medication regimen, she returns to your clinic complaining of chest pain and undergoes a stress test, which shows a large anterior ischemia. She undergoes catheterization and is found to have 85% stenosis of LAD. What should her antithrombotic regimen be?

(A) Heparin and GP IIb/IIIa inhibitor
(B) LMWH and GP IIb/IIIa inhibitor
(C) LMWH alone since she is already on clopidogrel
(D) Argatroban

8 A 78-year-old retired cardiologist with S/P CABG in 1990 and 1999 presents to your office with increasing chest pain with exertion. He undergoes a cardiac catheterization and is found to have severe ostial SVG to CX disease, patent LIMA to LAD, and patent SVG to PDA; however, there is distal SVG lesion. Other grafts are patent without significant disease including SVG to D1 and SVG to CX. His SVG to CX is from a 1990 surgery and SVG to PDA is from a 1999 surgery. You proceed to intervene upon SVG to CX and SVG to PDA. The patient wants to talk about his chances of final patency. In both lesions, there is diffuse disease but the lesions are not friable or degenerative. You state:

(A) Patency rates are the same for both grafts
(B) The older graft has less likelihood of patency
(C) Patency rates are equivalent since emboli protection devices will be used for both grafts
(D) The lesion location is a predictor of final patency—ostial lesion has lower likelihood patency
(E) The lesion location is a predictor of final patency—distal lesion has lower likelihood of patency

9 You are called to evaluate a 69-year-old woman in the surgical intensive care unit (ICU) who underwent CABG 3 days ago for ST elevation in the anterior leads. She underwent LIMA to LAD, SVG to OM2, SVG to PDA, and SVG to posterolateral (PL) 3 days ago and has been doing well until 3 hours ago when she started complaining of chest pain and was found to have ST elevation in leads V_2 through V_5. You take her to the catheterization laboratory and she is found to have severe 90% stenosis across suture line in her LIMA to LAD graft. You should:

(A) Proceed with balloon dilatation
(B) Proceed with balloon dilatation and stent placement
(C) Proceed with open native LAD
(D) Avoid PCI because it is not safe so soon after CABG

10 A 74-year-old woman in severe respiratory distress was taken to the ER by paramedics who intubated her in the field. According to her husband, she started experiencing chest pain 2 hours ago. She has a history of HTN and hyperlipidemia only and has been healthy until she experienced chest pain 2 hours ago. According to the ER physician, her BP is 80/60 on Levophed and her HR is 110. Her EKG shows 5 mm ST elevation in the anterior leads. The ER is located 3 hours from your hospital with catheterization laboratory. The ER physician is certified to place intra-aortic balloon pump (IABP). What should be done next?

(A) Fibrinolytic therapy if there are no contraindications and emergency transfer
(B) No fibrinolytic therapy, emergency transfer
(C) IABP and emergency transfer
(D) Fibrinolytic therapy, IABP, and emergency transfer

11 The patient referred in Question 10 is transferred to your hospital. You are waiting for her in the catheterization laboratory. She still has ST elevation and she is still on Levophed with a BP of 80/60 and an HR of 120. She undergoes emergent catheterization and is found to have multivessel disease with chronically occluded long RCA stenosis, 80% type A lesion in a moderate size CX artery and 100% LAD lesion. The proximal LAD is filled with thrombus but is a PCI approachable lesion. What should be done next?

(A) Proceed with multivessel PCI and plan on PCI to LAD and CX
(B) Proceed with infarct-related artery PCI only
(C) Refer to CABG
(D) Proceed with LAD PCI and if there is no improvement then PCI to CX

12 A 79-year-old man presented to an outside hospital 2 days ago with chest pain for 10 hours. At that time, he had ST elevation in the inferior leads and received fibrinolytic therapy because he did not want to be transferred to another hospital. At that time his BP was 130/80 with an HR of 94 and he did not have physical examination consistent with heart failure. With fibrinolytic therapy, there was no ST resolution and the patient continued to have chest pain. His chest pain resolved in 6 hours. His peak troponin was 6.5 ng per mL. Currently, he is doing well and denies any chest pain and there has been no ST depression on his monitor. His children want him to undergo catheterization. His general cardiologist performed an angiogram that showed 90% distal RCA lesion with TIMI III flow, moderate diffuse 50% lesion in LAD and CX, and inferior hypokinesis on LV gram. They would like you to intervene on his RCA. The patient's daughter who is a nurse wants to know if PCI will improve his prognosis.

(A) Extrapolating from non–ST-elevation myocardial infarction (NSTEMI) data, there is reason to believe that invasive therapy will decrease major adverse cardiac events in these patients

(B) There is no convincing data to support the routine use of late adjuvant PCI days after failed fibrinolysis in patients who are hemodynamically and electrically stable without any evidence of ischemia

(C) On the basis of observational and experimental data, infarct artery patency favorably influences LV remodeling and electrical stability; therefore, PCI to RCA is recommended

(D) On the basis of the recent DANAMI trial, PCI of infarct-related artery resulted in less major adverse cardiac events

13 You are contacted by a lawyer for the plaintiff of a case involving a 57-year-old female nurse with acute myocardial infarction (MI). She presented to the ER within 3 hours of chest pain and was found to have ST elevation inferiorly with reciprocal changes. She was given ASA 325 mg, 300 mg of clopidogrel, abciximab bolus and infusion, and 5,000 units of heparin in the ER. Her BP was 110/70 with a HR of 110. She was taken to the catheterization laboratory and was found to have 100% occlusion of a dominant CX artery. Her door-to-balloon time was 90 minutes. She underwent successful PCI to CX with a sirolimus stent. Subsequently she had retroperitoneal bleed, which required a 2-unit blood transfusion and 3 additional days of hospitalization. The claim is based on the fact that there is little data to support routine use of abciximab in ST-elevation myocardial infarction (STEMI). What is your response?

(A) You agree on the basis of the CADILLAC trial that there is little benefit of abciximab if stents are used in primary PCI

(B) There is evidence for small-molecule GP IIb/IIIa inhibitors like tirofiban or eptifibatide upstream but not for abciximab

(C) There is data to support early (before coronary angiography) administration of abciximab

(D) There is no data to support any GP IIb/IIIa inhibitor upstream

14 The patient referred in Question 13 is also stating that she should have received fibrinolytic therapy instead of primary PCI. She wants to know what evidence there is to support PCI versus fibrinolytic therapy in STEMI.

(A) Patients who underwent primary PCI have lower mortality, fewer reinfarction, and less bleeding

(B) Patients who underwent primary PCI have lower mortality, fewer reinfarction, and more bleeding

(C) Patients who underwent primary PCI have similar mortality, fewer reinfarction, and less bleeding

(D) Patients who underwent primary PCI have similar mortality, fewer reinfarction, and more bleeding

15 The patient referred in Question 13 also asks for clinical evidence regarding primary PCI with stent versus balloon angioplasty. Your response is that compared with balloon angioplasty:

(A) Primary PCI with stent has lower death and reinfarction rates

(B) Primary PCI with stent has similar death rates but lower reinfarction rates

(C) Primary PCI with stent has similar death and reinfarction rates

(D) Primary PCI with stent has lower bleeding rates

16 You have recently been elected to the quality assurance board of your hospital. They are reviewing protocol of cardiac biomarker (creatinine kinase [CK-MB], troponin I or T) blood draws after every PCI. They are being pressured from insurance companies to stop this procedure. On the basis of current data, what are the recommendations?

(A) Biomarkers should not be drawn since they add little value to prognosis or diagnosis of the patient

(B) All patients who have signs or symptoms suggestive of MI during or after PCI, and patients with complicated procedures should have biomarkers measured after the procedure only; routine measurement is not recommended

(C) Biomarkers should be measured only in patients who are admitted with STEMI, NSTEMI, or unstable angina

(D) In addition to patients who have signs or symptoms suggestive of MI during or after PCI, those with complicated procedures should have biomarkers measured after the procedure, and routine measurement in all patients undergoing PCI is a reasonable 8 to 12 hours after the procedure

17 A 61-year-old woman S/P CABG in 2003 undergoes SVG to D1 intervention owing to unstable angina. The intervention was performed with an emboli filter device, abciximab, and bare-metal 5.0/18 mm stent. PCI was uneventful: however, 3 hours after the case she complains of abdominal pain and her BP is 70/50 with a HR of 110. Her hemoglobin level, which was 14 g per dL at the start of PCI, is now 8.8 g per dL. Because of her profound hypotension, she requires a 2-unit blood transfusion. She stabilizes and is discharged home 3 days later. She does well; however, she is angry about her complication. She states that she bled from abciximab administration and that it should not have been used because abciximab is known to cause more major bleeding in women. Does abciximab cause more major bleeding in women?

(A) Abciximab causes more major and minor bleeding in women
(B) Abciximab causes more major bleeding but similar rates of minor bleeding in women
(C) Abciximab causes similar major bleeding but more minor bleeding in women
(D) Abciximab does not cause more major or minor bleeding in women

18 A 63-year-old hospital administrator with diabetes presents to your office for a second opinion. She has been experiencing increasing dyspnea on exertion and had a stress echo, which showed an EF of 55% and lateral ischemia. She exercised for only 6 minutes. She underwent catheterization and was found to have three-vessel disease with 90% focal proximal LAD bifurcation lesion which involves a large diagonal artery, CX has mild disease but is extremely angulated and comes off 110 degree from LMT, 90% moderately tortuous OM2 lesion and 95% distal diffuse RCA lesion which measures 15 mm, and 100% chronically occluded PDA and PL branch with bridging collaterals. She was offered CABG. However, she is adamant that she does not want CABG unless her lesions are high-risk lesions. Which of these lesions are high-risk?

(A) All of them
(B) All except OM2 lesion
(C) All except distal RCA lesion
(D) All except proximal LAD lesion

19 A 49-year-old trial lawyer presents to your office for a consultation. He has a family history of heart disease and has been on Zocor for several years. He is not a diabetic patient and does not have a history of CHF. He recently experienced chest pain at work and underwent a stress test, which showed inferior and lateral ischemia at peak stress. He underwent catheterization and was found to have single-vessel disease with normal LV function. He has 80% mid-LAD and 90% CX, and 95% RCA lesions. The lesions are amenable to PCI but he has heard about minimal invasive CABG and is interested in that as well. He has been emotionally debilitated since his catheterization and feels that he needs to proceed with whatever mode of revascularization that is going to make him live longer and with fewer heart attacks. What do you recommend?

(A) CABG because mortality and morbidity are lower with CABG in three-vessel disease
(B) CABG because there is no difference in mortality between CABG and PCI; however, PCI is associated with more MI later
(C) Either one because there is no difference in mortality or MI rate between the two
(D) CABG because it is superior to PCI in terms of lower mortality and morbidity when LAD is involved

20 A 76-year-old retired acupuncturist presents to your office with increasing SOB. The history of the patient is only remarkable for hyperlipidemia for which he uses red rice yeast. He undergoes a stress test and is found to have anterior ischemia and his catheterization shows a 90% mid-LAD lesion with no significant disease in other arteries and a normal EF. He states that he is willing to take "western medicine" but does not want PCI or CABG. His wife is very concerned about his risk and wants to know which modality, in your opinion, is best for long-term survival. You recommend:

(A) Medicine, since it is not a proximal LAD lesion
(B) CABG, for symptom relief as well as mortality benefit
(C) Either revascularization therapy since either one provides similar mortality benefit over medicine
(D) There is no mortality difference between medical therapy, PCI, or CABG

21 A 71-year-old retired executive presents to your office for a second opinion. She underwent a routine stress test on the persistence of her primary care provider (even though she had no symptoms) and was found to have inferior and posterior ischemia. She also underwent ambulatory electrocardiogram (EKG) monitoring, which also showed ST depression in the inferior and lateral leads. She then underwent cardiac catheterization and was found to have nondominant

RCA with minimal disease, hyperdominate CX with severe 95% proximal stenosis, and minimal disease in her LAD. She was offered PCI and now wants your opinion regarding the matter. What would you tell her?

(A) Angina-guided drug therapy is equivalent to PCI in major adverse cardiac event rates

(B) Angina plus ischemia-guided drug therapy is equivalent to PCI in major adverse cardiac event rates

(C) Revascularization with PCI lowers major adverse cardiac events

(D) There is no difference between either medical therapy or revascularization in terms of major adverse cardiac event rates

22 You are asked to provide an opinion regarding on-site PCI privileges for a colleague. He is an experienced interventional cardiologist who is Board certified and performs 130 PCI and 600 diagnostic angiograms a year. He had a recent disagreement with his partners and is opening his own practice at a local community hospital. The community hospital does not have on-site cardiac surgery and is located 40 minutes from the nearest high-volume hospital with on-site cardiac surgery. He wants to start performing diagnostic angiograms and elective PCIs. On the basis of current literature, what is the recommendation of performing elective PCI in a hospital without surgery backup?

(A) Elective, low-risk PCI may be performed in a hospital without on-site cardiac surgery if it is done by high-volume operators

(B) Elective low- or high-risk PCI may be performed in a hospital without on-site cardiac surgery if it is done by a high-volume operator in a high-volume center

(C) It is not recommended that elective PCI be performed at institutions that do not provide on-site cardiac surgery

(D) Elective PCI may be performed if there is a cardiac surgery program within 90 minutes of the hospital

23 The same colleague referred in Question 21 has been called by the state Medical Board for violation. He performed primary PCI at the community hospital without on-site cardiac surgery in a 64-year-old woman with acute lateral MI. She presented to the hospital with 2 hours of chest pain and was hemodynamically stable. Her catheterization showed 60% LMT, 50% mid-LAD, large CX with proximal 100% occlusion and nondominant RCA with minimal disease. During her CX PCI, she went into ventricular fibrillation and died. The patient's

family has filed a complaint to the state Medical Board and they have requested your opinion. What is the current recommendation regarding performing primary PCI without on-site cardiac surgery?

(A) Primary PCI may be performed in select cases by an experienced operator in a well-equipped lab with trained staff

(B) Primary PCI should never be performed without on-site cardiac surgery

(C) Primary PCI should be performed by a trained interventionalist on all patients with acute MI regardless of on-site cardiac surgery

24 A 46-year-old female physician presents to your office for a second opinion. She underwent a stress test for chest pain and was found to have lateral ischemia. She then underwent catheterization and was found to have diffuse proximal CX 90% stenosis. Her only risk factors are family history, early menopause, and hyperlipidemia. She is not a diabetic patient. She underwent successful PCI to CX with 3.5/33 mm bare metal stent. She then presented with in-stent restenosis and underwent β-radiation and balloon angioplasty. She has been taking clopidogrel and ASA and has been doing well until a month ago when she started experiencing exertional chest pain. Her stress test shows diffuse stenosis of her previously radiated CX lesion. She does not have CABG. What would you recommend?

(A) Balloon angioplasty and γ-radiation

(B) Drug-eluting stent (DES) without γ-radiation

(C) CABG is the only option

(D) DES with γ-radiation

25 A 68-year-old male nurse presents to your office for a fourth opinion. He underwent RCA PCI a year ago for exertional chest pain which was complicated by coronary artery dissection. He had a 3.5/18 mm paclitaxel stent placed for a mid-RCA lesion, which was postdilated with 4.5/15 mm noncompliant balloon because the reference diameter of the RCA was 4.4 mm. After the balloon dilatation, there was a long spiral dissection, which required three subsequent stents, a loss of PL branch and an increase in his troponin. Since then he has done well but has occasional chest pain with heavy exertion. His most recent stress thallium test does not show any signs of ischemia. Nevertheless, he is very upset and feels that they should never have placed a DES. In the trials of bare metal versus DESs (such as RAVEL, TAXUS, SIRIUS), what size vessels were intervened upon?

(A) 2.0 to 3.5 mm

(B) 2.5 to 4.0 mm

(C) 2.75 to 4.0 mm
(D) 2.75 to 3.75 mm

26 A 68-year-old man from Asia presents to your office to establish care. He comes with his son who is his interpreter. He has diabetes, hyperlipidemia, and HTN. He is on ASA 325 mg, clopidogrel 75 mg, Zocor 80 mg, Lopressor 75 mg b.i.d, and Vasotec 10 mg b.i.d. He underwent a catheterization last month where they found 70% proximal LMT disease with minimal disease in LAD, CX, and RCA. His EF was 65%. He underwent PCI to unprotected LMT with IVUS guidance with 5.0/12 mm bare-metal stent. He denies any chest pain or SOB and feels well. He was told by his physician that he should undergo a cardiac angiogram in 6 months. He does not want to do this since he has no symptoms and is feeling well. He seeks your opinion.

(A) In light of no symptoms and a good medical regimen, he does not need an angiogram. He can follow up in 6 months
(B) It is not reasonable to catheterize him. Obtain a stress test and if the result is positive, then catheterize him
(C) It is not reasonable to catheterize him. Obtain an echocardiogram if his EF is changed, then catheterize him
(D) It is reasonable to catheterize him in 6 months

27 The gentleman referred in Question 26 has been told by his outside physician to get a platelet aggregation study. He had this done at another hospital in your city and was told that there was <50% inhibitor of platelet aggregation. What should you do next?

(A) ASA 325 mg b.i.d.
(B) Switch to ticlopidine 250 mg b.i.d.
(C) Plavix 150 mg q.d.
(D) Nothing because this a device looking for an indication

28 A 63-year-old man presents for preoperative evaluation for back pain. His risk factors include hyperlipidemia, anemia, and HTN. He undergoes a stress test and has RCA ischemia with EF of 50%. He then undergoes catheterization, which shows a severe, diffuse RCA lesion which is amenable to PCI. This is a complicated type C lesion. He is a Jehovah's Witness and does not want any blood product. His baseline hemoglobin is 9. He had an aspirin load the day before catheterization and was given 60 u per kg of heparin and no GP IIb/IIIa inhibitor due to his anemia. His procedure activated clotting time (ACT) after heparin is 260 on a Hemochron device. On the basis of the literature, what is the optimal ACT for patients not on a GP IIb/IIIa inhibitor?

(A) Hemochron 300 to 350 seconds
(B) Hemochron 200 to 250 seconds
(C) Hemochron 250 to 300 seconds
(D) Optimal ACT studies have been done only with the HemoTec device and not with Hemochron

29 A 59-year-old CT surgeon with HTN, hyperlipidemia, and 20-year smoking history presents to the ER with chest pain for 5 hours. He is found to have nonspecific ST changes and is admitted. He is placed on enoxaparin, ASA, clopidogrel, Lipitor, and Lopressor. He no longer has chest pain. He refuses to have a stress test and just wants an angiogram. His catheterization shows severe proximal LAD stenosis. It is amenable to PCI and the decision is made to proceed. You ask for an abciximab bolus and IV and the nurse wants to know if you would like additional unfractionated heparin since the patient received his enoxaparin 7 hours ago. His ACT is 180 seconds.

(A) Yes, he needs an additional 50 u per kg of unfractionated heparin
(B) Yes, he needs to receive his enoxaparin IV now
(C) No, he is within 8 hours of his last enoxaparin dose
(D) No, he is within 12 hours of his last enoxaparin dose

30 A 49-year-old patient with diabetes and human immunodeficiency virus (HIV) is undergoing PCI to LAD for exertional chest pain. He is on ASA, Pravachol, Zetia, protease inhibitors, Lopressor, and received a 300-mg Plavix load yesterday. He had his diagnostic catheterization a week ago by a general cardiologist and presents to you now for PCI. He has a chronically occluded large CX, which is being fed by a diffusely diseased LAD. The mid-LAD lesion is tortuous and diffusely calcified and diseased. He is adamantly refusing CABG and wants you to be aggressive and fix his disease. You decide to use bivalirudin and GP IIb/IIIa infusion during PCI owing to the large myocardium at risk. You are able to cross the lesion after multiple attempts. The case is very time consuming. During the case, the nurse tells you his ACT is 450. You should:

(A) Hold bivalirudin infusion and recheck in 5 to 10 minutes
(B) Continue bivalirudin infusion but stop tirofiban infusion
(C) Stop both bivalirudin and GP IIb/IIIa infusion
(D) Continue both bivalirudin and tirofiban infusion

Answers and Explanations

1 **Answer A.** There is no data to support PCI in an asymptomatic patient with Class I angina. This patient has no evidence of ischemia in the moderate CX artery distribution and already had an exercise stress test, which showed no evidence of ischemia. Although adding Plavix therapy might seem reasonable, there is no evidence to support its routine use in asymptomatic patients. This is Class III indication for PCI.

2 **Answer C.** There is no data on IVUS and clinical event rates with normal FFR. There is evidence of low clinical event rates with normal FFR at 2 years. Therefore, PCI is not needed (Class III indication).

3 **Answer B.** This patient is not in cardiogenic shock. He does have heart failure but he does not have hemodynamic compromise. Therefore, elective PCI should not be performed in a noninfarct-related artery at the time of primary PCI of the infarct-related artery in patients without hemodynamic compromise. This is Class III indication for PCI in the 2005 American College of Cardiology (ACC)/American Heart Association (AHA) guidelines.

4 **Answer A.** According to the latest National Heart, Lung, and Blood Institute (NHLBI) dynamic (1997 to 1998) and ACC-National Cardiovascular Data Registry (NCDR) registries (1998 to 2000), the overall emergency CABG rate appears to be 1.9%, Q-wave mortality is 0.4% to 0.8% and clinical success was achieved in 91% to 97% of cases.

5 **Answer C.** This is a Class I indication for ASA and clopidogrel in the new ACC/AHA guidelines. Ideally, patients with DES without bleeding risk should be on 12 months of clopidogrel therapy; however, the minimal standard is 3 months with sirolimus stents and 6 months with paclitaxel stents. ASA 325 mg for 1 month, then reduction to 81 mg indefinitely is also a Class I indication.

6 **Answer B.** At the time of this writing (2006), the optimum loading dose and timing of clopidogrel appears to be 300 mg loading 6 hours before PCI. Currently there is little evidence to support clopidogrel 600 mg load at the time of PCI with GP IIb/IIIa inhibitor or bivalirudin. This patient is undergoing PCI for NSTEMI immediately without clopidogrel loading in the ER. Therefore, heparin and GP IIb/IIIa inhibitor administration is best. Currently, bivalirudin is not approved for patients with unstable angina (UA)/NSTEMI. This is a Class I recommendation.

7 **Answer D.** A serotonin assay for heparin-induced antibodies is more sensitive. The patient has a history of heparin-induced thrombocytopenia (HIT). Therefore, either bivalirudin or argatroban should be used in place of heparin. Although the incidence of LMWHs causing immune sensitization resulting in HIT is low, they can still develop anti-PF4 antibodies; therefore, LMWH should not be used. This is a Class I indication.

8 **Answer D.** Final patency after PCI is greater for distal SVG lesion than for ostial or mid-SVG lesions. Stenosis location appears to be a better determinant of final patency than graft age or the type of interventional device used.

9 **Answer A.** Balloon dilatation across suture lines has been accomplished safely within days of surgery. Recurrent ischemia that occurs early postoperatively reflects graft failure and may occur in both saphenous vein and arterial graft conduits. Urgent coronary angiography is indicated to define the anatomic cause of ischemia and to determine the best course of therapy. Emergency PCI of a focal graft stenosis may successfully relieve ischemia. This is a Level I indication.

10 **Answer D.** Fibrinolytic therapy is recommended if there is a >90-minute delay to PCI, 3 hours before onset of STEMI symptoms, and no contraindication to fibrinolytic therapy. IABP is recommended when shock is not quickly reversed with pharmacologic therapy, as a stabilizing measure for patients who are candidates for further invasive care.

11 **Answer C.** Early mechanical revascularization with PCI/CABG is a Class I recommendation for candidates younger than 75 years with ST elevation who develop shock <36 hours from STEMI and in whom revascularization can be performed within 18 hours of shock. In the SHOCK trial, the average patient underwent 2.3-vessel revascularization. A more thorough revascularization should be attempted in a patient who has shock. Therefore, in light of chronic total occlusion of RCA, CABG would provide more complete revascularization.

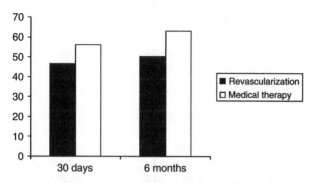

Mortality Rate (%) in the SHOCK trial at 30 days (46.7% vs. 56.0%) and at 6 months (50.3% vs. 63.1%).

12 Answer B. This is a Class III indication for PCI. There is no data at this time that support routine use of PCI days after failed fibrinolysis in patients who are hemodynamically and electrically stable and who do not have ischemia. The DANAMI trial tested PCI in patients who have spontaneous or inducible angina after STEMI. The patient does not fit the criteria.

13 Answer C. The results of a pooled analysis of CADILLAC, ADMIRAL, RAPPORT, ISAR-2, and ACE suggest that early administration of abciximab is associated with the most favorable clinical outcome. Therefore, in patients with STEMI undergoing PCI, it is reasonable to administer abciximab as early as possible and it is Level IIa recommendation.

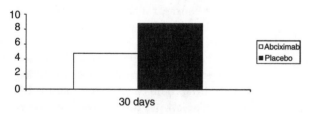

Death/MI/TVR rate at 30 days' abciximab (4.8%) versus placebo (8.8%) in acute MI patients.

14 Answer B. Patients with primary PCI have lower mortality, fewer reinfarction, and more bleeding. Moreover, they have fewer hemorrhagic strokes.

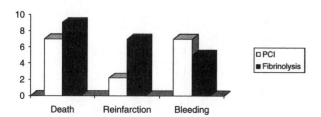

15 Answer C. Patients who underwent primary PCI with stent have similar death and reinfarction rates compared with patients who underwent primary balloon angioplasty.

16 Answer D. In all, patients who have signs or symptoms suggestive of MI during or after PCI and those with complicated procedures should have biomarkers measured after the procedure. This is a Class I indication. Routine measurement is a Class IIa indication.

17 Answer C. The patient had a major bleeding episode in the hospital. Major bleeding is defined as intracranial, intraocular, or retroperitoneal hemorrhage or any hemorrhage requiring a transfusion or surgical intervention or which results in a hematocrit decrease of >15% or hemoglobin decrease of >5 g per dL. Abciximab is not associated with an increased risk of major bleeding in women but does increase minor bleeding.

18 Answer C.

Anatomic Criteria for High-Risk Lesion

Diffuse disease—length >2 cm
Excessive tortuosity of proximal segment
Extremely angulated segments, >90 degree
Total occlusion for >3 months and/or bridging collateral
Inability to protect major side branches
Degenerated vein grafts with friable lesions

---

19 Answer C. ERACI, ARTS, SoS, and BARI have all addressed the question of PCI versus CABG. This patient does not have diabetes and has three-vessel disease without proximal LAD involvement. Therefore, totality of data suggests PCI or CABG would offer similar mortality and MI rate. PCI has a higher revascularization rate. The data on DES versus CABG for multivessel disease is pending.

20 Answer D. The MASS study tested medicine, PCI, or CABG in patients with isolated LAD disease. They found similar mortality rates in all groups. Proximal LAD lesions appear to benefit from revascularization; however, mid-LAD lesions such as in this patient generally have a good prognosis. Other trials, including ACME and RITA-2 have tested medical therapy versus PCI. They also found no difference in mortality.

21 Answer C. This scenario was tested in the ACIP study. Patients who underwent revascularization had lower death or MI rates. ACIP suggests that outcomes of revascularization with CABG surgery or PCI are very favorable compared with medical therapy in patients with asymptomatic ischemia with or without mild angina.

22 Answer C. This is a Class III indication. It is not recommended that elective PCI be performed by either low- or high-volume operators at low- or high-volume centers without on-site cardiac surgery.

23 Answer A. The guideline recommends that primary PCI for patients with STEMI might be considered in hospitals without on-site cardiac surgery provided it is done by high-volume operators, with an experienced catheterization team, in a well-equipped catheterization laboratory, and provided there is a proven plan for rapid transport to a cardiac surgery operating room in a nearby hospital with hemodynamic support capability for transfer. Also, they recommend avoiding intervention in STEMI hemodynamically stable patients with significant unprotected left main stenosis upstream from an acute occlusion in the left coronary system, extremely long or angulated infarct-related lesions with TIMI 3 flow, infarct-related lesions with TIMI 3 flow in stable patients with three-vessel disease, and infarct-related lesions of small or secondary vessels or hemodynamically significant lesions in sites other than the infarct artery.

24 Answer B. This is a Class IIa indication for DES stent. It is reasonable to perform repeat PCI for in-stent restenosis with a DES or a new DES for patients who develop in-stent restenosis if anatomic factors are appropriate.

25 Answer D. In RAVEL, TAXUS, and SIRIUS, patients with 2.75 to 3.75 mm reference diameter were intervened upon. A DES may be considered for use in anatomic settings in which the usefulness, effectiveness, and safety have not been fully documented in published trials. The use of DES post dilated with a much larger sized balloon for a large vessel PCI has not been studied. It is a Class IIb indication.

26 Answer D. It is reasonable that a patient undergoing PCI to unprotected left main be followed with coronary angiography between 2 and 6 months after PCI since they have higher rates of sudden cardiac death. This is a Class IIa indication. Unfortunately, the frequency and best method of follow-up is unknown. However, the ACC/AHA committee has recommended routine surveillance angiography at 2 to 3 months for all patients after unprotected left main PCI.

27 Answer C. In patients in whom stent thrombosis may be catastrophic or lethal, such as those with unprotected left main stent, bifurcating left main, or last patent coronary vessel stent, platelet aggregation studies may be considered and the dose of clopidogrel increased to 150 mg per day if <50% inhibition of platelet aggregation is demonstrated.

28 Answer A. In patients who do not receive a GP IIb/IIIa inhibitor, the recommendation based on the literature is ACT of 250 to 300 with the HemoTec device and 300 to 350 with the Hemochron device. With a GP IIb/IIIa inhibitor, it should be ACT in the 200 seconds with either the HemoTec or Hemochron device. The currently recommended target ACT for eptifibatide and tirofiban is <300 seconds during PCI.

29 Answer C. In patients who received the last subcutaneously administered dose of enoxaparin within 8 hours, no additional anticoagulant therapy is needed before PCI is performed. In patients who received the last subcutaneously administered dose of enoxaparin 8 to 12 hours before PCI an additional 0.3 mg per kg dose of enoxaparin should be administered intravenously before PCI.

30 Answer D. Ecarin clotting time provides a more accurate assessment of bivalirudin-mediated anticoagulation and bivalirudin concentration during PCI than the ACT. The lack of strong correlation between ACT and bivalirudin levels may be an explanation why previous studies have failed to show a relation between bleeding complications and the relatively high ACT values observed in the setting of direct thrombin inhibitors.

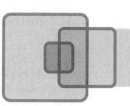

37

ST-Elevation Myocardial Infarction: American College of Cardiology/American Heart Association Guidelines

Ann O'Connor and David P. Faxon

Questions

1 A 57-year-old man with hypertension, who is a current tobacco user, presented to the emergency department with substernal chest pain. The chest pain started 90 minutes ago and is associated with nausea and diaphoresis. A prior electrocardiogram (EKG) from 1 year ago is shown below and his current EKG on presentation is shown in the figure in the next column. On physical examination his blood pressure (BP) is 146/84, with a pulse of 84 bpm. His lungs are clear to auscultation. His neck veins are flat. He has a regular rate and rhythm with no murmurs, rubs, or gallops. He has 2+ pulses in his distal extremities. He is placed on telemetry and is given aspirin 325 mg PO, nitroglycerin 0.4 mg SL, metoprolol 5 mg IV Q5$_{min}$ times three, and started

on an IV unfractionated heparin (UFH) drip. He has some relief in his chest pain. The most appropriate next step in this patient's management should include:

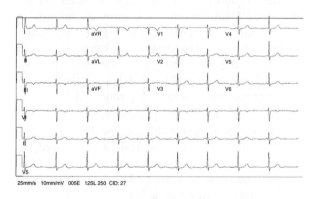

(A) Initiation of eptifibatide: 180 μg/kg IV bolus, followed by an infusion at 2 μg/kg/min IV
(B) Admission to the cardiac care unit for further monitoring while awaiting results of serial cardiac biomarkers
(C) Order a single photon emission computerized tomography (SPECT) radionuclide imaging stress test to further evaluate the etiology of the patient's chest pain
(D) Implement a strategy for early reperfusion

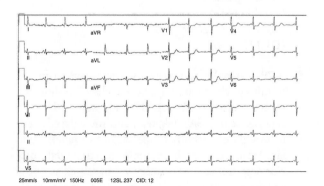

2 A 74-year-old woman presented with a posterolateral ST-elevation myocardial infarction (STEMI). She underwent emergent coronary angiography and primary percutaneous coronary intervention (PCI) of a totally occluded proximal left circumflex artery with percutaneous transluminal coronary angioplasty (PTCA) and stenting of the lesion with a sirolimus-eluting stent. At the conclusion of the case, the patient was administered an oral 300 mg loading dose of clopidogrel. On the basis of the current ACC/AHA guidelines, the most appropriate antiplatelet regimen at discharge for this patient is:

(A) Aspirin 162 mg PO daily for an indefinite period of time and clopidogrel 75 mg PO daily for at least 3 months
(B) Aspirin 162 mg PO daily for at least 12 months and clopidogrel 75 mg PO daily for at least 3 months
(C) Aspirin 325 mg PO daily for an indefinite period and clopidogrel 75 mg PO daily for at least 1 month
(D) Aspirin 162 mg PO daily for at least 12 months and clopidogrel 75 mg PO daily for at least 12 months

3 A 59-year-old woman with a history of hypertension and hypercholesterolemia presented with chest pain. The EKG demonstrated an inferolateral STEMI. She underwent early successful reperfusion with the administration of fibrinolytic agents. Her medications at the time of admission included hydrochlorothiazide, atenolol, simvastatin, and hormone replacement therapy (HRT) (estrogen/medroxyprogesterone combination pill). She has been taking HRT for 8 months for perimenopausal symptoms. In regard to her HRT, the most appropriate recommendation at this time is to:

(A) Continue the HRT indefinitely
(B) Discontinue the HRT indefinitely
(C) Continue the HRT while she is hospitalized, but discontinue it at discharge
(D) Discontinue the HRT while she is hospitalized, but continue it at discharge

4 A 49-year-old man with hypertension began experiencing chest "tightness" and shortness of breath while at work as a construction contractor. The patient's father died of a "massive heart attack" at age 52. His coworkers called 911 and the Emergency Medical Services (EMS) arrived on the scene within 10 minutes. Upon arrival, EMS gave the patient a chewable aspirin (325 mg), nitroglycerin SL (0.4 mg), and IV morphine (2 mg). He was started on oxygen 2 L through nasal cannula. Which of these

prehospital therapies has been shown to have the most benefit on mortality?

(A) Chewable aspirin (325 mg)
(B) Nitroglycerin SL (0.4 mg)
(C) IV morphine (2 mg)
(D) Oxygen 2 L through nasal cannula

5 EMS was called to the home of a 68-year-old woman with a history of diabetes and hypertension. Her initial complaint was chest discomfort that started 2 hours ago. On arrival, the paramedics find the patient to be minimally responsive with the following vital signs: Pulse of 104 bpm, respiration 24 to 28 breaths/minute, BP 95/60, oxygenation 91% on room air. She has bibasilar crackles on examination. The nearest hospital is 5 minutes away, but it does not have primary PCI capabilities. The nearest tertiary care center with primary PCI capabilities is 15 to 20 minutes away. The EMS team should ideally:

(A) Transfer the patient to the nearest hospital regardless of the facilities and capabilities of primary PCI
(B) Transfer the patient to the nearest hospital that utilizes fibrinolytic agents as the sole modality for treatment of STEMI
(C) Transfer the patient to the nearest hospital with primary PCI and coronary artery bypass grafting (CABG) capabilities
(D) Administer prehospital fibrinolytic therapy

6 A 69-year-old man is admitted to the emergency room with symptoms suggestive of an MI. The first cardiac biomarker that will be elevated in an acute MI is:

(A) Troponin I
(B) Troponin T
(C) Creatine kinase-MB
(D) Myoglobin

7 The most useful cardiac marker in the assessment of reinfarction after STEMI is:

(A) Troponin I
(B) Troponin T
(C) Creatine kinase–MB
(D) Myoglobin

8 A 79-year-old man presents to the hospital with intermittent chest pain for 6 hours. His EKG shows an evolving anterior STEMI. He is administered acetylsalicylic acid (ASA), heparin, and nitroglycerin and is brought emergently to the cardiac catheterization lab. He is found to have a 99% proximal left anterior descending (LAD) artery lesion as well as a 60% proximal right coronary artery (RCA) lesion and a

50% mid left circumflex artery lesion. After primary PCI of the proximal LAD lesion, he is clinically stable with no further chest pain. In regard to the other lesions, what therapy should be recommended at the time of the primary PCI?

(A) PCI of the proximal RCA lesion
(B) PCI of the proximal RCA lesion and the mid left circumflex lesions
(C) Fractional flow reserve evaluation of the RCA and LCx lesions
(D) No further assessment or intervention at this time

9 A 52-year-old woman with diabetes and hypertension presents to a rural hospital without primary PCI capabilities within 90 minutes of the onset of sudden crushing chest tightness. Her EKG reveals an anterolateral STEMI. She has no signs or symptoms of heart failure. Transfer to another facility for primary PCI is expected to take 90 minutes and transfer-to-balloon time is anticipated to be 120 minutes. In regard to the reperfusion therapy of the patient, the most appropriate plan of action is:

(A) Prompt administration of half-dose fibrinolytic agents with transfer for facilitated PCI
(B) Prompt administration of full-dose fibrinolytic agents
(C) Prompt transfer for primary PCI
(D) None of the above

10 A 68-year-old woman presented to the emergency department within 2 hours of chest discomfort described as an 8/10 "chest tightness." The EKG demonstrated a lateral STEMI with 4 to 5 mm ST elevation in V5, V6, I, and aVL. The patient received prompt reperfusion therapy with reteplase (in addition to ASA, heparin, metoprolol, and nitroglycerin) and was admitted to the coronary intensive care unit. Within 90 minutes of fibrinolytic administration, she has had some relief in her symptoms now describing the "chest tightness" as 3/10. Her EKG showed partial resolution of the ST elevations (now 3 mm). Her telemetry monitor showed several runs of nonsustained ventricular tachycardia (VT). What is the most appropriate management for this patient at this point?

(A) Continued monitoring in the coronary intensive care unit
(B) Transfer to a tertiary care center for rescue PCI
(C) Readministration of full-dose reteplase
(D) Readministration of half-dose reteplase

11 After primary PCI, which of the following findings is associated with the worst mortality?

(A) Thrombolysis in myocardial infarction (TIMI) 2 flow grade
(B) Transient no-reflow
(C) Persistent ST-segment elevation
(D) TIMI 2 myocardial perfusion grade

12 Immediate β-blockers should *not* be used in which of the following situations?

(A) Non–ST-segment elevation MIs
(B) Heart rate (HR) <70 bpm
(C) Systolic blood pressure (SBP) <100 mm Hg
(D) Patients undergoing primary PCI

13 Which of the following time delays in primary PCI is associated with the highest mortality?

(A) Door-to-balloon time
(B) Door-to-balloon time minus door-to-needle time
(C) Symptoms-to-balloon time
(D) Symptoms-to-door times

14 Goals for reperfusion therapy for STEMI are:

(A) Door-to-needle time <30 minutes and door-to-balloon time <120 minutes
(B) Door-to-needle time <60 minutes and door-to-balloon time <90 minutes
(C) Door-to-needle time <30 minutes and door-to-balloon time <90 minutes
(D) Door-to-needle time <60 minutes and door-to-balloon time <120 minutes

15 A 72-year-old man presents to a community hospital without cardiac catheterization facilities with a 6-hour history of severe substernal chest pain and shortness of breath. The initial EKG shows 3-mm ST elevations in the anterolateral leads (V2 to V6). On physical examination, his BP is 80/50 with an HR of 100 bpm and a pulse oximetery of 91% on room air. He has rales one third up the lung fields. The patient is given oxygen through nasal cannula, ASA, heparin, and morphine and is started on a dobutamine infusion with an increase in his BP to 85/55. The time to PCI in the nearest hospital is anticipated to be 90 minutes. The door-to-needle time for administration of fibrinolytics is anticipated to be 20 minutes. What strategy for reperfusion should be pursued?

(A) Place a pulmonary artery (PA) catheter and intra-aortic balloon pump (IABP) and give tenecteplase (TNK)
(B) Place PA catheter and IABP and transfer to primary PCI center
(C) Give TNK and transfer to primary PCI center
(D) Give TNK and abciximab and manage at the community hospital

16 A 67-year-old woman presents with confusion and shortness of breath that started 8 hours ago. Her EKG shows 3-mm ST elevation and Q waves in II, III, aVF, and V4 to V6. On physical examination, she has no focal neurologic signs. Her BP is 120/80 and pulse 90 bpm. She has minimal crackles at the base of the lung fields. She is given ASA, IV heparin, SL nitroglycerin, and IV reteplase. Within 30 minutes, the ST elevations have decreased. At 60 minutes, she becomes unresponsive. Her BP is 130/90 and pulse 100 bpm. What should you do now?

(A) Obtain transesophageal echocardiogram (TEE)
(B) Obtain head CT
(C) Take the patient to the catheterization laboratory emergently
(D) Stop heparin and obtain head CT

17 A 67-year-old man is admitted with 6 hours of chest pain similar to his previous MI pain. An EKG showed left bundle branch block (LBBB). There is no old EKG for comparison. Initial BP was 110/80 with an HR of 110 bpm and pulse oximetery of 87% on room air. He has rales over the lower half of the lung fields and the cardiovascular (CV) examination showed a II/IV holosystolic murmur at the LSB with an S3 gallop. Troponin T was elevated at 0.6 ng/dL. Transthoracic echocardiogram showed a reduced ejection fraction (EF) of 25% with anterior akinesis with thinning of the anterior wall and severe lateral hypokinesis with moderate to severe mitral regurgitation. He is taken to the catheterization laboratory. Coronary angiograms are shown. Following the angiogram the patient's BP falls to 70/50 and he becomes acutely short of breath. He is intubated, an IABP is placed, and dobutamine is started. There is some improvement in his BP (100/70) and oxygenation. What would you do now?

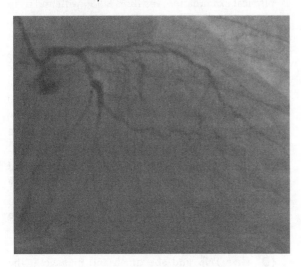

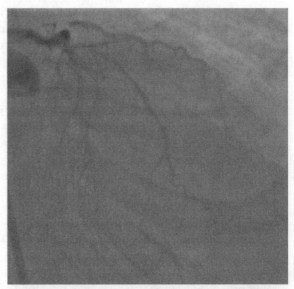

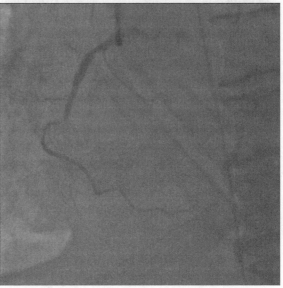

(A) Primary PCI of LAD artery
(B) Primary PCI of left circumflex artery
(C) PCI of all lesions
(D) Stabilization and urgent CABG

18 Ischemia/reperfusion injury is associated with which of the following?

(A) Decreased intracellular calcium
(B) Increased nitric oxide (NO)
(C) Opening of the ATP-dependent sodium-potassium channels
(D) Microvascular plugging

19 Which of the following interventions to reduce reperfusion injury have been shown to reduce infarct size in humans?

(A) Superoxide dismutase
(B) Glucose–insulin–potassium (GIK) infusion
(C) Pexelixumab (complement inhibitor)
(D) Ischemic preconditioning

20 Which of the following patients is most likely to have acute shortness of breath with no chest pain as their presenting symptoms of a STEMI?

(A) A 75-year-old white woman
(B) A 49-year-old white man
(C) A 49-year-old white woman
(D) A 75-year-old African American man

21 A 56-year-old man with a history of hyperlipidemia and cigarette smoking presents with severe substernal chest pain for the last 4 hours. EKG shows 3-mm ST-segment elevations in V1 to V4. BP is 130/70 and pulse is 82 bpm. His physical examination is otherwise unremarkable. He is given ASA, IV heparin, SL nitroglycerin, and IV morphine. The patient is taken to the catheterization laboratory for primary PCI. Which of the following additional medications is *not* indicated?

(A) IV β-blocker
(B) IV abciximab
(C) IV angiotensin-converting enzyme (ACE) inhibitor
(D) PO clopidogrel

22 A 49-year-old man with hypertension presents to the emergency department with 16 hours of severe substernal chest pain. The initial EKG shows Q waves and 1 mm ST-segment elevation in leads V1 to V4. He continues to have 3/10 chest discomfort despite nitroglycerine (NTG) and morphine. On physical examination, his BP is 110/60 with a pulse of 95 bpm. An S3 is present with rales half way up both lung fields. The monitor shows two 10-beat runs of nonsustained VT at 160 beats/minute. The patient is started on lidocaine. What would be the next step in the management of this patient?

(A) Immediate catheterization and possible PCI
(B) IV β-blocker and IV lasix with medical management
(C) IABP insertion with medical management
(D) PA catheter insertion and IV neseritide with medical management

23 A 67-year-old woman presents to the emergency department with 4 hours of substernal chest pain and shortness of breath. EKG shows 4-mm ST-segment elevation in II, III, and aVF. Physical examination shows a BP of 140/70 with a pulse of 80 bpm. An S4 is audible. The patient is given ASA, heparin, SL NTG, clopidogrel, and is taken to the catheterization laboratory. She is found to have a 99% lesion of the proximal RCA with large clot burden and TIMI 2 flow. The LAD has a 50% midlesion, and first obtuse marginal branch has an ostial 70% lesion. The patient had ventricular ectopy during the contrast injections. The patient is started on abciximab. What additional therapy is indicated?

(A) IV β-blocker
(B) IV lidocaine
(C) IC tissue plasminogen activator t-PA
(D) IC adenosine

24 A 64-year-old woman is seen in the emergency department with severe shortness of breath for the last hour. Her EKG shows ST-segment elevations with hyperacute T waves in leads II, III, and aVF. On physical examination, her BP is 140/70 with an HR of 85 bpm. The remainder of the physical examination is unremarkable. What is the best reperfusion strategy in this patient?

(A) Primary PCI
(B) Fibrinolytic therapy and facilitated PCI
(C) Fibrinolytic therapy
(D) Fibrinolytic therapy or primary PCI

25 A 65-year-old man presented to the emergency department with a 2-hour history of "indigestion" and shortness of breath. His EKG showed 2-mm ST-segment elevation in leads II, III, and aVF. He received prompt reperfusion therapy with fibrinolytic agents in addition to ASA, heparin, and β-blockers. Ninety minutes after the initiation of fibrinolytic agents, his chest pain has resolved and he has minimal residual ST-segment elevation on the repeat EKG. His vital signs have remained stable: BP 126/64 and pulse of 59 bpm. The following rhythm is observed on the telemetry monitor. What medical treatment should be added at this point?

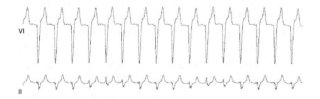

(A) IV amiodarone
(B) IV lidocaine

(C) IV procainamide

(D) Continue to observe

26 Primary stenting compared with primary angioplasty has been shown to:

(A) Reduce restenosis and target vessel revascularization

(B) Reduce restenosis and reinfarction

(C) Reduce restenosis and mortality

(D) Reduce mortality and congestive heart failure (CHF)

27 A 59-year-old woman with hypertension and diabetes presented with fatigue and a 4-hour history of chest discomfort. Her EKG demonstrated ST-segment elevations in V3 to V6. She was started on ASA, heparin, NTG, and metoprolol. Primary PCI was chosen as the strategy for reperfusion. En route to the catheterization laboratory, she became unresponsive. The monitor showed ventricular fibrillation (VF). She was successfully defibrillated with 150 J of biphasic energy. At catheterization, she had a total occlusion of the proximal to mid-LAD. The lesion was stented with good angiographic results. A transthoracic echo done 3 days after presentation showed an EF of 28% with hypokinesis of the anterior and lateral walls and apical akinesis. She has had no evidence of recurrent ischemia and no further ventricular arrhythmias. Her medical regimen now includes ASA, clopidogrel, metoprolol, lisinopril, and atorvastatin. What additional step should be taken in regard to the patient's episode of VF?

(A) Implantable cardioverter defibrillator (ICD) placement before discharge

(B) Electrophysiologic (EP) study before discharge

(C) ICD placement 1 month post discharge

(D) Reassessment of LV function at least 1 month post-STEMI

28 A 47-year-old man with hyperlipidemia, current tobacco use, and a significant family history of premature coronary artery disease presented to a community hospital with primary PCI capabilities with 5 hours of substernal chest pressure. The EKG showed 2- to 3-mm ST-segment elevations in V5, V6, aVL, and I. He received prompt therapy with fibrinolytic agents. Within 45 minutes, he had total resolution of his pain and his ST segments normalized. Three days after presentation, he had no recurrent chest discomfort. He had no events on the telemetry monitor and no signs of heart failure. A transthoracic echocardiogram was performed that showed a mild to moderately reduced EF of 43% with posterior wall and lateral hypokinesis and mild mitral

regurgitation. His post-STEMI medications include ASA, clopidogrel, metoprolol, and simvastatin. What should be done next?

(A) Perform diagnostic angiography

(B) Reassess EF at 1 month post-STEMI

(C) Perform functional evaluation

(D) Continue medical management

29 A 72-year-old woman with hypertension (HTN) presented to the emergency department of a community hospital (with no primary PCI capabilities) with sudden onset of chest pain and shortness of breath that began 90 minutes ago. Her EKG demonstrated a lateral ST-segment MI. On further review of her past medical history, it is found that she had pulmonary embolus 5 years earlier and remembers being treated with "clot busters." On physical examination, her BP is 147/86 with a pulse of 86 bpm. The remainder of the examination is unremarkable. She has no obvious contraindications to fibrinolytic agents. The estimated door-to-balloon time with transfer to a primary PCI center is 120 minutes. Fibrinolytic agents could be administered in the next 10 to 15 minutes. Which of the following is the most appropriate reperfusion strategy at this point?

(A) Full-dose streptokinase

(B) Transfer for primary PCI

(C) Full-dose tenecteplase (TNK)-tPA

(D) Half-dose tenecteplase (TNK)-tPA and transfer for facilitated PCI

30 In patients <75 years old receiving fibrin-specific fibrinolytic agents as the main strategy for reperfusion, which of the following is the most efficacious anticoagulation regimen?

(A) UFH IV 80 units/kg bolus followed by a continuous infusion at 18 units/kg/hour

(B) UFH SC 7,500 units b.i.d.

(C) Enoxaparin 1 mg/kg SC b.i.d.

(D) Enoxaparin 0.5 mg/kg SC b.i.d.

31 In patients undergoing elective, nonurgent coronary artery bypass surgery following a STEMI, which of the following is the most appropriate management of the antiplatelet regimen?

(A) Hold both aspirin and clopidogrel for 5 to 7 days before surgery

(B) Continue both aspirin and clopidogrel preoperatively

(C) Hold clopidogrel for 5 to 7 days before surgery, but continue aspirin preoperatively

(D) Hold aspirin for 5 to 7 days before surgery, but continue clopidogrel preoperatively

32 A 63-year-old man with hypertension and chronic persistent atrial fibrillation on chronic anticoagulation presented with chest pain. The EKG revealed a posterolateral STEMI and he underwent successful stenting of the proximal left circumflex artery with a paclitaxel-coated stent. His post-MI course has been uncomplicated. His discharge antithrombotic/antiplatelet regimen should include:

(A) Aspirin 81 mg q.d., clopidogrel 75 mg q.d., and warfarin (goal: INR 2 to 3)

(B) Clopidogrel 75 mg q.d. and warfarin (goal INR 2.5 to 3.5)

(C) Aspirin 325 mg q.d. and clopidogrel 75 mg q.d.

(D) Aspirin 325 mg q.d. and warfarin (goal INR 2 to 3)

Answers and Explanations

1 Answer D. The EKG demonstrates a true posterior MI with tall R waves and ST depressions in the right precordial leads (V1 to V2). In addition to standard medical treatment for acute STEMI (ASA, β-blocker, etc.), a strategy for early reperfusion should be implemented in a timely fashion. The pertinent American College Of Cardiology/American Heart Association (ACC/AHA) guidelines (*ACC/AHA 2004 guideline update.* 2004) are:

- Class I: All STEMI patients should undergo rapid evaluation for reperfusion therapy and have a reperfusion strategy implemented promptly after contact with the medical system (Level of Evidence B).
- Class I: If immediately available, primary PCI should be performed in patients with STEMI (including true posterior MI) or MI with new or presumably new LBBB who can undergo PCI of the infarct artery within 12 hours of symptom onset (Level of Evidence A).
- Class IIa: In the absence of contraindications, it is reasonable to administer fibrinolytic therapy to STEMI patients with symptom onset within the prior 12 hours and 12-lead EKG findings consistent with a true posterior MI (Level of Evidence: C).

2 Answer A. Aspirin should be given as soon as possible in patients with suspected STEMI regardless of reperfusion strategy and should be continued indefinitely for secondary prevention. A true aspirin allergy is the only contraindication to this recommendation. There is a dose-dependent increase in bleeding complications in patients on aspirin; therefore, low dose aspirin (75 to 162 mg) is preferred for long-term therapy. In regard to the combination antiplatelet regimen with clopidogrel 75 mg daily, the current recommendations after stent implantation are as follows: At least 1 month for bare-metal stents, at least 3 months for sirolimus-coated stents, and at least 6 months for pacilitaxel-coated stents. The pertinent ACC/AHA guidelines are:

- Class I: Aspirin 162 to 325 mg should be given on day 1 of STEMI and in the absence of contraindications should be continued on a daily basis thereafter at a daily dose of 75 to 162 mg. (Level of Evidence: A).
- Class I: For patients who have undergone diagnostic cardiac catheterization and for whom PCI

is planned, clopidogrel should be started and continued for at least 1 month after bare-metal stent implantation and for several months after drug-eluting stent implantation (3 months for sirolimus, 6 months for paclitaxel) and for up to 12 months in patients who are not at high risk for bleeding (Level of Evidence: B).

3 Answer B. Although estrogens have been shown to improve the lipid profile and observational studies demonstrated a potential CV benefit with HRT, data from the HERS (*JAMA.* 1998;280:605–613) and WHI (*JAMA.* 2002;288:321–333) studies have shown that HRT is associated with increased primary and secondary coronary events. HRT should not be initiated for secondary prevention. If a patient is already taking HRT at the time of STEMI, the HRT should be discontinued in nearly all cases. In a situation where the patient has a compelling indication for HRT and has been on therapy for over a year, continuation of HRT can be considered with the recognition of greater risk of CV events. In hospitalized patients, HRT should not be administered as it is associated with increased thromboembolic events. The pertinent ACC/AHA guidelines are:

- Class III: Hormone therapy with estrogen plus progestin should not be given *de novo* to postmenopausal women after STEMI for secondary prevention of coronary events. (Level of Evidence: A)
- Class III: Postmenopausal women who are already taking estrogen plus progestin at the time of a STEMI should not continue hormone therapy. However, women who are beyond 1 to 2 years after initiation of hormone therapy who wish to continue such therapy for another compelling indication should weigh the risks and benefits, recognizing a greater risk of CV events. Hormone therapy should not be continued while patients are on bed rest in the hospital (Level of Evidence: B).

4 Answer A. The use of prehospital aspirin is strongly encouraged in patients suspected of having a STEMI as its potential benefits outweigh the risks (*Arch Intern Med.* 1996;156:1506–1510). Although empiric treatment of patients with suspected STEMI with morphine, oxygen, nitroglycerin, and aspirin (MONA) is part of the recommended prehospital protocol, aspirin is the only therapy shown to decrease mortality. The sooner aspirin is administered, the greater impact on outcomes. The pertinent ACC/AHA guidelines are:

■ Class I: Prehospital EMS providers should administer 162 to 325 mg of aspirin (chewed) to patients with chest pain suspected of having STEMI unless contraindicated or already taken by the patient. Although some trials have used enteric-coated aspirin for initial dosing, more rapid buccal absorption occurs with non–enteric-coated formulations (Level of Evidence: C).

5 Answer C. This patient is most likely having a STEMI complicated by cardiogenic shock. In patients presenting with shock, rapid direct revascularization with PCI or CABG is preferred over fibrinolytic agents (in particular in patients <75 years of age based on data from the SHOCK trial) (*JAMA.* 2001;285:190–192). Although prehospital fibrinolytic therapy has been shown to be beneficial in some populations, this benefit has not been established in patients presenting with cardiogenic shock. The pertinent ACC/AHA guidelines are:

■ Class I: Patients with STEMI who have cardiogenic shock and are <75 years of age should be brought immediately or secondarily transferred to facilities capable of cardiac catheterization and rapid revascularization (PCI or CABG) if it can be performed within 18 hours of onset of shock (Level of Evidence: A).

6 Answer D. Myoglobin is found in cardiac and skeletal muscles. The initial elevation of myoglobin occurs at 1 to 4 hours and peaks at 6 to 7 hours. Myoglobin levels return to normal at 24 hours. Because myoglobin is not cardiac specific, it is infrequently used in clinical practice. Cardiac troponin levels are the preferred biomarker for the diagnosis of MI as these markers are very sensitive and are not normally detected in the blood of healthy individuals. The troponin I and troponin T levels are initially elevated at 3 to 12 hours. With no reperfusion therapy, the troponin I values peak at 24 hours, and the troponin T values peak at 12 to 48 hours. The troponin I level returns to normal at 5 to 10 days and the troponin T level returns to normal at 5 to 14 days. The initiation of reperfusion therapy should not be delayed while awaiting results of cardiac biomarkers in patients with STEMI.

7 Answer C. Troponin I and troponin T are continuously released from degenerating myocytes and levels can remain elevated for 7 to 14 days. Because CK-MB levels peak at 24 hours and return to normal range with 18 to 72 hours, CK-MB is the preferred biomarker to assess reinfarction. After reperfusion, a progressive fall in CK-MB levels is expected and a reelevation is highly suggestive of a reinfarction.

8 Answer D. The patient does not have any further ischemic symptoms and is hemodynamically stable. PCI of a noninfarct artery at the time of primary PCI in hemodynamically stable patients is a class III indication. The pertinent ACC/AHA guidelines are:

■ Class III: PCI should not be performed in a noninfarct artery at the time of primary PCI in patients without hemodynamic compromise (Level of Evidence: C).

9 Answer B. This patient is presenting within 3 hours of onset of symptoms. The patient does not have any high-risk features such as shock, heart failure, or rhythm instability. In this time frame (<3 hours from the onset of symptoms), the benefits of primary PCI versus fibrinolytic agents are similar in otherwise stable patients. Given that the expected door-to-balloon time with transfer exceeds the door-to-needle by >1 hour, the most appropriate therapy in this situation is to administer full-dose fibrinolytic agents. Facilitated PCI remains controversial. The pertinent ACC/AHA guidelines are:

■ Class I: Specific considerations: If symptom duration is within 3 hours and the expected door-to-balloon time minus the expected door-to-needle time is:

  ■ within 1 hour, primary PCI is generally preferred. (Level of Evidence: B)
  ■ >1 hour, fibrinolytic therapy (fibrin-specific agents) is generally preferred. (Level of Evidence: B)

Nallamothu, et al. in a recent analysis (*Am J Cardiol.* 2003;92:824–826) illustrated that the mortality benefit associated with primary PCI in STEMI is lost if door-to-balloon time is delayed by >1 hour as compared with fibrinolytic therapy door-to-needle time (see following figure).

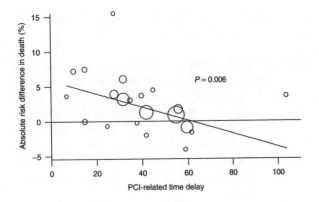

10   Answer B.   Rescue PCI is defined as PCI within 12 hours of failed fibrinolysis for patients with continuing or recurrent myocardial ischemia. Persistence of unrelenting ischemic chest pain, absence of resolution of the qualifying ST-segment elevation (loosely defined as >50% reduction in ST-segment elevation at 60 to 90 minutes after initiation of therapy), and hemodynamic or electrical instability are generally indicators of failed pharmacologic reperfusion. The pertinent guidelines regarding rescue PCI are:

- Class I: Rescue PCI should be performed in patients <75 years old with ST elevation or LBBB who develop shock within 36 hours of MI and are suitable for revascularization that can be performed within 18 hours of shock unless further support is futile because of the patient's wishes or contraindications/unsuitability for further invasive care (Level of Evidence: B).

- Class I: Rescue PCI should be performed in patients with severe CHF and/or pulmonary edema (Killip class 3) and onset of symptoms within 12 hours (Level of Evidence: B).

- Class IIa: Rescue PCI is reasonable for selected patients who are 75 years or older with ST elevation or LBBB or who develop shock within 36 hours of MI and who are suitable for revascularization that can be performed within 18 hours of shock. Patients with good prior functional status who are suitable for revascularization and who agree to invasive care may be selected for such an invasive strategy (Level of Evidence: B).

- Class IIa: It is reasonable to perform rescue PCI for patients with one or more of the following:

  - Hemodynamic or electrical instability (Level of Evidence: C)

  - Persistent ischemic symptoms (Level of Evidence: C).

- Class IIa: It is reasonable to monitor the pattern of ST elevation, cardiac rhythm, and clinical symptoms over the 60 to 180 minutes after initiation of fibrinolytic therapy. Noninvasive findings suggestive of reperfusion include relief of symptoms, maintenance or restoration of hemodynamic and/or electrical stability, and a reduction of at least 50% of the initial ST-segment elevation injury pattern on a follow-up EKG 60 to 90 minutes after initiation of therapy (Level of Evidence: B).

11   Answer D.   Despite TIMI 3 flow in an epicardial vessel after reperfusion, impaired myocardial perfusion may still be present and is associated with worse outcomes. The TIMI myocardial perfusion grading system (TMPG) or myocardial blush grade is a marker of myocardial perfusion and corresponds to higher mortality rates independent of epicardial flow (*Circulation.* 2000;101:125–130). TMPG grade 0 is defined as no apparent tissue-level perfusion (no ground-glass appearance of blush or opacification of the myocardium) in the distribution of the culprit artery. TMPG grade 1 indicates presence of myocardial blush but no clearance from the microvasculature (blush or a stain is present on the next injection). TMPG grade 2 blush clears slowly (blush is strongly persistent and diminishes minimally or not at all during three cardiac cycles of the washout phase). TMPG grade 3 indicates that blush begins to clear during washout (blush is minimally persistent after three cardiac cycles of washout). No-reflow is defined as a profound reduction in antegrade coronary blood flow despite vessel patency and the absence of dissection, spasm, or distal macroembolus. It is presumed to reflect microvascular dysfunction and appears to be more common in diabetic patients. TIMI myocardial perfusion grade is a stronger independent predictor of mortality outcomes in STEMI patients after reperfusion therapy than persistent ST-segment elevations, TIMI flow grade, or the presence of no-reflow. Patients with TIMI grade 2 flow may have a normal TMPG grade secondary to collateral circulation. Patients with both normal epicardial flow (TIMI grade 3 flow) and normal tissue-level perfusion (TMPG grade 3) have an extremely low risk of mortality (*Circulation.* 2002;105:1909–1913).

12   Answer C.   SBP <100 mm Hg. The current ACC/AHA guidelines in regard to immediate administration of β-blockers are:

- Class I: Oral β-blocker therapy should be administered promptly to those patients without a contraindication, irrespective of concomitant fibrinolytic therapy or performance of primary PCI (Level of Evidence: A).

■ Class IIa: It is reasonable to administer IV β-blockers promptly to STEMI patients without contraindications, especially if a tachyarrhythmia or hypertension is present (Level of Evidence: B).

The following are relative contraindications to β-blocker therapy: HR <60 bpm, systolic arterial pressure <100 mm Hg, moderate or severe left ventricular (LV) failure, signs of peripheral hypoperfusion, shock, PR interval >0.24 second, second- or third-degree atrioventricular (AV) block, active asthma, or reactive airway disease. The Clopidogrel and Metoprolol in Myocardial Infarction Trial/Second Chinese Cardiac Study (COMMIT/CCS-2) was the largest clinical study ever conducted in China (*Lancet.* 2005;366:1622–1632). The study enrolled 45,852 patients at 1,250 centers. COMMIT/CCS-2 was a randomized, parallel-controlled trial that used a 2 × 2 factorial design to assess the effects of adding 75 mg of clopidogrel (vs. placebo) and the effects of adding the β-blocker metoprolol (vs. placebo) in patients with acute MI on aspirin therapy (162 mg daily). The study enrolled patients with suspected acute MI (ST change or new LBBB) within 24 hours of symptom onset. Patients with shock, SBP <100 mm Hg, HR <50 bpm, or second- or third-degree AV block were excluded. The findings on metoprolol showed that giving three intravenous doses of 5 mg metoprolol followed by daily oral doses of 200 mg reduced the relative risks of reinfarction and vascular events by 15% to 20%, but increased the relative risk of cardiac shock by 30%, especially during the first day of treatment. This finding emphasizes that the β-blocker therapy in the setting of acute STEMI should be tailored to the individual patient. In patients at high risk of cardiogenic shock (borderline BP or those presenting in Killip class III), β-blockers should either be delayed until such patients are hemodynamically stable or they should be more slowly uptitrated.

13 **Answer C.** Symptoms-to-balloon time. Symptom onset to balloon inflation represents the true ischemic time in patients undergoing primary PCI. De Luca et al. demonstrated that for every 30-minute delay from the onset of symptoms to balloon inflation, the risk of 1-year mortality is increased by 7.5% (*Circulation.* 2004;109:1223–1225). The following figure depicts this relationship between ischemic time and 1-year mortality (the dotted line represents 95% confidence intervals of predicted mortality).

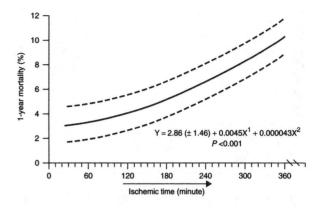

$$Y = 2.86 (\pm 1.46) + 0.0045X^1 + 0.000043X^2$$
$$P < 0.001$$

14 **Answer C.** The ACC/AHA guidelines recommend the following goals for time to reperfusion therapy: Door-to-needle time for initiation of fibrinolytic therapy of <30 minutes and door-to-balloon (or medical contact–to-balloon) time for PCI of <90 minutes.

15 **Answer B.** The patient described is a 72-year-old man with an anterolateral STEMI complicated by cardiogenic shock. Given his age (<75 years), time course of his chest pain symptoms (CP for >3 hours presenting with shock in <36 hours), and the anticipated time for PCI (90 minutes or less), the patient should be transferred for primary PCI after a PA catheter and IABP are placed. An IABP is recommended when shock is not rapidly reversed with pharmacologic therapy as is the case in this clinical scenario. The recommendations for the initial reperfusion therapy when cardiogenic shock complicates STEMI are outlined in the following figure (*Circulation.* 2003;107:2998–3002). Fibrinolytic therapy would be preferred if the anticipated PCI time was >90 minutes, symptoms had been present for <3 hours, and there were no contraindications.

The pertinent ACC/AHA guidelines are:

■ Class I: Primary PCI should be performed for patients <75 years old with ST elevation or LBBB who develop shock within 36 hours of MI and are suitable for revascularization that can be performed within 18 hours of shock unless further support is futile because of the patient's wishes or contraindications/unsuitability for further invasive care (Level of Evidence: A).

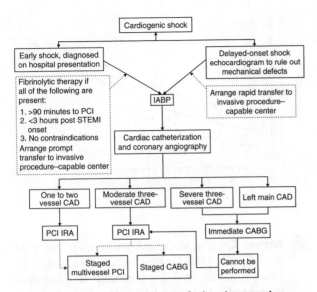

Recommendations for initial reperfusion therapy when cardiogenic shock complicates STEMI. Early mechanical revascularization with PCI/CABG is a class I recommendation for candidates younger than 75 years of age with ST elevation or LBBB who develop shock <36 hours from STEMI and in whom revascularization can be performed within 18 hours of shock, and a class IIa recommendation for patients 75 years of age or older with the same criteria. Eighty-five percent of shock cases are diagnosed after initial therapy for STEMI, but most patients develop shock within 24 hours. An IABP is recommended when shock is not quickly reversed with pharmacologic therapy, as a stabilizing measure for patients who are candidates for further invasive care. Dashed lines indicate that the procedure should be performed in patients with specific indications only. Recommendations for staged CABG and PCI are discussed in the text, as are definitions of moderate and severe three-vessel CAD. PCI, percutaneous coronary intervention; STEMI, ST-elevation myocardial infarction; IABP, intra-aortic balloon pump; CAD, coronary artery disease; IRA, infarct-related artery, CABG, coronary artery bypass graft surgery; LBBB, left bundle-branch block. Modified with permission from Hochman. Circulation 2003;107:2998–3002 (502).

16 **Answer D.**   This patient is likely suffering from an intracranial hemorrhage (ICH) after the administration of fibrinolytic agents. Any change in mental status in patients receiving fibrinolytics should be treated/managed as an ICH until proven otherwise. Recommendations for the management of ICH are outlined in the following figure from the ACC/AHA guidelines.

Before the administration of fibrinolytics, patients should be assessed for their risk of ICH. Absolute contraindications include the following: Any prior ICH, known structural cerebral vascular lesions, known malignant intracranial neoplasms, ischemia stroke within 3 months, suspected aortic

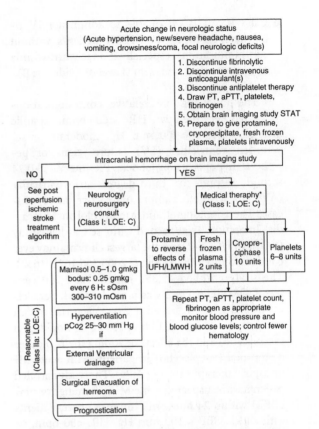

Algorithm for evaluation of intracranial hemorrhage complicating fibrinolytic therapy for ST-elevation myocardial infarction. PT, prothrombin time; aPTT, activated partial thromboplastin time; LOE, level of evidence; H, hours; sOsm, serum osmolality; mOsm, milliosmoles; UFH, unfractionated heparin; LMWH, low-molecular weight heparin. As dictated by clinical circumstances. Modified with permission from NINDS rt-PA Stroke Study Group. Stroke 1997;28:1530–1540 (370).

dissection, active bleeding or bleeding diathesis, and significant closed head trauma within 3 months. Relative contraindications include the following: History of chronic, severe, poorly controlled hypertension, severe uncontrolled hypertension on presentation, a history of prior ischemic stroke >3 months ago, traumatic or prolonged cardiopulmonary resuscitation (CPR), recent (2 to 4 weeks) internal bleeding, noncompressible vascular punctures, pregnancy, active peptic ulcer, and current use of anticoagulants. The pertinent ACC/AHA guidelines are:

■ Class I: Health care providers should ascertain whether the patient has neurologic contraindications to fibrinolytic therapy, including any history of ICH or significant closed head or facial trauma within the past 3 months, uncontrolled hypertension, or ischemic stroke within the past 3 months (Level of Evidence: A).

- Class I: STEMI patients at substantial (≥4%) risk of ICH should be treated with PCI rather than with fibrinolytic therapy (Level of Evidence: A).
- Class I: The occurrence of a change in neurologic status during or after reperfusion therapy, particularly within the first 24 hours of initiation of treatment, is considered to be due to ICH until proved otherwise. Fibrinolytic, antiplatelet, and anticoagulant therapies should be discontinued until brain-imaging scan shows no evidence of ICH (Level of Evidence: A).
- Class I: Neurology and/or neurosurgery or hematology consultations should be obtained for STEMI patients who have ICH, as dictated by clinical circumstances (Level of Evidence: C).
- Class I: In patients with ICH, infusions of cryoprecipitate, fresh frozen plasma, protamine, and platelets should be given, as dictated by clinical circumstances (Level of Evidence: C).

17 Answer C. In this patient presenting with cardiogenic shock and significant multivessel coronary artery, it is a reasonable approach to attempt PCI of all lesions. Although PCI in a noninfarct artery is not recommended in stable patients (Class III indication), it may be beneficial in hemodynamically compromised patients if the noninfarct artery supplies a significant area of myocardium and the procedure is fairly straight forward.

18 Answer D. Reperfusion injury refers to the myocardial, CV, and electrophysiologic dysfunction induced by the restoration of blood flow to previously ischemic tissue. The exact pathophysiology of reperfusion injury is still being defined, but there are several processes that have been proposed. First, endothelial cells become dysfunctional resulting in an excess of vasoconstrictors and a deficiency of vasodilators (such as NO). Endothelial dysfunction activates platelets, coagulation factors, and neutrophils promoting a proinflammatory and procoagulant state. Second, the oxidative stress promotes the generation of oxygen-free radicals and a relative reduction of free radical scavengers. Third, increased intracellular calcium is released from the compromised mitochondria and sarcoplasmic reticulum. The increased calcium levels promote damage to the myocyte myofibrils. Finally, embolization of thrombotic material with reperfusion therapy can result in plugging of the microvasculature (*Heart.* 2005;91:1530–1532). Increased intracellular calcium, decreased NO, and closing of the ATP-dependent sodium–potassium channels are all associated with reperfusion injury.

19 Answer D. Ischemic preconditioning is the phenomenon in which brief nonlethal episodes of ischemia protect the myocardium before a subsequent prolonged ischemic event through a variety of adaptive physiologic measures. This concept was initially described in animal models, but it has subsequently been described in humans and shown to decrease infarct size. Superoxide dismutase is an endogenous free radical scavenger that has been studied in a variety of animal models of reperfusion injury. To date, no human studies have shown a reduction in infarct size. The effects of GIK therapy were studied in the CREATE-ECLA trial (*JAMA.* 2005;293:437–446). Patients presenting with STEMI within 12 hours of symptom onset were randomized to GIK infusion or placebo. There was no difference in all-cause mortality, cardiac arrest, cardiogenic shock, or reinfarction. Pexelizumab is a monoclonal antibody against C5 complement and functions to inhibit the activation of the complement system. Complement activation is a mediator of inflammatory damage seen with reperfusion injury. In the recent COMMA trial (*Circulation.* 2003;108:1184–1190), pexelizumab was administered (bolus alone or bolus plus infusion) to patients with STEMI undergoing mechanical reperfusion. Administration of this monoclonal antibody failed to show a reduction in infarct size, but patients receiving the bolus plus infusion showed a significant reduction in 90-day mortality. Further clinical trials are ongoing (APEX MI). Other agents have also been unsuccessful in clinical trials. This includes monoclonal antibodies against white cell CD11/18 integrin receptors, calcium channel blockers, the Na/H exchange inhibitor, cariporide, the K_{ATP} channel opener, nicorandil, and adenosine. Whereas adenosine showed benefit following thrombolysis in initial trials, subsequent trials in patients undergoing primary PCI have been negative.

20 Answer A. McSweeney et al. (*Circulation.* 2003;108:2619–2623) retrospectively surveyed a group of women diagnosed with acute MI to determine the symptoms at presentation. In this cohort of predominantly white women, the most frequent presenting symptoms were shortness of breath (58%), weakness (55%), and fatigue (43%). Acute chest pain was absent in 43% of patients. In general, women and the elderly present with more atypical symptoms leading to delays in presentation and diagnosis.

21 Answer C. The use of IV ACE inhibitors within the first day of an acute MI is associated with adverse events, especially in the elderly (*Eur Heart J.*

1994;15(Suppl B):14–19; discussion 26–30). Oral ACE inhibitors, however, have been shown to be beneficial in this early period. The adverse events in the patients receiving IV ACE inhibitors are thought to be secondary to the risk of hypotension. The pertinent ACC/AHA guidelines regarding ACE inhibitor use in the early course of an acute STEMI are:

- Class I: An ACE inhibitor should be administered orally within the first 24 hours of STEMI to patients with anterior infarction, pulmonary congestion, or LVEF <0.40, in the absence of hypotension (SBP <100 mm Hg or <30 mm Hg below baseline) or known contraindications to that class of medications (Level of Evidence: A).

- Class I: An angiotensin receptor blocker (ARB) should be administered to STEMI patients who are intolerant of ACE inhibitors and who have either clinical or radiologic signs of heart failure or LVEF <0.40. Valsartan and candesartan have established efficacy for this recommendation (Level of Evidence: C).

- Class IIa: An ACE inhibitor administered orally within the first 24 hours of STEMI can be useful in patients without anterior infarction, pulmonary congestion, or LVEF <0.40 in the absence of hypotension (SBP <100 mm Hg or <30 mm Hg below baseline) or known contraindications to that class of medications. The expected treatment benefit in such patients is less (5 lives saved per 1,000 patients treated) than for patients with LV dysfunction (Level of Evidence: B).

- Class III: An intravenous ACE inhibitor should not be given to patients within the first 24 hours of STEMI because of the risk of hypotension (A possible exception may be patients with refractory hypertension.) (Level of Evidence: B).

22 **Answer A.** This patient is presenting >12 hours after his initial symptoms. However, he has evidence of heart failure, electric instability, and persistent symptoms. An emergent cardiac catheterization should be performed. The pertinent ACC/AHA guidelines are:

- Class IIa: It is reasonable to perform primary PCI for patients with onset of symptoms within the previous 12 to 24 hours and one or more of the following:
  - Severe CHF (Level of Evidence C)
  - Hemodynamic or electrical instability (Level of Evidence: C)
  - Persistent ischemic symptoms (Level of Evidence: C).

23 **Answer A.** Administration of β-blockers in the acute phase of a STEMI diminishes myocardial oxygen demand, reduces systemic arterial pressure, and reduces myocardial contractility. By a reduction in HR and prolongation of diastole, β-blockers are thought to augment myocardial perfusion. β-Blockers have been shown to decrease the size of infarction, decrease the rate of reinfarction, and decrease the frequency of life-threatening ventricular arrhythmias regardless of the reperfusion strategy. Several nonrandomized trials (e.g., PAMI and CADILLAC) have shown improved short- and long-term mortality with pretreatment with β-blockers in patients undergoing primary PCI. The pertinent ACC/AHA guidelines are:

- Class I: Oral β-blocker therapy should be administered promptly to those patients without a contraindication, irrespective of concomitant fibrinolytic therapy or performance of primary PCI (Level of Evidence: A).

- Class IIa: It is reasonable to administer IV β-blockers promptly to STEMI patients without contraindications, especially if a tachyarrhythmia or hypertension is present (Level of Evidence: B). In regard to the use of lidocaine, there is no convincing evidence that the routine prophylactic administration reduces mortality. The pertinent ACC/AHA guidelines are:

- Class III: The routine use of prophylactic antiarrhythmic drugs (i.e., lidocaine) is not indicated for suppression of isolated ventricular premature beats, couplets, runs of accelerated idioventricular rhythm, and nonsustained VT (Level of Evidence: B).

- Class III: The routine use of prophylactic antiarrhythmic therapy is not indicated when fibrinolytic agents are administered (Level of Evidence: B).

24 **Answer D.** The patient is presenting within 1 hour of the onset of symptoms and she has no evidence of CHF, shock, or rhythm instability. The efficacy of fibrinolytic agents decreases with the passage of time. However, in patients presenting within 3 hours of the onset of symptoms, mortality is equivalent in those patients treated with fibrinolytic agents and those treated with PCI. Provided that she has no contraindications, either primary PCI or fibrinolytic therapy would be appropriate in this patient. The following table from the ACC/AHA guidelines addresses the assessment of reperfusion options for patients with STEMI.

Assessment of reperfusion options for patients with STEMI

STEP 1: Assess time and risk
- Time since onset of symptoms
- Risk of STEMI
- Risk of fibrinolysis
- Time required for transport to a skilled PCI lab

STEP 2: Determine if fibrinolysis or an invasive strategy is preferred
If presentation is less than 3 hours and there is no delay to an invasive strategy, there is no preference for either strategy

Fibrinolysis is generally preferred if	An invasive strategy is generally preferred if
• Early presentation (≤3 hours from symptom onset and delay to invasive strategy) (see below) • Invasive strategy is not an option Catheterization lab occupied/not available Vascular access difficulties Lack of access to a skilled PCI lab *a,b* • Delay to invasive strategy Prolonged transport (Door-to-balloon)–(door-to-needle) is >1 hour *c,d* Medical contact-to-balloon or door-to-balloon is >90 minutes	• Skilled PCI lab available with surgical backup *a,b* Medical contact-to-balloon or door-to-balloon is <90 minutes (Door-to-balloon)–(door-to-needle) is <1 hour *c* • High risk from STEMI Cardiogenic shock Killip class is ≥ to 3 • Contraindications to fibrinolysis increased risk of bleeding and ICH • Late presentation The symptom onset was > 3 hours ago • Diagnosis of STEMI is in doubt

STEMI = ST-elevation myocardial infarction: PCI = percutaneous coronary intervention: ICH = intracranial hemorrhage.
*c*Applies to fibrin-specific agents
*a*Operator experience > a total of 75 primary PCI cases/layer
*b*Team experience > a total of 36 primary PCI cases/year
*d*This calculation implies that the estimated delay to the implementation of the invasive strategy is > one hour versus initiation of fibrinolytic therapy immediatly with a fibrin-specific agent.

25 **Answer D.** The rhythm is an accelerated idioventricular rhythm. This rhythm is frequently seen in the first 12 hours of infarction, but it is not a risk factor for the development of (VF). Accelerated idioventricular rhythms are thought to be related to reperfusion. They should be managed with observation rather than with antiarrhythmic agents.

26 **Answer A.** Compared with PTCA, intracoronary stents achieve better immediate angiographic results with a larger arterial lumen. No significant differences in mortality or reinfarction have been observed, but with primary stenting, there is less vessel reocclusion and restenosis, leading to less target vessel revascularization.

27 **Answer D.** This patient's VF event was in the setting of acute ischemia before revascularization. Although her EF is significantly reduced, she has had no further evidence of spontaneous VF or sustained VT. The LV function should be reassessed at least 1 month after her STEMI. Provided that she continues to have no further VF or sustained VT, if the EF remains <30%, ICD placement would be indicated. If the EF is >40%, an ICD is not indicated. With an EF between 31% and 40%, an EP study may be indicated. The following figure from the ACC/AHA guidelines is an algorithm for primary prevention of sudden cardiac death in post-STEMI patients without spontaneous VF or sustained VT at least 1 month post-MI.

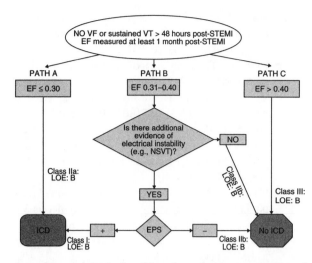

An evidence-based algorithm for primary prevention of sudden death in post-STEMI patients without spontaneous VF or sustained VT at least 1 month post-STEMI to aid in selection of implantable cardioverter/defibrillator (ICD) in patients with STEMI and diminished ejection fraction (EF). The appropriate management path is selected based on left ventricular ejection fraction (LVEF) measured at least 1 month after STEMI. These criteria, which are based on the published data, form the basis for the full-text guidelines. All patients, whether an ICD is implanted or not, should receive medical therapy as outlined in the full-text guidelines. VF, ventricular fibrillation; VT, ventricular tachycardia; STEMI, ST-elevation myocardial infarction; NSVT, nonsustained VT; LOE, level of evidence; EPS, electrophysiological study; LVEF, left ventricular EF.

The pertinent ACC/AHA guidelines are:

■ Class I: An ICD is indicated for patients with VF or hemodynamically significant sustained VT >2 days after STEMI, provided the arrhythmia is not judged to be due to transient or reversible ischemia or reinfarction (Level of Evidence: A).

■ Class I: An ICD is indicated for patients without spontaneous VF or sustained VT >48 hours after STEMI whose STEMI occurred at least 1 month previously, who have an LVEF between 0.31 and 0.40, demonstrate additional evidence of electrical instability (e.g., nonsustained VT), and have inducible VF or sustained VT on EP testing (Level of Evidence: B).

■ Class IIa: If there is reduced LVEF (0.30 or less) at least 1 month post-STEMI and 3 months after coronary artery revascularization, it is reasonable to implant an ICD in post-STEMI patients without spontaneous VF or sustained VT >48 hours after STEMI (Level of Evidence: B).

■ Class IIb: The usefulness of an ICD is not well established in STEMI patients without spontaneous VF or sustained VT >48 hours after STEMI who have a reduced LVEF (0.31 to 0.40) at least

1 month after STEMI but who have no additional evidence of electrical instability (e.g., nonsustained VT) (Level of Evidence: B).

■ Class IIb: The usefulness of an ICD is not well established in STEMI patients without spontaneous VF or sustained VT >48 hours after STEMI who have a reduced LVEF (0.31 to 0.40) at least 1 month after STEMI and additional evidence of electrical instability (e.g., nonsustained VT) but who do not have inducible VF or sustained VT on EP testing (Level of Evidence: B).

■ Class III: An ICD is not indicated in STEMI patients who do not experience spontaneous VF or sustained VT >48 hours after STEMI and in whom the LVEF is >0.40 at least 1 month after STEMI. (Level of Evidence: C).

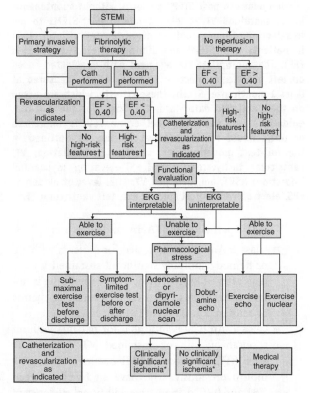

Evidence-based approach to need for catheterization (cath) and revascularization after ST-elevation myocardial infarction (STEMI). The algorithm shows treatment paths for patients who initially undergo a primary invasive strategy, receive fibrinolytic therapy, or do not undergo reperfusion therapy for STEMI. Patients who have not undergone a primary invasive strategy and have no high-risk features should undergo functional evaluation with one of the noninvasive tests shown. When clinically significant ischemia is detected, patients should undergo catheterization and revascularization as indicated; if no clinically significant ischemia is detected, medical therapy is prescribed after STEMI.

28 Answer C. STEMI patients who did not undergo a primary invasive strategy should have an early assessment of EF. If the EF is <40% and/or high-risk features (such as CHF or rhythm instability) are present, cardiac catheterization should be performed. The patient described has an EF >40% and no high-risk features. He should undergo a functional evaluation. The following figure from the ACC/AHA guideline outlines the risk stratification approach for patients post-STEMI.

29 Answer C. This patient is presenting early in her course of symptoms (<3 hours), and the estimated door-to-balloon time exceeds the door-to-needle time by >1 hour. She also has no high-risk features at this point (shock, CHF), so the preferred therapy would be fibrinolytic agents. The role of facilitated PCI is still being defined. Facilitated PCI refers to the strategy of planned immediate PCI after an initial pharmacologic regimen (such as full-dose fibrinolytics, half-dose fibrinolytics, or a combination of half-dose fibrinolytics with a platelet GPIIa/IIb inhibitor). In the trials to date, facilitated PCI has not shown any benefit in outcomes. Fibrinolytic agents work through the activation of plasmin. Plasmin then degrades fibrin, a major component of thrombi. With regard to the selection of fibrinolytic agent, streptokinase, and urokinase are the first generation fibrinolytic agents that promote systemic anticoagulation through plasmin activation throughout the circulation. Streptokinase is antigenic and can cause sensitization and allergic reactions, particularly with repeat administrations. The fibrin-specific agents (t-PA, reteplase, and TNK) promote targeted fibrinolysis in that the enzyme plasmin is activated when the drug is bound to fibrin within a thrombus. This targeted action theoretically improves clot lysis and lowers the risk of systemic bleeding. The fibrin-specific agents are more efficacious than the fibrin-nonspecific agents in head-to-head trials for the treatment of STEMI. Also, in the particular patient, there is a potential that she previously received streptokinase 5 years ago when she was administered a "clot buster" for her pulmonary embolus.

30 Answer C. In addition to promoting local clot lysis, the fibrin-specific agents are thought to exert a systemic procoagulant effect through increased thrombin production. Heparin agents act to inhibit the activation of thrombin and other clotting factors. In a recent meta-analysis published in December 2005, Eikelboom, et al. evaluated the efficacy of UFH versus low-molecular-weight heparin (LMWH) in acute STEMI patients undergoing fibrinolytic reperfusion therapy (*Circulation*. 2005;112:3855–3867). Their results demonstrated a 43% reduction in the rate of reinfarction in patients treated for 4 to 8 days with LMWH versus the UFH-treated group suggesting that LMWH heparin should be the preferred antithrombin in these patients. Enoxaparin is an LMWH agent. The dose of 1 mg/kg is a therapeutic dose while 0.5 mg/kg is a prophylactic dose. The use of LMWH heparin in patients older than 75 years has been associated with an increased risk of intracranial bleeding in some studies (*Lancet*. 2001;358:605–613). The routine use of LMWH in STEMI patients is not currently part of the ACC/AHA guidelines. The guidelines currently recommend the initial routine use of IV UFH in all patients regardless of the reperfusion strategy chosen.

31 **Answer C.** Aspirin therapy given perioperatively to patients after CABG reduces the rates of MI, stroke, and renal failure and bowel infarction, with no significant increase in bleeding complications. Clopidogrel use within 5 to 7 days of surgery is associated with increased bleeding complications and should be held if possible before surgery. The pertinent ACC/AHA guidelines are:

- Class I: Aspirin should not be withheld before elective or nonelective CABG after STEMI (Level of Evidence: C).
- Class I: Aspirin (75 to 325 mg/d) should be prescribed as soon as possible (within 24 hours) after CABG unless contraindicated (Level of Evidence: B).
- Class I: In patients taking clopidogrel in whom elective CABG is planned, the drug should be withheld for 5 to 7 days (Level of Evidence: B).

32 **Answer A.** This patient has a strong indication for antithrombotic agents (atrial fibrillation) and dual antiplatelet therapy (recently place intracoronary stent). The ACC/AHA recommendations for antiplatelet and antithrombotic therapy post-STEMI are:

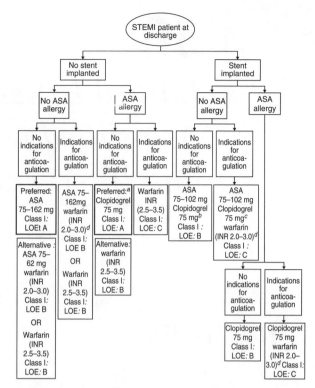

Long-term antithrombotic therapy at hospital discharge after ST-elevation myocardial infarction (STEMI). ASA, aspirin; INR, international normalized ratio; LEO, level of evidence. [a]**Clopidogrel is preferred over warfarin because of increased risk of bleeding and low patient compliance in warfarin trials.** [b]**For 12 months.** [c]**Discontinue clopidogrel 1 month after implantation of a bare-metal stent or several months after implantation of a drug-eluting stent (3 months after sirolimus and 6 months after paclitaxel) because of the potential increased risk of bleeding with warfarin and 2 antiplatelet agents. Continue aspirin and warfarin long term if warfarin is indicated for other reasons such as atrial fibrillation, LV thrombus, cerebral emboli, or extensive regional wall-motion abnormality.** [d]**An INR of 2.0 to 3.0 is acceptable with tight control, but the lower end of this range is preferable. The combination of antiplatelet therapy and warfarin may be considered in patients aged younger than 75 years with low bleeding risk who can be monitored reliably.**

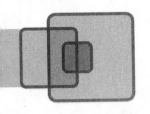

38

Ethical Issues and Risks Associated with Catheterization and Interventional Procedures

Christopher Walters and David C. Booth

Questions

1 A 65-year-old man presents to his local emergency department with 2 hours of severe substernal chest pain. The initial 12-lead electrocardiogram (EKG) reveals an acute injury pattern with 2 mm ST-segment elevation in leads II, III, aVF, as well as V_5 and V_6. His blood pressure is 125/75 mm Hg and his heart rate is 90 beats per minute and regular. The lung examination demonstrates rales throughout the lung fields. His pain is mostly relieved by intravenous nitroglycerin infusion. There is no on-site cardiac surgery capability at this facility, but a board-eligible interventional cardiologist has recently been added to the medical staff, and an acute interventional program has been initiated at the hospital. The nearest facility with on-site surgery is approximately 30 minutes away by ambulance. What is the appropriate management of this patient?

(A) Treat the patient with IV thrombolytic therapy along with routine medical therapy and observe for evidence of reperfusion

(B) Because the patient's discomfort has been largely relieved by intravenous nitroglycerin, admit the patient to the coronary care unit (CCU) for observation

(C) Proceed with urgent cardiac catheterization for possible coronary intervention

(D) Give thrombolytic therapy and immediately transfer to the nearest facility with both interventional and surgical backup

(E) Transfer immediately to the nearest facility with both interventional capability and surgical backup without initiating thrombolysis

2 Your catheterization laboratory is reviewing policy concerning which personnel are qualified to perform coronary interventions. Which of the following statements is *false*?

(A) A physician must be a full member of the hospital staff to be granted privileges to perform percutaneous coronary intervention (PCI) in the cardiac catheterization laboratory

(B) A primary operator must have completed an accredited fellowship in interventional cardiology and therefore be Board-eligible, or must have earned an American Board of Internal Medicine (ABIM) Certificate of Added Qualification in Interventional Cardiology

(C) The primary operator for PCI must have performed >250 coronary interventions in training, and must perform >75 PCI per year as primary operator

(D) An invasive cardiologist who has watched or participated in a total of 100 interventional procedures at a neighboring tertiary referral hospital, where the cardiologist drove once weekly to participate in cases, may be granted privileges to carry out interventional cardiology procedures

3 A 45-year-old man with a history of hypertension and cigarette smoking presents to the office of a Board-certified interventional cardiologist with coronary and peripheral artery expertise, with recent-onset exertional chest discomfort as well as pain in the right calf with walking. The cardiac exam and resting EKG are normal. Exercise echo stress test results are consistent with inferior ischemia. Coronary arteriography is subsequently performed and demonstrates important two-vessel involvement amenable to PCI, with a 90% unstable-appearing proximal right coronary artery stenosis and a 75% left anterior descending stenosis, but no significant left main or circumflex disease. There is difficulty noted in guidewire passage into the central aorta from the right iliac. Left ventriculography demonstrates normal wall motion. After completion of the diagnostic portion of the procedure, the patient reports he has been experiencing chest discomfort and discomfort in the right thigh that has worsened as the procedure has progressed. Right iliac and femoral angiography demonstrates a 90% right common iliac stenosis. On the basis of these findings, how best should the interventional cardiologist proceed?

(A) End the procedure and schedule the patient for left anterior descending and right coronary PCIs and right iliac intervention at three separate procedures

(B) Carry out PCI only for right iliac stenosis and have the patient return for coronary intervention at a later date

(C) Perform PCI for both coronary lesions and have the patient return at a later date for iliac intervention

(D) Carry out right coronary and right common iliac interventions and have the patient return for left anterior descending intervention

4 An 80-year-old woman with a history of chronic obstructive pulmonary disease is 2 days status post total arthroplasty following right hip fracture and develops respiratory distress that responds to continuous positive airway pressure with a mask, but from which the patient subsequently cannot be weaned. Cardiac markers include a troponin I of 6.25, and coronary arteriography is performed. From the outset of the procedure the patient is initially restive, then becomes agitated and combative and twice contaminates the femoral catheterization fields. Coronary arteriography has demonstrated serial severe left anterior descending lesions. The circumflex is left dominant and free of disease that appears to be hemodynamically significant. The patient's movement is compromising

the procedure. The interventional cardiologist does not have privileges for deep conscious sedation but feels that deeper sedation is the optimum means of managing the patient's combativeness. Which of the following is the optimal approach for managing the patient's sedation and airway during the procedure?

(A) Stop the procedure and refer the patient for emergency surgical revascularization

(B) Administer increasing doses of fentanyl and midazolam in an effort to sedate the patient

(C) Contact Anesthesiology for stat administration of propofol

(D) Use forcible restraints to prevent the patient from contaminating the field

(E) The interventional cardiologist should break scrub and administer a propofol 50 mg intravenous bolus and initiate 0.1 to 0.2 mg/kg/min continuous infusion, and then rescrub and perform PCI for the left anterior descending

5 An interventional cardiologist in a highly competitive environment is considering strategies to increase market share. Of the following options, which would constitute an ethical way of garnering more patient referrals?

(A) Contract with an advertising firm and for an Internet and billboard campaign that describes the physician as, "the Heavy Hitter in Interventional Cardiology in Our Area," and "the Sheriff Who'll Put Those Outlaw Stenoses Behind Bars for Good," and "Go to PlaqueBlaster.com"

(B) Have in practice a seasonal gift-giving plan in which physicians who refer five or more patients are sent a minimum of $1000 for professional development purposes, and monies for these payments are derived from the collections from the respective patients

(C) Initiate a system whereby in return for patient referrals, the interventional cardiologist will send the patient back to the referring physician for nonindicated procedures such as surveillance radionuclide stress testing

(D) Have in place a system whereby in return for referring friends and acquaintances, patients will be charged, "Insurance Only"

6 An interventional cardiologist utilizes samples provided by pharmaceutical firms as a means of providing medications at no cost to patients having difficulty paying the cost of drugs. One company provides more samples than any other firm. One of the company's drugs is the market leader for this indication, but other name-brand drugs that are sold by this company, although relatively effective, are much more expensive than generic drugs that are considered to be "top-tier" for these indications in most drug plans. In what way does the continued overstocking of the sample cabinet by the company create an ethical dilemma for the physician?

(A) Availability from the company of a surfeit of the superior therapy has the potential to engender ethical conflict in the physician's choice of other therapies, for example, generic drugs that may be equally or more effective than the company's products for other indications. In short, the dispensing of the one agent may lead to prescribing the other of the company's products, although less expensive alternatives of equal or greater efficacy exist. This prescribing pattern constitutes closure of a subtle *quid pro quo* situation that ultimately benefits the company

(B) Because the company markets the best drug for one indication, there is no ethical harm in prescribing the company's other drugs

(C) The interventional cardiologist worked 90 hours last week and is too tired to consider ethical issues

7 An 80-year-old woman with a history of age-related cognitive decline, who resides in an assisted living facility, has been admitted to hospital with a non–ST-segment elevation myocardial infarction (MI). The patient's husband is deceased. There are five children, all of whom frequently visit her. The eldest daughter has the power of attorney. There is a valid Living Will. The interventional cardiologist has been following up the patient and discusses treatment options with the siblings, who agree on an initial course of conservative management, with aspirin, clopidogrel, β blockade, and statin therapy, and reiterate the patient's request in the Living Will to not be resuscitated. The patient had been admitted to the CCU and has now been transferred to a nontelemetry floor bed. On the floor the patient has experienced two episodes of prolonged chest discomfort associated with ST-segment depression on the EKG. The children have met, and four out of the five, including the daughter with the power of attorney, wish to continue conservative management. The youngest son has demanded that the patient be taken for coronary arteriography and percutaneous coronary revascularization, and that the patient be resuscitated in the event of an arrest. What is the correct approach in this situation?

(A) The interventional cardiologist is supremely confident in his ability to see patients safely through complex, high-risk interventional procedures. The youngest son tells the physician

that he has spoken with the rest of the family, and that they now agree with him. Using an informed consent signed by the youngest son, the interventional cardiologist takes the patient to the cardiac catheterization laboratory

(B) The interventional cardiologist realizes the legal significance of power of attorney and recommends a joint meeting with all five siblings. The youngest son resists this suggestion and initially threatens to leave the hospital. Ultimately, with the intervention of an experienced, compassionate nurse, he agrees to join his brothers and sisters in a meeting

(C) Discuss the situation with the telemetry floor nursing staff, who have dealt with many such situations

(D) Because of the family strife, the interventional cardiologist notifies the family of his withdrawal from management of the patient

8 What, if any, federal regulation exists concerning self-referral?

(A) The Belmont Statute

(B) The Stark Law

(C) The Medicare-Medicaid Anti-Kickback Statute

(D) The Proxmire Designated Health Services Law, also referred to as the Golden Fleece Law

(E) There is no federal regulation regarding self-referral in medicine

9 You are actively enrolling patients at your institution in an ongoing clinical trial, and have provided valuable information to the study sponsor although at the same time ensuring that patient care is not negatively impacted by your financial relationship to the study. In addition to the study, you have begun to do continuing medical education (CME) presentations that are underwritten by the study. To date, you have received approximately $7500 in compensation for your participation in the CME activities. What level of compensation is considered significant?

(A) Any compensation is considered significant for CME activities

(B) Any compensation >$500

(C) Any compensation ≤$10,000

(D) Any compensation >$10,000

10 You are the medical director of a catheterization laboratory, which has just hired a female radiology technologist to assist with the increasing volume of cases. She is well-trained and eager to help. The catheterization laboratory nurse manager reports to you that a catheterization laboratory employee has recounted overhearing another male employee speak in overt sexual contexts both around and directly to the new female technician. The new female staff member confirms that these conversations took place, but she assures you that she is not affected by this environment. However, you feel that she is simply trying to protect her new job, and that such coworker behavior is inappropriate and unprofessional. What is the most appropriate way to handle this situation?

(A) Refer to the policy of your institution regarding sexual harassment in the workplace, then instruct the catheterization laboratory nurse or technical manager to address this issue directly with the coworker at the earliest opportunity, enforcing the principles of professionalism, and the consequences (both legal and professional) of sexual harassment either real or perceived

(B) Reassure the employee that this conduct is likely due to the predominance of men in the workplace, and that this behavior is a benign part of male-dominated workplaces

(C) Because the female technician stated that such conduct did not bother her, take no further action at this point

(D) See that the particular offending male staff members and physicians avoid working with the new female technician

11 You see a sedentary 35-year-old woman in the clinic with a chest pain syndrome, occurring once every 2 weeks. Risk factors include cigarette smoking. You recommend an exercise radionuclide stress test. The procedure is performed in your office. The patient walks 8:30 according to the Bruce protocol complains of sharp chest discomfort and breathlessness during the test, but there are no electrocardiographic changes. Perfusion scintigraphy performed immediately postexercise demonstrates a relatively small inferior defect. There is minimal reversibility noted on subsequent rest scintigraphy. You recommend and subsequently perform cardiac catheterization and PCI for what appears to be a 60% stenosis seen only in one angiographic view. What can be concluded regarding self-referral in this case?

(A) There is no self-referral issue of any kind in this case

(B) Given the good prognostic outcome of the stress test, as well as the incidence of false-positive radionuclide scintigraphic stress tests, particularly inferior perfusion defects that may occur as a result of attenuation artifact, you may have completed an unnecessary self-referral

(C) Because the radionuclide test demonstrates a perfusion abnormality, although subtle, you are on absolutely firm ethical ground in referring the patient to yourself for cardiac catheterization

(D) Cardiac catheterization is indicated in all patients presenting with chest pain syndromes

12 A 75-year-old man is known to have a history of diabetes mellitus, hypertension, dyslipidemia, and >50 pack-years of smoking. A high-risk stress test result is obtained, and the patient subsequently undergoes uncomplicated drug-eluting stent placement to the mid left anterior descending. One hour after the catheterization, the patient complains of severe pain at the femoral access site, and a 4-cm hematoma is noted. Of the clinical and/or procedural factors listed in the following text, which is most closely associated with the development of femoral catheterization site injury?

(A) Age >70 years

(B) Male gender

(C) Sheath size >6 French

(D) Use of a coronary stent during the procedure

(E) Use of mechanical clamp device for hemostasis

13 At a case conference with your colleagues, you discuss a 50-year-old patient who presented overnight with a non–ST-elevation acute coronary syndrome and was stabilized on medical therapy with Class I indications. The next morning the patient underwent uncomplicated primary stent placement in the circumflex, and 4 hours later developed ventricular fibrillation and died. What is the unadjusted in-hospital mortality from PCI?

(A) Less than 0.5%

(B) 0.5% to 1.5%

(C) 1.5% to 3.0%

(D) Greater than 3.0%

14 A 78-year-old woman undergoes elective PCI with a drug-eluting stent to the mid left anterior descending with no immediate complications. A glycoprotein IIb/IIIa inhibitor is used, and the patient received 600 mg of clopidogrel at the completion of the case. In the catheterization recovery area 30 minutes following the procedure, the patient develops back pain and becomes diaphoretic. A 12-lead EKG is normal. Acute retroperitoneal hemorrhage is suspected. What is the best clinical predictor of retroperitoneal hematoma (RPH) formation after PCI?

(A) Preexisting poorly controlled hypertension

(B) Arterial sheath size >7 French

(C) Female gender

(D) Glycoprotein IIb/IIIa use

(E) Body surface area (BSA) <1.73 m²

15 A 72-year-old woman with a history of hypertension, insulin-dependent diabetes mellitus, and chronic renal insufficiency (serum creatinine 2.2 mg per dL) is scheduled to undergo diagnostic coronary angiography and possible PCI, after presenting with a history consistent with Canadian Cardiovascular Society Class III angina. An exercise echo stress test demonstrated a large reversible anteroseptal wall motion abnormality. Should the patient develop acute renal failure (ARF) after a PCI procedure, what is the effect on her mortality?

(A) In-hospital mortality has been shown to increase dramatically in patients who develop ARF after PCI, and increases even more in patients who require hemodialysis (acute renal failure requiring dialysis [ARFD])

(B) In-hospital mortality is not impacted, but survival at 1 year is significantly decreased

(C) In-hospital mortality is only affected by development of ARFD, but not just development of ARF

(D) There are no data to suggest that development of ARFD after PCI affects overall mortality

16 A 73-year-old man with known coronary artery disease, severe left ventricular systolic dysfunction, and NYHA Class III heart failure symptoms presents by emergency medical transport to the emergency department with an unequivocal anterior ST-segment elevation myocardial infarction (STEMI). The patient has altered mental status, a blood pressure of 90 mm Hg palpable systolic, a heart rate of 100 beats per minute, and is unable to give informed consent. He is well known to you from follow-up in your clinic and has no living relatives. Recently, although in a better state of health, the patient told you that it is his desire to have no further cardiac interventions in the future, and he indicated that he had completed appropriate "Do Not Resuscitate (DNR) Orders" with his primary care provider. What option in the following text offers the most optimal and appropriate cardiovascular care for this patient?

(A) In addition to standard medical therapy, begin dopamine infusion due to hypotension, providing only bag-mask ventilation to see if he stabilizes

(B) Quickly confer with other medical professionals in the emergency room and proceed to the catheterization laboratory under an emergency informed consent signed by you

(C) Tell the patient that you feel he needs to go directly to the cath laboratory or he will likely die

(D) Consider thrombolytic therapy along with aspirin, oxygen, nitroglycerin, and heparin, and pressor support, if necessary, and move the patient to the CCU for further management and observation

17 A colleague consults you regarding a patient who has undergone diagnostic coronary angiography. Your colleague has identified a single lesion that he feels would benefit from PCI. Informed consent for possible PCI had been obtained before the procedure, and the patient is aware that you would be performing the procedure. You initially agree to perform the procedure, but as the equipment for the intervention is being pulled from electronic cabinets, your earlier doubt that the procedure is indicated intensifies because you in fact believe the stenosis is not hemodynamically significant. How do you proceed?

(A) Tell the patient you are uncertain of the potential benefit of the planned procedure, and ask if he chooses to proceed

(B) Tell the patient that assessment is that the procedure is not indicated and should be canceled, and that you will review his records further and discuss your findings with him

(C) Advise the patient that although you are unsure of the ultimate outcome, the potential risks of the procedure are low and proceed.

(D) Proceed without expressing your opinion to the patient in deference to both your colleague's opinion and the catheterization laboratory schedule

18 Before proceeding with a planned percutaneous mitral valvotomy, you explain the procedure to the patient, along with the risks, benefits, and alternatives. The patient is 75 years of age and has a history of "a touch of Alzheimer disease," according to a daughter who accompanies him. He is otherwise independent, and no separate provision such as a health care power of attorney has been established. What is the proper way to proceed with ensuring that informed consent is obtained?

(A) Ask your nurse to spend extra time assessing the patient's understanding of the procedure and let you know if the patient seems to understand the plan

(B) Ask the daughter if she understands the procedure and if she is agreeable to proceeding

(C) Have the daughter convince the patient to proceed and sign the consent form despite his reluctance

(D) Ensure that the patient displays competence, understanding, and autonomy in providing consent free of undue influence or coercion

19 You are carrying out a coronary intervention that has immediately followed the diagnostic procedure. The patient is a 68-year-old woman with no history of drug allergies who underwent an uncomplicated renal arteriogram several years ago, and since that procedure has been taking lisinopril for control of hypertension. For the procedure, the patient has received aspirin, clopidogrel, intravenous β-blocker, heparin, small doses of fentanyl and midazolam, and 150 mL of low-osmolality nonionic contrast material. The procedure has been going smoothly, but you have just encountered difficulty advancing a drug-eluting stent across a target lesion that was predilated with an appropriately sized balloon, when the patient complains of intense itching, queasy stomach, and a feeling of being unable to clear her throat, and the blood pressure has dropped to 80 mm Hg systolic. On examination the patient is found to have diffuse raised urticaria, including a 10-cm diameter right neck lesion extending from dorsal of the right ear lobe to the sternal notch. What is the most likely explanation for the patient's findings?

(A) The patient is having an immune-mediated reaction to contrast material

(B) The patient is having a delayed hypersensitivity reaction to the soft-shell crab she had for dinner the night before the procedure

(C) The patient is experiencing an anaphylactoid reaction to iodinated contrast material

(D) The episode constitutes evidence that the patient has a paraneoplastic syndrome in which a tumor is producing histamine

(E) The cutaneous findings are angioedema due to lisinopril

20 Several months after an acute coronary event, you are seeing a 40-year-old man in follow-up in the clinic. In the course of left leg trauma from a motor vehicular accident, the patient sustained an inferior MI, for which you performed PCI of the right coronary artery, including placement of a stent. You noted during the catheterization that the coronary arteries appeared smooth and normal, with the exception of the right coronary occlusion, which had the appearance of a meniscus convex in the direction of vessel origin (retrograde), suggesting an embolic coronary occlusion, which could have occurred as a result of the leg trauma, rather than the inferior infarction. Following the interventional procedure, you had ordered an echocardiogram including contrast study, that was performed in the catheterization laboratory holding area, but it was a busy day in the laboratory, and the patient passed to the care of trauma surgery without disposition on the echo findings. In fact, the echo contrast study had demonstrated passage of contrast from the right atrium into the left atrium, consistent with a patent foramen ovale (PFO). As a result of the leg trauma, the patient underwent left below-the-knee amputation, and now will require reconstructive knee surgery. In the clinic, now several months later, your adept midlevel associate has uncovered the echo contrast result. What is the best approach to convey the overlooked echo contrast result to the patient?

(A) The echo contrast result should be conveyed to the patient as having been an incidental finding on the echo during the hospitalization

(B) A personal policy of full disclosure should be held by the physician, and in this case, the physician should explicitly relate to the patient that the echo contrast result was overlooked, followed by a discussion of the test's potential significance

(C) The echo result need not be discussed with the patient, because the findings are not germane to the present illness

(D) The interventional cardiologist should disclose the echo finding to the patient and tell him that it was the responsibility of the trauma surgeon to notify the patient of the echo finding

Answers and Explanations

1 Answer C. The EKG is diagnostic for an acute inferolateral STEMI. The results of the ISIS-4 trial (*Lancet*. 1995;345:669–685) demonstrated no survival benefit of nitrates in STEMI, and, therefore B is incorrect. Option C is the most rapid option for reperfusion. On the basis of the DANAMI-2 trial (*Am Heart J*. 2003;146:234–241) and earlier smaller studies, there is now emerging guideline consensus (*ACC/AHA 2004 Guideline Update*. 2004) that PCI has superior efficacy to thrombolytic therapy even when the patient with STEMI is transferred from a non–cath-capable hospital. The issue of coronary intervention for STEMI at sites without surgical backup is less clear. Aversano et al. (*JAMA*. 2002;287:1943–1951) have reported superior outcome in the 6-month composite endpoint of death, recurrent MI, and stroke in patients with STEMI randomly assigned to PCI at 11 community hospitals without surgery backup, compared with patients assigned to thrombolytic therapy. The 2005 revision of the American College of Cardiology/American Heart Association/Society of Cardiac Angiography and Interventions (ACC/AHA/SCAI) Guidelines for Percutaneous Coronary Intervention (*ACC/AHA 2005 Guideline Update*. 2006) states that emergency PCI without surgical backup has Class IIb indication, and should only be done at facilities with a proven plan for rapid access (within 1 hour) to a cardiac surgery operating room. This indication assumes that the hospital without a cardiac surgery program performs high-quality acute interventional procedures. At a practical level, there should be virtually no "practice-makes-perfect interval" series of cases for the operator and the catheterization laboratory team that performs acute percutaneous intervention without immediate access to surgery backup. If a hospital with no backup facility is incapable of offering acute intervention 24 hours, 7 days a week, the program should be considered suboptimal. In acute PCI, the current standard for door-to-balloon time is quickly evolving from 90 to 60 minutes, and perhaps even less when the patient who is known to have STEMI and is moving to a cath-capable facility. To be considered qualified to perform such acute cases, the operator must perform >75 PCIs per year, and the facility >36 PCIs per year. A program of performance assessment and continuous improvement should be in place, as is afforded by a database such as the National Cardiovascular Data Registry of the American College of Cardiology. In the event the operator at the facility with no backup does not meet these criteria, for the physician who first encounters the patient with acute STEMI there can be no constraint with regard to transfer of the patient to a larger cardiac center, particularly a patient with Killip Class 3 or 4 as described in this scenario.

2 Answer D. The 2005 ACC/Society for Cardiac Angiography and Intervention (SCAI) guidelines (*ACC/AHA 2005 Guideline Update*. 2006) on PCI address the requirements for accreditation to perform PCI. To reach and maintain proficiency in performing PCI, formal training in interventional cardiology in an accredited program is considered a requirement. The ACC/SCAI has published guidelines for levels of proficiency in adult cardiac catheterization and coronary intervention. Level III proficiency includes 12 months of formal accredited interventional cardiology training with performance of at least 250 coronary interventions as the primary operator. Maintaining proficiency requires >75 PCI cases per year. It is recommended that a physician who is not a full member of the hospital staff should not be given privileges in the cardiac catheterization laboratory. Regarding professional certification to perform coronary interventions, eligibility for the interventional cardiology board examination through the "practice pathway," that is, without having completed an Accredited Council for Graduate Medical Education (ACGME)-accredited interventional training program, ended in 2002, and, therefore, physicians should not be privileged to perform coronary interventions unless Board-certified or Board-eligible.

3 Answer D. The ethical choice for managing the patient is to ameliorate the unstable coronary lesion, and as long as the coronary intervention is uncomplicated, to carry out right iliac intervention as well because the patient has experienced leg pain at rest during the procedure, and schedule the patient to return at a later date for left anterior descending intervention. Had not the right iliac lesion been present and produced symptoms during the procedure, two-vessel coronary intervention at the same setting may well have been appropriate. Detailing options for treatment is part of the informed consent process, and therefore it would also have been appropriate before catheterization to discuss surgical revascularization as an option for managing selected subsets of coronary anatomy. In some instances, reimbursement may be influenced by whether multiple coronary interventions are carried out at the same or in different settings. In these cases, it is essential for the well-being of the patient that the interventional cardiologist's efforts be directed solely toward what is most right for the patient. In the absence of the peripheral artery situation described in the preceding text, it can be argued persuasively that the ethical approach would have been to perform the diagnostic procedure and two-vessel PCI at the same setting.

4 Answer C.   Further narcotics and benzodiazepines in this patient may not result in the desired level of sedation, and apnea could result. The interventional cardiologist is confronted with the ethical dilemma presented by not having deep sedation privileges. Lacking these, the interventional cardiologist does not have the authority to administer propofol, although this is the most medically optimal approach. Forcible restraints may keep the patient from contaminating the field, but they will not stop the patient's movement. A valid Advanced Cardiac Life Support (ACLS) card may not constitute sufficient expertise in airway management to afford the interventional cardiologist deep conscious sedation privileges. Although deep sedation during interventional procedures is rarely necessary, in our experience most such patients can safely be administered propofol without resorting to elective intubation of the patient, utilizing the deep conscious sedation monitoring protocol of the catheterization laboratory; however, it is incumbent upon the interventional cardiologist to have the appropriate hospital privilege, as otherwise, to administer a drug that has the potential to result in apnea would be unethical. If the cardiac catheterization laboratory is staffed by a full-time certified nurse anesthetist, this individual may administer drugs such as propofol, but under current nurse professional guidelines, as well as Joint Accreditation of Hospital Organization assessments, nurses with critical care qualifications are not authorized to administer deep sedation unless the patient is already intubated. Therefore, were he or she to have the appropriate privilege in the present case, the interventional cardiologist could break scrub and personally administer therapy of deep sedation.

5 Answer A.   Although the Internet–billboard scheme may not be appealing, there would be nothing unethical about such an advertising campaign. The remaining options are either unethical, illegal, or both. Option B constitutes payola, or a kickback

to the primary physician in return for the referral of a patient and is a prosecutable offense under the Medicare-Medicaid Anti-Kickback provision in Chapter 42 of the United States Code. Similarly, charging "insurance only" is considered Medicare fraud and is a practice that is prohibited by the Commission for Medicare and Medicaid Services. Any such *quid pro quo* arrangements are unethical. Similarly, the practice of referring patients for any procedure that is not indicated is to be decried. For a Medicare patient, it would constitute fraud.

6 Answer A.   This question poses a subtle, "I give you this, you do this for me," situation for the care provider. Although there is no monetary compensation being provided by the company, there is the potential for the company to benefit inappropriately from the prescription pattern that may develop in the provider, who may feel obligated to prescribe the company's name-brand drugs to reward the company for keeping the sample cabinet stocked with its proven therapy. Should the physician curtail the provision of samples to patients? As long as the practitioner remains vigilant about the potential for this type of conflict, and realizes there is no obligation to dispense the company drugs, the practice of dispensing samples will not create an unethical situation. The physician should specify in the progress note the dose and exactly how many units of samples were dispensed, as a means of documenting therapy.

7 Answer B.   Continued communication with the youngest son is essential to the well-being of this individual, who is grief-stricken, and the well-being of the family unit. Regarding clinical decisions about the patient, the physician is legally obligated to follow the instructions of the power of attorney, and the law is clear in this situation that only the power of attorney's signature constitutes valid informed consent. Therefore, whether the procedure was successful, Option A would result in legal action by the family. Option D is unsavory and comes close to an abdication of the physician's covenant to care for the patient, who should never be abandoned in time of medical need. Repeated compassionate communication by care providers and family virtually never fails to aid bereaved relatives such as the youngest son, and an approach by the physician in concert with other providers such as the patient's nurse can gently move the process forward.

8 Answer B.   The Federal Physician Self-Referral Law, also known as the Stark Law, USC section 1395nn) prohibits referrals by a physician for "designated health services" covered by Medicare or Medicaid to entities in which the physician has a financial relationship (broadly defined as an ownership interest or compensation agreement). As the following figure demonstrates, there has been dramatic growth in the volume of both invasive and noninvasive procedures over the past decade.

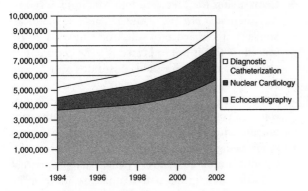

ACCF/AHA Consensus Conference Report on Professionalism and Ethics. 2004.

The Stark Law was conceived to curtail unnecessary usage of limited resources. The Medicare-Medicaid Anti-Kickback Statute (Chapter 42, United States Code Section 1320a–7b[b]) prohibits individuals or entities from knowingly and willfully offering, paying, soliciting, or receiving remuneration to induce referrals of items or services covered by Medicare or Medicaid. The Stark legislation is complex, but in essence is an attempt to control self-referrals motivated by personal or financial gain, hence creating overutilization of resources. The Stark Laws are distinct from the Anti-Kickback Statute in that Stark focuses on the financial aspects of referral relationships, and is a civil, rather than criminal statute (*J Am Coll Cardiol.* 2004;44:1740–1746).

9 **Answer A.** Transparency is the key to ensuring that the public and individual patients feel confident that we as cardiovascular clinician-researchers are keeping the public's best interests at the forefront of our activities. When activities such as the CME in the example present us with conflicts of interest, it is incumbent upon the physician to understand what the patient and fellow professionals expect regarding disclosure. The professional community has not been silent on these issues, and guidelines for conduct and disclosure are available. The 2004 ACC/AHA Consensus Conference Report on Professionalism and Ethics (*J Am Coll Cardiol.* 2004; 44:1722–1723) states that disclosure of financial arrangements should be mandatory for educational activities and scientific publications. The 2004 ACC/AHA guideline also states that relevant financial relationships between the clinical researcher and

industry should be defined in terms of levels of compensation and support: None, Modest (≤$10,000), and Significant (>$10,000). These levels are in keeping with previous guidelines offered by the NIH (*The National Institutes of Health.* 2004) and FDA (*The Food and Drug Administration.* 2000). In this case, the $7,500 the physician has been compensated, although considered "modest" under the guidelines, is clearly more than none and therefore should be disclosed by the physician when delivering talks, as well as when asking for patients' participation in the trial. It is required when enrolling subjects to ensure transparency of potential financial conflicts of interest to the trial participants and to the institutional review boards.

10 **Answer A.** Given your concerns regarding this conduct, it is most appropriate to first personally review your established policies regarding sexual harassment and promptly address the issue with the coworker and then perhaps with the entire catheterization laboratory staff. Stated succinctly, there should be zero tolerance for sexual harassment in the workplace. As the laboratory director, you have the obligation to ensure that all policies are current, available, and in practice on a daily basis in the catheterization laboratory. It is the supervisor's responsibility to provide a professional atmosphere and a safe, nonhostile working environment (*J Am Coll Cardiol.* 2001;37:2170–2214). Employees should participate in regular sexual harassment training and understand that harassment is a violation of federal, state, and local laws. The first federal guidelines regarding sexual harassment in the workplace were published by the Equal Employment Opportunity Commission (EEOC) in 1980. The EEOC is the federal organization that is responsible for enforcing and interpreting federal discrimination laws. The EEOC defines sexual harassment as:

■ Unwelcome sexual advances, requests for sexual favors, and other verbal or physical conduct of a sexual nature, where,

  ■ Submission to such conduct is made either implicitly or explicitly a term or condition of employment; or

  ■ Submission to or rejection of such conduct by an individual is used as a basis for employment decisions affecting the individual

■ Unwelcome sexual advances, requests for sexual favors, and other verbal or physical conduct of a sexual nature, where such conduct has the purpose or effect of unreasonably interfering with the individual's work performance or creating an intimidating, hostile, or offensive working environment. (*United States Equal Employment Opportunity Commission.* 2001:186–192).

In this case, it is reasonable to conclude that the explicit and suggestive behavior of the male colleague could interfere substantially with the ability of the female technician to carry out her work because the environment is offensive, hostile, and intimidating. Therefore such behavior must be considered inappropriate and a potential violation of federal antiharassment laws. If a "zero tolerance" policy is to be effective, there must be strict enforcement of the antiharassment policies and bylaws that are in place. Although in this scenario the female technician suggests that such explicit language and behavior does not excessively bother her, it is incumbent upon you as laboratory director to take the necessary actions to ensure that all staff members are free to work in a nonoffensive, nonhostile environment.

11 Answer B. Two ethical dilemmas arise from this patient scenario: (1) medical resource utilization and cost-containment, and (2) making recommendations that are in the best interest of the patient. In addition to the latter responsibility, the physician must be a steward of proper resource utilization, the use of which must never be based on personal financial gain or financial gain for his or her practice. Decisions should be made solely on medical merit, unless two or more equally effective modalities of diagnosis or treatment exist, and one is less expensive. "Self-referral" describes any situation in which a physician recommends a diagnostic or therapeutic plan from which the physician may personally benefit. Given that there is no way to eliminate all potential conflicts of interest from clinical practice, we must have strategies to ensure earnest and transparent practice to maintain the trust of patients as well as the trust of society. The 2004 ACC/AHA Consensus Conference on Professionalism and Ethics (*J Am Coll Cardiol.* 1995;44:1717–1761) outlines the following as part of an effective strategy to ensure appropriateness of testing and to minimize issues of self-referral:

- Use of evidence-based guidelines
- Physician and laboratory credentialing
- Periodic case conferences
- Oversight/review processes
- Consultation with other providers
- Full discussion with the patient regarding risks, benefit, alternatives, and the option for a second opinion
- Disclosure/transparency of ownership

Employing such a strategy, we can minimize potential abuses and maintain the trust of patients and colleagues. In the present scenario, the cardiologist appears to be following traditional practice patterns and available guidelines in the initial noninvasive portion of the evaluation. However, recent data regarding gender bias in invasive cardiovascular testing notwithstanding, the *a priori* odds of a positive test in this patient, based on age and gender, are very low, and there is significant risk of a false-positive test. One may argue that the physician was concerned enough about the patient that the original stress test was pursued. Given the absence of typical chest pain and electrocardiographic changes, the scintigraphic result probably should be interpreted as being due to diaphragmatic or breast attenuation. Certainly, the test cannot be interpreted as high risk by any criteria. Preauthorization of the catheterization by the patient's insurance carrier would be obtained by the physician's office because of the positive interpretation of test; however, such an indication for a procedure would be looked upon with skepticism in a cardiac catheterization conference with peers. Although there may be reasonable doubt about the merits of performing the catheterization, the PCI is probably not indicated. Further, during diagnostic procedures in which lesions of questionable severity are identified, the technique of Fractional Flow Reserve (*Circulation.* 1995;92:3183–3193) of Pijls et al. should be utilized to evaluate functional significance. It is at the point that the interventional cardiologist performs PCI on the nonhemodynamically significant lesion that he strays from a course that would pass a rigorous review or application of available guidelines. One could argue that the intervention would not be based on medical merit, but rather on the physician's personal and/or financial interests. It is in such cases that self-referral can work to the detriment of the patient, society, and the profession.

12 Answer D. The exact risks of coronary interventional procedures vary on a case-by-case basis according to a mix of clinical and procedural characteristics, which can be predicted with relative accuracy before the procedure, and these risks are part of the informed consent process for each patient. Peripheral vascular complications are the most common morbidity encountered in the setting of PCI and, arguably, although still relatively uncommon, have become more frequent in an era of potent antiplatelet and anticoagulant drugs. Serious vascular access complications include hematomas with significant blood loss, arterial pseudoaneurysm, and arteriovenous fistulas, and to this list, RPH should probably be added as an access complication. Data from trials such as CAVEAT-1 (*J Am Coll Cardiol*. 1995;26:922–930) indicate that the frequency of such complications ranges from 3% to 5% in noncomplex PCI. Results from the Evaluation of c7E3 for the Prevention of Ischemic Complications (EPIC) trial (*Am J Cardiol*. 1998;81:36–40) demonstrate that more potent anticoagulant and antiplatelet regimens do increase risk of minor and major bleeding. Konstance et al. (*J Interv Cardiol*. 2004;17:65–70) examined independent clinical and procedural risk factors for major vascular complications, and determined that *stent usage* is the strongest independent predictor of a vascular access complication in univariate and multivariate analysis. Age >65 and female gender are both independent risk predictors for vascular access complications as well. Sheath size has been shown to be associated with vascular complications, with studies showing up to fivefold increases in vascular access complication rates when upgrading from a 6F to an 8F sheath. Use of anticoagulants and procedure duration may play a role. The use of a mechanical clamp for hemostasis increases the risk of complication, but is not as strongly associated as is the use of stents, female sex, or sheath size.

13 Answer B. A review of the literature shows that unadjusted in-hospital mortality following PCI is approximately 0.5% to 1.5%. Abrupt coronary artery occlusion with associated left ventricular failure is noted as the primary cause of PCI-associated mortality. The clinical and angiographic variables associated with increased mortality include advanced age, female gender, diabetes, prior MI, multivessel disease, left main or equivalent coronary disease, a large area of myocardium at risk, preexisting impairment of left ventricular dysfunction or abnormal renal function, and collateral vessels supplying significant areas of myocardium that originate distal to the segment to be dilated. However, unadjusted mortality rates do not take into account the different settings in which PCI is performed or certain patient characteristics that may influence outcome. To date, six multivariate models have been published that can be utilized to estimate the mortality risk of PCI (*Circulation*. 1997;95:2479–2484, *JAMA*. 1997;277:892–898, *Circulation*. 2003;107:1871–1876, *J Am Coll Cardiol*. 1999;34:674–680, *Circulation*. 2001;104:263–268, *J Am Coll Cardiol*. 2002;39: 1104–1112). Findings from the American College of Cardiology National Cardiovascular Data Registry indicate a univariate mortality rate of 0.5% for patients undergoing elective PCI, a mortality rate of 5.1% for patients undergoing primary

PCI within 6 hours of the onset of STEMI, and a mortality rate of 28% for patients undergoing PCI for cardiogenic shock (*J Am Coll Cardiol*. 2002;39:1104–1112). Therefore, stratification by clinical setting of PCI is helpful in estimating individual patient mortality risk.

14 Answer E. A recent article by Farouque et al. from Stanford University Medical Center retrospectively evaluated the incidence, features, and risk factors for the formation of RPH in 3,508 patients undergoing PCI in which current techniques including glycoprotein IIb/IIIa receptor antagonists were utilized. Approximately one-third of these patients had presented with an acute coronary syndrome. The authors demonstrated that the variable, which conferred the most RPH formation was BSA <1.73 m^2. In multivariate analysis, relatively small BSA conferred an odds ratio of 7.1 ($p = 0.008$) for RPH formation. Female gender was also a significant factor, conferring an odds ratio of 5.4 for RPH ($p = 0.005$). The only other predictor showing statistical significance in multivariate analysis was high femoral puncture site, defined as above the middle third of the femoral head on fluoroscopy (OR 5.3, $p = 0.013$). Using linear regression analysis the authors also demonstrated a correlation between BSA and femoral artery size, and therefore, femoral artery size may have a role in RPH. The incidence of RPH in this study was 0.74%, and mortality associated with RPH 4%, similar to previous studies (*J Am Coll Cardiol*. 2005;45:363–368).

15 Answer A. The development of ARF or ARFD after PCI is a marker for poor outcomes. Multiple studies have now shown that both in-hospital and long-term mortality increase significantly in patients developing ARF, and even more in patients who require dialysis. The incidence of ARF after PCI is approximately 3%. Studies have demonstrated that preexisting renal insufficiency confers the highest risk for developing ARF after PCI. The incidence increases linearly with increasing baseline creatinine levels. A history of diabetes, congestive heart failure, and acute MI are among other risk factors that significantly increase the chance of developing ARF (*Circulation*. 2002;105:2259–2264). ARF is usually defined as a >25% rise in serum creatinine over baseline levels. In a retrospective analysis of the Mayo Clinic PCI registry, Rihal et al. evaluated the incidence and prognostic importance of ARF following PCI. Of the 7,586 patients included, there was a 22% in-hospital mortality rate in patients developing ARF compared with a mortality of 1.4% in patients who did not. The trend toward higher mortality was also noted at 1 and 5 years of follow-up (*Circulation.* 2002;105:2259–2264). Regarding preexisting renal insufficiency, Gruberg et al. evaluated 439 consecutive patients undergoing PCI in a tertiary facility who were not on dialysis but with a baseline serum creatinine >1.8 mg per dL. Patients developing a >25% increase over baseline creatinine had an in-hospital mortality of 14.9%, versus 4.9% in those with no such increase in creatinine. In patients requiring dialysis, the in-hospital mortality was 22.6%. The cumulative 1-year mortality was 45.2% for those who required dialysis, 35.4% for those who did not require dialysis, and 19.4% for patients with no creatinine increase ($p = 0.001$) (*J Am Coll Cardiol.* 2000;36:1542–1548). The development of ARF or the need for dialysis following PCI portends poorer outcomes both in-hospital and over time. Other than preprocedural shock, the strongest predictor of in-hospital death following PCI is the development of ARF (*Circulation.* 2002;105:2259–2264) (*Am J Med.* 1997;103:368–375).

16 Answer D. Situations such as this are relatively common for the interventional cardiologist. The issue of advance directives (ADs), advanced care plans (ACPs), Living Wills, and DNR orders will become increasingly prominent in cardiovascular medicine practice as the patient population continues to age and with the presentation of patients who have higher morbidity. Individuals have the right to forgo potentially life-sustaining treatment based on the principle of patient autonomy, which is the ethical centerpiece of the doctor–patient relationship. In this case, the patient, although in a competent state, has expressed directly to you that he desires not to have any further invasive procedures, even in an emergency. In patients who cannot make competent decisions, the issue of substitute decision making arises. The "substitute" decision maker must seek to approximate the patient's wishes. Who can legally assume the role of substitute decision maker and act as a proxy for the patient, as well as manage legal aspects of ADs, ACPs, Living Wills, and DNR orders, may vary by jurisdiction. However, the underlying ethical principles that guide therapy in this situation should not vary, and it is paramount to respect patient autonomy and decision making, recognizing that patients do have the right to refuse potentially life-saving therapies. In approximating the decision a patient would make if capable, one must consider in decreasing order of priority the patient's *wishes*, the patient's *values and beliefs*, and finally the patient's *best interests* (*J Am Coll Cardiol.* 1998;31:917–925). In the present scenario the patient's wishes are clear: He does not want any further invasive procedures, and he does not wish to be resuscitated in the event

of an emergency. Clearly, a key responsibility in the physician's job description is to inform, counsel, and guide patients and families through this process. The choice of starting pressor drugs and using bag-mask ventilation is not appealing, because these treatments are often precluded in the setting of a DNR order. Physicians should familiarize themselves with state law and advance directive policies in their practice settings. In the present case, there is ample information about the patient's prior wishes to proceed with more conservative noninvasive therapy, although we personally may feel that PCI is the best option. This approach ultimately respects the patient's autonomy and protects his trust.

17 Answer B. In this scenario, in which the first interaction with the patient is in the catheterization laboratory itself, the interventional cardiologist has a duty to advise the patient of his/her assessment of the findings and to cancel the procedure. It is ethically inappropriate for the interventional cardiologist to perform a procedure that he/she in fact judges to not be indicated, and in the present scenario would amount to a failure to take part in the clinical decision-making process. It would be better that the interventional physician does what he or she judges to be the right thing for the patient, than to later have to reconcile a complication during a nonindicated procedure. In our experience, colleagues will virtually always understand such a change in management when the physician's best judgment is the basis for taking the alternate approach. The interventional physician's responsibility is to be an advocate for the patient, to be free of avoidable conflicts of interest in decision making, and always use ethical judgment in providing patient care. The interventional physician must ultimately be responsible for determining the appropriateness and timing of any planned procedure, as well as ensuring that the patient is informed of the various options, risks, and benefits of any planned procedures. (*Catheter Cardiovasc Interv.* 2004;61:157–162).

18 Answer D. Neglect of ensuring proper informed consent can occur. The concept of informed consent is integral to the good clinical practice of any physician. Appropriate informed consent procedures must be maintained and constitute the main method of demonstrating respect for patient autonomy, and protecting the patient's trust in the physician. In the present scenario, the interventional cardiologist must spend adequate time to ensure that the patient possesses competence to understand the risks, benefits, and alternatives to the procedure, and does so with autonomy, that is, free of undue influence or coercion. Generally accepted essential elements of informed consent include (*Nurs Crit Care.* 1996;1:127–133):

- Documentation of full disclosure of the risks and benefits of the planned procedure
- Demonstration that the patient possesses the proper understanding of the planned procedure
- Demonstration of patient competence to understand the procedure as well as the risks and benefits it entails
- Demonstration of autonomy to make decisions regarding care without undo influence or coercion
- Documentation that the patient, after having displayed competence, understanding, and autonomy, has authorized the operator to proceed with the planned procedure

In the present scenario, the patient has been mentally capable of presenting a cogent history of exertional dyspnea, indicating that the patient should be considered competent to consent to a procedure intended to relieve these symptoms. As a general rule, the patient should be considered competent to provide informed consent unless there is a legally authorized health care power of attorney.

19 Answer C. Although it is possible that an individual could experience an anaphylactic reaction in response to iodinated contrast material, the incidence of immunoglobulin E (IgE) antibodies in patients who have sustained immediate hypersensitivity reactions in the cath laboratory is vanishingly low, and the likelihood is that the patient is experiencing an anaphylactoid reaction, probably to iodinated contrast material. Angioedema due to lisinopril would be in the differential, but is unlikely because the patient has been taking this drug for several years. So-called anaphylactoid reactions to contrast material are uncommon, especially in the era of low-osmolality and isosmolar contrast agents, but such reactions do occur and have manifestations similar to the classic anaphylactic reaction. Anaphylactoid reactions, as can be judged by the name, are non–immune mediated and are characterized by the release of vasoactive substances such as histamine and serotonin, presumably through a cytokine mechanism that is triggered by contrast administration, leading to the development of urticaria, indigestion, and hypotension that is usually manageable by volume expansion. Iodine contained in the contrast material is not necessarily the anaphylactoid trigger. The "queasy stomach" is a clinical sign of endogenous histamine release giving rise to secretion of stomach acid. If the patient in fact had IgE antibody to contrast material, an

anaphylactic reaction would have been likely to occur immediately upon the initial administration of contrast, and would have been associated with laryngeal edema and stridor, which the patient does not have. There is some delay in the development of a contrast reaction, as described in the scenario. Treatment consists of volume expansion, intravenous diphenhydramine and H2 receptor blocker, and intravenous glucocorticoid. Completion of the patient's interventional procedure might have to be delayed, but it would rarely be necessary to stop the procedure and reschedule to another sitting. It is possible that the patient is experiencing a delayed hypersensitivity reaction to the soft-shell crab, but such a reaction would most probably have awakened the patient in the middle of the night before the procedure.

20 Answer B. Honesty, coupled with full disclosure, is always the best policy when disclosing medical errors. The physician has only to fully disclose the echo contrast findings to the patient, explicitly take responsibility that the oversight was his error alone, and the patient, although perhaps briefly dismayed about this health history development, will immediately or soon see that the physician has the patient's best interest as his first priority. Any approach other than full disclosure constitutes dissembling, and there could be no other conclusion by the patient in that event other than the physician wishes to hide something. Fortunately in the present scenario, nothing untoward has occurred as a result of the patient's PFO, but the possibility of paradoxic embolism as a cause of MI must be introduced to the patient. Not only for situations such as the present scenario but also for serious errors of commission or omission, an approach of full disclosure allows the physician to proceed without emotional encumbrances, feelings of guilt for not having been forthcoming to the patient, and in the present case allows the physician to proceed with a positive discussion regarding management of the PFO, including the odds that the patient's left leg trauma resulted in either a thromboembolism or fat embolism that could have passed paradoxically to the right coronary artery. Lack of full disclosure leads down the path to repeated dissembling after dissembling, and, appropriately so, loss of the patient's trust, dissolution of the physician–patient relationship, and litigation. Litigation risk is not the reason to be honest, patient trust and care are. Breach of the physician–patient relationship as result of dishonesty will likely result in litigation (*Arch Intern Med.* 2005;165:1819–1824, *Ann Intern Med.* 1999;131:963–967, *Acta Anaesthesiol Scand.* 2005;49:728–734).

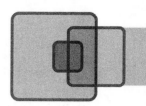

39

Statistics Related to Interventional Cardiology Procedures

Robert A. Harrington and Karen S. Pieper

Questions

1 You are the director of a community-based catheterization laboratory that performs approximately 500 percutaneous coronary interventions (PCIs) per year. As part of a quality improvement initiative, you have introduced a PCI database into practice that collects information at the time of the procedure and over the first year following discharge. One year ago, you introduced a new drug-eluting stent into the laboratory practice. It quickly became popular and now accounts for approximately one third of the procedures in the laboratory. One of your clinical colleagues is concerned that there have been several recent cases of subacute stent thrombosis and wonders if these events can be attributed to the new stent. What is the most appropriate study design to get information quickly in your practice setting that might be useful in addressing the question posed by your clinical colleague?

(A) Randomized clinical trial
(B) Case–control study
(C) Cohort study
(D) Nonrandomized observational registry

2 The Framingham Heart Study can best be described as what type of clinical study?

(A) Randomized clinical trial
(B) Case–control study

(C) Cohort study
(D) Community intervention study

3 One of your patients, who has been postmenopausal for several years and who suffered a non–ST-segment elevation myocardial infarction (NSTEMI) 2 years ago, asks you for a recommendation regarding hormone replacement therapy (HRT) to lower her risk of having a second heart attack. You review the literature on this topic and find divergent study results. Large observational databases such as the Nurses' Health Study suggest a very impressive reduction in the risk of ischemic events in women taking hormone therapies, but other data from large, well-powered randomized trials suggest that there is no benefit for this endpoint associated with HRT. What do you do?

(A) Recommend HRT since the effect reported in the observational studies is just too large to ignore
(B) Recommend HRT, because although the benefits are not clear, it likely does not cause harm
(C) Recommend against HRT because she is currently asymptomatic
(D) Recommend against HRT because there is no benefit seen in randomized controlled trials (RCTs), including in women with previously known ischemic heart disease

4 The following are all surrogate endpoints measured in recent clinical trials, *except*:

(A) Low-density lipoprotein (LDL) cholesterol levels
(B) High-density lipoprotein (HDL) cholesterol levels
(C) TIMI (thrombolysis in myocardial infarction) blood flow
(D) Systolic blood pressure
(E) Recurrent ischemia

5 Glycoprotein IIb/IIIa platelet inhibitors may be used as adjunctive pharmacotherapy during PCI. As you consider whether or not to use these therapies during a procedure, you review the available data from clinical studies. Eptifibatide has been shown to reduce the risk of which of these clinical events significantly, compared with placebo?

(A) All-cause mortality
(B) Cardiovascular mortality
(C) Bleeding
(D) Thrombocytopenia
(E) The composite of death, myocardial infarction (MI), urgent revascularization, or thrombotic bailout

6 You have been approached to help in the planning of a multicenter study that will examine a potential difference in the restenosis rate of two commonly used drug-eluting stents. The plan is to conduct a randomized controlled trial. As you begin discussions with your colleagues and the study sponsor, the first question that might arise is how many subjects will be needed for an adequate experiment. Which factor is *not* relevant to the ensuing scientific discussions?

(A) Anticipated event rate in the control group
(B) Estimated difference between the groups
(C) Amount of time required to complete enrollment
(D) Composition of the primary endpoint

7 A recently completed, randomized, active control clinical trial comparing new drug A with old drug B reports a 15% improvement with the new drug, $p = 0.06$. What is the most appropriate interpretation of these results?

(A) Drug A is comparable to Drug B
(B) Drug A is definitely inferior to Drug B
(C) Drug A is not statistically superior to Drug B
(D) Drug A is statistically superior to Drug B

8 You are part of a proposed study's steering committee that has been charged with designing a clinical trial to test whether new stent A is better than old stent B. The new stent has many attractive design features and your research group would like to be sure that the study is large enough to definitively conclude that stent A is truly superior to stent B if the rates hypothesized are seen. Which component of sample size calculation does this refer to?

(A) Type II error
(B) Type I error
(C) Number needed to treat (NNT)
(D) Study *p* value

9 In the following figure, which study demonstrates superiority of Drug X over Drug Y?

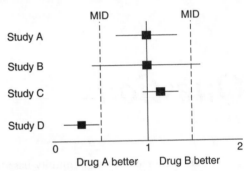

MID: Minimally important difference

(A) Study A
(B) Study B
(C) Study C
(D) Study D

10 In the figure in Question 9, which study demonstrates equivalence between Drug X and Drug Y?

(A) Study A
(B) Studies A and B
(C) Studies A and C
(D) Studies A, C, and D

11 In the figure in Question 9, which study demonstrates noninferiority between Drug X and Drug Y?

(A) Study A
(B) Studies A and B
(C) Studies A and C
(D) Studies A, C, and D

12 For which of the following reason(s) is blinding (or "masking") in a clinical trial important?

(A) It helps prevent introduction of treatment-specific biases
(B) It helps maintain objectivity in assessment of clinical events

(C) It preserves Type I error rate

(D) A and B

13 You are reviewing a manuscript reporting randomized clinical trial results for possible publication in a leading cardiovascular journal. As reported in the "Methods" section of the manuscript, the primary endpoint analysis was performed on the population who received the study medication "as intended." You read further and realize that the paper's primary analysis excludes all of the randomized patients whom the investigators felt did not meet the study's eligibility criteria. In your critique of the paper, which principle of good clinical research do you note that the authors may have violated?

(A) Avoiding Type II error

(B) Ensuring adequate sample size

(C) Blinding

(D) Conducting intention-to-treat (ITT) analysis

14 You are interpreting the results of a clinical trial that compared fibrinolysis with primary angioplasty for ST-segment elevation acute myocardial infarction. There were 6,600 patients randomly assigned to one of two treatments, with 3,300 patients in each group. If there were 300 deaths in the lysis group and 200 deaths in the PCI group, what is the odds ratio (OR) that most appropriately compares the two groups?

(A) 0.65

(B) 0.10

(C) 0.065

(D) 9.1%

15 In a clinical study, the absolute difference between a new drug and placebo for the endpoint of 30-day myocardial infarction is reported to be 2.0%. Your local formulary committee asks you to put this into clinical context and provide them the number needed to treat (NNT) with the new drug to prevent one myocardial infarction. In this example, the NNT is:

(A) 2

(B) Unable to calculate with the information provided

(C) 50

(D) 30

16 Some of the ways to describe continuous data include:

(A) Medians

(B) Means

(C) Interquartile ranges

(D) Standard deviations

(E) All of the above

17 As you read the medical literature, you note that p values are variously reported as being significant at very different levels, including ones listed as <0.05 and others listed as <0.01. Which of the following is most helpful in interpreting the reported clinical data?

(A) "Lower is better"

(B) "Higher is better"

(C) The pretest nominal p value

(D) Any p value <0.05 is considered significant

18 The 95% CI around a point estimate is identical to a study's p value. True or false?

(A) True

(B) False

19 A randomized clinical trial comparing two commonly used intracoronary stents was designed to test whether there were fewer adverse cardiac events with stent A than with stent B. The primary endpoint was a composite of death, MI, or target vessel revascularization at 9 months. The trial results showed that patients treated with stent A had a significant reduction in the occurrence of the primary endpoint compared with patients treated with stent B. Advocates of stent B point out that in a subgroup of patients with diabetes mellitus, there was no significant difference between the two stents with regard to the primary endpoint. You conclude the following:

(A) Diabetic patients can be treated with either stent

(B) The overall study results contain the most information

(C) Diabetic patients should be treated with stent B

(D) Neither stent reduces ischemic events among diabetic patients

20 The American College of Cardiology/American Heart Association (ACC/AHA) Practice Guidelines provide clinical practice recommendations on a variety of common diseases and cardiovascular procedures. Class I recommendations should only be followed if there are no reasonable alternatives for care. True or false?

(A) True

(B) False

21 A new device is introduced into the catheterization laboratory and is touted as "breakthrough" technology that will change the way you practice. The new device is quite expensive, and you, as the catheterization laboratory director, are worried about the effect that use of this new device will have on your catheterization laboratory budget. Cost-effectiveness is an important concept for you to consider when assessing the new technology. This might best be defined as:

(A) How much more expensive the new device is over standard therapies

(B) The laboratory's mix of privately insured patients versus Medicare patients

(C) The incremental amount of money required to produce additional clinical benefit

(D) The laboratory's negotiated price from the device vendor

Answers and Explanations

1 **Answer B.** The case–control study is well suited for providing preliminary information on a question using previously collected data (*Circulation*. 1996;93:667–671). Since you can identify patients who have experienced stent thrombosis and a matched group who have not, you should be able to get some preliminary information regarding the factors that are associated with the outcome. There are problems with the case–control study; most notably, bias that arises from the data already collected before occurrence of the event. Randomized trials provide the overall best method of evaluating and comparing treatments, but such studies are much larger and take longer than is practical to provide insight into this colleague's question.

2 **Answer C.** The Framingham Heart Study is an example of a cohort study (*Am J Public Health*. 1951;41:279–281). Patients are identified in a community and are followed for a long time, with periodic assessments to observe outcomes. Patients are examined as having some characteristic habits(e.g., smoking) and defined as an "exposed" group. They may be compared with a "nonexposed group" to allow insight into the effects of exposure over time. There are no attempts to introduce an intervention in this study, either randomized or nonrandomized.

3 **Answer D.** RCTs are preferred over observational studies when assessing the potential benefit of an intervention. Without randomization, there is no adequate way to balance the biases and confounders that exist in all observational assessments of a therapy. RCTs provide the strongest evidence of causation when evaluating a drug or device. Practice decisions regarding therapeutics are most appropriately made using RCT data, when available. This is why the ACC/AHA Guidelines give RCT data the highest weight of evidence when considering recommendations.

4 **Answer E.** Recurrent ischemia is a clinical endpoint, often measured in clinical trials of acute ischemic heart disease or those involving PCI. Surrogate endpoints typically refer to biomarkers, such as laboratory values or physical signs, which by their measurement are intended to provide information about actual clinical events. Validated surrogates have been shown repeatedly to be directly linked to clinical events of interest. An example of a validated surrogate is reduction in levels of LDL cholesterol with statin therapy (*Arch Intern Med*. 1999;159:1793–1802). In multiple studies, there is a highly predictable relationship between LDL cholesterol levels achieved through statin therapy and ischemic cardiac events, including death. Clinical studies typically use biomarkers for endpoints to learn about the biological effects of an intervention or, more frequently, because the measurement of biomarkers allows for the use of a smaller sample size, despite the less frequent occurrence of clinical events.

5 **Answer E.** Eptifibatide was shown in the Enhanced Suppression of the Platelet IIb/IIIa Receptor with Integrilin Therapy (ESPRIT) trial to significantly reduce the 48-hour composite endpoint of death, MI, or repeat revascularization compared with placebo (*Lancet*. 2000;356:2037–2044). There was no significant reduction in either mortality or cardiovascular mortality seen in ESPRIT with eptifibatide.

Composite endpoints are frequently used in clinical trials to capture many or most of the events of interest that might be affected with the therapy (drug or device) under investigation. The components are usually related events; for example, in this case they are all ischemic complications of PCI. More recently, composite endpoints have been constructed to combine both the ischemic and hemorrhagic events of interest, thereby creating a composite of "net clinical benefit." Examples of this include composite endpoints that include mortality plus intracranial hemorrhage in acute MI fibrinolytic trials.

On a practical level, composite endpoints are employed mostly because the larger number of events may allow a smaller sample size to be used in the study. When interpreting a potential treatment effect upon composite endpoints, it is a good practice always to examine the individual composites with an eye to consistency of the effect, recognizing that it is unlikely that there will be a significant effect found on any individual component due to statistical power issues.

6 **Answer C.** While the length of time required to enroll patients into the study is an important part of feasibility discussions and considerations, it does not affect the total number of patients required to adequately answer the question of interest.

Calculation of sample size depends on multiple factors, including the Type I error rate, the Type II error rate, the endpoint to be analyzed, the estimated value for the endpoint occurring in the control arm, the estimated improvement in the treatment arm, the amount of variation in the endpoint measured, and the statistical method to be used in analyzing the endpoint. Sample size is also influenced by the decision to undertake a superiority, noninferiority, or equivalence trial.

7   Answer C. Trials that compare therapeutic strategies frequently are designed to test whether the new or experimental therapy is better than (superior to) a control therapy. The control therapy might be a placebo or it might be an established therapy, often referred to as an active control. Sample size calculation for clinical trials requires that the investigator consider the acceptable Type I error (α). A Type I error is when an effect is observed when in truth no effect exists. By convention, in most cardiovascular clinical experiments the Type I error rate is set at 5% (0.05) (*Ann Epidemiol.* 1998;8:351–357). For example, if the same experiment was repeated 1,000 times, then by chance alone there would be 50 studies that demonstrated that the experimental agent was superior to the control therapy even if there was no difference between the therapies. Nominal statistical significance requires the testing procedure to have a significance level less than or equal to this ($p \leq 0.05$). In the example above, although there is a measured difference between the treatments, the conventional Type I error has been exceeded; therefore, we cannot conclude that A is superior to B. Although the reported p value is very close to 0.05, we cannot conclude comparability of the treatments without more information on aspects such as formal testing for noninferiority.

8   Answer A. The Type II error (β) occurs when no effect is seen between the studied treatments when in fact a treatment effect truly exists. One minus the Type II error ($1 - \beta$) is also known as the *trial's power*. By understanding the risk of a Type II error, or conversely, the importance of power in examining clinical trial results, one can appreciate whether a study actually had adequate power or was truly large enough in size to answer the desired question. Many studies that fail to show a statistical difference between therapies suffer from a lack of power; that is, the study design accepted a large potential Type II error (*Prog Cardiovasc Dis.* 1985;27:335–371). By convention, a well-powered clinical trial accepts a potential β error of <10% to no more than 20%. In the example given, one would want to be sure that the planned trial had a minimum of 80% power (but preferably $\geq$90%) to definitively conclude that stent A was truly superior to stent B.

9   Answer D. In Study D, all of the values of the CI fall on the side of the chart where Drug A is better than Drug B, thereby showing statistical superiority. A superiority trial tests for statistically and clinically significant improvement (or harm) resulting from the use of the experimental treatment compared with the standard of care. By contrast, an equivalence trial is designed to assess whether the difference in outcome for the experimental treatment compared with the standard treatment lies within the boundary of a clinically defined minimally important difference (MID).

10   Answer C. Both Studies A and C fall within the bounds of the MID. The MID represents the largest difference in outcome between the experimental and standard groups that can be accepted while still considering them clinically comparable. The results of a noninferiority trial are assessed under the assumption that the experimental treatment is not worse than the standard of care by some clinically meaningful amount. Noninferiority studies, unlike equivalence studies, are not designed to identify incremental improvements over the experimental therapy, although the MID is still utilized in fixing the noninferiority boundary. This can be viewed as a one-sided test, as opposed to the two-sided evaluation that is the hallmark of equivalence.

11   Answer D. We are interested in whether the CI falls below the bound for Drug B being better than Drug A. Even though Study D is statistically superior, if the study had been designed for noninferiority, noninferiority would have been met. As therapies for acute cardiovascular disease proliferate, equivalence and noninferiority trials are becoming critical in assessing the therapeutic value of new drugs and devices. Noninferiority and equivalence trials are most useful when the experimental therapy is unlikely to prove superior to established therapy, but may provide incremental benefit. These benefits may include a reduction in adverse events, easier administration of the therapeutic agent, or reduced cost. For both noninferiority and equivalence studies, establishing the MID boundary is of primary importance.

12   Answer D. Blinding in a clinical trial can reduce the likelihood of biased behavior on the part of investigators, patients, or other study personnel. For example, knowledge of the treatment assignment might cause an investigator to look harder for certain drug effects, both expected and unexpected. For trials that include an independent assessment of the study's endpoint events, such as review by a clinical events committee, blinding is essential to maintain the integrity of a process that relies on a completely objective determination of suspected endpoint events (*Curr Control Trials Cardiovasc Med.* 2001;2:180–186).

13 Answer D. An important concept in the evaluation of clinical studies is analysis according to the ITT principle. This means that patients are analyzed according to the group to which they were randomly assigned. Most strictly defined, any patient who gives informed consent and who is randomly assigned to a treatment remains in that treatment arm for the purpose of analysis, even if that patient drops out before receiving treatment or receives a treatment other than the one allocated.

A variation on this is the ITT-treated analysis. In this frequently performed adaptation of the ITT analysis, patients remain in the group to which they were randomly assigned for the purpose of analysis, but only those patients who actually received the treatment are considered in the primary analysis. The investigator must be blinded to the treatment the patient is to receive when deciding to withhold treatment, if the analysis is to remain valid. In the example described, additional patients believed to be ineligible for the study were removed from the primary analysis. Although these types of analyses are sometimes performed as a "per protocol" analysis, they lack the rigor provided by adherence to the ITT principle and should be reserved for secondary, hypothesis-generating analyses.

14 Answer A. ORs and risk ratios are two of the more common ways to display comparative data in the medical literature. To calculate the odds of having an event in any one group, we divide the number of events in that group by the number of patients in that group who did not have an event. The OR is the ratio of those two odds. Risk is calculated by dividing the number of events by the total number of patients in a group. Risk ratios are then calculated by dividing the risks of the individual groups. In the example given, the odds of dying in the lysis group are 0.10 (300/3,000) and 0.065 (200/3,100) in the PCI group. This provides an OR of 0.65 (0.064/0.10).

15 Answer C. The NNT refers to the number of patients who would need to be treated with a therapy to prevent one adverse outcome. We can calculate the NNT by dividing 1 by the absolute risk reduction. In this case, a 2% absolute reduction means that on average 2 out of every 100 patients receiving the new drug had fewer events than 100 patients without the new drug. In our example, we divide 1.0 by 0.02. Therefore, 50 patients must be treated with this new therapy to prevent one MI.

16 Answer E. To describe continuous data, we can calculate measures of the center of the distribution. For example, the mean is the average of the measures and the median is the middle value, or 50th percentile, of the distribution. Measures of the variability around the center might be described as the range of the data (maximum value–minimum value), the standard deviation or variance, or percentile (e.g., 25th to 75th).

17 Answer C. A *p* value is the probability of obtaining the results (or even more extreme results) observed, if the effect is really due to random chance alone. For example, a *p* value of ≤0.05 indicates that a difference of at least the amount observed in the experiment would occur in ≤50 out of 1,000 similar experiments if the treatment studied had no effect on the measured outcome.

Before conducting a clinical study, one must prospectively state the hypothesis being tested, the statistical test that will be used on this hypothesis (to reject the null hypothesis, meaning the rejection of the statement that there is no difference between the treatment groups), and the critical (or nominal) value for declaring significance (the Type I error rate). By convention, the nominal value for declaring significance in much medical research is set at 0.05. However, it is appropriate for certain types of studies to set a different level of nominal significance, for example at 0.025 or 0.001. The key concept is that the level of significance is determined by the pretest establishment of the Type I error (*Ann Epidemiol.* 1998;8:351–357).

18 Answer B. Although CIs are complementary to a study's *p* value, they are not the same. The 95% CI that surrounds a study's point estimate of effect (perhaps an OR or risk ratio) suggests that if one were to perform this same experiment an infinite number of times, then 95% of the estimates of the effect would fall within the bounds of that interval. Because a ratio of two identical rates gives a value of 1, a CI that overlaps 1 implies that any treatment difference is not statistically different or significant. An interval that does not include 1 implies statistical significance.

19 Answer B. Clinical trials are typically designed and powered to answer one question, represented by the primary endpoint. Subgroups of patients, defined by patient or disease characteristics, are best viewed for consistency. If there is a positive treatment effect in favor of one therapy over another, there may well be *quantitative* differences in the magnitude of the observed treatment effect that favor certain subgroups, but it is unlikely that there will be important *qualitative* differences among subgroups. The most appropriate way to view randomized clinical trial results is from the perspective of the overall trial results.

20 Answer B. Class I recommendations describe interventions believed, on the basis of the preponderance of current scientific evidence, to be useful and effective; Class III recommendations are given to interventions that are considered useless or ineffective,

or even potentially harmful. Class II recommendations describe intermediate circumstances, where evidence for or against a therapy is equivocal. Class IIa recommendations denote conflicting evidence, but with an overall tilt toward benefit; Class IIb recommendations also indicate conflicting evidence or opinion, but in this case the evidence leans against benefit (*Circulation*. 2003;107:2979–2986).

21 Answer C. Cost-effectiveness is best defined as the incremental amount of money required to produce additional clinical benefit. It is typically defined in terms of added life years or quality-adjusted life years (QALY). At least one societal benchmark that has been used in assessing the economic feasibility in the adoption of new therapies is whether the therapy is in the range of $50,000/QALY gained (*Am Heart J*. 1999;137:S38–S40).

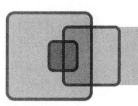

40

Approach to Interventional Boards and Test-Taking Strategies

Joseph Babb and Steven R. Daugherty

Questions

1 You have just finished reading through all of your study materials for the Board examination and you have some additional time before the date at which you are scheduled to take the same. To make the best use of this remaining preparation time you should:

(A) Do as many practice questions as possible in the time you have left
(B) Do some practice questions and let the ones you get wrong tell you what to go back and study again
(C) Find and review new study material to give you an alternative perspective on the core concepts for the examination
(D) Read over your study materials again
(E) Take a break from study so you will be fresh for the examination itself

2 Once you gather the material you need to study for the Board examination, you are ready to start your preparation. After acquiring your study material you should organize your study plan to:

(A) Begin with the subject matter you know best to build your confidence
(B) Focus on doing practice questions
(C) Focus on the content you have heard is most important for the examination
(D) Map out how many pages of material you will cover each day
(E) Start by focusing on the content area where you are least confident

3 There is a lot of information to commit to memory for the Board examination. The most efficient way to commit critical study material to memory is to:

(A) Copy the details from your study material into a personal study notebook
(B) Do a lot of practice questions
(C) Organize the material into clusters
(D) Read over it repeatedly
(E) Talk it over with a friend or colleague

4 There is a lot of material to study for the Board examination, and many people feel frustration at some point in the study process. When you feel frustrated in the middle of your study process, the best thing to do is:

(A) Find a different source to study from
(B) Shift to a different topic area
(C) Stop studying for the day and come back to look at the material the next day
(D) Take a 10-minute break from study
(E) Take a deep breath and focus your attention on the material before you

5 When answering questions during the Board examination, if you are able to eliminate all but two of the presented options, but cannot come up with a reason to select one or the other, the best strategy is to:

(A) Go back and reread the questions to check for important details you might have missed

(B) Make an argument to yourself about why one, then the other, option must be right

(C) Read each option again and think about what it reminds you of

(D) Read each option again and think carefully about the exact wording

(E) Take a guess

6 Taking time to do practice questions is an important part of preparation for the Board examination. The best strategy for getting the most benefit out of practice questions is to:

(A) Do as many practice questions as you can from as many different sources as possible

(B) Focus on a particular set of questions and do them repeatedly until you get them all correct

(C) Save your practice questions until you have completed your study of the content material

(D) Take your time when doing practice questions to give yourself a chance to think clearly about each one

(E) Use the questions you get wrong to guide you as to what to go back and review again

7 In medical practice, experts often disagree as to the proper course of action in a given circumstance. When confronting a presented situation in an examination question where you know there may be some difference of opinion among practitioners in the field, the best way to decide on an answer is:

(A) Become familiar with clinical findings and research published in the last year

(B) Consider what you think most of the colleagues you know would do in a similar situation

(C) Select an answer based on existing practice guidelines

(D) Think about how you would handle the situation in your own practice

(E) Think back to the direction you received in handling similar situations when you were in residency and fellowship training

8 People have a lot of different advice as to how to best prepare for the Board examination. Some of this advice is good and some is not. Most people find that the best way to understand and remember important information for the Board examination is to:

(A) Focus on linking the material you study to real-life patients you have encountered

(B) Rearrange study materials to focus on differences among concepts

(C) Reread the details to reinforce their importance

(D) Try hard to remember the material exactly as it was presented

(E) Write everything out long-hand in parallel with your study material

9 Preparation for the examination usually does not occur all at once, but in a series of study sessions across several weeks or months. The best thing to do at the end of each of these study sessions is to:

(A) Chart your progress in covering the material you will need to master for the examination

(B) Look ahead at the study material you have left for the specific topic you are studying

(C) Map out what you will study next

(D) Summarize for yourself the key concepts covered during your study session

(E) Think about something besides the study material to give yourself a mental break

10 To do well in the Board examination you have to apply the knowledge you have learned to the questions presented. During the actual examination, after first reading through the clinical information presented in the stem of a question, the next thing you should do is

(A) Focus on the question at the end of the clinical case

(B) Go back over the presented content and check on relevant details

(C) Read down over the presented options to see what comes to mind

(D) Take a moment and think about the issues that the presentation brings to mind

(E) Try to connect what you have read to a real-life patient you have encountered

11 Practice questions are usually a part of everyone's preparation for the Board examination. The best way to integrate practice questions into the weeks and months of your study is to:

(A) Begin by doing a few questions early and increase the number as the examination gets closer

(B) Do not limit practice questions to study time, but do them whenever you have a spare moment in you day

(C) Hold off doing practice questions until you have completed your content study

(D) Spend most of your study time on practice questions and reading the annotated answers

(E) Start your study by doing a lot of questions to guide you as to what to study

12 Different people need to take different amounts of time to prepare for the Board examination depending on their general familiarity with the material. The best way to decide how much time you need to prepare for your Board examination is to:

(A) Assume you will need approximately 2 weeks of preparation for every year you are out of your fellowship

(B) Begin preparation early to get a sense of what is familiar and how comfortable you are with the material

(C) Check with people who took the examination in the past few years and see how long they took

(D) Decide how many pages of study material you can cover in a week and project the time needed to complete the material

(E) Take a practice examination and see how well you do

13 The way we learn should be different for different types of material and different kinds of tests. The best way to get ready for a multiple-choice examination is to:

(A) Focus on memorizing important details just as they are presented in study materials

(B) Organize material in modules, and modules in clusters that emphasize differentiation

(C) Read your study material aloud to make sure you cover it all and to help with memorization

(D) Talk to colleagues who have taken the examination in the past and focus your study on the things that were featured prominently in their examination

(E) Write or type out explanations of important concepts in sentence form to get familiar with the essential details

14 Some of the material you have to learn for the Board examination will be relatively easy and simple memorization will suffice. Other material is more complex and will require more sophisticated techniques to master. When trying to master difficult or complex material for the Board examination, the best strategy is to:

(A) Block out time and sit studying the material until you have mastered it

(B) Focus on practice questions so you will now know how it will appear in the examination

(C) Gather all the reference material you can on the subject and work your way through all of it

(D) Look at it for a little bit of time every day until you feel comfortable with it

(E) Skip it completely and hope that it will not account for much of the examination

15 For people who have recently completed a relevant fellowship before taking the Interventional Boards,

the best suggestion for planning how to spend study time would be:

(A) Feel confident that your fellowship has given you exposure to the best and most recent information, and work on maintaining confidence and getting well rested

(B) Organize a study group of colleagues whom you know from your fellowship program

(C) Plan an extensive review based on the notes and materials collected from the recently completed fellowship

(D) Select study material independent of your fellowship and organize your time for a complete review of all of it

(E) Wait to study until right before the examination so that your knowledge will be as fresh as possible

16 The best motto for helping yourself remember and understand the material at the level you will need for the Board examination is:

(A) Be consistent: Doing the same study procedures every day is the key to success

(B) Follow your nose: Trust your instincts as to what is important and what you need to learn

(C) Nose to the grindstone: Keep at it and do not stop until you have completed the task

(D) Repetition is best: Reading over material again is always a good use of time

(E) Variety is the spice of life: Doing different things with the material will give better results than getting stuck on one approach

17 In the week immediately leading up to the examination, the best strategy to maximize performance in the examination would be to:

(A) Maintain your clinical schedule, but do as many practice questions as possible in the evening

(B) Maintain your clinical schedule, but meet with colleagues in the evening to have them grill you on essential concepts

(C) Stick with your regular professional routine to maintain the appropriate clinical perspective

(D) Take time off from clinical work and spend all the time possible in intensive reading and study

(E) Take time off from clinical work and spend the day alternating between doing practice questions and reviewing material as you decide you need to

18 Because the Board examination is a timed test, it is important to have a developed strategy for managing time over the course of the examination. For this examination, the best strategy to manage your time would be:

(A) Answer easy questions and very hard questions quickly so you will have time to think about other questions when you need it

(B) Go slow and concentrate in the beginning of the examination and pick up the pace if you find you run short of time

(C) Practice allocating time evenly and spending the same amount of time on each question

(D) Relax and proceed at a measured pace without focusing on the time issue

(E) Work as quickly as possible from the very beginning to be sure that there is enough time

19 When you feel short of time during the Board examination, the best strategy to pick up speed would be to read:

(A) The first line and the last line of the question stem and then move to the options

(B) The last line of the stem, the actual question, and take your best guess at an answer after looking at the options

(C) The presented options first so you will know what the key issues are as you read through the question stem

(D) Through the question stem carefully and spend just enough time on the presented options to make a decision

(E) Through the question stem quickly so you will have time to think about the answer options

20 Some people are concerned that the makeup of the Board examination is unknown and obscure and this makes it difficult for them to study for the examination correctly. This concern is often heightened as they discover that few of their colleagues who have previously taken the examination have been helpful in telling them what questions were asked and what types of material were covered other than to say "everything." In the face of this uncertainty, the best strategy for getting a clear sense of what is tested in the Board examination is to:

(A) Buy a couple of large textbooks on interventional cardiology and read each one cover to cover, focusing on memorizing as much as possible

(B) Contact the College of Education at a local University for insight and advice on how to prepare for these examinations

(C) Hire an educational/testing consultant to assist you in preparation

(D) Rely on your developed clinical instincts as to what is most important and most likely to be tested

(E) Visit the American Board of Internal Medicine (ABIM) website for guidance

21 The ABIM website states that "the examination will assess the candidate's knowledge and clinical judgment in aspects of interventional cardiology required to perform at a high level of competence." Because performing at a high level of competence demands current knowledge, good clinical judgment, and awareness of the latest thinking and trends, your best sources of information for studying will be:

(A) Controversies and debates at the most recent appropriate annual professional meetings

(B) Materials for a Board review course run last year

(C) Recent ACCEL and other media releases

(D) Recent issues of major cardiovascular journals dealing with interventional cardiology

(E) Textbooks and practice guideline documents published at least 6 months before the examination

Answers and Explanations

1 **Answer B.** Do some practice questions and let the ones you get wrong tell you what to go back and study again. Questions benefit you in two ways. First, they give you experience in the behaviors and thought processes you need for the examination. Second, they can uncover weaknesses in your knowledge and understanding before the real examination. Your task is to take the information provided by questions you miss and do something about it. If you find that you do not understand a concept, go back and look at it again. And do not just look at the exact issue you missed. If you missed one issue in a subject area, the odds are you have other weaknesses there are well. Just doing a lot of questions provides no real benefit. All you are doing is retesting yourself, but doing nothing to improve and increase your chances of success. Looking at brand new study material will simply expand the amount of material you have to master and likely result in you feeling confused or overloaded. Rereading repetitiously increases boredom, but does little to give you a better grasp or increased understanding of the material. Replowing the same field over and over again does not give you a better crop. You have time to prepare more. The issue now is to move from simple repetition to something that will help direct your study efforts; question-guided study will do that.

2 **Answer E.** Start by focusing on the content area where you are least confident. Most people like to spend the most time on things that they already know fairly well. Although this might make you feel good, it does little to identify and correct deficits, which should be the main goal of your examination preparation. Starting with the weakest subject ensures that you will give it the time and attention it deserves. It is simply easier to bring your worst subject area to average than to try to make your best subject areas even better. Doing practice questions too early is like hunting without ammunition. You need to have a good sense of the material already before the practice questions can really guide your further review. Focusing on what others have told you can be dangerous. First, memory of examination takers is selective and what people remember is often not a good representation of what was really on the examination. In addition, what was on the examination last year may not be your best guide as to what will be on the examination you take. Trying

to cover a set number of pages each day misses the fact that some content will be easy for you and some will be hard. You need to spend as much time on a subject as you need, but not waste time on content you already know fairly well. Covering a set number of pages per day means you are not tailoring your study time to your specific needs.

3 **Answer C.** Organize the material into clusters. Our minds are not wired to learn lists, but classes of things. You must organize the study to take advantage of this fact. Group similar content together. What are key differentials? How will you decide when to choose among a select set of procedures or techniques? These are the questions you will be called upon to address in the examination. Organize your study to anticipate this. Copying details from your study material takes quite a bit of time and does not provide much return. Keeping things in the format of your study material does not render it in a form that has the most resonance with you and focusing on all the details risks having you overwhelmed by the weight of the particulars. Questions test what you know, but do not help you with the process of memorization. Rereading gets boring and eventually results in diminishing returns. Mechanically rereading means that you must cover a lot of material you already know just to uncover a few nuggets of new insight. Talking with a friend can really help you sort out and learn to articulate your understanding of difficult concepts, but memorization is an individual process done in private.

4 **Answer D.** Take a break from study. Nothing fuels frustration as much as to keep pushing on the thing that is frustrating you. Walk away briefly and take a mental break. When you return to the material, you will find you have a different perspective and what was obscure before now makes sense. Changing to a different source risks increasing the volume of material you have to study and can result in overload. There is no reason that a break should be 24 hours. A short time away from the content is usually all it takes. Shifting topics can make your study schedule choppy, make it hard to track what you have and have not studied, and often means that you never do return to the point of frustration to clarify it and achieve resolution.

5 **Answer E.** If you are able to eliminate all but two options and you do not know which one to select, you have taken the question as far as you can. You now have a 50% shot. Take it and run. It's time to guess and move on to the next question. Most people get less than half of these questions correct because they use one of several bad strategies. Rereading the question takes time and usually does not clarify. Making an argument usually means inventing a different question and losing track of exactly what it is you are supposed to answer. Reading each option again and reflecting usually makes you think about things not anticipated by the question writer. And looking carefully at the wording of options often makes you overinterpret simple wording and talk yourself out of a right answer. When you get to two options and you are through, it's time to guess.

6 **Answer E.** Questions test you, but do not teach you. The learning occurs when you respond to the deficit uncovered by the questions by fixing it. Usually, this means returning to your primary study materials and reexamining the sections relevant to the question you just got incorrect. Doing a lot of questions from a lot of different sources will have you spending your time getting comfortable doing questions, but will not help you improve your score. Doing more questions without additional review simply gives a more reliable assessment of your current level of expertise. Doing the same questions over and over will help you memorize those questions, but will not help you learn the material in a way you will need for the new questions you will face in the Board examination. Saving practice questions until the end of studying means you will not have the benefit of a reminder of what it is you are preparing for. You need to be reminded of the task at hand to help you focus on what is essential rather than what is simply interesting. And because the examination is timed, you should do your practice questions under timed conditions to get used to the pressures of the examination. Doing well in the examination means not just being able to answer the questions, but being able to answer them within the given timeframe.

7 **Answer C.** Select an answer based on existing practice guidelines. Established practice guidelines represent the consensus of the best minds in the field. When question writers are constructing questions, they are very likely to use existing guidelines as templates for writing questions and as arbiters for what makes the best answer. The most recently published clinical work is likely too new and was not available when the questions for your examination were written. What everyone thinks is right is not always what objective research tells us is correct. Consider that questions are especially likely to be written about topics in which what many practitioners actually do is not supported by the empirical research. When everyone knows the right thing to do, it simply does not make a very good question. And keep in mind that the field is constantly undergoing changes. What was state-of-the-art several years ago may not be so today. In residency, the right answer is whatever your current attending physician says it is. In the Board examination, the right answer is what the committee of experts relying on empirical research says it is.

8 **Answer B.** One of the most important strategies for efficient study is rearranging materials to focus on differences among concepts. Your task in a multiple-choice examination is to select among presented options. To do your best you need to study the same way. Focus on learning set options and then how to choose among those options. Learning all the details of something will not be nearly as useful as knowing which clinical detail makes one option better than another. Differential diagnosis should be your template. You need to be able to do more than recognize a patient with a certain condition. You need to be able to tell yourself why it is that condition and not something similar. The same logic holds for choosing among procedures, techniques, and patient management options. Real-life cases may not offer the type of choices you will be given at the actual examination. Rereading and remembering something exactly as presented helps memorize the text, but does not give you an understanding of the material in your own words and on your own terms. Material memorized does not help you decide. Material you have organized in your head for that purpose does. And writing everything out long-hand just takes too much time given the amount of material you have to master for your examination.

9 **Answer D.** Summarize for yourself the key concepts covered during your study session. A quick mental review of what you have covered is the best way to get closure for your study session, to facilitate remembering key concepts, and forcing you to think about things in your own terms rather than just mimicking the words you have studied. Focusing on where you are in your progress tends to make the task seem longer. Each time you focus on looking ahead, you risk your inner child asking, "Are we there yet?" Before you look ahead, be sure of what you have just covered. Looking ahead to the next topic can make it hard to concentrate on and retain the current issues under study. And at the end of your study session, you will have a mental break as you move on to other things in your life. Just be sure to summarize and reinforce what you have just done before moving on.

10 Answer A. Focus on the question at the end of the clinical case. One of the most common, and avoidable, mistakes in a multiple-choice examination is to answer the question you wanted or expected rather than the one you were actually asked. This error costs otherwise well prepared people valuable points they deserve to have. After reading the case, you must pay careful attention to what it is that has been asked about the case. Learn this when you are doing your practice questions and you will not make the mistake during the real examination when it counts. Going back over the case takes time you do not have. You must get key information on the first reading. Looking at options before you focus on the question is really putting the "cart before the horse." Without the guidance of the questions, options tend to only confuse you. And thinking in general or about a real-life patient takes you away from that matter at hand. Focus on the questions asked and let your thinking be about that!

11 Answer A. Begin by doing a few questions early and increase the number as the examination gets closer. Questions are the target that you are in training to hit. You need to be reminded of why you are studying. Start doing practice questions, just a few, early in your study. As you progress through the material, day by day you can increase the number of questions you do and the time you spend reviewing them. Do not do questions haphazardly in spare moments, but keep your practice as close as you can to the real examination situation. This means questions should be done in a cluster and with a clock. Do a set of questions before looking up the answer to any one question. But also remember that questions themselves will not get you where you need to be. The hard work of study is how you learn what you need to learn. Questions just help you refine your knowledge and gain perspective on how an issue might be approached in an examination question. Study is first. Questions are second. Just do not leave them until the end.

12 Answer B. There is no magic number of days, weeks, or months required to prepare for the examination. You simply need to make sure you have the time that *you* need, which may be different than that of other people. By starting early you will ensure that you have the time if you need it, and will be able to get a real concrete sense of how

familiar or unfamiliar the material might be. The key is not to adopt some formula like a set number of weeks or a certain number of pages per day, but to select a solution and study schedule that meets your particular needs. A practice examination is always a nice idea, if possible, and can pinpoint areas of weakness, but it cannot tell you how long you, personally, need to prepare. When are you ready to take the examination? When you *get it*! You should be at the level of being able to argue and explain the material to others. Most people have pretty good gut instincts as to when they have reached this level.

13 Answer B. Organize material in modules, and modules in clusters that emphasize differentiation. The two most important issues for study are organizing the material in a way that makes sense to you, and making sure you focus on being able to make choices among presented options. If you can lay out everything that is known about a procedure or a technique, this will not help you. You will not be asked to lay out everything you know. Instead, you will have to be able to say why "this" and not "that." Details that help you make these kinds of decisions are essential. Details that do not are mere knowledge ornamentation with no value for improving your examination performance. Not all the details matter. Everything in your study material is not important. Make choices and focus on what matters. Review courses help you with this, but you can also give yourself guidance by remembering the type of decisions the examination will ask you to make. Reading aloud is a good way to reinforce memory regarding difficult concepts, but simply takes too long given the body of material you have to master, nor does reading someone else's words help get concepts framed in the way that makes the most sense to you. Studying what was in the examination last year can be a recipe for disaster. Board examinations tend to shift content year to year. Study for *this* examination, not for the one last year. Outlines and tales showing similarities and differences among concepts are much better choices than writing out content in full sentences.

14 Answer D. Sequential study sessions over a period of days are by far the most effective and efficient way to master complex materials. Learning theory tells us that "spaced practice is better than massed practice," which means that sitting and trying to grasp content all at once is not nearly as effective as looking at it repeatedly over time. Trying to get it all in one day is a residual of the days when you had to cram for an examination in only a day or two. Preparing for the Board examination is different. You will be studying over weeks and months and will have the time to take when you need it. Practice questions are an excellent vehicle to get you to think about the examination and to break you from the monotony of rote rereading of material, but they will likely not show you the material just as you will encounter it in the examination. Most people walk out of the examination surprised that although practice questions do cover much of the same information as the examination, they do so in a different and, sometimes, surprising way. You cannot anticipate all the questions, but you can arm yourself with the information you need and train yourself to be able to think with it and solve whatever problem you are presented with. Gathering all the reference material available is a sure way to end up overloaded and overwhelmed. Do not skip over complex material. Complex material is more likely than easier material to be the source of questions. Take the time you need, look at it repeatedly, and you will find you are able to master now what you could not master before.

15 Answer D. No matter how well known and structured the program and how compulsive the fellow, it is unlikely that any program will impart all of the possible testable knowledge in an ABIM examination. In each program, there is an intended curriculum (objectives, examination blueprint, etc.) and an informal curriculum (content emphasized during lectures and small group discussions, etc.) (*BMC Education.* 2005;5:69). Frequently, it is the informal curriculum that flavors a trainee's data retention and clinical practice patterns. However, the examiners for the ABIM-sponsored examinations are focused on assessing core knowledge of generally accepted practice standards. Therefore, it is important to recognize that the examiners' perception of core knowledge may not be consonant with the examination-taker's experience with an informal curriculum. All programs have strengths and weaknesses, and it is the latter components in which it is particularly important to study and increase your knowledge. A casual attitude of preparation is likely to lead to disappointing results in testing.

16 Answer E. Effective study requires a series of steps in which you do different things with the material as your familiarity with it changes. Step 1 is to decide what you will study. Step 2 requires repetition and reading over the essential material. Step 3 requires fostering recall by doing something active with the material such as making outlines, drawing pictures, talking to yourself about it, or talking with others. Step 4 moves on to practice using the material as you focus on practice questions. Doing the exact

same thing everyday does not make sense as your understanding changes and improves. Following your instincts will likely have you study what you like, but avoid what you hate. You need guidance as to what to study beyond your personal preferences. Pushing on for weeks at a time without a break is emotionally damaging and cognitively ineffective. Schedule some pauses in your study. You will come back to it fresher, with more insight and more motivation. Rereading helps to get the content into your head, but does not help you get it out when you need it. At some point you need to change from repetition to active processes that promote recall.

17 Answer E. The Board examination will require different mental processes and a different perspective than daily clinical work. Taking a break from your clinical duties will aid you in making this transition. It will also help ensure that you do not walk into the examination sleep deprived by trying to do your usual work and your examination preparation at the same time. When you take time off, do not spend every waking moment in preparation. Instead, set up each day like a job, put in the time you planned, and then stop and allow yourself some time to relax.

18 Answer A. The essential notion here is to have the time when you need it by not wasting it on difficult questions you do not know or lingering over easy questions when the answer is obvious to you. Going slow and focusing on concentration will result in you having too little time at the end. Not all questions take the same amount of time. Spend just what is needed on each one and then move on. If you do not think about time at all, you will be ambushed by a shortage of time at the end of the examination period. The trick is to track the time without being panicked by the ticking of the clock. Working as quickly as possible makes most people feel rushed and unable to have that moment of reflection that makes the difference. Questions will require you to think. You need to move efficiently through the examination. But not at the expense of giving up applying your intelligence and thinking through to the best answer.

19 Answer D. The question stem is your friend. It must, by the rules, give you everything that you need to analyze the question and come up with the best answer. The options are the enemy. Their task is to confuse you and con you into picking the wrong answer. Time spent reading the question is time well spent. Focus on reading what is presented and thinking about the issues involved. Spend as little time on the options as possible. Make a choice and move on! Skipping over parts of the question stem is a high-risk strategy. It may work for you sometimes, but usually you will miss some key detail or some essential clue and, therefore, not converge on the correct answer. We all tend to like the options because options are the way out of the question. But be careful. Getting to the options before reading and processing the clues given in the question is essentially hunting in the dark. You will pick an option and get out of the questions all right. But, you are unlikely to get the right option that gives you the point and improves your chances of passing.

20 **Answer E.** To get specific information about the examination you are preparing for, go right to the source. An educational consultant or the local College of Education at the university will provide useful information about the broad field of study techniques, improving data retention, and the like. They will not be knowledgeable about the structure of the ABIM Certification of Added Qualification (CAQ) in Interventional Cardiology, however. Knowing that structure can help you target your preparation better. It is available at the ABIM website (www.abim.org) and currently has the web address www.abim.org/cert/aqic.shtm. The primary content areas and their relative proportions in the examination as of April 2006 are:

- Case selection and management, 25%
- Procedural technique, 25%
- Basic science, 15%
- Pharmacology, 15%
- Imaging, 15%
- Miscellaneous, 5%

The website provides additional information as to what the specific contents are within each of these broad areas. Merging this information with your own awareness of strengths and weaknesses in your own knowledge base allows you to tailor your study, spending more time on relatively weaker areas of knowledge and slightly less in areas of greater proficiency.

21 **Answer E.** Board questions are focused on the core knowledge required to support excellent clinical judgment. As such, the boards do not examine the examination takers on the latest and greatest theories, ideas, and personal opinions of interventional thought leaders. Guidelines are a rich source of information as they are robust, amply referenced, and based on levels of evidence. Because they are evidence based, they provide a rich source of potential examination material with "single best answers." Textbooks are also excellent sources of information but this information is often a bit outdated. Nonetheless, such information is often highly relevant and "testable." Remember that the Board questions are written, vetted, and "put to bed" several months before the actual examination. The ABIM has never given an exact cut-off date for inclusion of information in the examination, but a general time frame of 6 to 9 months preexamination has been suggested as reasonable. Data more recent than that is not felt to be known widely enough, disseminated, and incorporated to provide valid test material. Also, the debates at large annual meetings, recent reports, opinions of interventional cardiology leaders, and other such opinion-based materials are not the core information used for ABIM testing. Board review courses are rich sources of information for preparation as they are focused on core knowledge and not the latest, hottest new topics.

Index

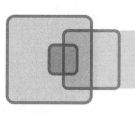